Mammography Centers Directory

HOSPITAL

Registered Trademark

Your guide to over 8,700 mammography facilities, including name, address, telephone and fax numbers

HENRY A. ROSE, Editor

All information published herein is gathered from sources which are considered reliable by the editor. We have tried our best to record all the information correctly, any errors or omissions will be corrected in a subsequent edition.

The publisher does not assume responsibility for errors, omissions, or interpretations.

Published by:

UNICOL, Inc.
P.O. Box 260550
Pembroke Pines, Florida 33026
PHONE: (954) 430-7271
FAX: (954) 430-7227
WEB: Unicol-Publishing.com

Mammography Centers Directory

Registered Trademark

Your guide to over 8,700 mammography facilities, including name, address, telephone and fax numbers

Published by:

UNICOL, INC.
P.O. Box 260550
Pembroke Pines, Florida 33026-7550
PHONE: (954) 430-7271
FAX: (954) 430-7227
WEB: Unicol-Publishing.com

ISBN 978-1-880973-37-0

Printed in U.S.A.
Manufactured in U.S.A.

Product Stock #301-J
Federal ID Number 65-0288668

Preface

Mammography Centers Directory

Registered Trademark

Your guide to over 8,700 mammography facilities, including name, address, telephone and fax numbers

The MAMMOGRAPHY CENTERS DIRECTORY is your guide to over 8,700 mammography facilities, including name, address, telephone and fax numbers.

The most current information available at the time of publication.

Published by:

UNICOL, Inc.
P.O. Box 260550
Pembroke Pines, Florida 33026
PHONE: (954) 430-7271
FAX: (954) 430-7227
WEB: Unicol-Publishing.com

Area Codes – Alphabetically by Location

205	Alabama
251	Alabama
256	Alabama
334	Alabama
907	Alaska
480	Arizona
520	Arizona
602	Arizona
623	Arizona
928	Arizona
479	Arkansas
501	Arkansas
870	Arkansas
209	California
213	California
310	California
323	California
408	California
415	California
424	California
442	California
510	California
530	California
559	California
562	California
619	California
626	California
650	California
657	California
661	California
707	California
714	California
747	California
760	California
805	California
818	California
831	California
858	California
909	California
916	California
925	California
949	California
951	California
303	Colorado
719	Colorado
720	Colorado
970	Colorado
203	Connecticut
860	Connecticut
302	Delaware
202	District of Columbia
239	Florida
305	Florida
321	Florida
352	Florida
386	Florida
407	Florida
561	Florida
727	Florida
754	Florida
772	Florida
786	Florida
813	Florida
850	Florida
863	Florida
904	Florida
941	Florida
954	Florida
229	Georgia
404	Georgia
478	Georgia
678	Georgia
706	Georgia
762	Georgia
770	Georgia
912	Georgia
808	Hawaii
208	Idaho
217	Illinois
224	Illinois
309	Illinois
312	Illinois
331	Illinois
618	Illinois
630	Illinois
708	Illinois
773	Illinois
779	Illinois
815	Illinois
847	Illinois
872	Illinois
219	Indiana
260	Indiana
317	Indiana
574	Indiana
765	Indiana
812	Indiana
319	Iowa
515	Iowa
563	Iowa
641	Iowa
712	Iowa
316	Kansas
620	Kansas
785	Kansas
913	Kansas
270	Kentucky
502	Kentucky
606	Kentucky
859	Kentucky
225	Louisiana
318	Louisiana
337	Louisiana
504	Louisiana
985	Louisiana
207	Maine
240	Maryland
301	Maryland
410	Maryland
443	Maryland
339	Massachusetts
351	Massachusetts
413	Massachusetts
508	Massachusetts
617	Massachusetts
774	Massachusetts
781	Massachusetts
857	Massachusetts
978	Massachusetts
231	Michigan
248	Michigan
269	Michigan
313	Michigan
517	Michigan
586	Michigan
616	Michigan
734	Michigan
810	Michigan
906	Michigan
947	Michigan
989	Michigan
218	Minnesota
320	Minnesota
507	Minnesota
612	Minnesota
651	Minnesota
763	Minnesota
952	Minnesota
228	Mississippi
601	Mississippi
662	Mississippi
769	Mississippi
314	Missouri
417	Missouri
573	Missouri
636	Missouri
660	Missouri
816	Missouri
406	Montana
308	Nebraska
402	Nebraska
702	Nevada
775	Nevada
603	New Hampshire
201	New Jersey
551	New Jersey
609	New Jersey
732	New Jersey
848	New Jersey
856	New Jersey
862	New Jersey
908	New Jersey
973	New Jersey
505	New Mexico
575	New Mexico
212	New York
315	New York
347	New York
516	New York
518	New York
585	New York
607	New York
631	New York
646	New York
716	New York
718	New York
845	New York
914	New York
917	New York
252	North Carolina
336	North Carolina
704	North Carolina
828	North Carolina
910	North Carolina
919	North Carolina
980	North Carolina
701	North Dakota
216	Ohio
234	Ohio
330	Ohio
419	Ohio
440	Ohio
513	Ohio
567	Ohio
614	Ohio
740	Ohio
937	Ohio
405	Oklahoma
580	Oklahoma
918	Oklahoma
503	Oregon
541	Oregon
971	Oregon
215	Pennsylvania
267	Pennsylvania
412	Pennsylvania
484	Pennsylvania
570	Pennsylvania
610	Pennsylvania
717	Pennsylvania
724	Pennsylvania
814	Pennsylvania
878	Pennsylvania
787	Puerto Rico
939	Puerto Rico
401	Rhode Island
803	South Carolina
843	South Carolina
864	South Carolina
605	South Dakota
423	Tennessee
615	Tennessee
731	Tennessee
865	Tennessee
901	Tennessee
931	Tennessee
210	Texas
214	Texas
254	Texas
281	Texas
325	Texas
361	Texas
409	Texas
430	Texas
432	Texas
469	Texas
512	Texas
682	Texas
713	Texas
806	Texas
817	Texas
830	Texas
832	Texas
903	Texas
915	Texas
936	Texas
940	Texas
956	Texas
972	Texas
979	Texas
385	Utah
435	Utah
801	Utah
802	Vermont
276	Virginia
434	Virginia
540	Virginia
571	Virginia
703	Virginia
757	Virginia
804	Virginia
206	Washington
253	Washington
360	Washington
425	Washington
509	Washington
304	West Virginia
262	Wisconsin
414	Wisconsin
608	Wisconsin
715	Wisconsin
920	Wisconsin
307	Wyoming

Operator Information can be dialed direct.
First dial "0" or "1", then the area code as shown above, then 555-1212.

Toll-Free Prefixes – 800, 866, 877, and 888.

Area Codes – Numerically

203	Connecticut
205	Alabama
206	Washington
207	Maine
208	Idaho
209	California
210	Texas
212	New York
213	California
214	Texas
215	Pennsylvania
216	Ohio
217	Illinois
218	Minnesota
219	Indiana
224	Illinois
225	Louisiana
228	Mississippi
229	Georgia
231	Michigan
234	Ohio
239	Florida
240	Maryland
248	Michigan
251	Alabama
252	North Carolina
253	Washington
254	Texas
256	Alabama
260	Indiana
262	Wisconsin
267	Pennsylvania
269	Michigan
270	Kentucky
276	Virginia
281	Texas
301	Maryland
302	Delaware
303	Colorado
304	West Virginia
305	Florida
307	Wyoming
308	Nebraska
309	Illinois
310	California
312	Illinois
313	Michigan
314	Missouri
315	New York
316	Kansas
317	Indiana
318	Louisiana
319	Iowa
320	Minnesota
321	Florida
323	California
325	Texas
330	Ohio
331	Illinois
334	Alabama
336	North Carolina
337	Louisiana
339	Massachusetts
347	New York
351	Massachusetts
352	Florida
360	Washington
361	Texas
385	Utah
386	Florida
401	Rhode Island
402	Nebraska
404	Georgia
405	Oklahoma
406	Montana
407	Florida
408	California
409	Texas
410	Maryland
412	Pennsylvania
413	Massachusetts
414	Wisconsin
415	California
417	Missouri
419	Ohio
423	Tennessee
424	California
425	Washington
430	Texas
432	Texas
434	Virginia
435	Utah
440	Ohio
442	California
443	Maryland
469	Texas
478	Georgia
479	Arkansas
480	Arizona
484	Pennsylvania
501	Arkansas
502	Kentucky
503	Oregon
504	Louisiana
505	New Mexico
507	Minnesota
508	Massachusetts
509	Washington
510	California
512	Texas
513	Ohio
515	Iowa
516	New York
517	Michigan
518	New York
520	Arizona
530	California
540	Virginia
541	Oregon
551	New Jersey
559	California
561	Florida
562	California
563	Iowa
567	Ohio
570	Pennsylvania
571	Virginia
573	Missouri
574	Indiana
575	New Mexico
580	Oklahoma
585	New York
586	Michigan
601	Mississippi
602	Arizona
603	New Hampshire
605	South Dakota
606	Kentucky
607	New York
608	Wisconsin
609	New Jersey
610	Pennsylvania
612	Minnesota
614	Ohio
615	Tennessee
616	Michigan
617	Massachusetts
618	Illinois
619	California
620	Kansas
623	Arizona
626	California
630	Illinois
631	New York
636	Missouri
641	Iowa
646	New York
650	California
651	Minnesota
657	California
660	Missouri
661	California
662	Mississippi
678	Georgia
682	Texas
701	North Dakota
702	Nevada
703	Virginia
704	North Carolina
706	Georgia
707	California
708	Illinois
712	Iowa
713	Texas
714	California
715	Wisconsin
716	New York
717	Pennsylvania
718	New York
719	Colorado
720	Colorado
724	Pennsylvania
727	Florida
731	Tennessee
732	New Jersey
734	Michigan
740	Ohio
747	California
754	Florida
757	Virginia
760	California
762	Georgia
763	Minnesota
765	Indiana
769	Mississippi
770	Georgia
772	Florida
773	Illinois
774	Massachusetts
775	Nevada
779	Illinois
781	Massachusetts
785	Kansas
786	Florida
787	Puerto Rico
801	Utah
802	Vermont
803	South Carolina
804	Virginia
805	California
806	Texas
808	Hawaii
810	Michigan
812	Indiana
813	Florida
814	Pennsylvania
815	Illinois
816	Missouri
817	Texas
818	California
828	North Carolina
830	Texas
831	California
832	Texas
843	South Carolina
845	New York
847	Illinois
848	New Jersey
850	Florida
856	New Jersey
857	Massachusetts
858	California
859	Kentucky
860	Connecticut
862	New Jersey
863	Florida
864	South Carolina
865	Tennessee
870	Arkansas
872	Illinois
878	Pennsylvania
901	Tennessee
903	Texas
904	Florida
906	Michigan
907	Alaska
908	New Jersey
909	California
910	North Carolina
912	Georgia
913	Kansas
914	New York
915	Texas
916	California
917	New York
918	Oklahoma
919	North Carolina
920	Wisconsin
925	California
928	Arizona
931	Tennessee
936	Texas
937	Ohio
939	Puerto Rico
940	Texas
941	Florida
947	Michigan
949	California
951	California
952	Minnesota
954	Florida
956	Texas
970	Colorado
971	Oregon
972	Texas
973	New Jersey
978	Massachusetts
979	Texas
980	North Carolina
985	Louisiana
989	Michigan

Operator Information can be dialed direct.
First dial "0" or "1", then the area code as shown above, then 555-1212.

Toll-Free Prefixes – 800, 866, 877, and 888.

TABLE OF CONTENTS

ALABAMA

Alabaster

Shelby Baptist Medical Center
PO Box 488, 1004 First St N Suite 100
Alabaster, AL 35007-2043
(205)620-8027
FAX: (205)620-8193

Shelby Ob/Gyn Pc
408 1st St N, Ste 200B
Alabaster, AL 35007-9271
(205)664-9995
FAX: (205)664-9907

Alexander City

Russell Medical Women's Center
3316 Highway 280 Bldg Su W Professional
Alexander City, AL 35010-3369
(256)329-7246
FAX: (256)329-7374

Andalusia

Andalusia Health
849 S Three Notch St
Andalusia, AL 36420-5399
(334)428-7080
FAX: (334)222-6996

Anniston

Advanced Imaging Of Alabama
1699 Golden Springs Rd
Anniston, AL 36207-7097
(256)835-0835
FAX: (256)835-1939

Anniston Ob-Gyn Associates, P.A.
901 Leighton Ave Ste 502
Anniston, AL 36207-5765
(256)237-6755
FAX: (256)237-4966

Barbara L. Moersch, M.D. - Obgyn
825 Keith Ave
Anniston, AL 36207-4760
(256)238-0448
FAX: (256)238-1685

North East Alabama Regional Medical Center
400 E 10th St
Anniston, AL 36207-4716
(256)235-5141
FAX: (256)235-5058

Northeast Alabama Regional Medical Center-Tyler Center
731 Leighton Ave
Anniston, AL 36207-5761
(256)235-5141
FAX: (256)235-5058

Ashland

Clay County Hospital And Nursing Home
83825 Highway 9
Ashland, AL 36251-7981
(256)354-1169
FAX: (256)354-1191

Athens

Athens Limestone Hospital
700 W Market St
Athens, AL 35611-2422
(256)216-9696
FAX: (256)233-9573

Athens-Limestone Hospital Limestone Medical Village
15243 Greenfield Dr
Athens, AL 35613-2899
(256)216-9696
FAX: (256)233-9573

Diaghlth Mri Of Gasden Llc Dba Outpatient Diag Ctr Athens
22281 US Highway 72 Ste B & C
Athens, AL 35613-2601
(256)532-2404
FAX: (256)532-2404

Atmore

Atmore Community Hospital
401 Medical Park Dr
Atmore, AL 36502-3091
(251)368-6378
FAX: (251)446-6410

Auburn

Auburn Diagnostic Imaging
1527 Professional Pkwy
Auburn, AL 36830-2858
(334)826-2500
FAX: (334)502-6736

Bridgeway Diagnostic Radiology, Llc
2415 Moores Mill Rd Unit 265
Auburn, AL 36830-8484
(334)408-2854
FAX: (334)384-9274

Bridgeway Diagnostics Radiology, Llc
1910 E Samford Ave
Auburn, AL 36830-6386
(334)539-5700
FAX: (334)539-5704

Bay Minette

North Baldwin Infirmary
PO Box 131, 1815 Hand Ave
Bay Minette, AL 36507-0131
(251)580-1747
FAX: (251)580-1768

Bessemer

Medical West Hospital Authority,An Affiliate Of Uab Health S
995 9th Ave SW
Bessemer, AL 35022-4527
(205)481-7170
FAX: (205)481-7971

Birmingham

Birmingham Ob/Gyn, Pc
800 Saint Vincents Dr, Ste 500
Birmingham, AL 35205-1629
(205)933-8334
FAX: (205)933-8466

Birmingham Radiological Group, P.C.
50 Medical Park Dr E, Ste 162
Birmingham, AL 35235-3401
(205)838-3134
FAX: (205)838-3540

Brookwood Women's Health, P.C.
2006 Brookwood Medical Ctr Dr Ste
Birmingham, AL 35209-6899
(205)397-8850
FAX: (205)397-8855

Complete Womens Care Of Alabama
4600 Highway 280, Ste 230
Birmingham, AL 35242-5185
(205)664-9995
FAX: (205)582-7520

Cooper Green Mercy Health Svc. Authority An Affiliate Of Uab
1515 6th Ave S
Birmingham, AL 35233-1601
(205)930-3280
FAX: (205)930-3647

Eastern Ob Gyn
48 Medical Park Dr E Ste 355
Birmingham, AL 35235-3470
(205)838-3036
FAX: (205)838-5832

Grandview Imaging Trussville
5890 Valley Rd Ste 100
Birmingham, AL 35235-8669
(205)655-7896
FAX: (205)655-5637

Henderson And Walton Women's Center
806 Saint Vincents Dr Ste 500
Birmingham, AL 35205-1617
(205)930-1800
FAX: (205)930-1851

Ob-Gyn South, P.C.
2006 Brookwood Medical Ctr Dr, Ste 402
Birmingham, AL 35209-6823
(205)397-9006
FAX: (205)397-9013

Ob/Gyn Associates Of Alabama
800 Saint Vincents Dr Ste 600, St Vincent's North Tower
Birmingham, AL 35205-1630
(205)271-1600
FAX: (205)271-3167

Princeton Baptist Medical Center
833 Princeton Ave SW Pob III
Birmingham, AL 35211-1323
(205)783-7107
FAX: (205)783-7120

Simon-Williamson Clinic, P.C.
832 Princeton Ave SW
Birmingham, AL 35211-1320
(205)206-8386
FAX: (205)206-8381

Sparks And Favor, P.C.
2006 Brookwood Medical Ctr Dr Ste 700
Birmingham, AL 35209-6899
(205)397-1286
FAX: (205)397-1343

St. Vincent's Hospital Comprehensive Breast Center
800 Saint Vincents Dr Ste 400, North Tower, 4th Flr
Birmingham, AL 35205-1632
(205)939-7003
FAX: (205)930-2848

St. Vincent's One Nineteen Health & Wellness
7191 Cahaba Valley Rd
Birmingham, AL 35242-6443
(205)408-6508
FAX: (205)408-6501

The Women's Imaging Center At Grandview
3686 Grandview Pkwy Ste 210, Grandview Physicians Plaza
Birmingham, AL 35243-3391
(205)971-1477
FAX: (205)971-1476

University Of Alabama At Birmingham-The Kirklin Clinic
2000 6th Ave S, 3rd Floor Mammography
Birmingham, AL 35233-2110
(205)801-7735
FAX: (205)801-7403

Women's Care Specialists, P.C.
3686 Grandview Pkwy Ste 800
Birmingham, AL 35243-3408
(205)858-0900
FAX: (205)858-0901

Women's Diagnostic Center, Inc.
2006 Brookwood Medical Ctr Dr, Ste 112
Birmingham, AL 35209-6823
(205)877-5200
FAX: (205)877-2680

Boaz

Marshall Medical Center South
2505 US Highway 431
Boaz, AL 35957-5908
(256)840-4704
FAX: (256)840-4611

Brewton

D. W. McMillan Hospital
1301 Belleville Ave
Brewton, AL 36426-1391
(251)809-8127
FAX: (251)809-8167

Camden

J. Paul Jones Hospital
317 McWilliams Ave
Camden, AL 36726-1623
(334)682-4131
FAX: (334)682-4131

Centreville

Bibb Medical Center
208 Pierson Ave
Centreville, AL 35042-2918
(205)926-3257
FAX: (205)928-3448

Chatom

Washington County Hospital And Nursing Home
14600 Saint Stephens Ave
Chatom, AL 36518-6711
(251)847-4284
FAX: (251)847-6349

Clanton

St. Vincent's Chilton
2030 Lay Dam Rd
Clanton, AL 35045-8344
(205)258-4351
FAX: (205)258-4401

Cullman

Cullman Internal Medicine, P.C.
1890 Alabama Hwy 157, Ste 300
Cullman, AL 35058
(256)737-8000
FAX: (256)737-8060

Cullman Primary Care Diagnostics
501 Clark St NE
Cullman, AL 35055-1921
(256)739-9898
FAX: (256)739-9556

Cullman Regional Medical Center Women's Diagnostic Ctr
1912 Alabama Highway 157
Cullman, AL 35058
(256)737-2667
FAX: (256)737-2133

Henderson And Walton Women's Center Cullman
212 4th Ave SE
Cullman, AL 35055-3673
(256)739-2626
FAX: (256)739-6588

Dadeville

Lake Martin Community Hospital
201 Mariarden Rd
Dadeville, AL 36853-6251
(256)825-3245
FAX: (256)827-0811

Daphne

Thomas Medical Center
27961 US Highway 98
Daphne, AL 36526-4702
(251)990-1042
FAX: (251)279-1022

Decatur

Decatur Med-Surg. Clinic, Llc
2828 Highway 31 S
Decatur, AL 35603-1538
(256)353-2000
FAX: (256)686-2151

Decatur Morgan Hospital Decatur General Campus
PO Box 2239, 1215 7th St SE
Decatur, AL 35609-2239
(256)973-6722
FAX: (256)973-3682

Demopolis

Tombigbee Healthcare Authority Operating Bwwmh
105 US Highway 80 E
Demopolis, AL 36732-3605
(334)287-2662
FAX: (334)287-2614

Dothan

Flowers Hospital Breast Health Center
4370 W Main St Ste 101
Dothan, AL 36305-1056
(334)671-4908
FAX: (334)615-8482

Southeast Health
1108 Ross Clark Cir
Dothan, AL 36301-3024
(334)712-3241
FAX: (334)712-3451

Enterprise

Medical Center Enterprise
400 N Edwards St
Enterprise, AL 36330-2584
(334)339-8780
FAX: (334)348-8859

Eufaula

Medical Center Barbour
820 W Washington St
Eufaula, AL 36027-1899
(334)688-7070
FAX: (334)688-7080

Evergreen

Evergreen Medical Center
101 Crestview Ave
Evergreen, AL 36401-3396
(251)578-0146
FAX: (251)578-0262

Fairhope

Thomas Hospital
750 Morphy Ave
Fairhope, AL 36532-1899
(251)279-1042
FAX: (251)279-1483

Women's Imaging Specialists - Fairhope, Llc
7540 Cipriano Ct, Ste A
Fairhope, AL 36532-3029
(404)775-4228
FAX: (800)613-8386

Fayette

Fayette Medical Center
1653 Temple Ave N
Fayette, AL 35555-1314
(205)932-1246
FAX: (205)932-1108

Florence

Ob-Gyn Associates Of Northwest Alabama P.C.
2407 Helton Dr
Florence, AL 35630-1067
(256)718-5900
FAX: (256)718-5918

Tri-State Center For Breast Health At Ecm East
2111 Cloyd Blvd
Florence, AL 35630-1503
(256)768-8181
FAX: (256)768-8066

Foley

The Women's Imaging Ctr At S. Baldwin Regional Medical Ctr
161 W Peachtree Ave
Foley, AL 36535-2239
(251)949-3784
FAX: (251)943-2035

Women's Imaging Specialists - Foley, Llc
2508 S McKenzie St
Foley, AL 36535-3406
(251)255-6262
FAX: (800)899-0010

Fort Payne

Dekalb Regional Medical Center
200 Medical Center Dr SW
Fort Payne, AL 35968-3458
(256)997-2844
FAX: (256)997-2511

Fultondale

Norwood Clinic, Inc.
339 Walker Chapel Plz, Ste 101
Fultondale, AL 35068-3402
(205)250-6830
FAX: (205)250-6560

Gadsden

Advanced Imaging Of Gadsden
820 S 4th St
Gadsden, AL 35901-5223
(256)549-0008
FAX: (256)543-0514

Gadsden Regional Medical Center
1026 Goodyear Ave Ste 102
Gadsden, AL 35903-1194
(256)492-0337
FAX: (256)492-7656

The Women's Diagnostic Center
303 Bay St, Ste 403
Gadsden, AL 35901-5203
(256)543-5815
FAX: (256)549-1120

Gardendale

North Jefferson Imaging
2217 Decatur Hwy Ste 115
Gardendale, AL 35071-2301
(205)418-1280
FAX: (205)418-1281

Uab Medicine Gardendale Primary & Specialty Care
960 Rocket Way Ste 110
Gardendale, AL 35071-4750
(205)443-1714
FAX: (205)443-1717

Geneva

Wiregrass Medical Center
1200 W Maple Ave
Geneva, AL 36340-1694
(334)684-3655
FAX: (334)684-1297

Greenville

Regional Medical Center Of Central Alabama
29 L V Stabler Dr
Greenville, AL 36037-3850
(334)383-2327
FAX: (334)383-2339

Grove Hill

Grove Hill Memorial Hospital
295 S Jackson St
Grove Hill, AL 36451-3231
(251)275-3191
FAX: (251)275-3551

Gulf Shores

Foley Hospital Corp Dba South Baldwin Regional Med Ctr Gs
3590 Gulf Shores Pkwy
Gulf Shores, AL 36542-2804
(251)949-3784
FAX: (251)968-5905

Guntersville

Marshall Medical Center North
8000 Hwy. 69
Guntersville, AL 35976
(256)571-8130
FAX: (256)571-8104

Haleyville

Lakeland Community Hospital
42024 Highway 195
Haleyville, AL 35565-7054
(205)485-7140
FAX: (205)485-7265

Hoover

Baptist Imaging Hoover
5295 Preserve Pkwy Ste 110
Hoover, AL 35244-4702
(205)949-4900
FAX: (205)949-4902

Brookwood Baptist Diagnostic Center-119
7131 Cahaba Valley Rd, Suite101
Hoover, AL 35242-6402
(205)725-6901
FAX: (205)715-8905

Camellia Imaging
2068 Valleydale Rd
Hoover, AL 35244-2092
(205)544-2828
FAX: (205)783-1208

Uab Medicine At Hoover Primary And Specialty Care
501 Emery Dr W
Hoover, AL 35244-4625
(205)801-8317
FAX: (205)801-7625

Huntsville

Crestwood Womens Center - Breast Care At Crestwood
185 Chateau Dr SW, Ste 200
Huntsville, AL 35801-7414
(256)429-4888
FAX: (256)883-7140

Huntsville Hospital Breast Center
910 Adams St SE Ste 110
Huntsville, AL 35801-3751
(256)801-6283
FAX: (256)265-7126

Melanie H Scott MD Pc
204 Lowe Ave SE Ste 8
Huntsville, AL 35801-4254
(256)539-0085
FAX: (256)539-0082

Outpatient Diagnostic Center Of Huntsville
115 Saint Clair Ave SE
Huntsville, AL 35801-4343
(256)534-5600
FAX: (256)532-2420

The Center Of Imaging Excellence Women's Center
2003A Whitesburg Dr SE
Huntsville, AL 35801-4543
(256)536-3550
FAX: (256)536-3554

Jackson

Jackson Medical Center
220 Hospital Dr
Jackson, AL 36545-2459
(251)246-9021
FAX: (251)246-3238

Jasper

Bbh -Walker Breast Center
3400 Highway 78 E, Ste 218
Jasper, AL 35501-8954
(205)387-4750
FAX: (205)387-4753

Leeds

Uab-Medicine Leeds
1141 Payton Way
Leeds, AL 35094-1116
(205)699-4180
FAX: (205)699-4186

Madison

Crestwood Outpatient Diagnostics Madison
20 Hughes Rd Ste 102
Madison, AL 35758-2435
(256)429-4888
FAX: (256)883-7140

Madison Hospital Breast Center
8337 US Hihgway 72, Ste. 202
Madison, AL 35758
(256)801-6283
FAX: (256)265-5954

Outpatient Diagnostic Center Of Madison
398 Hughes Rd
Madison, AL 35758-1102
(256)534-5600
FAX: (256)532-2420

Mobile

Alabama Medical Group, P.C.
101 Memorial Hospital Dr Ste 200
Mobile, AL 36608-1787
(251)410-3083
FAX: (251)459-8964

Franklin Primary Health Center, Inc.-Mobile
1303 Dr Martin L King Jr Ave
Mobile, AL 36603-5341
(251)432-4117
FAX: (251)436-7773

Infirmary Imaging Hillcrest
845 Hillcrest Rd
Mobile, AL 36695-3909
(251)435-5090
FAX: (251)435-5091

Mobile Obstetrics And Gynecology, P.C.
6701 Airport Blvd Ste B321
Mobile, AL 36608-6703
(251)633-0793
FAX: (251)633-0736

Springhill Medical Center Women's Diagnostic Center
3715 Dauphin St Bldg 2 Ste 2C, Women's Diagnostic Center
Mobile, AL 36608-1771
(251)460-5258
FAX: (251)460-5463

The Breast Center - Outpatient Diagnostic
6801 Airport Blvd
Mobile, AL 36608-3709
(251)266-1196
FAX: (251)266-2879

The Breast Center At Mobile Infirmary
1720 Spring Hill Ave
Mobile, AL 36604-1410
(251)435-5090
FAX: (251)435-5091

USA Children's And Women's Hospital Breast Center
1601 Center St, Clinic 2 G
Mobile, AL 36604-1541
(251)415-1660
FAX: (251)415-1016

Monroeville

Monroe County Hospital
2016 S Alabama Ave
Monroeville, AL 36460-3096
(251)743-7468
FAX: (251)743-7356

Montgomery

Baptist Breast Health Center
6880 Winton Blount Blvd
Montgomery, AL 36117-3506
(334)747-4490
FAX: (334)747-4486

Jackson Imaging Ctr
1825 Park Pl
Montgomery, AL 36106-1149
(334)834-3671
FAX: (334)834-2185

Montgomery Breast Center
4145 Carmichael Rd
Montgomery, AL 36106-2803
(334)387-1120
FAX: (334)387-1121

Ob-Gyn Associates Of Montgomery
7045 Sydney Curv
Montgomery, AL 36117-3509
(334)279-9333
FAX: (334)279-9057

Moulton

Lawrence Medical Center
202 Hospital St
Moulton, AL 35650-1254
(256)974-2230
FAX: (256)974-0640

Muscle Shoals

Shoals Hospital
201 Avalon Ave
Muscle Shoals, AL 35661-2805
(256)386-1624
FAX: (256)386-1527

Northport

Northport Medical Center - Dch
2700 Hospital Dr
Northport, AL 35476-3380
(205)750-5572
FAX: (205)750-5935

Oneonta

St. Vincent's Blount
150 Gilbreath Dr
Oneonta, AL 35121-2827
(205)274-3170
FAX: (205)274-3171

Opelika

East Alabama Medical Center
2000 Pepperell Pkwy
Opelika, AL 36801-5422
(334)528-1155
FAX: (334)528-2109

Opp

Mizell Memorial Hospital
702 N Main St
Opp, AL 36467-1626
(334)493-3541
FAX: (334)493-5519

Oxford

Regional Medical Center Mediplex - Oxford
1400 Highway Dr
Oxford, AL 36203-1951
(256)235-5141
FAX: (256)235-5058

Ozark

Dale Medical Center
2126 W Roy Parker Rd
Ozark, AL 36360-8566
(334)774-2601
FAX: (334)445-2263

Pelham

Cahaba Valley Imaging
201 Racquet Club Ln
Pelham, AL 35124-6271
(205)620-3830
FAX: (205)620-3831

Pell City

Birmingham Internal Medicine, Llc Dba Complete Health
70 Plaza Dr
Pell City, AL 35125-9314
(205)814-7437
FAX: (205)338-0461

St. Vincent's St. Clair
7063 Veterans Pkwy
Pell City, AL 35125-5114
(205)814-2124
FAX: (205)814-2129

Prattville

Med Tech Imaging Center
102 Medical Center Dr
Prattville, AL 36066-7286
(334)358-1666
FAX: (334)777-1811

Prattville Imaging Center
635 McQueen Smith Rd N, Ste B
Prattville, AL 36066-5662
(334)358-6282
FAX: (334)358-1026

Red Bay

Red Bay Hospital
211 Hospital Rd
Red Bay, AL 35582-3858
(256)356-9532
FAX: (256)356-1188

Reform

Pickens County Primary Care, Pc
108 4th Ave SW
Reform, AL 35481-8018
(205)375-6251
FAX: (205)375-9064

Russellville

Russellville Hospital
15155 Highway 43
Russellville, AL 35653-1975
(256)332-8643
FAX: (256)331-4138

Saraland

Infirmary Imaging Saraland
95 Shell St Ste 100
Saraland, AL 36571-2202
(251)435-7500
FAX: (251)435-7501

Scottsboro

Mmi Breast Center Pc
1108 S Broad St B
Scottsboro, AL 35768-2514
(256)574-2883
FAX: (256)259-9397

Selma

Vaughan Regional Medical Center Llc
1015 Medical Center Pkwy
Selma, AL 36701-6748
(334)418-4388
FAX: (334)418-3545

Sheffield

Helen Keller Hospital
101 W Saywell St
Sheffield, AL 35660-6356
(256)386-4150
FAX: (256)386-4516

Sylacauga

Coosa Valley Medical Center
315 W Hickory St
Sylacauga, AL 35150-2996
(256)401-4024
FAX: (236)401-4505

Talladega

Citizens Baptist Medical Center
604 Stone Ave
Talladega, AL 35160-2217
(256)761-4618
FAX: (256)761-4087

Tallassee

Community Hospital
805 Friendship Rd
Tallassee, AL 36078-1225
(334)283-3772
FAX: (334)283-3834

Thomasville

Thomasville Regional Medical Center
300 Park Med Drive
Thomasville, AL 36784
(334)636-2525
FAX: (334)635-4111

Troy

Troy Regional Medical Center
1330 Highway 231 S
Troy, AL 36081-3067
(334)670-5000
FAX: (334)670-5369

Trussville

St. Vincent's Trussville
7201 Happy Hollow Rd
Trussville, AL 35173-2458
(205)508-6259
FAX: (205)508-6252

Tuscaloosa

Dch Regional Medical Center
809 University Blvd E
Tuscaloosa, AL 35401-2071
(205)750-5572
FAX: (205)750-5935

The Radiology Clinic, Llc
208 McFarland Cir N
Tuscaloosa, AL 35406-1800
(205)345-7000
FAX: (205)345-2494

Union Springs

Bullock County Hospital
102 Conecuh Ave W
Union Springs, AL 36089-1300
(334)738-1428
FAX: (334)738-5514

Valley

Eamc-Lanier
4800 48th St, Radiology Department
Valley, AL 36854-3666
(334)756-1429
FAX: (334)756-5678

Wetumpka

Elmore Community Hospital
500 Hospital Dr
Wetumpka, AL 36092-1600
(334)514-3835
FAX: (334)514-3822

Winfield

Northwest Medical Center
1530 US Highway 43
Winfield, AL 35594-5056
(205)487-7748
FAX: (205)487-7199

ALASKA

Anchorage

Alaska Native Medical Center
4315 Diplomacy Dr, Imaging Services
Anchorage, AK 99508-5926
(907)729-2347
FAX: (907)729-2376

Alaska Regional Hospital
1200 Airport Heights Dr Ofc Bui Medical, Alaska Regional Imaging Alliance-Alaska
Anchorage, AK 99508-2965
(907)264-1074
FAX: (907)264-2944

Anchorage Native Primary Care Clinic
4320 Diplomacy Dr, Imaging Services
Anchorage, AK 99508-5925
(907)729-2347
FAX: (907)729-2376

Anchorage Neighborhood Health Center
4951 Business Park Blvd
Anchorage, AK 99503-7174
(907)743-7388
FAX: (907)743-7249

Diagnostic Health Center Of Anchorage, Llc
4100 Lake Otis Pkwy Ste 102
Anchorage, AK 99508-5230
(907)729-5800
FAX: (907)729-5889

Imaging Associates
3650 Piper St Ste A
Anchorage, AK 99508-4692
(907)222-4624
FAX: (907)222-4651

Providence Imaging Center
3340 Providence Dr, Ste 101
Anchorage, AK 99508-4663
(907)212-3151
FAX: (907)212-5828

Barrow

Samuel Simmonds Memorial Hospital
PO Box 29, 7000 Uula St
Barrow, AK 99723-0029
(907)852-9225
FAX: (907)852-2375

Bethel

Yukon-Kuskokwim Delta Regional Hospital
700 Chief Eddie Hoffman Hwy, Ste 3000, Diagnostic Imaging Department
Bethel, AK 99559
(907)543-6238
FAX: (907)543-6314

Dillingham

Bristol Bay Area Health Corporation
PO Box 130 6000 Kanakanak Rd, Kanakanak Hospital
Dillingham, AK 99576-0130
(907)842-9365
FAX: (907)842-9476

Fairbanks

Breast Cancer Detection Center Of Alaska
1905 Cowles St
Fairbanks, AK 99701-5914
(907)479-3909
FAX: (907)479-2215

Chief Andrew Isaac Health Center
1717 W Cowles St
Fairbanks, AK 99701-5926
(907)451-6682
FAX: (907)459-3913

Fairbanks Memorial Hospital
1650 Cowles St
Fairbanks, AK 99701-5907
(907)458-6900
FAX: (907)458-6929

Ft Wainwright

Bassett Army Community Hospital
1060 Gaffney Rd, Usa-Meddac-Ak Attention: McUc-Ra
Ft Wainwright, AK 99703-5002
(907)361-5023
FAX: (907)361-5577

Homer

South Peninsula Hospital
4300 Bartlett St
Homer, AK 99603-7000
(907)235-0362
FAX: (907)235-0278

Jber

Elmendorf Air Force Base, 673d Medical Group
5955 Zeamer Ave
Jber, AK 99506-3702
(907)580-2523
FAX: (907)580-2521

Juneau

Bartlett Regional Hospital
3260 Hospital Dr
Juneau, AK 99801-7808
(907)796-8802
FAX: (907)796-8467

Searhc Elmc, Juneau
1200 Salmon Creek Lane
Juneau, AK 99801
(907)463-4029
FAX: (907)463-3719

Ketchikan

Peacehealth Ketchikan Medical Center
3100 Tongass Ave
Ketchikan, AK 99901-5746
(907)228-7644
FAX: (907)228-8337

Klawock

Searhc, Alicia Roberts Medical Center
7300 Klawock Hollis Hwy
Klawock, AK 99925
(907)755-4800
FAX: (907)755-4908

Kodiak

Providence Health & Services-Washington Dba Prov Ki Med Ctr
1915 E Rezanof Dr
Kodiak, AK 99615-6602
(907)486-9520
FAX: (907)486-9523

Kotzebue

Maniilaq Health Center
436 5th Ave & Ted Stevens Way
Kotzebue, AK 99752
(907)442-7222
FAX: (907)442-7310

Nome

Norton Sound Health Corporation
PO Box 996, 1000 Greg Kruschek Ave
Nome, AK 99762-0996
(907)443-3227
FAX: (907)443-9688

Palmer

Imaging Associates
2280 S Woodworth Loop
Palmer, AK 99645-7412
(907)746-4646
FAX: (907)746-4640

Mat-Su Regional Medical Center
2500 S Woodworth Loop
Palmer, AK 99645-8984
(907)861-6677
FAX: (907)861-6765

Petersburg

Petersburg Medical Center
PO Box 589, 103 Fram St
Petersburg, AK 99833-0589
(907)772-4291
FAX: (907)772-9271

Sitka

Searhc Mt. Edgecumb Hospital
222 Tongass Dr, Radiology Department
Sitka, AK 99835-9416
(907)966-8327
FAX: (907)966-8810

Soldotna

Central Peninsula Hospital
250 Hospital Pl
Soldotna, AK 99669-6999
(907)714-4542
FAX: (907)714-4995

Wasilla

Alaska Imaging
261 E Park Ave Ste 3
Wasilla, AK 99654-8022
(907)373-3700
FAX: (907)373-3799

Valley Native Primary Care Center
1001 S Knik Goose Bay Rd
Wasilla, AK 99654-8083
(907)631-7321
FAX: (907)631-7621

Wrangell

Searhc Wrangell Medical Center
232 Wood Street
Wrangell, AK 99929
(907)874-7128
FAX: (907)874-7122

ARIZONA

Anthem

Smi Imaging, Llc- Anthem
3618 W Anthem Way, Suite D-104-108
Anthem, AZ 85086-0419
(623)879-3740
FAX: (602)302-5865

Apache Junction

Arizona Diagnostic Radiology Group, Llc.
1840 W Apache Trl
Apache Junction, AZ 85120-3728
(480)455-1850
FAX: (480)288-4079

Smi Imaging, Llc - Apache Junction
2080 W Southern Ave, Bldg C
Apache Junction, AZ 85120-7653
(480)747-5960
FAX: (602)302-5861

Avondale

Smi Imaging, Llc - Avondale
10815 W McDowell Rd Ste 102
Avondale, AZ 85392-5009
(623)433-0121
FAX: (602)302-5902

Valleywise Community Health Center-Avondale
950 E Van Buren St
Avondale, AZ 85323-1506
(602)344-1300
FAX: (602)344-1313

Bisbee

Copper Queen Community Hospital
101 Cole Ave
Bisbee, AZ 85603-1399
(520)432-6541
FAX: (520)432-3173

Buckeye

Smi Imaging, Llc - Buckeye
818 S Watson Rd, Ste 102
Buckeye, AZ 85326-3423
(623)302-9080
FAX: (602)302-5864

Bullhead City

Western Arizona Regional Medical Center - Imaging Ctr.
1245 Hancock Rd
Bullhead City, AZ 86442-5940
(928)704-8889
FAX: (928)763-2735

Casa Grande

Arizona Diagnostic Radiology Group, Llc.
1669 E McMurray Blvd
Casa Grande, AZ 85122-6010
(520)876-0297
FAX: (520)876-0167

Banner Imaging, Casa Grande
1828 E Florence Blvd, Bldg B Spc 118
Casa Grande, AZ 85122-4783
(520)381-6745
FAX: (623)842-5936

Smi Imaging, Llc - Casa Grande
1664 E Florence Blvd, Ste 18
Casa Grande, AZ 85122-4779
(520)421-4875
FAX: (520)421-4876

Chandler

Banner Imaging Chandler
1076 W Chandler Blvd Ste 120
Chandler, AZ 85224-5224
(480)610-7400
FAX: (623)842-5936

Chandler Regional Medical Center
1727 W Frye Rd Ste 110
Chandler, AZ 85224-5296
(480)728-2008
FAX: (480)728-5562

Smi Imaging, Llc Dba Simonmed Imaging - Dobson Women's Center
1960 W Frye Rd, Ste 1
Chandler, AZ 85224-6238
(480)306-7340
FAX: (602)302-5812

Smi Imaging, Llc Dba Simonmed-New Horizons
1900 W Frye Rd, Ste 1
Chandler, AZ 85224-6235
(480)895-9555
FAX: (480)895-9494

Solis Benora Mammography
2081 W Frye Rd Bldg E Ste 110
Chandler, AZ 85224-6278
(623)419-3770
FAX: (602)234-3183

Chinle

Chinle Comprehensive Health Care Facility
Highway 191, Hospital Turnoff
Chinle, AZ 86503
(928)674-7137
FAX: (928)674-7583

Cottonwood

Nah Medical Imaging Center
340 S Willard St
Cottonwood, AZ 86326-4126
(928)649-1260
FAX: (928)649-3182

Nah Verde Valley Medical Center
269 S Candy Ln
Cottonwood, AZ 86326-4170
(928)639-6580
FAX: (928)639-6677

Flagstaff

Northern Arizona Radiology, P.C.
77 W Forest Ave Ste 101
Flagstaff, AZ 86001-1482
(928)773-2515
FAX: (928)846-8888

Smi Imaging, Llc- Flagstaff
1000 N Humphreys St, Ste 100
Flagstaff, AZ 86001-3124
(928)223-0200
FAX: (602)302-5991

Fort Mohave

Valley View Medical Center
5330 S Highway 95
Fort Mohave, AZ 86426-9225
(928)788-7228
FAX: (928)788-4919

Fountain Hills

Southwest Medical Imaging
16838 E Palisades Blvd, Ste 151
Fountain Hills, AZ 85268-3790
(480)425-5030
FAX: (480)657-3461

Gilbert

Arizona Diagnostic Radiology Group, Llc.
4915 E Baseline Rd Ste 116
Gilbert, AZ 85234-2966
(815)901-6919
FAX: (480)354-9201

Banner Imaging Gilbert
665 N Gilbert Rd Ste 154
Gilbert, AZ 85234-3395
(480)610-7400
FAX: (623)842-5936

Banner M.D. Anderson Cancer Center
2940 E Banner Gateway Dr Ste 150
Gilbert, AZ 85234-2170
(480)543-6900
FAX: (480)543-6985

Ma'am Exams
1684 E Boston St
Gilbert, AZ 85295-6219
(480)448-2411
FAX: (480)476-8718

Mercy Gilbert Medical Center Women's Imaging Center
3686 S Rome St, Ste 200
Gilbert, AZ 85297-7341
(480)728-7465
FAX: (480)728-5562

Smi Imaging Llc - Spectrum
2680 S Val Vista Dr Bldg 7, Ste 135
Gilbert, AZ 85295-2152
(480)584-4900
FAX: (623)322-7683

Smi Imaging, Llc
875 N Greenfield Rd, Ste 107
Gilbert, AZ 85234-5044
(480)813-8700
FAX: (602)302-5928

Southwest Medical Imaging
3645 S Rome St Ste 101
Gilbert, AZ 85297-7337
(480)425-5030
FAX: (480)425-5033

Glendale

Banner Imaging Management Services Llc, Arrowhead Commons
18275 N 59th Ave Bldg K-168
Glendale, AZ 85308-1260
(623)847-2000
FAX: (623)842-5936

Banner Imaging Management Services Llc, New River Trails
7701 W Aspera Blvd Ste 101
Glendale, AZ 85308-7947
(623)847-2000
FAX: (623)842-5936

Banner Imaging Management Services Llc, Sunwest Breast
5757 W Thunderbird Rd Ste W100
Glendale, AZ 85306-5612
(623)847-2000
FAX: (623)842-5936

Smi Imaging Llc - Arrowhead
6320 W Union Hills Dr, Ste 120
Glendale, AZ 85308-7237
(602)535-2840
FAX: (602)302-5966

Smi Imaging, Llc
5620 W Thunderbird Rd Ste A
Glendale, AZ 85306-4636
(602)863-9729
FAX: (602)993-5634

Smi Imaging, Llc - Thunderbird
5410 W Thunderbird Rd, Ste 221
Glendale, AZ 85306-4711
(602)682-5000
FAX: (602)682-5010

Solis Benora Mammography
18699 N 67th Ave Ste 110
Glendale, AZ 85308-7141
(602)234-2601
FAX: (602)234-3183

Sun Radiology
16222 N 59th Ave Ste C150
Glendale, AZ 85306-1747
(623)815-8200
FAX: (623)815-8299

Globe

Cobre Valley Regional Medical Center
5880 S Hospital Dr
Globe, AZ 85501-9447
(928)425-3261
FAX: (928)425-3566

Goodyear

Smi Imaging, Llc - Litchfield
1325 N Litchfield Rd, Ste 115
Goodyear, AZ 85395-1214
(602)584-4944
FAX: (602)302-5779

Valley Radiologists, Ltd Palm Valley
13555 W McDowell Rd, Ste 106
Goodyear, AZ 85395-2625
(623)847-2000
FAX: (623)842-5936

Western Regional Medical Center Inc
14200 W Celebrate Life Way
Goodyear, AZ 85338-3007
(623)207-3617
FAX: (623)207-3611

Green Valley

Radiology Ltd. Green Valley Casa Verde
400 W Camino Casa Verde Ste 170
Green Valley, AZ 85614-3564
(520)733-7226
FAX: (520)290-8377

Radiology Ltd. Green Valley Continental
450 W Continental Rd
Green Valley, AZ 85622-3551
(520)733-7226
FAX: (520)290-8377

Santa Cruz Valley Regional Hospital
4455 S I 19 Frontage Rd
Green Valley, AZ 85614-5884
(520)393-4813
FAX: (520)393-4910

Kayenta

Kayenta Health Center
Mp 394.3 Highway 160
Kayenta, AZ 86033
(928)697-4315
FAX: (928)697-4107

Kingman

Krmc Imaging Center
1033 Sycamore Ave
Kingman, AZ 86409-3580
(928)681-8604
FAX: (928)263-3735

Lake Havasu City

Havasu Regional Medical Center
101 Civic Center Ln
Lake Havasu City, AZ 86403-5683
(928)302-5411
FAX: (928)505-5772

Laveen

Smi Imaging, Llc - Laveen
7205 S 51st Ave, Ste 101
Laveen, AZ 85339-7399
(602)627-0170
FAX: (602)627-0171

Luke Afb

56th Medical Group/Sgss, Luke Afb
7219 N Litchfield Rd, Luke Air Force Base
Luke Afb, AZ 85309-1529
(623)856-7618
FAX: (623)856-4009

Marana

Marana Health Center
13395 N Marana Main St
Marana, AZ 85653-7008
(520)682-4111
FAX: (520)682-9746

Maricopa

Arizona Diagnostic Radiology Group, Llc.
21300 N John Wayne Pkwy Ste 113
Maricopa, AZ 85139-8964
(520)568-6411
FAX: (520)568-6312

Banner Health Center-Maricopa
17900 N Porter Rd
Maricopa, AZ 85138-4228
(520)233-2500
FAX: (520)233-2688

Smi Imaging, Llc -Maricopa
44555 W Edison Rd, Ste B
Maricopa, AZ 85138-6409
(520)666-7960
FAX: (602)302-5819

Mesa

Banner Baywood Medical Center - Women's Services
6644 E Baywood Ave
Mesa, AZ 85206-1797
(480)321-4444
FAX: (480)321-4445

Banner Imaging Baywood Breast Center
6553 E Baywood Ave Ste 102
Mesa, AZ 85206-1753
(480)610-7400
FAX: (480)610-7401

Banner Imaging Dobson Breast Center
1450 S Dobson Rd, Ste A100
Mesa, AZ 85202-4709
(480)610-7400
FAX: (623)842-5936

Cigna Healthcare Of Arizona Superstition Springs
6811 E Superstition Springs Blvd
Mesa, AZ 85209-4001
(602)282-9828
FAX: (855)502-5460

Mountain Vista Medical Center
1301 S Crismon Rd, Imaging Services
Mesa, AZ 85209-3767
(480)358-6450
FAX: (480)358-6451

Smi Imaging Llc - Baywood
130 S 63rd St Ste 123
Mesa, AZ 85206-1604
(480)264-4900
FAX: (602)302-5707

Smi Imaging, Llc
1425 S Greenfield Rd, Ste. 112 &114 Bldg. 2
Mesa, AZ 85206-5529
(480)584-3400
FAX: (480)324-8038

Smi Imaging, Llc - McKellips
1345 E McKellips Rd, Ste 106
Mesa, AZ 85203-2721
(480)265-8101
FAX: (602)302-5728

Smi Imaging, Llc - Mesa Desert
1111 S Dobson Rd
Mesa, AZ 85202-3902
(623)271-4830
FAX: (602)302-5797

Southwest Medical Imaging
1052 E McKellips Rd
Mesa, AZ 85203-2625
(480)425-5030
FAX: (480)425-5033

Nogales

Holy Cross Hospital
1171 W Target Range Rd
Nogales, AZ 85621-2415
(520)287-8092
FAX: (520)285-8097

Mariposa Community Health Center, Inc.
1852 N Mastick Way
Nogales, AZ 85621-1063
(520)281-1550
FAX: (520)377-5467

Oro Valley

Oro Valley Womens Imaging
1521 E Tangerine Rd, Ste 283
Oro Valley, AZ 85755-6220
(520)901-3600
FAX: (520)818-2020

Radiology Ltd., Rancho Vistoso Diagnostic Imaging
2551 E Vistoso Commerce Loop
Oro Valley, AZ 85755-9124
(520)825-1990
FAX: (520)545-1888

Page

Page Hospital
501 N Navajo Dr
Page, AZ 86040-0959
(928)645-0157
FAX: (928)645-0184

Paradise Valley

Southwest Medical Imaging
10575 N Tatum Blvd Ste C128
Paradise Valley, AZ 85253-1070
(480)425-5000
FAX: (480)425-4196

Parker

La Paz Regional Hospital
1200 W Mohave Rd, Radiology Department
Parker, AZ 85344-6349
(928)669-7325
FAX: (928)669-7324

Payson

Banner Payson Medical Center
127 E Main St Ste B
Payson, AZ 85541-5646
(928)474-7762
FAX: (928)472-3424

Peoria

Banner Imaging Management Services Llc, Peoria
13640 N Plaza Del Rio Blvd
Peoria, AZ 85381-4846
(623)876-3920
FAX: (623)842-5936

Cigna Healthcare Of Arizona - Sun City Facility
9069 W Thunderbird Rd
Peoria, AZ 85381-4412
(602)282-9828
FAX: (855)502-5460

Smi Imaging, Llc
9139 W Thunderbird Rd Ste 112
Peoria, AZ 85381-4271
(623)875-1637
FAX: (623)875-3068

Valleywise Comprehensive Health Center-Peoria
8088 W Whitney Dr
Peoria, AZ 85345-6564
(602)344-1300
FAX: (602)655-9553

Peridot

San Carlos Apache Healthcare Corporation
103 Medicine Way Rd
Peridot, AZ 85542-5000
(928)475-1200
FAX: (928)475-7349

Phoenix

Arizona Diagnostic Radiology Group, Llc.
4530 E Ray Rd Ste 160
Phoenix, AZ 85044-6097
(480)893-1004
FAX: (480)893-0306

Arizona Diagnostic Radiology Group, Llc.
444 W Osborn Rd Ste 105
Phoenix, AZ 85013-3816
(602)277-4111
FAX: (602)277-1333

Banner Imaging Management Serviced Llc, Estrella Breast
9305 W Thomas Rd Ste 200
Phoenix, AZ 85037-3447
(623)847-2000
FAX: (623)842-5936

Banner Imaging Management Services Llc, Paradise Valley
16641 N 40th St Ste 1
Phoenix, AZ 85032-3343
(623)847-2000
FAX: (623)465-6762

Banner Imaging Management Services Llc, Union Hills
18444 N 25th Ave Ste 140
Phoenix, AZ 85023-1263
(623)847-2000
FAX: (623)842-5936

Camelback Women's Health
11209 N Tatum Blvd Ste 255
Phoenix, AZ 85028-6061
(602)319-9176
FAX: (602)234-3183

Cigna Healthcare Of Az Inc Dba Cigna Med Group Phoenix Cntrl
3003 N 3rd St
Phoenix, AZ 85012-3031
(602)282-9870
FAX: (877)752-3087

Ctca-Outpatient Care Center North Phoenix
20950 N 29th Ave, Ste 110
Phoenix, AZ 85027-3110
(623)932-8960
FAX: (623)258-4152

Dignity Health Cancer Institute
625 N 6th St
Phoenix, AZ 85004-2155
(602)406-0420
FAX: (602)798-9656

Honorhealth Breast Health And Research Center - Jcl
9250 N 3rd St Ste 1002
Phoenix, AZ 85020-2402
(623)780-4673
FAX: (623)434-2788

Honorhealth Breast Health And Research Center- Dv
19646 N 27th Ave Ste 205
Phoenix, AZ 85027-4026
(623)780-4673
FAX: (623)434-2789

Honorhealth Breast Health And Research Center- Sonoran
33423 N 32nd Ave
Phoenix, AZ 85085-8874
(623)780-4673
FAX: (623)434-2783

Laura Dreier Breast Center
1111 E McDowell Rd
Phoenix, AZ 85006-2612
(602)839-2617
FAX: (602)839-6541

Maricopa Integrated Health System Chc Mammography
2525 E Roosevelt St
Phoenix, AZ 85008-4948
(602)344-1300
FAX: (602)344-1313

Mayo Clinic Arizona - Phoenix Campus
5881 E Mayo Blvd
Phoenix, AZ 85054-4504
(480)301-8016
FAX: (480)301-4303

Mountain Park Health Center
635 E Baseline Rd, Radiology Dept: Melanie Ortiz
Phoenix, AZ 85042-6583
(602)243-7277
FAX: (602)243-1356

Phoenix Indian Medical Center
4212 N 16th St
Phoenix, AZ 85016-5389
(602)263-1524
FAX: (602)263-1627

Smi Imaging Llc
2620 N 3rd St, Ste 102
Phoenix, AZ 85004-1153
(602)648-6570
FAX: (623)322-7683

Smi Imaging Llc - Deer Valley
20414 N 27th Ave, Ste 150
Phoenix, AZ 85027-3246
(623)234-2520
FAX: (623)322-7683

Smi Imaging, Llc
4045 E Bell Rd Ste 143
Phoenix, AZ 85032-2239
(602)867-5780
FAX: (602)302-5761

Smi Imaging, Llc - 19th Ave
6707 N 19th Ave, Ste 101
Phoenix, AZ 85015-1105
(602)688-6200
FAX: (602)688-6201

Smi Imaging, Llc - Ahwatukee
15810 S 45th St Ste 110
Phoenix, AZ 85048-7695
(480)753-6161
FAX: (623)322-7683

Smi Imaging, Llc - Desert Ridge
20830 N Tatum Blvd Ste 190
Phoenix, AZ 85050-7253
(480)614-8555
FAX: (623)322-7683

Smi Imaging, Llc - Estrella
8921 W Thomas Rd, Ste 101
Phoenix, AZ 85037-3244
(602)651-1945
FAX: (602)302-5707

Smi Imaging, Llc - Paradise Valley
4219 E Bell Rd
Phoenix, AZ 85032-3366
(480)428-5660
FAX: (602)302-5860

Smi Imaging, Llc Biltmore
2502 E Camelback Rd, Ste 167
Phoenix, AZ 85016-9316
(480)428-5980
FAX: (602)302-5980

Solis Benora Mammography
11220 N Tatum Blvd Ste 105
Phoenix, AZ 85028-1629
(602)319-9176
FAX: (602)234-3183

Solis Mammography
1661 E Camelback Rd, Ste 140
Phoenix, AZ 85016-3957
(480)499-6001
FAX: (602)234-3183

Southwest Medical Imaging
2222 E Highland Ave Ste 120
Phoenix, AZ 85016-4874
(480)425-5000
FAX: (480)657-3461

Vhs Of Phoenix Inc. Dba Abrazo Central Campus
2000 W Bethany Home Rd
Phoenix, AZ 85015-2443
(602)246-5550
FAX: (602)433-6623

Prescott

Prescott Medical Imaging
810 Whipple St
Prescott, AZ 86301-1606
(928)771-7577
FAX: (928)771-7616

Smi Imaging, Llc - Prescott
790 Gail Gardner Way
Prescott, AZ 86305-2337
(928)776-9900
FAX: (928)776-1444

Prescott Valley

Smi Imaging Llc
3033 N Windsong Dr, Ste 102
Prescott Valley, AZ 86314-2296
(928)772-5250
FAX: (928)772-5709

Yavapai Regional Medical Center Breast Care Center
7700 E Florentine Rd
Prescott Valley, AZ 86314-2245
(928)442-8900
FAX: (928)442-8833

Queen Creek

Smi Imaging , Llc - Queen Creek
36297 N Gantzel Rd, Ste 101
Queen Creek, AZ 85140-7324
(480)804-4400
FAX: (623)322-7683

Safford

Mt Graham Regional Medical Center
1600 S 20th Ave
Safford, AZ 85546-4011
(928)348-4251
FAX: (928)348-3806

Scottsdale

Arizona Breastnet, L.L.C.
8896 E Becker Ln Ste 101
Scottsdale, AZ 85260-6281
(480)314-7600
FAX: (480)767-7601

Assured Imaging Women's Wellness Of Southern Az, Llc
9180 E Desert Cove Ave Ste 102
Scottsdale, AZ 85260-6254
(888)233-6121
FAX: (520)572-7138

Smi Imaging, Llc
6740 E Camelback Rd, Ste 100
Scottsdale, AZ 85251-2096
(480)478-8400
FAX: (623)322-7683

Smi Imaging, Llc
9201 E Mountain View Rd, Ste 112
Scottsdale, AZ 85258-5140
(623)371-4830
FAX: (602)302-5797

Southwest Medical Imaging
9220 E Mountain View Rd Ste 214
Scottsdale, AZ 85258-5136
(480)425-5030
FAX: (480)657-3461

Southwest Medical Imaging
7301 E 2nd St Ste 112
Scottsdale, AZ 85251-5609
(480)425-5030
FAX: (480)657-3484

Southwest Medical Imaging
9700 N 91st St Ste C200
Scottsdale, AZ 85258-5064
(480)425-5030
FAX: (480)425-5033

Southwest Medical Imaging
20201 N Scottsdale Healthcare Dr Ste
Scottsdale, AZ 85255-4134
(480)425-5050
FAX: (480)425-5033

Sedona

Nah Sedona Campus
3700 W State Route 89A
Sedona, AZ 86336-4937
(928)639-6580
FAX: (928)204-4194

Show Low

Summit Healthcare Regional Medical Center
2200 E Show Low Lake Rd
Show Low, AZ 85901-7831
(928)537-6554
FAX: (928)532-1411

Sierra Vista

Canyon Vista Medical Center
151 Colonia De Salud
Sierra Vista, AZ 85635-8223
(520)263-2653
FAX: (520)263-2664

Southern Arizona Rad Associates,Dba Sierra Vista Diagnostics
155 Calle Portal, Ste 500
Sierra Vista, AZ 85635-2973
(520)459-5227
FAX: (520)459-2191

Snowflake

Summit Healthcare Reg Med Ctr Snowflake Outpatient Ctr
1121 S Main St
Snowflake, AZ 85937-5645
(928)537-6554
FAX: (928)537-4701

Sun City

Womens's Diagnostic Svcs At Banner Lakes Imaging Ctr
10474 W Thunderbird Blvd Ste 100
Sun City, AZ 85351-3015
(480)684-7500
FAX: (623)842-5936

Sun City West

Banner Del E Webb Women's Diagnostic Services
14502 W Meeker Blvd
Sun City West, AZ 85375-5282
(623)524-4462
FAX: (623)524-4179

Banner Imaging Management Services Llc, Camino Del Sol
13909 W Camino Del Sol Ste 101
Sun City West, AZ 85375-1413
(623)847-2000
FAX: (623)842-5936

Smi Imaging , Llc - Sun City West
13624 W Camino Del Sol, Ste 300
Sun City West, AZ 85375-3402
(623)214-6609
FAX: (623)374-2506

Sun Lakes

Smi Imaging, Llc
10440 E Riggs Rd, Ste 110
Sun Lakes, AZ 85248-7751
(480)338-6860
FAX: (602)302-5862

Surprise

Smi Imaging, Llc - Surprise Stadium Village
14823 W Bell Rd Ste 110
Surprise, AZ 85374-7604
(623)302-7900
FAX: (623)322-7683

Tempe

Arizona Diagnostic Radiology Group
2501 E Southern Ave Ste 8
Tempe, AZ 85282-7666
(480)455-1860
FAX: (480)467-3252

Banner Imaging Tempe
1840 E Warner Rd Ste 114
Tempe, AZ 85284-3445
(480)610-7400
FAX: (623)842-5936

Cigna Hlthcare Of Az Dba Cigna Med Grp Cj Harris Fac
1920 E Baseline Rd
Tempe, AZ 85283-1595
(602)282-9828
FAX: (855)502-5460

Smi Imaging, Llc Dba Simonmed Imaging-Mom
8380 S Kyrene Rd, Ste 105
Tempe, AZ 85284-2120
(480)967-3767
FAX: (480)967-3787

Southwest Contemporary Women's Care
6301 S McClintock Dr, Ste 215
Tempe, AZ 85283-3394
(480)820-6657
FAX: (480)730-0803

Tuba City

Tuba City Regional Health Care Corporation
167 North Main
Tuba City, AZ 86045
(928)283-2702
FAX: (928)283-1312

Tucson

Acp Northwest Imaging Center
2191 W Orange Grove Rd
Tucson, AZ 85741-3175
(520)547-3940
FAX: (520)547-3945

Arizona Community Physicians- Eastside Imaging Center
5515 E 5th St
Tucson, AZ 85711-2415
(520)298-1138
FAX: (520)547-6091

Assured Imaging Women's Wellness Of Southern Arizona, Llc
6261 N La Cholla Blvd, Ste 151A
Tucson, AZ 85741-3565
(888)233-6121
FAX: (520)572-7138

Assured Imaging Women's Wellness Of Southern Az Llc-Mobile
7717 N Hartman Ln
Tucson, AZ 85743-5800
(520)233-6121
FAX: (520)572-7138

Assured Imaging Womens Wellness Of California Inc - Mobile
7717 N Hartman Ln
Tucson, AZ 85743-5800
(888)233-6121
FAX: (520)572-7138

Banner University Medicine - Advanced Breast Imaging
4291 N Campbell Ave
Tucson, AZ 85719-1117
(520)694-4034
FAX: (520)874-7118

Davis Monthan Afb 355th Medical Group
4175 S Alamo Ave, Radiology Element/Hcos/Sgga
Tucson, AZ 85707
(520)228-2870
FAX: (520)228-2869

El Rio Health Center
6950 E Golf Links Rd
Tucson, AZ 85730-1017
(520)670-3750
FAX: (520)309-3279

El Rio Health Center
1230 S Cherrybell Stra
Tucson, AZ 85713-1907
(520)670-3750
FAX: (520)670-3799

El Rio Health Center
839 W Congress St
Tucson, AZ 85745-2819
(520)670-3747
FAX: (520)670-3799

Genesis Ob/Gyn La Cholla
6261 N La Cholla Blvd, Ste 277
Tucson, AZ 85741-3564
(520)795-0771
FAX: (520)795-0354

Genesis Ob/Gyn Wyatt
2424 N Wyatt Dr, Ste 260
Tucson, AZ 85712-6118
(520)795-0771
FAX: (520)795-0354

Northwest Women's Imaging
6060 N Fountain Plaza Dr Ste 100
Tucson, AZ 85704-7871
(520)877-4185
FAX: (520)498-0711

Radiology Ltd La Cholla Center For Diagnostic Imaging
5960 N La Cholla Blvd
Tucson, AZ 85741-3535
(520)797-3439
FAX: (520)326-7989

Radiology Ltd Midvale Imaging Center
1598 W Commerce Ct A
Tucson, AZ 85746-6015
(520)290-4842
FAX: (520)318-6145

Radiology Ltd Wilmot Ctr For Women's Imaging
677 N Wilmot Rd
Tucson, AZ 85711-2701
(520)733-7226
FAX: (520)290-8377

Radiology Ltd. St. Mary's Medical Plaza
395 N Silverbell Rd Ste 185
Tucson, AZ 85745-2721
(520)733-7226
FAX: (520)290-8377

Radiology Ltd., Rincon Imaging Center
10350 E Drexel Rd Unit 160
Tucson, AZ 85747-9411
(520)733-7226
FAX: (520)290-4847

Smi Imaging, Llc
4566 N 1st Ave Ste 100
Tucson, AZ 85718-5686
(520)498-2095
FAX: (520)498-2099

Smi Imaging, Llc - Orange Grove
1845 W Orange Grove Rd, Ste 105/103
Tucson, AZ 85704-1134
(520)230-4900
FAX: (520)230-4910

Smi Imaging, Llc- Wilmot
310 N Wilmot Rd, Ste 302
Tucson, AZ 85711-2628
(520)459-8001
FAX: (520)449-8010

Southern Arizona Radiology Associates
2492 E River Rd
Tucson, AZ 85718-9552
(520)777-1860
FAX: (520)300-8070

Tucson Medical Center
2625 N Craycroft Rd Ste 111
Tucson, AZ 85712-2254
(520)324-1286
FAX: (520)324-1309

Wickenburg

Wickenburg Community Hospital
520 Rose Ln
Wickenburg, AZ 85390-1447
(928)684-4382
FAX: (928)684-0653

Willcox

Northern Cochise Community Hospital
901 W Rex Allen Dr
Willcox, AZ 85643-1009
(520)766-6461
FAX: (520)384-3974

Yuma

Smi Imaging , Llc - Yuma
2500 S 8th Ave, Ste 103
Yuma, AZ 85364-7132
(928)304-7801
FAX: (602)302-5769

Womens Health Services
2911 S 8th Ave
Yuma, AZ 85364-8000
(928)336-7306
FAX: (928)336-1208

Yuma Regional Foothills Imaging Center
11142 S Scottsdale Dr
Yuma, AZ 85367-5616
(928)336-7751
FAX: (928)336-7384

Yuma Regional Outpatient Diagnostic Imaging Ctr.
2460 S Parkview Loop Ste 2
Yuma, AZ 85364-5357
(928)336-7306
FAX: (928)336-7384

ARKANSAS

Arkadelphia

Baptist Health Medical Center-Arkadelphia
3050 Twin Rivers Dr, Radiology Department
Arkadelphia, AR 71923-4218
(870)245-1240
FAX: (870)245-1181

Ashdown

Little River Memorial Hospital
451 W Locke St
Ashdown, AR 71822-3325
(870)898-5011
FAX: (870)898-4666

Batesville

White River Medical Center
PO Box 2197, 1710 Harrison St
Batesville, AR 72503-2197
(870)262-3229
FAX: (870)262-1092

Benton

Baptist Health Imaging Center - Saline County
829 W Carpenter St
Benton, AR 72015-3349
(501)776-2006
FAX: (501)776-2153

Saline Memorial Hospital
1 Medical Park Dr
Benton, AR 72015-3354
(501)776-6616
FAX: (501)776-6188

Bentonville

Imaging Associates Of Nw Ar At Fountain Plaza
801 SE Plaza Ave Ste 5
Bentonville, AR 72712-7925
(479)271-0084
FAX: (479)271-7148

Mercy Clinic Highway 102
3101 SE 14th St
Bentonville, AR 72712-4900
(479)338-2797
FAX: (479)986-6115

Northwest Medical Center- Bentonville
3000 Medical Center Pkwy
Bentonville, AR 72712-3217
(479)553-4253
FAX: (479)553-1932

Berryville

Mercy Hospital Berryville
214 Carter St
Berryville, AR 72616-4303
(870)423-5263
FAX: (870)423-5227

Blytheville

Great River Medical Center
1520 N Division St
Blytheville, AR 72315-1448
(870)838-7371
FAX: (870)838-7301

Camden

Ouachita County Medical Center
638 California Ave SW
Camden, AR 71701-4699
(870)836-1220
FAX: (870)836-1445

Cherokee Village

White River Medical Center-North Complex Imaging Center
195 Hospital Dr, Ste C
Cherokee Village, AR 72529-7330
(870)257-6040
FAX: (870)257-7667

Clarksville

Johnson Regional Medical Center
1100 E Poplar St
Clarksville, AR 72830-4419
(479)754-5304
FAX: (479)754-5325

Clinton

Ozark Health Medical Center
PO Box 206, 2500 Highway 65 S
Clinton, AR 72031-0206
(501)745-9542
FAX: (501)745-9544

Conway

Baptist Health Medical Center-Conway
1555 Exchange Ave
Conway, AR 72032-7824
(501)202-1922
FAX: (501)585-2906

Conway Regional Health System Women's Center
2302 College Ave
Conway, AR 72034-6297
(501)513-5116
FAX: (501)513-5175

Crossett

Ashley County Medical Center
PO Box 400, 1015 Unity Rd
Crossett, AR 71635-0400
(870)364-1283
FAX: (870)364-1233

Danville

Chambers Memorial Hospital
PO Box 639, 719 Detroit Ave
Danville, AR 72833-0639
(479)495-6267
FAX: (479)495-6295

Dumas

Delta Memorial Hospital
PO Box 887, 811 Hwy 65 S
Dumas, AR 71639-0887
(870)382-8228
FAX: (870)382-8152

El Dorado

McSa Outpatient Imaging Center
2401 W Hillsboro St, P O Box 1998
El Dorado, AR 71730-6815
(870)862-4624
FAX: (870)862-4626

Medical Center Of South Arkansas
700 W Grove St, P O Box 1998
El Dorado, AR 71730-4416
(870)864-3366
FAX: (870)864-3593

Fayetteville

The Breast Center Of Northwest Arkansas
55 W Sunbridge Dr
Fayetteville, AR 72703-1825
(479)442-6266
FAX: (479)582-2710

Forrest City

Forrest City Medical Center
1601 New Castle Rd
Forrest City, AR 72335-2218
(870)261-0228
FAX: (870)261-0018

Fort Smith

Baptist Health Services-Women's Imaging
PO Box 2406, 1500 Dodson Ave Suite 140
Fort Smith, AR 72902-2406
(479)709-1913
FAX: (479)573-7869

Mercy Hospital Fort Smith, Mobile Mammography
PO Box 17000, 7301 Rogers Ave
Fort Smith, AR 72917-7000
(479)314-5264
FAX: (479)314-5299

Mercy Hospital Fort Smith-Women's Imaging Center
7301 Rogers Ave
Fort Smith, AR 72903-4100
(479)314-5264
FAX: (479)314-5299

Harrison

North Arkansas Regional Medical Center
620 N Main St
Harrison, AR 72601-2926
(870)414-4209
FAX: (870)414-4917

The Breast Center Of Northwest Arkansas-Harrison
502 N Walnut St
Harrison, AR 72601-3616
(479)442-6266
FAX: (479)271-7148

Heber Springs

Baptist Medical Center Heber Springs
1800 By Pass Rd
Heber Springs, AR 72543-9135
(501)887-3245
FAX: (501)887-3396

Helena

Helena Regional Medical Center
PO Box 788, 1801 Martin Luther King Dr
Helena, AR 72342-0788
(870)816-3920
FAX: (870)816-3931

Hope

Wadley Regional Medical Center At Hope
2001 S Main St, Radiology Dept.
Hope, AR 71801-8124
(870)722-3980
FAX: (870)722-3989

Hot Springs

Chi St. Vincent Hot Springs Breast Center
1 Mercy Ln Ste 107
Hot Springs, AR 71913-6474
(501)622-4589
FAX: (501)622-4541

Chi St. Vincent Hot Springs Mobile Mammography Van
1 Mercy Ln Ste 107, 300 Werner Drive
Hot Springs, AR 71913-6474
(501)622-2277
FAX: (501)622-4541

The Breast Center Of National Park Medical Center
1900 Malvern Ave, Ste 101
Hot Springs, AR 71901-7776
(501)620-2377
FAX: (501)321-9407

Hot Springs Village

Chi St. Vincent Hot Springs Imaging Services-H S Village
4419 N Highway 7
Hot Springs Village, AR 71909-9301
(501)984-5039
FAX: (501)984-5043

Jonesboro

Nea Baptist Memorial Hospital Breast Imaging Center
4802 E Johnson Ave
Jonesboro, AR 72405-8413
(870)936-8038
FAX: (870)936-8081

St. Bernard's Imaging Center
1144 E Matthews Ave
Jonesboro, AR 72401-4314
(870)207-8000
FAX: (870)207-0541

St. Bernard's Medical Center - Mobile
225 E Washington Ave
Jonesboro, AR 72401-3111
(870)207-8000
FAX: (807)207-0541

Lake Village

Chicot Memorial Medical Center
PO Box 512, 2729 Highway 65 & 82 S
Lake Village, AR 71653-0512
(870)265-5351

Little Rock

Baptist Health Breast Center
9500 Kanis Rd, Ste 250
Little Rock, AR 72205-6371
(501)202-1922
FAX: (501)202-7002

Central Clinic For Women
9601 Baptist Health Dr, Ste 500
Little Rock, AR 72205-6341
(501)227-5885
FAX: (877)584-0426

Cornerstone Clinic For Women, Pa
9500 Baptist Health Dr, Ste 100
Little Rock, AR 72205-6340
(501)224-5500
FAX: (877)464-0229

St. Vincent Breast Center
500 S University Ave Ste 114
Little Rock, AR 72205-5314
(501)661-9766
FAX: (501)975-4666

St. Vincent Breast Center-West
16115 Saint Vincent Way, Uppr 200
Little Rock, AR 72223-3002
(501)975-5470
FAX: (501)975-4666

The Breast Center Carti
PO Box 55050, 8901 Carti Way
Little Rock, AR 72215-5050
(501)537-6266
FAX: (501)906-2698

The Womans Clinic Pa
9601 Baptist Health Dr, Ste 1200
Little Rock, AR 72205-6334
(877)455-1491
FAX: (877)211-4393

Uams Breast Center
4018 W. Capitol Ave, Cancer Institute 3rd Floor
Little Rock, AR 72205
(501)526-7300
FAX: (501)526-6789

Uams Breast Center At Midtown
6119 Midtown Ave First Floor
Little Rock, AR 72205-5313
(501)526-7300
FAX: (501)526-6789

Uams Rockefeller Cancer Institute Mobile Mammography
4301 West Markham, Slot 125
Little Rock, AR 72205
(501)258-6564
FAX: (501)603-1441

Magnolia

Magnolia Regional Medical Center
PO Box 629, 101 Hospital Dr
Magnolia, AR 71754-0629
(870)235-3165
FAX: (870)235-3404

Malvern

Baptist Health Medical Center Hot Spring County
1001 Schneider Dr
Malvern, AR 72104-4811
(501)332-7373
FAX: (501)332-7376

Mena

Mena Regional Health System
311 Morrow St N
Mena, AR 71953-2516
(479)394-6100
FAX: (479)243-4598

Monticello

Drew Memorial Hospital
778 Scogin Dr
Monticello, AR 71655-5729
(870)367-2411
FAX: (870)460-3502

Morrilton

Chi St. Vincent Morrilton
4 Hospital Dr
Morrilton, AR 72110-4510
(501)977-2433
FAX: (501)977-2259

Mountain Home

Baxter Regional Medical Center
624 Hospital Dr
Mountain Home, AR 72653-2955
(870)508-1154
FAX: (870)508-1696

Imaging Center Of Baxter Regional Medical Center-Mobile
624 Hospital Dr
Mountain Home, AR 72653-2955
(870)508-1164
FAX: (870)508-1696

Regional Family Medicine, Pa
630 Burnett Dr
Mountain Home, AR 72653-2941
(870)425-6971
FAX: (870)508-8901

Mountain View

Stone County Medical Center
PO Box 510, 2106 Main St
Mountain View, AR 72560-0510
(870)269-4361
FAX: (870)269-8265

Nashville

Howard Memorial Hospital
130 Medical Cir
Nashville, AR 71852-8606
(870)845-8070
FAX: (870)845-8259

Newport

Unity Hospital - Newport
1205 McLain St
Newport, AR 72112-3533
(870)512-3004
FAX: (870)523-0374

North Little Rock

Baptist Health Breast Center North Little Rock
3401 Springhill Dr Ste 265
North Little Rock, AR 72117-2936
(501)202-3401
FAX: (501)202-4979

The Breast Center @ Carti - North
3400 Springhill Dr.
North Little Rock, AR 72117
(501)537-6266
FAX: (501)906-2698

Paragould

Arkansas Methodist Medical Center
900 W Kingshighway
Paragould, AR 72450-5942
(870)239-7820
FAX: (870)239-7212

Pine Bluff

Jefferson Regional Medical Center
1600 W 40th Ave
Pine Bluff, AR 71603-6301
(870)541-7104
FAX: (870)541-3289

Pocahontas

Pocahontas Medical Clinic
2901 Medical Center Dr
Pocahontas, AR 72455-9438
(870)892-4467
FAX: (501)712-1392

Russellville

Carti Cancer Center Russellville
209 S Portland Ave
Russellville, AR 72801-2339
(501)296-3221

St. Mary's Regional Medical Center
1808 W Main St
Russellville, AR 72801-2724
(501)964-9150
FAX: (501)968-6965

Searcy

Radiology Associates P.A.-Searcy
415 Rodgers Dr, Ste B
Searcy, AR 72143-7434
(501)278-3298
FAX: (501)278-3298

Sherwood

Chi St. Vincent Medical Center North
2215 Wildwood Ave
Sherwood, AR 72120-5089
(501)552-7395
FAX: (501)552-7493

Siloam Springs

Siloam Springs Regional Hospital
603 N Progress Ave
Siloam Springs, AR 72761-4352
(479)215-3420
FAX: (479)215-3429

Springdale

Northwest Breast Imaging Center At Willow Creek
5501 Willow Creek Dr Ste 103
Springdale, AR 72762-8707
(479)750-6660
FAX: (479)757-1645

The Breast Center Of Northwest Arkansas-Springdale
3901 Parkway Cir Ste 125
Springdale, AR 72762-6362
(479)332-6420
FAX: (479)442-6266

Stuttgart

Baptist Health Medical Center-Stuttgart
1703 N Buerkle St
Stuttgart, AR 72160-3153
(870)674-6381
FAX: (870)672-6875

Walnut Ridge

Lawrence Memorial Health Foundation, Inc
PO Box 839, 1309 W Main St
Walnut Ridge, AR 72476-0839
(870)886-1244

Warren

Bradley County Medical Center
404 S Bradley St
Warren, AR 71671-3459
(870)226-4165
FAX: (870)226-4168

West Memphis

Baptist Memorial Hospital Crittenden
2100 N 7th St
West Memphis, AR 72301-2017
(870)394-7842

Outpatient Radiology Clinic P.A.
200 S Rhodes St, Ste B
West Memphis, AR 72301-4213
(870)735-5555
FAX: (870)735-5660

White Hall

Family Medicine Of White Hall
7245 Sheridan Rd
White Hall, AR 71602-3214
(870)850-8055
FAX: (870)850-8056

Wynne

Crossridge Community Hospital
PO Box 590, 310 South Fls
Wynne, AR 72396-0590
(870)208-2139
FAX: (870)208-2157

CALIFORNIA

Alameda

Alameda Health System Dba Alameda Hospital
2070 Clinton Ave
Alameda, CA 94501-4399
(510)814-4314
FAX: (510)814-4314

The Permanente Medical Group - Alameda
2424 Central Ave
Alameda, CA 94501-4516
(510)752-1255
FAX: (510)752-2783

Alhambra

Calvin Yang MD
235 S Garfield Ave
Alhambra, CA 91801-3885
(626)943-9985
FAX: (626)943-7679

Pacific Medical Imaging & Oncology Ctr
707 S Garfield Ave Ste B001
Alhambra, CA 91801-5864
(626)227-2727
FAX: (626)227-2799

Aliso Viejo

Hoag Imaging Center Aliso Viejo
26671 Aliso Creek Rd, Ste 106
Aliso Viejo, CA 92656-4807
(949)764-7555
FAX: (949)425-1779

Anaheim

Breast Center - Ahmc Anaheim Regional Medical Center
1211 W La Palma Ave Ste 104
Anaheim, CA 92801-2810
(714)999-6134
FAX: (714)999-6007

Cancer Treatment Medical Center Inc.
2571 W La Palma Ave
Anaheim, CA 92801-2619
(714)827-9797
FAX: (714)827-5377

Dynamic Medical Imaging - Anaheim
408 S Beach Blvd, Ste 106
Anaheim, CA 92804-1873
(714)995-5471
FAX: (714)995-5815

Pacific Coast Medical Services - Mobile
1440 S State College Blvd Ste 3K
Anaheim, CA 92806-5721
(714)758-0660
FAX: (714)758-0770

S Khf Euclid Medical Offices
1188 N Euclid St
Anaheim, CA 92801-1900
(714)223-3028
FAX: (949)932-6330

Skfh Kraemer 2
3430 E La Palma Ave Mob2
Anaheim, CA 92806-2020
(714)223-3028
FAX: (949)932-6330

United Medical Imaging Of Anaheim
1801 W Romneya Dr Ste 104
Anaheim, CA 92801-1824
(714)678-4000
FAX: (714)678-4022

Antioch

Antioch Health Center
2335 Country Hills Dr
Antioch, CA 94509-7319
(925)431-2370
FAX: (925)431-2373

Antioch Medical Imaging
3450 Hillcrest Ave
Antioch, CA 94531-8238
(925)757-2100
FAX: (925)757-2101

Kaiser Foundation Hospital, Antioch Medical Ctr
4501 Sand Creek Rd, Radiology Department
Antioch, CA 94531-8687
(925)813-6276
FAX: (925)813-7063

Sutter Delta Medical Center
3901 Lone Tree Way
Antioch, CA 94509-6200
(925)756-1146
FAX: (925)779-3096

The Permanente Medical Group, Delta Fair Medical Offices
3400 Delta Fair Blvd
Antioch, CA 94509-4004
(925)779-5286
FAX: (925)779-5408

Arcadia

Arcadia Radiology Imaging
612 W Duarte Rd, Ste 101
Arcadia, CA 91007-9220
(626)447-0035
FAX: (626)447-2924

Arcadia Radiology Women's Imaging
622 W Duarte Rd Ste 104
Arcadia, CA 91007-9269
(626)447-0035
FAX: (626)447-2924

Diagnostic Medical Group Of Southern California
25 N Santa Anita Ave, Ste C
Arcadia, CA 91006-3168
(626)282-2802
FAX: (626)282-3159

Huntington-Hill Breast Center
301 W Huntington Dr Ste 617
Arcadia, CA 91007-1518
(626)701-5850
FAX: (626)701-5854

Keck Medical Center Of Usc-Arcadia
125 W Huntington Dr, Bldg B Suite B100
Arcadia, CA 91007-3050
(626)574-2800
FAX: (323)865-0114

Arcata

Mad River Community Hospital
3800 Janes Rd
Arcata, CA 95521-4788
(707)822-7220
FAX: (707)825-4928

Atwater

Castle Family Hlth Ctrs Inc
3605 Hospital Rd, Ste H
Atwater, CA 95301-5173
(209)381-2000
FAX: (209)349-8221

Auburn

Sutter Valley Medical Foundation - Sutter Imaging Auburn
3123 Professional Dr Ste 100
Auburn, CA 95603-2400
(530)888-8878
FAX: (530)887-8255

Bakersfield

Adventist Health Bakersfield
2615 Chester Ave
Bakersfield, CA 93301-2014
(661)869-6260
FAX: (661)869-6966

Adventist Health Bakersfield
9602 Stockdale Hwy
Bakersfield, CA 93311-3618
(661)633-5001
FAX: (661)633-2500

Adventist Health- Bakersfield
2700 Chester Ave
Bakersfield, CA 93301-2017
(661)637-8708
FAX: (661)633-2500

Comprehensive Blood And Cancer Center
6501 Truxtun Ave
Bakersfield, CA 93309-0633
(661)322-2206
FAX: (661)616-1694

Kern Medical Center
1700 Mount Vernon Ave
Bakersfield, CA 93306-4018
(661)326-2886
FAX: (661)326-2888

Kern Radiology
3838 San Dimas St Ste A120
Bakersfield, CA 93301-2281
(661)326-9600
FAX: (661)395-0871

Kern Radiology
9330 Stockdale Hwy Ste 100
Bakersfield, CA 93311-3615
(661)326-9600
FAX: (661)654-8543

Kern Radiology Medical Group
9900 Stockdale Hwy Ste 100
Bakersfield, CA 93311-3633
(661)325-6800
FAX: (661)362-0129

Kern Radiology Medical Group
4500 Morning Dr Ste 202
Bakersfield, CA 93306-7277
(661)326-7000
FAX: (661)873-0011

Kern Radiology Medical Group
1817 Truxtun Ave
Bakersfield, CA 93301-5008
(661)616-1488
FAX: (661)616-3509

Kern Radiology Medical Group, Inc.
2301 Bahamas Dr
Bakersfield, CA 93309-0663
(661)326-9600
FAX: (661)332-8041

Mercy Womens' Imaging Center
500 Old River Rd Ste 200
Bakersfield, CA 93311-9505
(661)663-6429
FAX: (661)663-6041

S Kfh Discovery
1200 Discovery Dr Ste 150
Bakersfield, CA 93309-7034
(661)412-6767
FAX: (661)664-3766

S Kfh Ming
8800 Ming Ave
Bakersfield, CA 93311-1308
(661)412-6767
FAX: (661)664-3766

S Kfh Stockdale
3501 Stockdale Hwy
Bakersfield, CA 93309-2150
(661)412-6767
FAX: (661)664-3766

San Dimas Medical Group
100 Old River Rd
Bakersfield, CA 93311-8823
(661)663-4800
FAX: (877)237-2905

Stockdale Radiology
4000 Empire Dr, Ste 100
Bakersfield, CA 93309-0401
(661)631-8000
FAX: (661)631-8005

Baldwin Park

Skfh Baldwin Park-Kaiser Permanente Baldwin Park Medical Ctr
1011 Baldwin Park Blvd
Baldwin Park, CA 91706-5806
(626)851-5130
FAX: (626)851-5461

Banning

San Gorgonio Memorial Hospital
600 N Highland Springs Ave, Radiology Department
Banning, CA 92220-3090
(951)769-2142
FAX: (951)769-4803

Barstow

Barstow Community Hospital
820 E Mountain View St
Barstow, CA 92311-3086
(760)256-1761
FAX: (760)957-3385

Bellflower

Pioneer Medical Group - Artesia Facility
10251 Artesia Blvd
Bellflower, CA 90706-6719
(562)862-4566
FAX: (562)862-4638

United Medical Imaging Of Bellflower
10230 Artesia Blvd, Ste 100
Bellflower, CA 90706-6763
(562)461-3400
FAX: (562)216-7207

Berkeley

The Permanente Medical Group - Berkeley
2610 10th Street, Berkeley Medical Office Building - 2nd F
Berkeley, CA 94710
(510)752-1255
FAX: (510)752-2783

Ucsf-John Muir Health Imaging Center Berkeley
3100 San Pablo Ave
Berkeley, CA 94702-2498
(415)353-3900
FAX: (510)985-5062

Beverly Hills

Bedford Breast Center
436 N Bedford Dr, Ste 105
Beverly Hills, CA 90210-4323
(310)278-8590
FAX: (424)202-3759

Beverly Radiology Medical Group At Tower Womens Ctr
465 N Roxbury Dr Ste 101
Beverly Hills, CA 90210-4230
(310)385-7747
FAX: (310)385-9144

Lsg Imaging
9675 Brighton Way Ste 240
Beverly Hills, CA 90210-5138
(310)859-8104
FAX: (310)859-2592

Big Bear Lake

Bear Valley Community Hospital
41870 Garstin Dr
Big Bear Lake, CA 92315-2088
(909)878-8226
FAX: (909)878-8280

Bishop

Northern Inyo Hospital Healthcare District
150 Pioneer Ln
Bishop, CA 93514-2599
(760)873-2155
FAX: (760)873-6393

Bonita

S Kfh - Bonita
3955 Bonita Rd
Bonita, CA 91902-1230
(800)290-5000
FAX: (619)528-6588

Brawley

Pioneers Memorial Healthcare District
207 W Legion Rd
Brawley, CA 92227-7780
(760)351-3281
FAX: (760)344-5325

Brea

United Medical Imaging Of Brea
380 W Central Ave, Ste 210
Brea, CA 92821-3066
(714)482-2121
FAX: (714)482-2120

Brentwood

John Muir Medical Imaging Brentwood
2400 Balfour Rd
Brentwood, CA 94513-4945
(925)952-2701
FAX: (925)941-4065

Brownsville

Sutter Valley Medical Foundation - Sutter Imaging North
16911 Willow Glen Rd
Brownsville, CA 95919
(530)749-3609
FAX: (530)675-0530

Buena Park

Shin Imaging Center
5832 Beach Blvd Unit 104
Buena Park, CA 90621-5500
(714)578-8882
FAX: (714)578-8886

United Medical Imaging Of Buena Park
6131 Orangethorpe Ave, Ste 130
Buena Park, CA 90620-4905
(714)522-2077
FAX: (714)522-2474

Burbank

Providence Saint Joseph Breast Health Center
181 S Buena Vista St, Ste 300
Burbank, CA 91505-4504
(818)847-4999
FAX: (818)847-6732

The Burbank Breast Care Center
2601 W Alameda Ave, Ste 101
Burbank, CA 91505-4810
(800)378-5597
FAX: (818)843-4148

Ucla Eimg Toluca Lake Health Center
4323 W Riverside Dr
Burbank, CA 91505-4044
(310)301-6800
FAX: (818)295-3357

Camarillo

Rolling Oaks Radiology - Camarillo
3801 Las Posas Rd Ste 111
Camarillo, CA 93010-1477
(805)357-0067
FAX: (805)389-3218

St. John's Pleasant Valley Hospital
2309 Antonio Ave
Camarillo, CA 93010-1401
(805)389-5655
FAX: (805)389-5671

Cameron Park

Marshall Medical Center-Cameron Park
3581 Palmer Dr Ste 301
Cameron Park, CA 95682-8238
(530)626-2770
FAX: (530)344-5434

Camp Pendleton

Naval Hospital - Camp Pendleton
200 Mercy Circle H-200
Camp Pendleton, CA 92055
(760)719-3742
FAX: (760)725-1355

Campbell

Nk Tpmg Campbell Mob
220 E Hacienda Ave
Campbell, CA 95008-6617
(408)851-5054
FAX: (408)851-3669

Carlsbad

S Kfh - Carlsbad
6860 Avenida Encinas
Carlsbad, CA 92011-3201
(800)290-5000
FAX: (619)528-3297

Carmichael

Mercy Imaging Ctrs A Service Of Dignity Hlth Med Foundation
6305 Coyle Ave
Carmichael, CA 95608-0438
(916)434-7600
FAX: (916)966-5063

Sutter Valley Medical Foundation - Sutter Imaging Carmichael
6620 Coyle Ave Ste 110
Carmichael, CA 95608-6336
(916)961-4910
FAX: (916)965-6855

Carson

Torrance Memorial Breast Diagnostic Center II
824 E Carson St Ste 208
Carson, CA 90745-2262
(310)233-3230
FAX: (310)233-3233

Castro Valley

Eden Medical Center
20103 Lake Chabot Rd
Castro Valley, CA 94546-5305
(510)727-3020
FAX: (510)727-3358

Sutter East Bay Medical Foundation
20101 Lake Chabot Rd 1st Fl
Castro Valley, CA 94546-5305
(510)247-6350
FAX: (510)247-6392

Ceres

Life Saving Images
PO Box 544
Ceres, CA 95307-0544
(209)689-3211
FAX: (209)554-8315

Cerritos

Kaiser Permanente Medical Offices - Cerritos
10820 183rd St
Cerritos, CA 90703-8010
(800)823-4040
FAX: (562)657-7228

Chico

Halo Medical Group Dba Halo Breast Care Center
1720 Esplanade
Chico, CA 95926-3315
(530)209-9066
FAX: (530)898-0533

Mangrove Medical Group
1040 Mangrove Ave
Chico, CA 95926-3509
(530)345-0064
FAX: (530)343-2612

Chino

Centrelake Imaging & Oncology
5562 Philadelphia St, Ste 100
Chino, CA 91710-2482
(909)242-7300
FAX: (909)784-3760

Chino Valley Medical Center
5451 Walnut Ave
Chino, CA 91710-2672
(909)464-8643
FAX: (909)464-8886

Chino Hills

Pomona Valley Imaging Center At Chino Hills
2140 Grand Ave Ste 115
Chino Hills, CA 91709-6801
(909)865-9897
FAX: (909)865-9794

Chowchilla

Central California Women's Facility
23370 Road 22
Chowchilla, CA 93610-8504
(559)665-5531
FAX: (559)665-8188

Chula Vista

Imaging Healthcare Specialists - South Bay
333 H St Ste 1095
Chula Vista, CA 91910-5557
(866)558-4320
FAX: (866)558-4329

San Diego Imaging, Chula Vista, Llc
765 Medical Center Ct
Chula Vista, CA 91911-6600
(619)397-6577
FAX: (619)502-8585

Scripps Mercy Imaging Center
480 Fourth Ave, Ste 212
Chula Vista, CA 91910-4412
(619)691-7295
FAX: (619)862-6670

Sharp Rees - Stealy Otay Ranch
1400 E Palomar St, Radiology
Chula Vista, CA 91913-1800
(858)586-6730
FAX: (619)446-1630

City Of Industry

Diagnostic Medical Group Of Southern California
18575 Gale Ave Ste 105
City Of Industry, CA 91748-1382
(626)363-1733
FAX: (626)363-1735

Pacific Medical Imag. & Oncology Ctr - City Of Industry
1661 Hanover Rd Ste 102
City Of Industry, CA 91748-1734
(626)965-8118
FAX: (626)965-8114

Claremont

Pomona Valley Imaging Ctr Claremont
1601 Monte Vista Ave Ste 170
Claremont, CA 91711-6603
(909)865-9583
FAX: (909)865-9794

Clearlake

Adventist Health Clear Lake Hospital
15322 Lakeshore Dr Ste 204
Clearlake, CA 95422-9815
(707)995-5760
FAX: (707)994-8917

Clovis

Clovis Community Medical Center
2755 Herndon Ave
Clovis, CA 93611-6801
(559)324-4848
FAX: (559)324-4777

Nk Tpmg Clovis
2071 Herndon Ave
Clovis, CA 93611-6101
(559)324-5025
FAX: (559)324-5026

Colton

Arrowhead Regional Medical Center
400 N Pepper Ave
Colton, CA 92324-1819
(909)580-2231
FAX: (909)580-1561

Concord

John Muir Health Medical Imaging, Cmc
2540 East St
Concord, CA 94520-1906
(925)952-2701
FAX: (925)674-2934

Norcal Imaging - Concord
2300 Clayton Rd Ste 160
Concord, CA 94520-2128
(925)825-7777
FAX: (925)288-8719

Corona

California Institution For Women
16756 Chino Corona Rd
Corona, CA 92880-9507
(909)597-1771
FAX: (909)393-8678

Corona Community Health Clinic
2813 S Main St
Corona, CA 92882-5942
(951)955-0151
FAX: (951)272-5452

Corona Comprehensive Imaging Center
801 S Main St, Ste 101
Corona, CA 92882-3410
(951)238-6071
FAX: (951)238-6044

Corona Regional Medical Center
800 S Main St
Corona, CA 92882-3420
(951)736-6270
FAX: (951)736-4888

Kaiser Permanente Medical Offices - Corona
2055 Kellogg Ave
Corona, CA 92879-3111
(951)353-4000
FAX: (951)353-5797

Coronado

Sharp Coronado Hospital
250 Prospect Pl
Coronado, CA 92118-1999
(619)522-3721
FAX: (619)502-8552

Costa Mesa

Hoag Imaging Center - Costa Mesa
1190 Baker St Ste 102
Costa Mesa, CA 92626-4105
(949)764-1888
FAX: (714)668-0378

Pacific Breast Care Center
1640 Newport Blvd Ste 200
Costa Mesa, CA 92627-3786
(949)515-3544
FAX: (949)515-3644

Covina

Centrelake Medical Group
1433 N Hollenbeck Ave, Ste 105
Covina, CA 91722-1558
(909)242-7300
FAX: (909)784-3764

Emanate Health Inter-Community Hospital
315 N 3rd Ave Ste 203
Covina, CA 91723-1915
(626)915-6266
FAX: (626)339-0903

Magan Medical Clinic, Part Of Optumcare
420 W Rowland St
Covina, CA 91723-2943
(626)251-1350
FAX: (626)251-1484

Crescent City

Sutter Coast Hospital
800 E Washington Blvd
Crescent City, CA 95531-8359
(707)464-8844
FAX: (707)464-8935

Cudahy

Kaiser Permanente Medical Offices-Cudahy
7825 Atlantic Ave
Cudahy, CA 90201-5022
(800)823-4040
FAX: (562)657-7228

Daly City

Chinese Hospital Outpatient Center
386 Gellert Blvd
Daly City, CA 94015-2611
(415)677-2320
FAX: (415)677-2444

Health Diagnostics Of California, A Professional Corporation
455 Hickey Blvd Ste 200
Daly City, CA 94015-2630
(650)757-2030
FAX: (650)757-2036

Seton Breast Health Center Dba Ahmc Healthcare Inc.
1850 Sullivan Ave Ste 110
Daly City, CA 94015-2204
(650)991-6030
FAX: (650)756-1116

Tpmg Daly City
395 Hickey Blvd, Radiology Dept - 3rd Floor
Daly City, CA 94015-2770
(650)301-4700
FAX: (650)742-2085

Danville

Palo Alto Medical Foundation — Danville
915 San Ramon Valley Blvd, Ste 100
Danville, CA 94526-4063
(650)853-2902
FAX: (650)853-6099

Davis

Sutter Valley Medical Foundation - Sutter Imaging Davis
2020 Sutter Pl Ste 102
Davis, CA 95616-6217
(530)747-5030
FAX: (530)747-5031

The Permanente Medical Group, Davis
1955 Cowell Blvd
Davis, CA 95618-6325
(916)973-5720
FAX: (916)497-4210

Delano

Adventist Health Delano
1401 Garces Hwy Bldg A
Delano, CA 93215-3699
(661)721-5788
FAX: (661)375-5373

Diamond Bar

Providence Medical Foundation
1514 Valley Vista Dr
Diamond Bar, CA 91765-3929
(909)860-1144
FAX: (909)860-9304

Skfh Diamond Bar Kaiser Permanente - Diamond Bar
1336 Bridgegate Dr
Diamond Bar, CA 91765-3955
(626)851-5130
FAX: (626)851-5461

Downey

Centrelake Imaging And Oncology
10226 Lakewood Blvd
Downey, CA 90241-2742
(562)287-7205
FAX: (909)786-4391

Downey Breast Diagnostic Clinic
8301 Florence Ave Ste 101
Downey, CA 90240-3946
(562)862-2778
FAX: (562)862-7649

Kaiser Permanente Downey Medical Center
9333 Imperial Hwy
Downey, CA 90242-2812
(800)823-4040
FAX: (562)657-7228

Kaiser Permanente Medical Offices-Downey/Orchard Mob
9449 Imperial Hwy Ste D233
Downey, CA 90242-2814
(800)823-4040
FAX: (562)657-7228

Pih Health Hospital-Downey
11500 Brookshire Ave
Downey, CA 90241-4917
(562)904-5293
FAX: (562)904-5102

Umi Of Downey
11411 Brookshire Ave, Ste 101
Downey, CA 90241-5008
(562)923-5521
FAX: (562)923-1604

Duarte

City Of Hope National Medical Center
1500 Duarte Rd, Mammography Department/Women's Center
Duarte, CA 91010-3000
(626)256-8692
FAX: (626)471-7118

Dublin

Federal Bureau Of Prisons Fci Dublin-Hsa
5701 8th St. Camp Parks
Dublin, CA 94568
(925)833-7500
FAX: (925)833-7595

Nk Tpmg Dublin
3100 Dublin Blvd
Dublin, CA 94568-4363
(925)556-4747
FAX: (925)295-6334

Palo Alto Medical Foundation - Dublin
4050 Dublin Blvd
Dublin, CA 94568-3112
(925)875-6144
FAX: (925)875-6210

East Los Angeles

Kaiser Permanente - East Los Angeles
5119 Pomona Blvd
East Los Angeles, CA 90022-1711
(323)783-2662
FAX: (323)783-6908

East Palo Alto

Ravenswood Family Health Center
1885 Bay Rd
East Palo Alto, CA 94303-1312
(650)330-7400
FAX: (650)321-4009

El Cajon

Kaiser Permanente - Bostonia
1630 E Main St
El Cajon, CA 92021-5204
(800)290-5000
FAX: (619)528-6588

El Centro

Clinicas De Salud Del Pueblo Inc
852 Danenberg Dr
El Centro, CA 92243-8517
(760)879-0989
FAX: (760)352-9999

El Centro Regional Medical Center
1271 Ross Ave
El Centro, CA 92243-4304
(760)339-7241
FAX: (760)339-7249

El Monte

Centrelake Imaging And Oncology- El Monte
11436 Garvey Ave Ste D
El Monte, CA 91732-3304
(909)242-7300
FAX: (909)784-3828

El Monte Comprehensive Health Center
10953 Ramona Blvd
El Monte, CA 91731-2629
(626)434-2830
FAX: (626)527-6947

Elk Grove

Diagnostic Radiological Imaging Elk Grove
7911 Laguna Blvd
Elk Grove, CA 95758-7920
(916)585-8990
FAX: (916)478-3719

Dignity Health Advanced Imaging, A Service Of Dhmf
8220 Wymark Dr Ste 101
Elk Grove, CA 95757-6298
(916)464-7600
FAX: (916)689-5897

Nk Tpmg Elk Grove
9201 Big Horn Blvd
Elk Grove, CA 95758-1240
(916)688-2355
FAX: (916)688-6103

Nk Tpmg Elk Grove - Promenade
10305 Promenade Pkwy
Elk Grove, CA 95757-9400
(916)688-2355
FAX: (916)688-6103

Sutter Valley Medical Foundation - Sutter Imaging Elk Grove
8170 Laguna Blvd Ste 112
Elk Grove, CA 95758-7902
(916)691-5922
FAX: (916)691-5911

Emeryville

Stanford Health Care Emeryville
5800 Hollis St
Emeryville, CA 94608-2016
(650)723-6855
FAX: (650)736-9859

Encinitas

Imaging Healthcare Specialists - Encinitas
477 N El Camino Real, Ste A102
Encinitas, CA 92024-1329
(866)558-4320
FAX: (619)694-1144

Scripps Encinitas Imaging Center
320 Santa Fe Dr Ste Ll8
Encinitas, CA 92024-5100
(760)633-7770
FAX: (760)633-7335

Escondido

Graybill Medical Group, Inc.
225 E 2nd Ave Ste 104
Escondido, CA 92025-4212
(760)291-6766
FAX: (760)737-7348

Kaiser Permanente-Escondido
732 N Broadway
Escondido, CA 92025-1897
(800)290-5000
FAX: (619)528-6588

San Diego Imaging
1955 Citracado Pkwy, Ste 100
Escondido, CA 92029-4111
(760)743-3873
FAX: (760)743-3874

Vrc Holdings, Llc Escondido
255 N Elm St, Ste 102
Escondido, CA 92025-3431
(760)739-5400
FAX: (760)739-8440

Eureka

St. Joseph Hospital Outpatient Imaging Center
2330 Buhne St
Eureka, CA 95501-3237
(707)269-4211
FAX: (855)677-5550

Fairfield

Solano Diagnostics Imaging
1101 B Gale Wilson Blvd Ste 100
Fairfield, CA 94533-3771
(707)646-4646
FAX: (707)646-4949

Sutter Valley Medical Foundation - Sutter Imaging Fairfield
2700 Low Ct, Frnt
Fairfield, CA 94534-9713
(707)432-2500
FAX: (707)432-2583

The Permanente Medical Group - Fairfield
1550 Gateway Blvd
Fairfield, CA 94533-6901
(707)427-4228
FAX: (707)427-4229

Fallbrook

Graybill Medical Group Inc
1035 S Main Ave, Radiology Department
Fallbrook, CA 92028-3338
(760)291-6766
FAX: (760)737-7348

Folsom

Dignity Health Advanced Imaging, A Service Of Dhmf
1625 Creekside Dr Ste 101
Folsom, CA 95630-3819
(916)434-7600
FAX: (916)858-3292

Sutter Valley Medical Foundation - Sutter Imaging Folsom
1661 Creekside Dr
Folsom, CA 95630-3489
(916)984-0739
FAX: (916)865-1491

The Permanente Medical Group, Folsom
2155 Iron Point Rd
Folsom, CA 95630-8707
(916)474-6736
FAX: (916)474-6701

Uc Davis Medical Group-Folsom
1370 Prairie City Rd
Folsom, CA 95630-9554
(916)985-9300
FAX: (916)355-1216

Fontana

Kaiser Foundation Hospital
9961 Sierra Ave, Mammography Dept
Fontana, CA 92335-6794
(909)427-7650
FAX: (909)427-4668

Foothill Ranch

Hoag Health Center-Foothill Ranch
26672 Portola Pkwy, Ste 106
Foothill Ranch, CA 92610-1773
(949)557-0780
FAX: (949)557-0781

Fort Bragg

Adventist Mendocino Coast Hospital
700 River Dr
Fort Bragg, CA 95437-5495
(707)961-4665
FAX: (707)961-4780

Fortuna

Redwood Memorial Hospital
3300 Renner Dr, Mammography Dept.
Fortuna, CA 95540-3198
(707)725-3361
FAX: (707)725-7215

Fountain Valley

Medizen Advanced Imaging, Inc.
17305 Brookhurst St
Fountain Valley, CA 92708-3721
(714)968-8998
FAX: (714)968-8628

Memorial Care Breast Center At Orange Coast
9900 Talbert Ave Ste 102
Fountain Valley, CA 92708-5153
(714)378-7955
FAX: (714)378-7954

Newhope Imaging Center
11190 Warner Ave Ste 110
Fountain Valley, CA 92708-4028
(714)431-0303
FAX: (714)431-0393

Umi Of Fountain Valley
11160 Warner Ave, Ste 105
Fountain Valley, CA 92708-4010
(714)619-7500
FAX: (714)619-7519

Fremont

Inview Medical Imaging
39465 Paseo Padre Pkwy Ste 1000
Fremont, CA 94538-5347
(510)490-0961
FAX: (510)490-0971

Nk-Kfh Fremont
39400 Paseo Padre Pkwy
Fremont, CA 94538-2310
(510)248-3155
FAX: (510)248-3899

Norcal Imaging Fremont
2201 Walnut Ave Ste 150
Fremont, CA 94538-2355
(510)713-1234
FAX: (510)713-1236

Palo Alto Medical Foundation-Fremont Center
3200 Kearney St
Fremont, CA 94538-2299
(510)498-2812
FAX: (510)498-2887

Washington Hospital
2000 Mowry Ave
Fremont, CA 94538-1746
(510)608-6103
FAX: (510)608-1387

French Camp

San Joaquin General Hospital
500 W Hospital Rd
French Camp, CA 95231-9693
(209)468-6221
FAX: (209)468-6038

Fresno

Advanced Medical Imaging Northpointe
6771 N Palm Ave
Fresno, CA 93704-1082
(559)835-0700
FAX: (559)835-0728

Dynamic Imag Assoc Of Ca Inc Cntrl Valley Med & Womens Imag
Suite 103
Fresno, CA 93720
(559)878-4510
FAX: (559)878-4515

Fresno Diagnostic Center
2210 E Illinois Ave Ste 106
Fresno, CA 93701-2184
(559)324-4750
FAX: (559)324-4773

N Kfh Fresno
7300 N Fresno St
Fresno, CA 93720-2941
(559)448-4055
FAX: (559)448-5191

St. Agnes Breast Center At The Plaza
7202 N Millbrook Ave Ste 206
Fresno, CA 93720-3341
(559)450-5656
FAX: (559)450-5206

Wish Fresno Breast Center
6107 N Fresno St Ste 101
Fresno, CA 93710-5275
(559)435-4433
FAX: (559)435-0846

Fullerton

Shin Imaging Llc
1955 Sunny Crest Dr, Ste 110
Fullerton, CA 92835-3653
(714)578-8882
FAX: (714)578-8886

St. Jude Breast Center
2151 N Harbor Blvd Ste 2100
Fullerton, CA 92835-3824
(714)446-5650
FAX: (714)446-5674

Garberville

Jerold Phelps Community Hospital
733 Cedar St
Garberville, CA 95542-3201
(707)923-3921
FAX: (707)923-2578

Garden Grove

Breastlink Women's Imaging Center-Garden Grove
9191 Westminster Ave, Ste 210
Garden Grove, CA 92844-2751
(714)784-1657
FAX: (714)583-6326

Excel Imaging Center
13071 Brookhurst St Ste 185
Garden Grove, CA 92843-5500
(714)583-8126
FAX: (714)583-8148

S Kfh Garden Grove
12100 Euclid St
Garden Grove, CA 92840-3304
(714)223-3028
FAX: (949)932-6330

United Medical Imaging Healthcare Inc Dbaumi Of Garden Grove
12665 Garden Grove Blvd, Ste 103
Garden Grove, CA 92843-1915
(714)620-8200
FAX: (714)620-8211

Gardena

Kaiser Permanente Medical Office-Gardena
15446 S Western Ave, Diagnostic Imaging/Mammography
Gardena, CA 90249-4319
(800)780-1230
FAX: (310)257-6193

Kaiser Permanente Medical Offices Carson
18600 S Figueroa St
Gardena, CA 90248-4505
(800)780-1230
FAX: (310)257-6193

United Medical Imaging Of Gardena
1141 W Redondo Beach Blvd, Ste 105
Gardena, CA 90247-3585
(310)436-1730
FAX: (310)436-1731

Gilroy

St Louise Regional Hospital Breastcare Center
9460 N Name Uno Ste 225
Gilroy, CA 95020-3532
(408)848-8640
FAX: (408)848-2561

Tpmg Gilroy Medical Offices
7520 Arroyo Cir
Gilroy, CA 95020-7303
(408)362-4365
FAX: (408)972-7163

Valley Health Center At Gilroy
7475 Camino Arroyo
Gilroy, CA 95020-7348
(408)885-6350
FAX: (408)885-6360

Glendale

Adventist Health Glendale
1509 Wilson Ter
Glendale, CA 91206-4007
(818)409-8444
FAX: (818)863-4990

Broadway Imaging Center
140 N Glendale Ave
Glendale, CA 91206-4451
(818)548-0022
FAX: (818)548-8385

Central Diagnostic Imaging Network
800 S Central Ave Ste 100B
Glendale, CA 91204-4375
(818)548-8333
FAX: (818)986-4215

Kaiser Permanente - Glendale
444 W Glenoaks Blvd
Glendale, CA 91202-2917
(323)783-7662
FAX: (323)783-7397

Marcia Ray Breastlink Women's Imaging Center
222 W Eulalia St
Glendale, CA 91204-2849
(818)502-2323
FAX: (818)502-4747

Optum [glendale]
225 W Broadway Ste 100
Glendale, CA 91204-1393
(818)545-7117
FAX: (323)728-0697

United Medical Imaging Of Glendale
624 S Central Ave, Ste 230
Glendale, CA 91204-2009
(818)241-3369
FAX: (818)485-2213

Usc Verdugo Hills Hospital Breast Healthcare Center
1818 Verdugo Blvd Ste 103
Glendale, CA 91208-1429
(818)952-2267
FAX: (818)952-4611

Glendora

Emanate Health -Foothill Presbyterian Hospital
250 S Grand Ave
Glendora, CA 91741-4218
(626)857-3118
FAX: (626)857-3110

Emanate Health Medical Group
315 E Route 66
Glendora, CA 91740-6244
(626)963-4124
FAX: (626)963-6773

Hill Imaging Center, Inc.
130 W Route 66 Ste 110
Glendora, CA 91740-6250
(626)698-7266
FAX: (626)914-6254

Grand Terrace

San Manuel Indian Health
11980 Mount Vernon Ave
Grand Terrace, CA 92313-5172
(951)864-1097
FAX: (909)503-1970

Grass Valley

Insight Imaging Inc
117 Neal St Ste A
Grass Valley, CA 95945-6705
(530)273-2720
FAX: (530)273-2770

Sierra Nevada Women's Imaging Center
155 Glasson Way Bldg 4
Grass Valley, CA 95945-5723
(530)274-6262
FAX: (530)274-6646

Greenbrae

Breast Health Center
100A Drakes Landing Rd Ste 140
Greenbrae, CA 94904-2438
(415)925-7301
FAX: (415)925-7317

Gridley

Orchard Hospital
284 Spruce St
Gridley, CA 95948-2216
(530)846-9052
FAX: (530)846-9053

Hacienda Heights

Pih Health Mammography Hacienda Heights
1850 S Azusa Ave Ste 88
Hacienda Heights, CA 91745-6813
(626)225-4905
FAX: (626)225-4911

Hanford

Adventist Health Breast Care Center - Hanford
125 Mall Dr, Ste 203
Hanford, CA 93230-5794
(559)537-2300
FAX: (559)537-2303

Harbor City

Kaiser Permanente Kaiser Foundation Hospital
25825 Vermont Ave
Harbor City, CA 90710-3599
(800)780-1230
FAX: (310)257-6193

Kaiser Permanente Medical Office-Normandie North
25965 Normandie Ave
Harbor City, CA 90710-3416
(800)780-1230
FAX: (310)257-6193

Hayward

Bay Valley Medical Group, Inc.
27212 Calaroga Ave
Hayward, CA 94545-4349
(650)498-4672
FAX: (510)785-0690

Healdsburg

Healdsburg Hospital OP Services
1540 Healdsburg Ave
Healdsburg, CA 95448-3253
(707)473-4400
FAX: (707)473-4408

Hemet

California Imaging And Diagnostics Medical Group, Inc
850 E Latham Ave Ste 101
Hemet, CA 92543-4391
(866)419-3372
FAX: (951)766-1269

Hemet Valley Imaging Medical Group, Inc.
1001 E Latham Ave Ste G
Hemet, CA 92543-4435
(951)658-9243
FAX: (951)658-5083

Hesperia

S Kfh Hesperia
9550 Escondido Ave
Hesperia, CA 92345-9120
(909)427-3914
FAX: (909)427-4668

Highland

Beaver Medical Group, L.P.
7000 Boulder Ave, Highland Radiology
Highland, CA 92346-3348
(909)425-3133
FAX: (909)862-1064

Hollister

Hazel Hawkins Memorial Hospital
911 Sunset Dr, San Benito Hospital District
Hollister, CA 95023-5695
(831)636-2656
FAX: (831)636-2605

Huntington Beach

Hoag Imaging Center Huntington Beach
19582 Beach Blvd Ste 150
Huntington Beach, CA 92648-5949
(714)378-4992
FAX: (714)968-7235

Huntington Beach Diagnostic Imaging And Breast Center
17822 Beach Blvd Ste 101
Huntington Beach, CA 92647-7179
(714)842-5337
FAX: (714)847-6597

Memorialcare Breast Center Huntington Beach
7055 Yorktown Ave Ste 102
Huntington Beach, CA 92648-6468
(714)378-7556
FAX: (714)378-7407

United Medical Imaging Of Huntington Beach
16161 Gothard St, Ste C
Huntington Beach, CA 92647-3603
(714)843-6255
FAX: (714)842-6957

Imperial

Imperial Radiology
2407 Marshall Ave Ste A
Imperial, CA 92251-9504
(760)545-0340
FAX: (760)545-0341

Indio

Desert Advanced Imaging Center
81880 Doctor Carreon Blvd, Ste A102
Indio, CA 92201-5583
(760)863-3857
FAX: (760)863-5249

Inglewood

Centinela Hospital Medical Center
575 E Hardy St, Ste 207
Inglewood, CA 90301-4000
(310)680-8186
FAX: (310)412-4568

Inglewood Imaging Center, Llc
211 N Prairie Ave
Inglewood, CA 90301-1412
(310)672-9729
FAX: (310)672-9720

Kaiser Permanente Medical Offices - Inglewood
110 N La Brea Ave
Inglewood, CA 90301-1708
(323)857-3766
FAX: (323)857-2292

Umi Of Inglewood
110 S La Brea Ave, Ste 150
Inglewood, CA 90301-8771
(310)671-6000
FAX: (310)671-6302

Irvine

Breast Center Of Irvine
16100 Sand Canyon Ave, Ste 100
Irvine, CA 92618-3721
(949)502-3489
FAX: (949)417-1165

Hoag Clinic-Irvine
16105 Sand Canyon Ave, Ste 200
Irvine, CA 92618-3779
(949)829-5533
FAX: (949)581-9155

Hoag Health Center Irvine - Sand Canyon
16305 Sand Canyon Ave Ste 160
Irvine, CA 92618-3790
(800)309-9729
FAX: (949)557-0181

Hoag Imaging Center Irvine
4870 Barranca Pkwy Ste 100
Irvine, CA 92604-4787
(949)451-6000
FAX: (949)551-8115

Kaiser Alton - Sand Canyon
6650 Alton Pkwy
Irvine, CA 92618-3734
(714)223-3028
FAX: (714)284-4499

Memorialcare Breast Center At Saddleback, Irvine
4040 Barranca Pkwy, Ste 110
Irvine, CA 92604-4772
(949)425-7207
FAX: (949)699-0532

Memorialcare Breast Center At Saddleback, Sand Canyon Irvine
15500 Sand Canyon Ave Ste 120
Irvine, CA 92618-7708
(949)452-7207
FAX: (949)699-0532

University Of California, Irvine
1 Medical Plaza Dr
Irvine, CA 92697-0001
(714)456-6175
FAX: (714)456-6908

Jackson

Sutter Amador Hospital
100 Mission Blvd
Jackson, CA 95642-2536
(209)223-7560
FAX: (209)257-5836

Joshua Tree

Hi-Desert Medical Center
6601 White Feather Rd, Medical Imaging Dept
Joshua Tree, CA 92252-6607
(760)366-6175
FAX: (760)366-6242

King City

George L. Mee Memorial Hospital
300 Canal St
King City, CA 93930-3457
(831)385-7130
FAX: (831)386-7378

La Jolla

Green Hospital Of Scripps Clinic
10666 N Torrey Pines Rd
La Jolla, CA 92037-1027
(858)554-4900
FAX: (858)554-2788

Imaging Healthcare Specialists - Golden Triangle
4150 Regents Park Row Ste 195
La Jolla, CA 92037-9139
(866)558-4320
FAX: (866)558-4329

Scripps Polster Breast Care Center
9850 Genesee Ave Ste 170, Scripps Ximed Building
La Jolla, CA 92037-1226
(858)626-5200
FAX: (858)626-5230

Uc San Diego Health Koman Family Outpatient Pavilion
9400 Campus Point Dr, Mail Code 7316
La Jolla, CA 92093-1350
(619)543-3405
FAX: (858)822-6124

La Mesa

Grossmont Imaging Llc
8881 Fletcher Pkwy Ste 102
La Mesa, CA 91942-3129
(619)461-1830
FAX: (619)797-1484

Scripps Clinic Rancho San Diego
10862 Calle Verde
La Mesa, CA 91941-7387
(619)660-1814
FAX: (619)660-1851

Skfh - La Mesa
8080 Parkway Dr
La Mesa, CA 91942-2104
(800)290-5000
FAX: (619)528-6588

La Quinta

Desert Regional Medical Ctr - Comprehensive Cancer Ctr
47647 Caleo Bay Dr Ste 260
La Quinta, CA 92253-8859
(760)416-4700
FAX: (760)416-4715

Eisenhower Health Schnitzer/Novack Breast Center
45280 Seeley Dr
La Quinta, CA 92253-6834
(760)773-4338
FAX: (760)773-8840

La Verne

Pomona Valley Imaging Center At Laverne
2333 Foothill Blvd
La Verne, CA 91750-3027
(909)469-9472
FAX: (909)865-9794

Lafayette

Alta Bates Summit Med. Ctr-Lafayette Womens Hlth
3595 Mt Diablo Blvd Ste 350
Lafayette, CA 94549-3849
(510)869-8387
FAX: (510)869-8323

Inview Imaging Dba Tom H Piatt MD Inc
970 Dewing Ave, Suite100
Lafayette, CA 94549-4291
(925)297-6460
FAX: (925)297-6459

Laguna Beach

Providence Mission Hospital-Laguna Beach
31872 Coast Hwy
Laguna Beach, CA 92651-6773
(949)364-1400
FAX: (949)347-8104

Laguna Hills

Health Diagnostics Of California, Pc - Laguna Hills
24022 Calle De La Plata, Ste 100
Laguna Hills, CA 92653-3627
(949)330-8996
FAX: (949)330-8997

Hoag Clinic
24411 Health Center Dr, Ste 200C
Laguna Hills, CA 92653-3633
(949)829-5533
FAX: (949)763-7379

Memorialcare Breast Center At Saddleback Memorial
24401 Calle De La Louisa Ste 200
Laguna Hills, CA 92653-3624
(949)452-7207
FAX: (949)380-4513

Lake Arrowhead

Mountains Community Hospital
29101 Hospital Rd
Lake Arrowhead, CA 92352-9706
(909)436-3130
FAX: (909)336-2048

Lakeport

Sutter Lakeside Hospital
5176 Hill Rd E
Lakeport, CA 95453-6357
(707)262-5000
FAX: (707)573-5370

Lakewood

Lakewood Regional Medical Center
3700 South St
Lakewood, CA 90712-1498
(562)602-6810
FAX: (562)630-3594

Lancaster

High Desert Regional Health Center
335 E Avenue I
Lancaster, CA 93535-1916
(661)471-4120
FAX: (661)524-2911

Lancaster Imaging
44725 10th St W Ste 150
Lancaster, CA 93534-3000
(661)945-5855
FAX: (661)945-7568

Renaissance Imaging Ctr At Antelope Valley Hospital [avoic]
44105 15th St W Ste 100
Lancaster, CA 93534-4090
(661)726-6399
FAX: (661)949-5759

S Kfh Lancaster
43112 15th St W
Lancaster, CA 93534-6219
(818)375-1755
FAX: (818)815-5156

Lemoore

Naval Health Clinic Lemoore
937 Franklin Blvd
Lemoore, CA 93246-4700
(559)998-2596
FAX: (559)998-4653

Lincoln

The Permanente Medical Group, Lincoln
1900 Dresden Dr
Lincoln, CA 95648-8803
(916)201-7499
FAX: (916)746-4597

Livermore

The Permanente Medical Group, Livermore
3000 Las Positas Rd, Radiology Dept.
Livermore, CA 94551-9627
(925)243-4501
FAX: (925)243-4514

Valleycare Medical Plaza At Livermore
1133 E Stanley Blvd
Livermore, CA 94550-4200
(925)734-3376
FAX: (925)416-6758

Lodi

Advanced Imaging Center At Adventist Health Lodi Memorial
1031 S Fairmont Ave
Lodi, CA 95240-5112
(209)339-7505
FAX: (209)333-8263

Valley Mri And Radiology, Inc.
801 S Ham Ln
Lodi, CA 95242-7501
(209)467-1000
FAX: (209)467-7335

Loma Linda

Loma Linda University Medical Center Faculty Med Office
11370 Anderson St Ste 1700
Loma Linda, CA 92354-3450
(909)558-5385
FAX: (909)558-2431

Lompoc

Lompoc Valley Medical Center
1515 E Ocean Ave
Lompoc, CA 93436-7092
(805)737-3375
FAX: (805)875-8566

Professional Imaging Of Lvmc
1111 E Ocean Ave, Ste 2
Lompoc, CA 93436-2500
(805)735-9229
FAX: (805)735-8540

Long Beach

Kaiser Permanente Long Beach Medical Offices
3900 E Pacific Coast Hwy, Diagnostic Imaging/Mammography
Long Beach, CA 90804-2000
(800)780-1230
FAX: (310)257-6193

Lakewood Open Mri
3715 E South St
Long Beach, CA 90805-4521
(562)602-0700
FAX: (562)420-9883

Long Beach Comprehensive Health Center
1333 Chestnut Ave
Long Beach, CA 90813-2944
(562)753-2440
FAX: (562)218-2816

Long Beach Memorial Breast Center
2810 Long Beach Blvd
Long Beach, CA 90806-1558
(562)933-7880
FAX: (562)933-7807

Los Coyotes Medical Group
3320 N Los Coyotes Diagonal Ste 260
Long Beach, CA 90808-3939
(562)627-0903
FAX: (562)627-0923

Pro-Life Imaging Llc
5450 N Paramount Blvd, Spc 133 133
Long Beach, CA 90805-8325
(661)713-8720
FAX: (855)940-1565

The Imaging Ctr At St Mary Medical Ctr/Dignity Hlth
1045 Atlantic Ave, Ste 105
Long Beach, CA 90813-3404
(562)432-0079
FAX: (562)437-6982

United Medical Imaging Of Central Long Beach
701 E 28th St, Ste 318
Long Beach, CA 90806-2785
(562)426-7000
FAX: (562)426-7099

United Medical Imaging Of South Long Beach
1040 Elm Ave, Ste 102
Long Beach, CA 90813-3265
(562)285-1000
FAX: (562)285-1019

Los Alamitos

Los Alamitos Medical Center - Totalcare
3951 Katella Ave
Los Alamitos, CA 90720-3303
(562)799-3195
FAX: (562)799-3469

Memorialcare Breast Center In Los Alamitos
11121 Los Alamitos Blvd Ste B
Los Alamitos, CA 90720-3603
(562)933-7880
FAX: (562)933-7807

Los Altos

Palo Alto Medical Foundation - Los Altos Center
370 Distel Cir
Los Altos, CA 94022-1404
(650)254-5259
FAX: (650)254-5287

Los Angeles

Arroyo Vista Family Health Center
6000 N Figueroa St
Los Angeles, CA 90042-4232
(323)254-5221
FAX: (323)254-4618

California Hospital Medical Center
1513 S Grand Ave Ste 400
Los Angeles, CA 90015-3075
(213)742-6400
FAX: (213)765-4080

Cedars Sinai Medical Center
8631 W 3rd St Ste 120
Los Angeles, CA 90048-5904
(310)423-9317
FAX: (310)423-9400

Cedars Sinai Medical Center
310 N San Vicente Blvd
Los Angeles, CA 90048-1810
(310)423-9317
FAX: (310)423-0143

Cedars-Sinai Medical Center
8700 Beverly Blvd
Los Angeles, CA 90048-1865
(310)423-9317
FAX: (310)423-9400

Cha Hollywood Presbyterian Medical Center
1300 N Vermont Ave
Los Angeles, CA 90027-6098
(213)913-4835
FAX: (323)913-4205

Edward R. Roybal Chc
245 S Fetterly Ave
Los Angeles, CA 90022-1605
(323)362-1112
FAX: (323)362-1367

Grand Avenue Imaging
1400 S Grand Ave Ste 608
Los Angeles, CA 90015-3068
(213)746-5800
FAX: (213)746-5802

H. Claude Hudson Comprehensive Health Center
2829 S Grand Ave
Los Angeles, CA 90007-3304
(323)865-3226
FAX: (323)224-7830

Hubert H. Humphrey Comprehensive Health Center
5850 S Main St
Los Angeles, CA 90003-1215
(323)897-6300
FAX: (323)232-0764

Iris Cantor Breast Imaging Center At Ucla
200 Ucla Medical Plaza, Ste B165-26
Los Angeles, CA 90095-6952
(310)301-6800
FAX: (310)825-3205

Kaiser Foundation Hospital West Los Angeles Medical Center
6041 Cadillac Ave
Los Angeles, CA 90034-1702
(323)857-3766
FAX: (323)857-2292

Kaiser Permanente -Lamc
1505 N Edgemont St
Los Angeles, CA 90027-5299
(323)783-7880
FAX: (323)783-7397

Kaiser Permanente Medical Offices - Culver Marina
12001 W Washington Blvd
Los Angeles, CA 90066-5801
(323)857-2421
FAX: (323)857-2312

Kaiser Permanente Medical Offices - S Los Angeles
1550 W Manchester Ave
Los Angeles, CA 90047-5424
(323)857-3766
FAX: (323)857-2292

Keck Medical Center Of Usc-Downtown
830 S Flower St Ste A-100
Los Angeles, CA 90017-4608
(213)486-8646
FAX: (323)865-9322

Kfh- Playa Vista Medical Offices
5300 McConnell Ave
Los Angeles, CA 90066-7026
(323)857-3766
FAX: (323)857-2292

Kfh-Baldwin Hills Crenshaw
3782 W Martin Luther King Jr Blvd
Los Angeles, CA 90008-1703
(323)857-3766
FAX: (323)857-2292

Lac Usc Medical Center
1100 N State St, Diagnostic And Treatment Tower 3rd Floor
Los Angeles, CA 90033-5000
(323)409-5167
FAX: (323)441-8233

Martin Luther King, Jr. Outpatient Center
1670 E 120th St
Los Angeles, CA 90059-3026
(424)338-2007
FAX: (310)223-1392

Optum
1120 W Washington Blvd
Los Angeles, CA 90015-3316
(213)623-2225
FAX: (213)741-2011

Renaissance Imaging Medical Associates, Inc.
500 S Virgil Ave Ste 102
Los Angeles, CA 90020-1447
(323)375-3950
FAX: (323)375-3945

Shin Mri Llc
266 S Harvard Blvd Ste 180
Los Angeles, CA 90004-4885
(213)387-3002
FAX: (213)387-3057

Skfh Hollywood Romaine
7007 Romaine St
Los Angeles, CA 90038-2438
(800)954-8000
FAX: (323)783-7397

Sun Imaging,Inc.
824 N Hill St
Los Angeles, CA 90012-2321
(213)626-7816
FAX: (213)621-7787

Ucla Health Department Of Radiology Century City Bi
10250 Santa Monica Blvd Ste 2450
Los Angeles, CA 90067-6593
(310)301-6800
FAX: (310)825-3205

Ucla Health Department Of Radiology Dtla-Bloc Breast Imaging
700 W 7th St, Ste S270A
Los Angeles, CA 90017-3768
(310)301-6800
FAX: (310)267-5601

Umi Of Century City
2080 Century Park E, Ste 104
Los Angeles, CA 90067-2004
(310)432-8000
FAX: (310)432-8019

Umi Of East Los Angeles
3513 Whittier Blvd
Los Angeles, CA 90023-1765
(323)262-1814
FAX: (323)262-1699

United Medical Imaging Of Los Angeles
1127 Wilshire Blvd, Ste 100
Los Angeles, CA 90017-3902
(213)202-5785
FAX: (213)202-5709

Usc Norris Cancer Hospital-Norris Healthcare Center 3
1516 San Pablo St 3rd Fl
Los Angeles, CA 90033-5313
(323)865-3463
FAX: (323)865-0114

Valley Breast Care At Olympia
5901 W Olympic Blvd Ste 105
Los Angeles, CA 90036-4680
(323)879-9792
FAX: (323)938-1089

Watts Health Care Corporation
10300 Compton Ave
Los Angeles, CA 90002-3628
(323)564-4331
FAX: (323)357-9477

Westchester Advanced Imaging Center Med Group
8540 S Sepulveda Blvd Ste 111
Los Angeles, CA 90045-3810
(310)854-7722
FAX: (310)645-1256

Women's Imaging Center
1700 E Cesar E Chavez Ave Ste 1800
Los Angeles, CA 90033-2468
(323)881-8800
FAX: (323)307-8554

Los Banos

Memorial Hospital Los Banos
1253 W I St
Los Banos, CA 93635-3930
(209)826-0591
FAX: (209)827-1201

Merced Mri Medical Group Dba El Portal Imaging Los Banos
245 H St Ste 3
Los Banos, CA 93635-4150
(209)710-5630
FAX: (209)826-2921

Padres Medical Imaging, Inc.
311 W I St
Los Banos, CA 93635-3479
(209)826-6444
FAX: (209)826-6464

Los Gatos

Breast Imaging Specialists, Inc.
15195 National Ave Ste 201
Los Gatos, CA 95032-2631
(408)800-5247
FAX: (408)356-5526

El Camino Hospital Los Gatos
815 Pollard Rd
Los Gatos, CA 95032-1438
(650)940-7050
FAX: (408)866-4082

Good Samaritan Breast Care Center
15400 National Ave Ste 200
Los Gatos, CA 95032-2433
(408)358-8414
FAX: (408)356-2740

Mammography Specialists Medical Group, Inc.
14651 S Bascom Ave, Ste 210
Los Gatos, CA 95032-2045
(408)356-6611
FAX: (408)356-9001

Palo Alto Medical Foundation - Los Gatos
15400 Los Gatos Blvd
Los Gatos, CA 95032-2502
(650)934-7700
FAX: (650)934-7790

Lynwood

Primehealtcare Services- St Francis, Llc Dba St. Francis Med
3630 E Imperial Hwy, Mammography Dept.
Lynwood, CA 90262-2609
(310)900-4514
FAX: (310)900-4505

Madera

Madera Community Hospital Outpatient Center
1270 E Almond Ave
Madera, CA 93637-5606
(559)675-5534
FAX: (559)675-5517

Madera Mri
360 E Almond Ave
Madera, CA 93637-5688
(559)206-9901
FAX: (559)512-2329

Mammoth Lakes

Mammoth Hospital
85 Sierra Park Rd
Mammoth Lakes, CA 93546-2073
(760)924-4070
FAX: (760)924-4207

Manhattan Beach

Torrance Memorial Breast Diagnostic Center III
855 Manhattan Beach Blvd Ste 208
Manhattan Beach, CA 90266-4965
(310)939-7864
FAX: (310)939-7865

Ucla Health System Department Of Radiology Manhattan Beach
2200 N Sepulveda Blvd
Manhattan Beach, CA 90266-2910
(310)301-6800
FAX: (310)825-0429

Manteca

Doctor's Hospital Of Manteca
1205 E North St
Manteca, CA 95336-4900
(209)239-8370
FAX: (209)824-4950

The Permanente Medical Group- Manteca Mob
1721 W Yosemite Ave
Manteca, CA 95337-5130
(209)824-6269
FAX: (209)825-3615

Marina Del Rey

Cedars Sinai Marina Del Rey Hospital
4650 Lincoln Blvd
Marina Del Rey, CA 90292-6306
(310)577-5559
FAX: (310)577-5660

Mink Radiologic Imaging
13160 Mindanao Way, Ste 175
Marina Del Rey, CA 90292-7907
(310)305-4500
FAX: (310)305-4611

Mink Radiologic Imaging Medical Associates, Inc
4640 Admiralty Way Ste 102
Marina Del Rey, CA 90292-6629
(310)287-4000
FAX: (310)773-3606

Mariposa

John C. Fremont Healthcare District
5189 Hospital Rd
Mariposa, CA 95338-9524
(209)966-3631
FAX: (209)966-2972

Martinez

Contra Costa Regional Medical Center
2500 Alhambra Ave
Martinez, CA 94553-3152
(925)370-5320
FAX: (925)370-5344

Nk Tpmg Martinez
200 Muir Rd
Martinez, CA 94553-4614
(925)372-1960
FAX: (925)372-1633

Maywood

United Medical Imaging Healthcare, Inc. Dba Umi Of Maywood
4316 Slauson Ave
Maywood, CA 90270-2838
(323)771-9867
FAX: (323)771-6094

Menifee

Temecula Valley Imaging Ctr Medical Group
27168 Newport Rd Ste 2
Menifee, CA 92584-7383
(951)600-2839
FAX: (951)600-2863

Menlo Park

University Healthcare Alliance
321 Middlefield Rd
Menlo Park, CA 94025-3500
(650)498-6530
FAX: (650)329-0586

University Healthcare Alliance
1300 Crane St
Menlo Park, CA 94025-4260
(650)498-6530
FAX: (650)329-0586

Welch Rd. Imaging
401 Burgess Dr Ste D
Menlo Park, CA 94025-3476
(650)323-1343
FAX: (650)323-1352

Merced

Dignity Health
315 Mercy Ave Ste 102
Merced, CA 95340-8363
(209)564-3161
FAX: (209)564-3199

El Portal Imaging Center
3365 G St Ste 200
Merced, CA 95340-0995
(209)384-4250
FAX: (209)722-1975

Milpitas

Nk Tpmg Milpitas Mob
770 E Calaveras Blvd, Mammography Department
Milpitas, CA 95035-5491
(408)851-5054
FAX: (408)851-3669

Valley Health Center Of Milpitas
143 N Main St
Milpitas, CA 95035-4322
(408)885-6350
FAX: (408)885-6360

Mission Hills

Facey Medical Foundation Mission Hills
11333 Sepulveda Blvd
Mission Hills, CA 91345-1116
(818)869-7034
FAX: (818)869-7219

Outpatient Diagnostic Center Providence Holy Cross Med Ctr
11570 Indian Hills Rd
Mission Hills, CA 91345-1238
(818)496-4686
FAX: (818)365-7891

Mission Viejo

Providence Mission Imaging Center
26732 Crown Valley Pkwy Ste 171A
Mission Viejo, CA 92691-6306
(949)364-1400
FAX: (949)347-8104

S Kfh Mission Viejo
23781 Maquina
Mission Viejo, CA 92691-2716
(714)223-3028
FAX: (714)284-4499

Modesto

Kaiser Foundation Hospital-Modesto Mmo
4601 Dale Rd
Modesto, CA 95356-9718
(209)476-3875
FAX: (209)476-5203

Modesto Advanced Imaging Center
157 E Coolidge Ave
Modesto, CA 95350-4565
(209)524-6800
FAX: (209)524-1286

Modesto Radiology Imaging Inc. Breast Health Center
1524 McHenry Ave Ste 100
Modesto, CA 95350-4566
(209)577-4444
FAX: (209)522-2984

Stanislaus Surgical Hospital Precision Imaging
1239 McHenry Ave Ste A
Modesto, CA 95350-5330
(209)491-5200
FAX: (209)526-0935

Sutter Gould Medical Foundation
600 Coffee Rd
Modesto, CA 95355-4276
(209)550-4755
FAX: (209)521-3970

The Permanente Medical Group- Modesto Mob
3800 Dale Rd
Modesto, CA 95356-8627
(209)476-3875
FAX: (209)476-5203

Montebello

Beverly Hospital Plaza Radiology
101 E Beverly Blvd Ste 104
Montebello, CA 90640-4314
(323)725-5017
FAX: (323)725-5098

Optum
2601 Via Campo
Montebello, CA 90640-1807
(323)837-7238
FAX: (323)728-0697

Skfh Montebello Kaiser Permanente-Montebello
1550 Town Center Dr, X-Ray/Mammography Department
Montebello, CA 90640-2173
(626)851-5130
FAX: (626)851-5461

Monterey

Carol Hatton Breast Care Center-Chomp
2 Upper Ragsdale Dr, Ste C100 Suite 100
Monterey, CA 93940-7871
(831)622-2760
FAX: (831)622-2766

Mammography Center Of Monterey
700 Cass St Ste 120
Monterey, CA 93940-2921
(831)373-8932
FAX: (831)373-5465

Monterey Park

Chieh-Jen Calvin Yang, Md. A Professional Corporation
312 N Garfield Ave
Monterey Park, CA 91754-1707
(626)572-2889
FAX: (626)572-2989

Diagnostic Medical Group Of Southern California
208 N Garfield Ave
Monterey Park, CA 91754-1705
(626)288-8029
FAX: (626)288-7056

Julie K. Sun, M.D., Inc.
223 N Garfield Ave Ste 100
Monterey Park, CA 91754-1700
(626)571-6177
FAX: (626)571-7144

Moorpark

Los Robles Imaging Center
865 Patriot Dr Ste 100
Moorpark, CA 93021-3407
(805)523-8062
FAX: (805)523-8403

Moreno Valley

Kaiser Permanente Medical Offices Moreno Valley
12815 Heacock St
Moreno Valley, CA 92553-2836
(951)353-4449
FAX: (951)353-5797

Riverside University Health System - Medical Center
26520 Cactus Ave
Moreno Valley, CA 92555-3911
(951)486-4053
FAX: (951)486-4286

Ruhs Medical Surgical Center
26600 Cactus Ave
Moreno Valley, CA 92555-3901
(951)486-4100
FAX: (951)486-4310

Morgan Hill

Mammography Specialists Medical Group, Morgan Hill
18525 Sutter Blvd Ste 260
Morgan Hill, CA 95037-2899
(408)356-6611
FAX: (408)356-9001

Morgan Hill Diagnostics
18550 De Paul Dr Ste 104
Morgan Hill, CA 95037-2911
(408)782-2570
FAX: (408)778-6497

Mount Shasta

Mercy Medical Center Mt. Shasta
635 Lassen Ln
Mount Shasta, CA 96067-9003
(530)926-7158
FAX: (530)926-3032

Mountain View

El Camino Hospital Women's Imaging Center
2500 Grant Rd, Sobrato Pavilion MS 1F63
Mountain View, CA 94040-4302
(650)962-4954
FAX: (650)988-7542

Nk Tpmg Mountain View Mob
555 Castro St, Mammography Department
Mountain View, CA 94041-2009
(408)851-5054
FAX: (408)851-3669

Palo Alto Med Foundation - Mountain View
701 E El Camino Real
Mountain View, CA 94040-2833
(650)934-7700
FAX: (650)934-7790

Murrieta

Breastlink Women's Imaging Center-Temecula
25455 Medical Center Dr Ste 210
Murrieta, CA 92562-1500
(951)587-8956
FAX: (951)600-2863

California Imaging & Diag. Medical Group
25470 Medical Center Dr Ste 101
Murrieta, CA 92562-4901
(866)419-3372
FAX: (951)894-1842

Kaiser Permanente Medical Offices Murrieta
28150 Keller Rd
Murrieta, CA 92563-2432
(951)353-4449
FAX: (951)353-5797

Loma Linda University Medical Center - Murrieta
28078 Baxter Rd Ste 220, Women's Diagnostic Center
Murrieta, CA 92563-1403
(951)290-4360
FAX: (951)290-4995

Rancho Springs Medical Center
25500 Medical Center Dr
Murrieta, CA 92562-5965
(951)677-9797
FAX: (951)696-6193

N Hollywood

S Kfh North Hollywood Medical Offices
5250 Lankershim Blvd, Kaiser Permanente Medical Offices
N Hollywood, CA 91601-3186
(818)375-1755
FAX: (818)815-5156

Napa

Nk Tpmg Napa Mob2
16975 Permanente Way
Napa, CA 94558
(707)258-4414
FAX: (707)258-4451

Queen Of The Valley Medical Center
3421 Villa Ln, Ste E
Napa, CA 94558-3056
(707)257-4047
FAX: (707)251-1811

National City

Imaging Healthcare Specialists - National City
2427 Transportation Ave
National City, CA 91950-6664
(858)658-6500
FAX: (866)558-4329

Newark

Newark Wellness Center
6066 Civic Terrace Ave
Newark, CA 94560-3746
(510)437-4157
FAX: (510)535-7315

Newport Beach

Breastlink Women's Imaging Center-Newport Beach
1441 Avocado Ave, Ste 301
Newport Beach, CA 92660-7704
(949)272-2095
FAX: (949)272-2096

Care Connectors Medical Group Inc - Mobile
520 Superior Ave, Ste 255
Newport Beach, CA 92663-3668
(310)927-0919
FAX: (949)402-0042

Elizabeth Pusey Md, Inc Dba Women's Medical Imaging
361 Hospital Rd Ste 528
Newport Beach, CA 92663-3526
(949)645-2321
FAX: (949)645-2039

Hoag Breast Care And Imaging Center
1 Hoag Dr
Newport Beach, CA 92663-4162
(949)764-5573
FAX: (949)764-5463

Memorialcare Breast Center Newport Beach
2001 Westcliff Dr Ste 103
Newport Beach, CA 92660-5552
(714)378-7955
FAX: (714)378-7474

Newport Diagnostic Center - Women's Center
1605 Avocado Ave
Newport Beach, CA 92660-7725
(949)467-3150
FAX: (949)467-3183

Newport Imaging Center
360 San Miguel Dr Ste 106
Newport Beach, CA 92660-7833
(949)721-8191
FAX: (949)721-1206

Northridge

Dignity Community Care, Northridge Hospital Medical Center
18300 Roscoe Blvd
Northridge, CA 91325-4167
(818)885-8500
FAX: (818)409-5346

Facey Medical Foundation: Northridge-Corbin
9111 Corbin Ave
Northridge, CA 91324-2402
(818)869-7034
FAX: (818)869-7219

Renaissance Imaging Medical Associates, Inc.
18436 Roscoe Blvd
Northridge, CA 91325-4107
(818)435-1400
FAX: (818)435-1490

United Medical Imaging Of Northridge
18250 Roscoe Blvd, Ste 135
Northridge, CA 91325-4263
(818)701-7111
FAX: (818)701-7841

Novato

Nk Tpmg Novato
97 San Marin Dr
Novato, CA 94945-1100
(415)444-2280
FAX: (415)444-4948

Sutter Bay Hospitals Dba Novato Community Hospital
180 Rowland Way
Novato, CA 94945-5009
(415)209-1524
FAX: (415)209-1513

Oakdale

Oak Valley District Hospital
350 S Oak Ave
Oakdale, CA 95361-3581
(209)848-4171
FAX: (209)847-4558

Oakhurst

Adventist Health Medical Imaging Oakhurst
48677 Victoria Ln
Oakhurst, CA 93644-9216
(559)692-8651
FAX: (559)692-8693

Oakland

Eastmont Wellness Center
6955 Foothill Blvd, Ste 200
Oakland, CA 94605-2426
(510)437-4211
FAX: (510)535-7318

Highland Hospital
1411 E 31st St
Oakland, CA 94602-1092
(510)437-4157
FAX: (510)535-7315

Inview Imaging Dba Tom H. Piatt, M.D., Inc.
1300 Clay St, Ste 165
Oakland, CA 94612-1421
(510)823-2211
FAX: (925)297-6459

Norcal Imaging Oakland
3200 Telegraph Ave
Oakland, CA 94609-3016
(510)663-1950
FAX: (510)663-1951

Sbh Dba Absmc Carol Ann Read Breast Health Center
3100 Summit St
Oakland, CA 94609-3412
(510)869-8377
FAX: (510)869-8378

Sbh Dba Absmc Imaging & Mammography-5730 Telegraph
5730 Telegraph Ave
Oakland, CA 94609-1710
(510)204-1880
FAX: (510)204-1049

The Permanente Medical Group - Oakland
3801 Howe St, Fabiola Building - Ground Floor
Oakland, CA 94611-5312
(510)752-6031
FAX: (510)752-2783

Oceanside

Imaging Healthcare Specialists - Tri City
3601 Vista Way Ste 101
Oceanside, CA 92056-4559
(866)558-4320
FAX: (866)558-4329

San Diego Imaging
3909 Waring Rd Ste C
Oceanside, CA 92056-4455
(760)630-0014
FAX: (760)630-0015

Scripps Medical Center Jefferson
2205 Vista Way
Oceanside, CA 92054-5661
(760)806-5458
FAX: (760)806-5636

Tri-City Medical Center Women's Diagnostic Center
4002 Vista Way, Women's Center
Oceanside, CA 92056-4506
(760)940-7470
FAX: (760)940-4070

Ojai

Ojai Valley Community Hospital
1306 Maricopa Hwy
Ojai, CA 93023-3163
(805)640-2250
FAX: (805)640-2283

Ontario

Centrelake Imaging & Oncology
3115 E Guasti Rd
Ontario, CA 91761-7853
(909)242-7300
FAX: (909)212-6252

Kaiser Foundation Hospital - Ontario
2295 S Vineyard Ave, Ste A
Ontario, CA 91761-7926
(909)427-7650
FAX: (909)427-4668

Orange

Breastlink Women's Imaging Center-Orange
230 S Main St Ste 100
Orange, CA 92868-3851
(714)541-0101
FAX: (714)619-3317

Providence Medical Foundation C/O St Joseph Heritage Medical
2501 E Chapman Ave Ste 102
Orange, CA 92869-3204
(714)628-3223
FAX: (714)628-0451

The Center For Breast Imaging And Diagnosis
1010 W La Veta Ave Ste 400
Orange, CA 92868-4305
(714)734-6280
FAX: (714)734-6281

University Of California, Irvine
101 The City Dr S Bldg 30 Pavilion 1 Br
Orange, CA 92868-3201
(714)456-6175
FAX: (714)456-6908

Women's Imaging Center
431 S Batavia St, Ste 100
Orange, CA 92868-3937
(714)771-8360
FAX: (714)771-8364

Orinda

John Muir Medical Imaging Orinda
140 Brookwood Rd, Ste 100
Orinda, CA 94563-3043
(925)254-9850
FAX: (925)941-4046

Oroville

Valley Womens Imaging
2809 Olive Hwy Ste 120
Oroville, CA 95966-6132
(530)532-8676
FAX: (530)538-3272

Oxnard

Grossman Imaging Center
2151 E Gonzales Rd Ste 101
Oxnard, CA 93036-3712
(805)988-0616
FAX: (805)983-2681

Kaiser Permanente Medical Offices - Oxnard
2200 E Gonzales Rd
Oxnard, CA 93036-0619
(818)719-4173
FAX: (818)719-3251

Palms Imaging Medical Group
1901 Outlet Center Dr, Ste 120
Oxnard, CA 93036-0664
(805)604-9500
FAX: (805)604-9559

Rolling Oaks Radiology Oxnard
1901 N Rice Ave Ste 155
Oxnard, CA 93030-7912
(805)604-3370
FAX: (805)981-4623

Rolling Oaks Radiology-St. John's
1700 N Rose Ave Ste 110
Oxnard, CA 93030-7630
(805)983-0883
FAX: (805)983-1029

Palm Springs

Desert Advanced Imaging Center
2601 E Tahquitz Canyon Way
Palm Springs, CA 92262-7015
(760)318-2980
FAX: (760)327-7835

Desert Comprehensive Breast Center
1180 N Indian Canyon Dr Ste E150
Palm Springs, CA 92262-4835
(760)416-4700
FAX: (760)416-4715

Palmdale

Advanced Imaging Center
607 W Avenue Q, Ste A
Palmdale, CA 93551-3872
(661)456-2020
FAX: (661)456-2021

S Kfh Palmdale
4502 E Avenue S
Palmdale, CA 93552-4480
(661)729-4431
FAX: (661)726-2202

Palo Alto

Northern California Women's Imaging Center
2421 Park Blvd Ste B202
Palo Alto, CA 94306-1956
(650)617-8655
FAX: (650)322-3416

Palo Alto Medical Foundation - 49 Wells
49 Wells Ave
Palo Alto, CA 94301-2313
(650)853-2955
FAX: (650)853-6099

Stanford Health Care
875 Blake Wilbur Dr, Mc5828 Rm Cc1226
Palo Alto, CA 94304-2205
(650)736-2304
FAX: (650)736-9859

Stanford Health Care
900 Blake Wilbur Dr W130
Palo Alto, CA 94304-2201
(650)723-6855
FAX: (650)736-9859

Stanford Health Care Hoover
211 Quarry Rd Rm 1201
Palo Alto, CA 94304-1416
(650)723-6855
FAX: (650)736-9859

Panorama City

Kaiser Foundation Hospital - Panorama City
13652 Cantara St
Panorama City, CA 91402-5423
(818)375-1755
FAX: (818)375-2632

Kaiser Permanente Medical Offices - Panorama City
13640 Roscoe Blvd
Panorama City, CA 91402-3904
(888)778-5000
FAX: (818)815-6849

Rj Imaging
14500 Roscoe Blvd Fl 4
Panorama City, CA 91402-4194
(818)714-2043
FAX: (747)529-4592

Pasadena

Huntington Hill Imaging
751 Corvoda St.
Pasadena, CA 91101
(626)698-7226
FAX: (626)577-2986

Jim And Eleanor Randall Breast Center
625 S Fair Oaks Ave Ste 140
Pasadena, CA 91105-2650
(626)698-7210
FAX: (626)445-1124

Kaiser Permanente
3280 E Foothill Blvd
Pasadena, CA 91107-3103
(323)783-2662
FAX: (323)783-6908

Madison Radiology Medical Group, Inc
65 N Madison Ave Lowr Level
Pasadena, CA 91101-2035
(626)793-8189
FAX: (626)795-3975

Women's Diagnostic Imaging Medical Center Inc
333 S Fair Oaks Ave
Pasadena, CA 91105-2541
(626)405-8070
FAX: (626)405-8804

Petaluma

Nk Tpmg Petaluma
3900 Lakeville Hwy
Petaluma, CA 94954-5698
(415)444-2360
FAX: (415)444-4948

Norcal Healthconnect Dba Petaluma Valley Hospital
400 N McDowell Blvd
Petaluma, CA 94954-2339
(833)789-6802
FAX: (707)781-1436

Pinole

Nk Tpmg Pinole
1301 Pinole Valley Rd
Pinole, CA 94564-1384
(510)243-4056
FAX: (510)243-4058

Pismo Beach

Coastal Diagnostic Center
921 Oak Park Blvd Ste 100B
Pismo Beach, CA 93449-3400
(805)481-4705
FAX: (805)481-7279

Pittsburg

Pittsburg Health Center
2311 Loveridge Rd
Pittsburg, CA 94565-5117
(925)431-2370
FAX: (925)431-2373

Placentia

Imaging Center Placentia Linda Hospital
1325 N Rose Dr Ste 101
Placentia, CA 92870-3800
(714)961-5990
FAX: (714)961-5997

Placerville

Marshall Hospital
1100 Marshall Way
Placerville, CA 95667-6599
(530)626-2861
FAX: (530)672-7089

Pleasanton

Norcal Imaging Pleasanton
5924 Stoneridge Dr Ste 105
Pleasanton, CA 94588-5400
(925)463-0554
FAX: (925)463-0497

Pleasanton Diagnostic Imaging
5860 Owens Dr, Ste 150
Pleasanton, CA 94588-3980
(925)467-1400
FAX: (925)467-1409

Stanford Health Care-Valleycare Breast Imaging Center
5725 W Las Positas Blvd, Ste 120
Pleasanton, CA 94588-4016
(925)734-3376
FAX: (925)416-6758

The Permanente Medical Group, Pleasanton
7601 Stoneridge Dr
Pleasanton, CA 94588-4501
(925)847-5178
FAX: (925)847-5200

Pomona

Alinea Medical Imaging
2475 N Garey Ave
Pomona, CA 91767-2139
(909)622-3166
FAX: (909)622-8046

Alinea Medical Imaging-Mobile
2475 N Garey Ave
Pomona, CA 91767-2139
(909)622-3166
FAX: (909)622-8046

Breast Health Center
1910 Royalty Dr
Pomona, CA 91767-3021
(909)865-9583
FAX: (909)865-9794

Centrelake Medical Group
1555 N Orange Grove Ave
Pomona, CA 91767-3811
(909)242-7000
FAX: (909)212-6252

Claremont Imaging Associates
255 E Bonita Ave, Bldg 3A
Pomona, CA 91767-1923
(909)450-0393
FAX: (909)450-0394

Porter Ranch

Providence Holy Cross Health Ctr - Porter Ranch
19950 Rinaldi St
Porter Ranch, CA 91326-4141
(818)496-7535
FAX: (818)496-7535

Porterville

Sequoia Mri - California Medical Imaging Inc
462 W Putnam Ave
Porterville, CA 93257-3321
(559)713-6050
FAX: (559)713-6321

Sierra View Medical Center Womens Imaging Dept
263 Pearson Dr Ste 104
Porterville, CA 93257-3333
(559)791-3941
FAX: (559)791-3978

Portola

Eastern Plumas Health Care
500 1st Ave
Portola, CA 96122-9406
(530)832-6516
FAX: (530)832-5829

Poway

Imaging Healthcare Specialists Poway
12620 Monte Vista Rd Ste A
Poway, CA 92064-2531
(866)558-4320
FAX: (866)558-4329

Jean McLaughlin Women's Center For Health And Healing
15611 Pomerado Rd Ste 106 1st Floor, Pomerado Outpatient Pavilion
Poway, CA 92064-2437
(858)613-6154
FAX: (858)613-6140

Vrc Holdings, Llc Rb/Poway
15725 Pomerado Rd Ste 101
Poway, CA 92064-2057
(858)485-6500
FAX: (858)485-6059

Quincy

Plumas District Hospital
1065 Bucks Lake Rd
Quincy, CA 95971-9599
(530)283-7155
FAX: (530)283-1838

Rancho Cordova

The Permanente Medical Group, Rancho Cordova
10725 International Dr
Rancho Cordova, CA 95670-7967
(916)973-5720
FAX: (916)614-4991

Rancho Cucamonga

Breast Care And Imaging Center Of Grove
8805 Haven Ave Ste 220
Rancho Cucamonga, CA 91730-5157
(909)450-0688
FAX: (909)450-0650

Kaiser Permanente Medical Offices - Rancho Cucamonga
10850 Arrow Rte
Rancho Cucamonga, CA 91730-4833
(909)427-3914
FAX: (909)427-4668

Rancho San Antonio Medical Center
7777 Milliken Ave, Ste A
Rancho Cucamonga, CA 91730-7489
(909)920-4726
FAX: (909)579-6797

Rancho Mirage

Breast Care Center Of The Desert
35800 Bob Hope Dr, Ste 150B
Rancho Mirage, CA 92270-1740
(760)318-2980
FAX: (760)323-9654

Eisenhower Medical Center-Breast Center
39000 Bob Hope Dr, Lucy Curci Cancer Center Building
Rancho Mirage, CA 92270-3221
(760)773-4338
FAX: (760)837-8840

Rancho Mission Viejo

Memorialcare Breast Center At Saddleback, R.M.V.
30492 Gateway Pl Ste 100
Rancho Mission Viejo, CA 92694-1862
(949)452-7200
FAX: (949)699-0532

Red Bluff

Dignity Health Sech Lassen Medical Clinic
2450 Sister Mary Columba Dr
Red Bluff, CA 96080-4356
(530)527-0414
FAX: (530)528-7933

St. Elizabeth Imaging Center
2580 Sister Mary Columba Dr
Red Bluff, CA 96080-4327
(530)529-7880
FAX: (530)529-7828

Redding

MD Imaging Womens Imaging Center
2020 Court St
Redding, CA 96001-1822
(530)243-1249
FAX: (530)243-0372

North Valley Breast Clinic
1335 Buenaventura Blvd Ste 204
Redding, CA 96001-0160
(530)243-5551
FAX: (530)245-0572

Redlands

Beaver Medical Group, L.P.
2 W Fern Ave
Redlands, CA 92373-5971
(909)425-3313
FAX: (909)862-1064

Kaiser Foundation Hospital Redlands
1301 California St
Redlands, CA 92374-2910
(909)427-3914
FAX: (909)427-4668

Nancy Varner Center For Women's Health
255 Terracina Blvd Ste 104A
Redlands, CA 92373-4870
(909)793-4399
FAX: (909)793-3302

Redondo Beach

Optum
601 Torrance Blvd
Redondo Beach, CA 90277-3416
(310)792-8316
FAX: (310)543-5142

Redwood City

Nk Tpmg Redwood City Marshall Mob
905 Maple Street
Redwood City, CA 94063
(650)299-2015
FAX: (650)299-4865

Sequoia Whipple Radiology
2900 Whipple Ave, Ste 100
Redwood City, CA 94062-2844
(650)367-5536
FAX: (650)261-2301

Reedley

Adventist Health Reedley Dba Adventist Med Ctr Reedley
372 W Cypress Ave, Medical Imaging Department
Reedley, CA 93654-2113
(800)990-7607
FAX: (800)537-2313

Reseda

Northridge Diagnostic Med Group
8227 Reseda Blvd
Reseda, CA 91335-1247
(800)378-5597
FAX: (818)701-5936

Rialto

Pinnacle Medical Group
1851 N Riverside Ave
Rialto, CA 92376-8069
(909)874-2371
FAX: (909)874-1230

Richmond

Nk Kfh Richmond
901 Nevin Ave
Richmond, CA 94801-3143
(510)307-2357
FAX: (510)307-2566

Ridgecrest

Ridgecrest Regional Hospital Womens Imaging
1111 N China Lake Blvd
Ridgecrest, CA 93555-3131
(760)499-3551
FAX: (760)499-7471

Riverside

Breastlink Women's Imaging Riverside
3900 Sherman Dr Ste 110
Riverside, CA 92503-4006
(951)238-6050
FAX: (951)238-6044

Good Shepherd Healthcare Llc
9395 Magnolia Ave
Riverside, CA 92503-3747
(714)801-8878
FAX: (714)801-8878

Healthcare Imaging Center At Day Street
6485 Day St, Ste 101
Riverside, CA 92507-0930
(951)682-1099
FAX: (951)656-6068

Kaiser Permanente Medical Offices Meridian
14305 Meridian Pkwy
Riverside, CA 92518-3034
(951)353-4000
FAX: (951)353-5797

Kaiser Permanente Medical Offices Riverside
10800 Magnolia Ave
Riverside, CA 92505-3043
(951)353-4000
FAX: (951)353-5797

Parkview Outpatient Radiology
9041 Magnolia Ave Ste 101
Riverside, CA 92503-3942
(951)687-5755
FAX: (951)687-2832

Riverside Community Hospital Breast Imaging Center
4500 Brockton Ave Ste 219
Riverside, CA 92501-4027
(951)276-7550
FAX: (951)276-9883

Riverside Medical Clinic
6405 Day St
Riverside, CA 92507-0901
(951)697-5678
FAX: (951)784-5572

Riverside Medical Clinic
7117 Brockton Ave
Riverside, CA 92506-2658
(951)782-3714
FAX: (951)784-3274

Riverside Medical Clinic
3660 Arlington Ave
Riverside, CA 92506-3912
(951)493-6909
FAX: (951)784-5572

Rocklin

Placer Center For Health
550 W Ranch View Dr Ste 1200
Rocklin, CA 95765-5398
(916)295-5810
FAX: (916)295-5815

Rohnert Park

Nk Tpmg Rohnert Park
5900 State Farm Dr
Rohnert Park, CA 94928-2149
(707)566-5560
FAX: (707)566-5887

Rolling Hills Estates

Torrance Memorial Breast Diagnostic Center IV
65 Peninsula Ctr
Rolling Hills Estates, CA 90274-3506
(310)891-6630
FAX: (310)377-9141

Ucla Radiology Palos Verdes Women's Imaging Center
501 Deep Valley Dr Ste 300
Rolling Hills Estates, CA 90274-7620
(310)301-6800
FAX: (310)825-3205

Rosemead

Advanced Radiology Medical Group, Inc.
7715 Garvey Ave
Rosemead, CA 91770-3003
(626)280-0431
FAX: (626)280-6840

Roseville

Dignity Health Advanced Imaging, A Service Of Dhmf
1380 Lead Hill Blvd Ste 100
Roseville, CA 95661-2941
(916)535-2030
FAX: (916)771-5770

Kaiser Permanente Roseville Riverside Mob
1011 Riverside Ave
Roseville, CA 95678-5134
(916)474-6684
FAX: (916)474-6648

Sutter Valley Medical Foundation - Sutter Imaging Roseville
1640 E Roseville Pkwy Ste 100
Roseville, CA 95661-3922
(916)784-2277
FAX: (916)784-7771

Sutter Valley Medical Foundation-Sutter Imaging Roseville II
2 Medical Plaza Dr Ste 105
Roseville, CA 95661-3042
(916)878-3490
FAX: (916)865-1461

The Permanente Medical Group, Roseville-Mob II
1600 Eureka Rd
Roseville, CA 95661-3027
(916)201-7499
FAX: (916)746-4597

Sacramento

Diagnostic Radiological Imaging
79 Scripps Dr Ste 100
Sacramento, CA 95825-6208
(916)921-1300
FAX: (916)921-1095

Dignity Health Medical Foundation
3301 C St Ste 500
Sacramento, CA 95816-3372
(916)434-7600
FAX: (916)325-2125

Nk Kfh South Sacramento
6600 Bruceville Rd
Sacramento, CA 95823-4671
(916)688-2355
FAX: (916)688-6103

Nk Tpmg Sacramento Point West
1650 Response Rd
Sacramento, CA 95815-4807
(916)614-4982
FAX: (916)614-4991

Sutter Valley Medical Foundation - Campus Commons
2 Scripps Dr Ste 110
Sacramento, CA 95825-6207
(916)929-3393
FAX: (916)929-1568

Sutter Valley Medical Foundation - Capitol Pavilion
2725 Capitol Ave Ste 104
Sacramento, CA 95816-6004
(877)515-0053
FAX: (916)262-9525

Sutter Valley Medical Foundation - Sutter Imaging Sacramento
3161 L St First Fl
Sacramento, CA 95816-5234
(916)451-3344
FAX: (916)457-5847

Sutter Valley Medical Foundation - Sutter Imaging South
8118 Timberlake Way Ste 110
Sacramento, CA 95823-5400
(916)681-8852
FAX: (916)682-9562

The Permanente Medical Group, Fair Oaks
2345 Fair Oaks Blvd, Diagnostic Imaging
Sacramento, CA 95825-4708
(916)973-5720
FAX: (916)614-4991

Tpmg Sacramento Downtown Commons
501 J St
Sacramento, CA 95814-2325
(916)973-5720
FAX: (916)497-4210

University Of California Davis Imaging Center
4860 Y St Ste 0500
Sacramento, CA 95817-2307
(916)734-0655
FAX: (916)734-0650

Saint Helena

Adventist Health Physicians Network 821 S St. Helena Hwy 2
821 Saint Helena Hwy S Ste 2
Saint Helena, CA 94574-2266
(707)963-1912
FAX: (707)963-3439

Salinas

Natividad Medical Center
1441 Constitution Blvd Bldg 400
Salinas, CA 93906-3100
(831)772-7610
FAX: (831)755-4269

The Nancy Ausonio Mammography Ctr
240 San Jose St
Salinas, CA 93901-3901
(831)759-1908
FAX: (831)758-6437

San Andreas

Mark Twain Medical Center
768 Mountain Ranch Rd
San Andreas, CA 95249-9710
(209)754-2517
FAX: (209)754-2508

San Bernardino

Arrowhead McKee Family Health Center
1499 E Highland Ave
San Bernardino, CA 92404-4611
(909)777-0834
FAX: (909)580-1720

Center For Imaging At St. Bernardine
401 E Highland Ave
San Bernardino, CA 92404-3803
(909)881-4568
FAX: (909)881-4438

Health Diagnostics Of California, A Professional Corporation
225 W Hospitality Ln, Ste 100/102
San Bernardino, CA 92408-3237
(909)890-5856
FAX: (909)890-5725

Inland Family Community Health Center
665 N D St
San Bernardino, CA 92401-1109
(909)708-8158
FAX: (909)380-7030

Loma Linda University Health-Palm Imaging Sb
399 E 21st St
San Bernardino, CA 92404-4815
(909)882-2266
FAX: (909)474-4760

Redlandsfamilypracticemedicalgroup,Inc.
1700 N Waterman Ave
San Bernardino, CA 92404-5115
(909)883-8611
FAX: (909)881-5707

San Bernardino Advanced Imaging - Highland
800 E Highland Ave
San Bernardino, CA 92404-4006
(909)450-0640
FAX: (909)881-5745

Women's Diag Ctr-Community Hosp Of San Bernardino
1800 Western Ave Ste 102
San Bernardino, CA 92411-1352
(909)887-6333
FAX: (909)887-3254

San Carlos

Palo Alto Medical Foundation - San Carlos Center
301 Industrial Rd
San Carlos, CA 94070-2603
(650)853-2902
FAX: (650)853-6099

San Clemente

Hoag Clinic- San Clemente
1031 Avenida Pico, Ste 203
San Clemente, CA 92673-6356
(949)829-5500
FAX: (949)461-5163

San Diego

Community Health Imaging Centers
4060 Fairmount Ave Ste 120
San Diego, CA 92105-1608
(619)269-1299
FAX: (619)961-0812

Imaging Healthcare Specialists - Alvarado
6386 Alvarado Ct Ste 121
San Diego, CA 92120-4906
(866)558-4320
FAX: (866)558-4329

Imaging Healthcare Specialists-150 West Washington
150 W Washington St
San Diego, CA 92103-2005
(866)558-4320
FAX: (866)558-4329

Infertility, Gynecology And Obstetrics
9339 Genesee Ave Ste 220, Medical Group Of San Diego
San Diego, CA 92121-2121
(858)455-7520
FAX: (858)642-1728

Kaiser Permanente - Vandever
4405 Vandever Ave
San Diego, CA 92120-3315
(800)290-5000
FAX: (619)229-7551

Kaiser Permanente Point Loma
3250 Fordham St
San Diego, CA 92110-5397
(800)290-5000
FAX: (619)528-6588

Kaiser Permanente-Hospital Zion
4647 Zion Ave
San Diego, CA 92120-2507
(800)290-5000
FAX: (619)528-6588

Kaiser Permanente-Otay Mesa
4652 Palm Ave
San Diego, CA 92154-8404
(800)290-5000
FAX: (619)528-6588

Naval Branch Health Clinic Kearny Mesa
8808 Balboa Ave
San Diego, CA 92123-1592
(619)532-7394
FAX: (619)645-0193

Naval Medical Center San Diego
34800 Bob Wilson Dr Ste 204, Mammography Section
San Diego, CA 92134-1204
(619)532-7394
FAX: (619)532-5024

S Kfh Clairemont Mesa
6911 Convoy Ct
San Diego, CA 92111-1014
(800)290-5500
FAX: (619)528-6588

Scripps Clinic Carmel Valley Gooding Imaging Center
3811 Valley Centre Dr
San Diego, CA 92130-3318
(858)764-3400
FAX: (858)764-3395

Scripps Clinic Mission Valley
7425 Mission Valley Rd Ste 202
San Diego, CA 92108-4409
(619)245-2385
FAX: (619)245-2383

Scripps Clinic Rancho Bernardo
15004 Innovation Dr
San Diego, CA 92128-3491
(858)554-7844
FAX: (858)605-7878

Scripps Mercy O'Toole Breast Care Center
550 Washington St, Ste 200
San Diego, CA 92103-2243
(619)260-7225
FAX: (619)686-4103

Sharp Memorial Outpatient Pavilion Imaging
3075 Health Center Dr, 2nd Floor - Women's Imaging
San Diego, CA 92123-2773
(858)939-5100
FAX: (858)939-5066

Sharp Rees - Stealy/ Sorrento Mesa
10243 Genetic Center Dr, Radiology Dept.
San Diego, CA 92121-6310
(858)586-6730
FAX: (858)262-6200

Sharp Rees Stealy - Downtown
300 Fir St, Radiology
San Diego, CA 92101-2393
(858)586-6730
FAX: (858)262-6200

Sharp Rees Stealy Rancho Bernardo
16899 W Bernardo Dr
San Diego, CA 92127-1603
(858)586-6730
FAX: (619)446-1630

Sharp Rees-Stealy Breast Imaging Center
8933 Activity Rd
San Diego, CA 92126-4427
(858)586-6730
FAX: (858)262-6200

Skfh - Carmel Valley
3851 Shaw Ridge Rd
San Diego, CA 92130-2807
(800)290-5000
FAX: (619)528-6588

Skfh - San Diego Medical Center
9455 Clairemont Mesa Blvd
San Diego, CA 92123-1297
(800)290-5000
FAX: (619)528-6588

Uc San Diego Health Rancho Bernardo At Via Tazon
16950 Via Tazon
San Diego, CA 92127-1607
(619)543-3405
FAX: (858)249-5723

Ucsd Center For Women's Health
330 Lewis St Ste 202
San Diego, CA 92103-2108
(858)249-3060
FAX: (858)249-3070

San Dimas

San Dimas Community Hospital
1350 W Covina Blvd
San Dimas, CA 91773-3219
(909)599-6811
FAX: (909)305-5681

Skfh - San Dimas Kaiser Permanente - San Dimas
1255 W Arrow Hwy Bldg B
San Dimas, CA 91773-2340
(626)851-5130
FAX: (626)851-5461

San Francisco

Chinese Hospital
845 Jackson St
San Francisco, CA 94133-4899
(415)677-2328
FAX: (415)217-4196

Health Diagnostics Of California, A Professional Corporation
1180 Post St
San Francisco, CA 94109-5505
(415)248-3700
FAX: (650)257-6233

Health Diagnostics Of California, A Professional Corporation
325 Sacramento St
San Francisco, CA 94111-3601
(415)321-4674
FAX: (415)321-4677

Nk The Permanente Medical Group San Francisco
2238 Geary Blvd, Radiology Department, 3rd Floor
San Francisco, CA 94115-3416
(415)833-3700
FAX: (415)833-0132

Nk Tpmg San Francisco Mission Bay
1600 Owens St
San Francisco, CA 94158-2261
(415)833-3700
FAX: (415)833-0132

North East Medical Services
1422 Noriega St
San Francisco, CA 94122-4432
(415)352-5073
FAX: (415)644-5588

North East Medical Services
1520 Stockton St
San Francisco, CA 94133-3354
(415)391-9686
FAX: (415)644-5588

Spmf Breast Health Center St. Luke's Campus
1580 Valencia St, Ste 237M28
San Francisco, CA 94110-4423
(415)641-3360
FAX: (415)647-7514

St. Mary's Medical Center
1 Shrader St, Ste 490
San Francisco, CA 94117-1016
(415)750-4377
FAX: (415)750-5744

Sutter Bay Hospitals Dba Cpmc - Phoc
2333 Buchanan St 2/F
San Francisco, CA 94115-1925
(415)600-2700
FAX: (415)375-4883

Ucsf Medical Center - Montgomery Street
1725 Montgomery St Ste 250
San Francisco, CA 94111-1018
(415)353-2573
FAX: (415)353-7299

Ucsf Medical Center Mission Bay
1825 4th St 3rd Floor Mammography
San Francisco, CA 94143-2350
(415)353-2573
FAX: (415)353-7299

Ucsf Medical Center Mt Zion
2356 Sutter St, Box 1667
San Francisco, CA 94115-3006
(415)353-2573
FAX: (415)353-7299

Zuckerberg San Francisco General Hospital
1001 Potrero Ave, Avon Breast Ctr- Bldg 4
San Francisco, CA 94110-3594
(415)206-4965
FAX: (415)206-5844

San Gabriel

Diagnostic Medical Group Of Southern California
1129 S San Gabriel Blvd
San Gabriel, CA 91776-3114
(626)287-6746
FAX: (626)248-9314

San Jacinto

San Jacinto Imaging
1695 S San Jacinto Ave Ste B
San Jacinto, CA 92583-5103
(951)665-1500
FAX: (951)655-1550

Soboba Indian Health
607 Donna Way
San Jacinto, CA 92583-5517
(951)654-0803
FAX: (951)654-9053

San Jose

County Of Sta. Clara Dba O'Connor Hospital Radiology
2105 Forest Ave
San Jose, CA 95128-1425
(408)947-2808
FAX: (408)947-3475

Nk Tpmg San Jose - Skyport
1721 Technology Dr, Mob - Dept 145 - Radiology/Imaging Servi
San Jose, CA 95110-1305
(408)851-5020
FAX: (408)851-3669

North East Medical Services
1870 Lundy Ave
San Jose, CA 95131-1826
(415)352-5073
FAX: (415)644-5588

Santa Clara Valley Medical Center
751 S Bascom Ave
San Jose, CA 95128-2699
(408)885-6372
FAX: (408)885-6360

Santa Clara Valley Medical Center - Tully
500 Tully Rd
San Jose, CA 95111-1917
(408)885-6350
FAX: (408)885-6360

Silicon Valley Medical Development
625 Lincoln Ave
San Jose, CA 95126-3785
(408)278-3370
FAX: (408)278-3378

Silver Creek Radiology
2365 Quimby Rd, Ste 100
San Jose, CA 95122-1337
(669)888-0001
FAX: (669)888-0551

Stanford Cancer Center, South Bay
2589 Samaritan Dr
San Jose, CA 95124-4102
(650)736-2304
FAX: (650)617-4066

The Permanente Med. Group, San Jose Women's Health
276 Hospital Pkwy
San Jose, CA 95119-1103
(408)972-7100
FAX: (408)972-7163

University Healthcare Alliance Imaging San Jose
798 S Winchester Blvd
San Jose, CA 95128-2928
(408)313-1131
FAX: (408)984-7225

Valley Health Center At Bascom
750 S Bascom Ave
San Jose, CA 95128-2639
(408)885-6350
FAX: (408)885-6360

Valley Health Center At Downtown
777 E Santa Clara St
San Jose, CA 95112-1934
(408)885-6350
FAX: (408)885-6360

Valley Health Center At East Valley
1993 McKee Rd
San Jose, CA 95116-1406
(408)885-6372
FAX: (408)885-6360

Valley Radiology Imaging
125 Ciro Ave Ste 220
San Jose, CA 95128-1671
(408)272-2873
FAX: (408)272-7784

Valley Radiology Imaging
2323 McKee Rd Ste 40
San Jose, CA 95116-1609
(408)964-1005
FAX: (408)964-1038

Vri Samaritan Women's Center
2581 Samaritan Dr Ste 206
San Jose, CA 95124-4112
(408)358-6881
FAX: (408)356-8785

San Leandro

Kaiser Foundation Hospital-San Leandro
2500 Merced St, First Floor - Radiology
San Leandro, CA 94577-4201
(510)454-6290
FAX: (510)454-6280

Norcal Imaging Sanleandro
2450 Washington Ave Ste 120
San Leandro, CA 94577-5943
(510)351-7734
FAX: (510)351-7742

San Leandro Hospital
13855 E 14th St, Atten: Radiology
San Leandro, CA 94578-2600
(510)814-4003
FAX: (510)357-9510

San Luis Obispo

Dignity Community Care - San Luis Diagnostic Center
1100 Monterey St Ste 210
San Luis Obispo, CA 93401-3102
(805)542-9700
FAX: (805)542-9060

Dignity Community Care-French Hospital Medical Center
1911 Johnson Ave
San Luis Obispo, CA 93401-4131
(805)597-6700
FAX: (805)614-5873

Selma A. Carlson Diagnostic Center
77 Casa St Ste 102
San Luis Obispo, CA 93405-5804
(805)546-7733
FAX: (805)549-9217

San Marcos

S Kfh - San Marcos
400 Craven Rd
San Marcos, CA 92078-4201
(800)290-5000
FAX: (619)528-6588

San Mateo

Mills-Peninsula Medical Center
100 S San Mateo Dr
San Mateo, CA 94401-3805
(650)696-4140
FAX: (650)696-4159

Nk Tpmg San Mateo Mob
1000 Franklin Pkwy
San Mateo, CA 94403-1922
(650)299-3851
FAX: (650)299-4865

Peninsula Diagnostic Imaging, Inc.
101 S San Mateo Dr Ste 201
San Mateo, CA 94401-3843
(650)343-1655
FAX: (650)343-1686

San Mateo Medical Center
222 W 39th Ave, Radiology Department
San Mateo, CA 94403-4364
(650)573-2681
FAX: (650)573-2122

San Pablo

Alliance Medical Group
100 San Pablo Towne Center, A
San Pablo, CA 94806
(510)237-2802
FAX: (866)601-1562

West County Health Center
13601 San Pablo Ave
San Pablo, CA 94806-3858
(510)231-9494
FAX: (510)231-9493

San Pedro

Providence Little Company Of Mary San Pedro
1300 W 7th St
San Pedro, CA 90732-3505
(855)353-3910
FAX: (855)359-6330

San Rafael

Nk - Kfh - San Rafael
99 Montecillo Rd
San Rafael, CA 94903-3308
(415)444-2966
FAX: (415)444-4948

Nk Tpmg San Rafael Park Medical Center
1650 Los Gamos Dr
San Rafael, CA 94903-1850
(415)444-2280
FAX: (415)444-4948

Nktpmg San Rafael
1033 3rd St
San Rafael, CA 94901-3107
(415)444-2280
FAX: (415)444-4948

San Ramon

John Muir Medical Imaging San Ramon
2305 Camino Ramon Ste 108
San Ramon, CA 94583-1394
(925)952-2701
FAX: (925)941-4065

San Ramon Regional Medical Center
7777 Norris Canyon Rd, Radiology Dept
San Ramon, CA 94583-5404
(925)275-8273
FAX: (925)275-8361

The Permanente Medical Group, San Ramon
2300 Camino Ramon
San Ramon, CA 94583-1354
(925)244-7250
FAX: (924)244-7256

Santa Ana

Breastlink Women's Imaging Center-Santa Ana
1100 N Tustin Ave Ste A
Santa Ana, CA 92705-3509
(714)784-1643
FAX: (714)550-7130

Kaiser Permanente Medical Offices Tustin Santa Ana
1900 E 4th St
Santa Ana, CA 92705-3910
(714)223-3028
FAX: (949)932-6330

S Khf Santa Ana Harbor Macarthur Facility
3401 S Harbor Blvd
Santa Ana, CA 92704-7933
(714)223-3028
FAX: (949)932-6330

United Medical Imaging Of Santa Ana
800 N Tustin Ave, Ste M
Santa Ana, CA 92705-3605
(714)450-1410
FAX: (714)450-1429

Santa Barbara

California Managed Imaging Medical Group, Inc Dba Sbwic
2320 Bath St Ste 113
Santa Barbara, CA 93105-4339
(805)682-7744
FAX: (805)682-3321

Goleta Valley Cottage Hospital
351 S Patterson Ave
Santa Barbara, CA 93111-2496
(805)681-6459
FAX: (805)681-6482

Sansum Clinic
215 Pesetas Ln
Santa Barbara, CA 93110-1416
(805)681-7675
FAX: (805)681-7579

Santa Barbara Cottage Hospital
2410 Fletcher Ave
Santa Barbara, CA 93105-4828
(805)569-7279
FAX: (805)569-8279

Santa Clara

Nk Tpmg Santa Clara M.O.B.
710 Lawrence Expy, Dept. 396 - Women's Imaging
Santa Clara, CA 95051-5173
(408)851-5054
FAX: (408)851-3669

Santa Clarita

Facey Medical Group Canyon Country
14550 Soledad Canyon Rd, Radiology, 1st Floor
Santa Clarita, CA 91387-2200
(818)869-7201
FAX: (818)869-7219

S Kfh Santa Clarita
27107 Tourney Rd
Santa Clarita, CA 91355-1860
(818)375-1755
FAX: (818)815-6849

Ucla Health Santa Clarita Women's Imaging Center
27235 Tourney Rd
Santa Clarita, CA 91355-5904
(310)301-6800
FAX: (310)825-3205

Santa Cruz

Palo Alto Medical Foundation - Santa Cruz
2025 Soquel Ave
Santa Cruz, CA 95062-1323
(831)458-4877
FAX: (831)458-6285

Radiology Medical Group Of Santa Cruz County, Inc.
1661 Soquel Dr Ste G
Santa Cruz, CA 95065-1790
(831)476-7711
FAX: (831)476-5495

Santa Maria

Digital Medical Imaging
522 Plaza Dr
Santa Maria, CA 93454-6908
(805)928-3673
FAX: (805)928-9588

Marian Breast Imaging Center
1325 E Church St Ste 201
Santa Maria, CA 93454-5915
(805)346-3490
FAX: (805)349-0271

Santa Monica

Barbara Kort Women's Imaging Ctr. At Ucla Santa Monica
1260 15th St Ste 111
Santa Monica, CA 90404-1136
(310)301-6800
FAX: (310)825-3205

Lsg Imaging
2730 Wilshire Blvd Ste 110
Santa Monica, CA 90403-4724
(310)394-2761
FAX: (310)394-2766

Medical Imaging Center Of Southern California
2811 Wilshire Blvd
Santa Monica, CA 90403-4803
(310)829-9788
FAX: (310)696-0102

Providence Saint John's Health Center
2121 Santa Monica Blvd, Providence Saint John's Health Center
Santa Monica, CA 90404-2303
(310)582-7100
FAX: (310)582-7110

Tower Saint John's Imaging
2202 Wilshire Blvd
Santa Monica, CA 90403-5706
(310)264-9000
FAX: (310)264-4092

Ucla Health Breast Imaging Santa Monica Surgery Center
1223 16th St Ste 3100
Santa Monica, CA 90404-1275
(310)310-6800
FAX: (310)825-3205

Santa Paula

Santa Paula Hospital
825 N 10th St
Santa Paula, CA 93060-1309
(805)933-8674
FAX: (805)933-8668

Santa Rosa

Nk Tpmg Santa Rosa Mob5
3975 Old Redwood Hwy
Santa Rosa, CA 95403-1719
(707)566-5560
FAX: (707)566-5067

Nk Tpmg Santa Rosa Mob6
2240 Mercury Way, Medical Imaging
Santa Rosa, CA 95407-5413
(707)566-5560
FAX: (707)566-5823

Santa Rosa Memorial Hospital Outpatient Imaging
121 Sotoyome St
Santa Rosa, CA 95405-4823
(707)525-4027
FAX: (707)525-4097

Sutter Bay Medical Foundation
3883 Airway Dr Ste 100
Santa Rosa, CA 95403-1672
(707)521-4480
FAX: (707)521-4460

Santee

Sharp Rees-Stealy Medical Centers-Santee
8701 Cuyamaca St
Santee, CA 92071-4253
(858)586-6730
FAX: (858)262-6200

Scotts Valley

Nk Tpmg Scotts Valley
5615 Scotts Valley Dr
Scotts Valley, CA 95066-3492
(408)972-4365
FAX: (408)972-7163

Selma

Adventist Medical Center-Selma
1141 Rose Ave
Selma, CA 93662-3241
(559)856-7330
FAX: (559)856-7332

Nk Tpmg Selma
2651 Highland Ave
Selma, CA 93662-3392
(559)448-4055
FAX: (559)448-5191

Sherman Oaks

Diagnostic Imaging Network
4910 Van Nuys Blvd, Ste 110
Sherman Oaks, CA 91403-1782
(818)986-8215
FAX: (818)986-9582

Signal Hill

Liberty Pacific Advanced Imaging Long Beach
2708 E Willow St
Signal Hill, CA 90755-2217
(562)216-5120
FAX: (562)733-5880

Simi Valley

Adventist Health Simi Valley Nancy Reagan Breast Center
2750 Sycamore Dr, Ofc
Simi Valley, CA 93065-1500
(805)955-8115
FAX: (805)955-8146

Kaiser Permanente Medical Office - Simi Valley
3900 Alamo St
Simi Valley, CA 93063-2111
(818)719-4173
FAX: (818)719-3251

Soledad

Soledad Women's Health Center
600B Main St
Soledad, CA 93960-2533
(831)678-2665
FAX: (831)678-1355

Solvang

Santa Ynez Valley Cottage Hospital
2050 Viborg Rd
Solvang, CA 93463-2295
(805)686-3967
FAX: (805)749-2858

Sonoma

Sonoma Valley Hospital Diag. Imaging Anx.
347 Andrieux St
Sonoma, CA 95476-6863
(707)935-5233
FAX: (707)935-5271

Sonora

Adventist Health Sonora Health Pavilion
900 Mono Way
Sonora, CA 95370-5229
(209)536-3437
FAX: (209)536-3509

Sonora Community Hospital Dba Sonora Regional Med Ctr
1000 Greenley Rd
Sonora, CA 95370-5200
(209)536-3459
FAX: (209)536-3509

South Lake Tahoe

Barton Memorial Hospital
2170 South Ave
South Lake Tahoe, CA 96150-7008
(530)542-3000
FAX: (530)542-9550

Stockton

Sgmf Stockton Medical Plaza Imaging Center
2505 W Hammer Ln
Stockton, CA 95209-2839
(209)954-4019
FAX: (209)954-9442

St. Joseph's Women's Imaging Ctr
3439 Brookside Rd Ste 107
Stockton, CA 95219-1754
(209)466-5027
FAX: (209)466-5461

St. Joseph's Imaging Center
1617 N California St, Ste 1A
Stockton, CA 95204-6117
(209)944-1223
FAX: (209)948-2661

Stockton Diagnostic Imaging
1801 E March Ln Ste A130
Stockton, CA 95210-6650
(209)475-9871
FAX: (209)474-9620

The Permanente Medical Group - Stockton Mob
7373 West Ln
Stockton, CA 95210-3377
(209)476-2111
FAX: (209)476-3875

Valley Mri And Radiology Inc
3031 W March Ln, Ste 336
Stockton, CA 95219-6577
(209)952-9300
FAX: (209)952-9191

Sun City

California Imaging And Diagnostics Medical Group
26870 Cherry Hills Blvd
Sun City, CA 92586-2568
(866)419-3372
FAX: (951)677-7839

Sun Valley

Serra Community Medical Clinic, Inc.
9375 San Fernando Rd
Sun Valley, CA 91352-1418
(818)504-4540
FAX: (818)504-4685

Sunnyvale

Valley Radiology Sunnyvale Radnet Inc
696 W El Camino Real
Sunnyvale, CA 94087-1211
(650)967-1331
FAX: (650)691-6794

Susanville

Banner Lassen Medical Center
1800 Spring Ridge Dr
Susanville, CA 96130-6100
(530)252-2121
FAX: (530)252-2122

Sylmar

Olive View - Ucla Medical Center
14445 Olive View Dr, Rm 1D-102
Sylmar, CA 91342-1438
(747)210-4096
FAX: (747)210-3597

Tarzana

Breastlink Women's Imaging Center Tarzana
18133 Ventura Blvd, Ste 200
Tarzana, CA 91356-3641
(800)378-5597
FAX: (818)342-0303

Providence Cedars-Sinai Tarzana Outpatient Women's Center
18344 Clark St Ste 110
Tarzana, CA 91356-3565
(818)881-9814
FAX: (818)881-3424

Tehachapi

Adventist Health Tehachapi Valley
1100 Magellan Dr
Tehachapi, CA 93561-1380
(661)771-8885
FAX: (661)771-8393

Temecula

Kaiser Permanente Medical Offices Temecula
27309 Madison Ave
Temecula, CA 92590-5685
(951)353-4000
FAX: (951)353-5797

Temecula Valley Advanced Imaging- Temecula Parkway
31775 De Portola Rd, Ste 100
Temecula, CA 92592-2742
(951)238-6070
FAX: (951)238-6069

Templeton

Radiology Diagnostic Center
1310 Las Tablas Rd Ste 103
Templeton, CA 93465-9746
(805)434-0829
FAX: (805)434-0826

Templeton Imaging, Inc
262 Posada Ln Ste C
Templeton, CA 93465-4057
(805)434-1491
FAX: (805)434-3591

Thousand Oaks

Kaiser Permanente Medical Offices-Thousand Oaks
365 E Hillcrest Dr
Thousand Oaks, CA 91360-5820
(818)719-4173
FAX: (818)719-3251

Rolling Oaks Imaging Center
415 Rolling Oaks Dr Ste 230
Thousand Oaks, CA 91361-1029
(805)778-1513
FAX: (805)494-1620

Thousand Oaks Radiology Group
227 W Janss Rd Ste 150
Thousand Oaks, CA 91360-1859
(805)496-7755
FAX: (805)379-3913

Torrance

Harbor Ucla Medical Center
1000 W Carson St, Department Of Radiology
Torrance, CA 90502-2059
(424)306-8178
FAX: (310)782-6323

Harbor-Ucla Diagnostic Imaging
21828 Normandie Ave, Radiology Department Ste 3
Torrance, CA 90502-2047
(424)306-4835
FAX: (310)782-6323

Kaiser Permanente Torrance Medical Offices
20790 Madrona Ave
Torrance, CA 90503-3777
(800)780-1230
FAX: (310)517-6193

Optum [torrance]
3565 Del Amo Blvd
Torrance, CA 90503-1637
(424)350-3657
FAX: (323)728-0697

Providence Little Co. Of Mary Women's Imaging Center
20929 Hawthorne Blvd
Torrance, CA 90503-4611
(310)303-6500
FAX: (310)303-7049

Torrance Memorial Breast Diagnostic Center
3275 Skypark Dr, Ste A
Torrance, CA 90505-5027
(310)517-4709
FAX: (310)784-6377

United Medical Imaging Of Torrance D.B A. Umi Of Torrance
3640 Lomita Blvd, Ste 105
Torrance, CA 90505-3936
(310)375-8088
FAX: (310)375-8659

Tracy

Sutter Tracy Imaging Center
1530 Bessie Ave Ste 109
Tracy, CA 95376-3080
(209)832-6022
FAX: (209)833-2362

The Permanente Medical Group- Tracy Mob
2185 W Grant Line Rd
Tracy, CA 95377-7309
(209)839-6277
FAX: (209)839-6275

Travis Afb

David Grant Medical Center 60th Mdts Sgqx
101 Bodin Cir
Travis Afb, CA 94535-1809
(707)423-7593
FAX: (707)423-7207

Truckee

Tahoe Forest Hospital District
10121 Pine Ave
Truckee, CA 96161-4856
(530)582-6510
FAX: (530)582-3599

Tulare

Adventist Health Tulare
869 N Cherry St, Medical Imaging Department
Tulare, CA 93274-2207
(559)366-1121
FAX: (559)685-3828

Turlock

Ruby E Bergman Women's Diagnostic Center
880 E Tuolumne Rd Ste 202
Turlock, CA 95382-1550
(209)669-4620
FAX: (209)664-2834

Sgmf Turlock Medical Clinic
3100 W Christoffersen Pkwy
Turlock, CA 95382-9547
(209)550-4755
FAX: (209)634-4338

Tustin

Tustin Imaging Center
15000 Kensington Park Dr Ste 150
Tustin, CA 92782-1836
(714)477-8340
FAX: (714)477-8341

Twentynine Palms

Naval Hospital Twentynine Palms
1145 Sturgis Road
Twentynine Palms, CA 92277
(760)830-2155
FAX: (760)830-2156

Ukiah

Adventist Health Ukiah Valley
245 Hospital Dr
Ukiah, CA 95482-4531
(707)463-7342
FAX: (707)463-7392

Adventist Health Ukiah Valley
1165 S Dora St, Ste C2 Ste D
Ukiah, CA 95482-6353
(707)468-9335
FAX: (707)468-0302

Union City

Nk Tpmg Union City Mob B
3553 Whipple Rd
Union City, CA 94587-1507
(510)454-4645
FAX: (510)454-4652

Upland

San Antonio Regional Women's Breast & Imaging Center
1100 San Bernardino Rd, 2nd Fl
Upland, CA 91786-4952
(909)579-6700
FAX: (909)579-6797

Vacaville

Nk Kfh Vacaville Mob B
1 Quality Dr
Vacaville, CA 95688-9494
(707)624-3610
FAX: (707)624-1805

Solano Diagnostics Imaging
1020 Nut Tree Rd, Ste 150
Vacaville, CA 95687-4100
(707)646-4646
FAX: (707)646-4977

Sutter Valley Medical Foundation - Sutter Imaging Vacaville
770 Mason St
Vacaville, CA 95688-4646
(707)427-4900
FAX: (707)454-5922

Valencia

Facey Medical Foundation-Valencia Specialty
23803 McBean Pkwy, Radiology/Suite 101
Valencia, CA 91355-4462
(818)869-7034
FAX: (818)869-7219

Santa Clarita Imaging
25775 McBean Pkwy, Ste 100
Valencia, CA 91355-3702
(800)378-5597
FAX: (661)255-9563

Sheila R.Veloz Breast Imaging Ctr- H. M. Newhall Mem. Hosp.
23929 McBean Pkwy Ste 101
Valencia, CA 91355-4467
(661)200-1099
FAX: (661)200-1098

Vallejo

Kaiser Foundation Hospital - Vallejo
975 Sereno Dr
Vallejo, CA 94589-2441
(707)651-1315
FAX: (707)651-2353

Sutter Solano Medical Center
300 Hospital Dr, Imaging Department/Mammo
Vallejo, CA 94589-2594
(707)554-5153
FAX: (707)554-5108

Sutter Valley Medical Foundation - Sutter Imaging Vallejo
100 Hospital Dr
Vallejo, CA 94589-2580
(707)432-2500
FAX: (707)432-2583

Van Nuys

Mid-Valley Comprehensive Health Center
7515 Van Nuys Blvd
Van Nuys, CA 91405-1949
(818)627-3115
FAX: (818)902-4474

Valley Breast Care And Women's Health Center
15211 Vanowen St Ste 202
Van Nuys, CA 91405-3625
(818)782-4232
FAX: (818)782-4802

Ventura

Grossman Imaging Center
2705 Loma Vista Rd Ste 100
Ventura, CA 93003-1595
(805)988-0616
FAX: (805)983-2681

Kaiser Permanente Medical Offices-Ventura
888 S Hill Rd
Ventura, CA 93003-8400
(888)515-3500
FAX: (818)719-3251

Rolling Oaks Radiology Ventura
4516 Market St
Ventura, CA 93003-8087
(805)644-7300
FAX: (805)644-8614

The Breast Center Of Community Memorial Hospital
168 N Brent St Ste 401
Ventura, CA 93003-2824
(805)948-5093
FAX: (805)641-3965

Ventura County Medical Center
300 Hillmont Ave
Ventura, CA 93003-1651
(805)652-6815
FAX: (805)652-3399

Victorville

Desert Valley Medical Group, Inc.
12276 Hesperia Rd Ste 2
Victorville, CA 92395-5838
(760)241-8000
FAX: (760)962-8563

Kaiser Permanente Victorville Medical Offices
14011 Park Ave
Victorville, CA 92392-2413
(909)427-3914
FAX: (909)427-4668

St. Joseph Heritage Healthcare
12602 Amargosa Rd Suites F & G
Victorville, CA 92392-7640
(760)261-5000
FAX: (760)243-1123

Victor Valley Global Medical Center
15203 Eleventh St Ste G
Victorville, CA 92395-3737
(760)245-4555
FAX: (760)245-4231

Victor Valley Womens Center
12276 Hesperia Rd, Ste 5
Victorville, CA 92395-5838
(760)951-2867
FAX: (760)951-7473

Visalia

California Medical Imaging Associates
3610 W Packwood Ave
Visalia, CA 93277-5010
(559)713-6050
FAX: (559)713-6321

Kaweah Delta Health Care Inc.Dba Kaweah Health Medical Group
5400 W Hillsdale Ave
Visalia, CA 93291-8222
(559)738-7500
FAX: (559)738-7527

Kaweah Health Imaging & Breast Center
4949 W Cypress Ave
Visalia, CA 93277-1591
(559)624-3200
FAX: (559)625-7412

Visalia Womens Imaging Specialists
1700 S Court St Ste C
Visalia, CA 93277-4931
(559)734-5674
FAX: (559)734-4283

Vista

Optum
145 Thunder Dr
Vista, CA 92083-6010
(760)630-5485
FAX: (760)630-5455

Scripps Coastal Medical Center
130 Cedar Rd Ste 101
Vista, CA 92083-5102
(760)806-5450
FAX: (760)806-5636

Walnut Creek

Bass Imaging
2637 Shadelands Dr
Walnut Creek, CA 94598-2512
(925)329-3710
FAX: (925)329-3711

John Muir Medical Imaging
133 La Casa Via Ste 100
Walnut Creek, CA 94598-3005
(925)952-2701
FAX: (925)947-3228

Norcal Imaging - Walnut Creek
114 La Casa Via Ste 100
Walnut Creek, CA 94598-3044
(925)937-6100
FAX: (925)947-0130

The Permanente Medical Group, Park Shadelands
320 Lennon Ln, Yosemite Building
Walnut Creek, CA 94598-2419
(925)295-5020
FAX: (925)906-2414

The Permanente Medical Group, Walnut Creek
1425 S Main St, Radiology Dept.
Walnut Creek, CA 94596-5318
(925)295-5448
FAX: (925)295-6326

Watsonville

Nk Tpmg Watsonville
1931 Main St
Watsonville, CA 95076-3027
(408)362-4365
FAX: (408)972-7163

Watsonville Community Hospital
75 Neilson St
Watsonville, CA 95076-2468
(831)761-5626
FAX: (831)763-6057

West Covina

Centrelake Imaging
1700 W West Covina Pkwy
West Covina, CA 91790-2706
(909)242-7300
FAX: (909)786-4397

S Kfh West Covina Kaiser Permanente-West Covina
1249 S Sunset Ave
West Covina, CA 91790-3960
(626)851-5130
FAX: (626)851-5461

United Medical Imaging Of West Covina
1401 W Merced Ave, 102
West Covina, CA 91790-3401
(626)813-6100
FAX: (626)813-0075

West Hills

West Hills Hospital & Medical Center/Women's Diagn. Ctr.
7325 Medical Center Dr Ste 106
West Hills, CA 91307-4109
(855)500-6674
FAX: (818)227-6768

Westlake Village

Renaissance Imaging Medical Associates, Inc.
2 Dole Dr
Westlake Village, CA 91362-7300
(818)575-8000
FAX: (818)575-8067

Ucla Health Westlake Village Women's Imaging Center
30700 Russell Ranch Rd, Ste 110
Westlake Village, CA 91362-9500
(310)301-6800
FAX: (310)825-3205

Westminster

Bolsa Medical Group
10362 Bolsa Ave, Ste 100
Westminster, CA 92683-6763
(714)531-2091
FAX: (714)531-7926

Magnolia Medical Imaging Center, Inc.
14571 Magnolia St Ste 101
Westminster, CA 92683-5575
(714)893-1915
FAX: (714)898-8142

Whittier

Dynamic Medical Imaging - Whittier
8135 Painter Ave Ste 101
Whittier, CA 90602-3160
(562)789-9770
FAX: (562)789-0484

Kaiser Permanente Medical Offices - Whittier
12470 Whittier Blvd
Whittier, CA 90602-1017
(800)823-4040
FAX: (562)657-7228

Pih Health Breast Center Whittier
12393 Washington Blvd
Whittier, CA 90606-2502
(562)907-0667
FAX: (562)789-4411

Willits

Willits Hospital, Inc., Dba Adventist Health Howard Memorial
1 Marcela Dr
Willits, CA 95490-5769
(707)456-3090
FAX: (707)459-7306

Woodland

Dignity Health Medical Foundation
2081 Bronze Star Dr
Woodland, CA 95776-5423
(530)668-2632
FAX: (530)662-7436

Woodland Clinic, A Service Of Dignity Health Medical Fdn
632 W Gibson Rd
Woodland, CA 95695-5169
(530)668-2632
FAX: (530)662-7436

Woodland Hills

Kaiser Foundation Hospital - Woodland Hills
5601 De Soto Ave
Woodland Hills, CA 91367-6701
(818)719-4173
FAX: (818)719-3251

Yorba Linda

St Jude Imaging Center Yorba Linda
4300 Rose Dr
Yorba Linda, CA 92886-2026
(714)446-5650
FAX: (714)446-5216

Uci Health-Yorba Linda
18639 Yorba Linda Blvd
Yorba Linda, CA 92886-4136
(714)456-6175
FAX: (714)456-6908

Yreka

Fairchild Medical Center
444 Bruce St
Yreka, CA 96097-3450
(530)841-6265
FAX: (530)841-6262

Yuba City

Adventist Health And Rideout Center For Women's Imaging
945 Shasta St Ste 150
Yuba City, CA 95991-4124
(530)751-5410
FAX: (530)751-5414

Precise Radiological Associates, Inc.
470 Plumas Blvd Ste 101
Yuba City, CA 95991-5077
(530)673-6674
FAX: (530)673-3335

Sutter Valley Medical Foundation - Sutter Imaging Yuba
440 Plumas Blvd
Yuba City, CA 95991-5071
(530)749-3609
FAX: (530)749-3496

COLORADO

Alamosa

San Luis Valley Regional Medical Center
106 Blanca Ave
Alamosa, CO 81101-2340
(719)587-1231
FAX: (719)587-1370

Aspen

Aspen Valley Hospital
401 Castle Creek Rd
Aspen, CO 81611-1159
(970)544-7386
FAX: (970)544-1594

Aurora

Colorado Breast Care At The Medical Center Of Aurora
1444 S Potomac St Ste 160
Aurora, CO 80012-4508
(303)338-7292
FAX: (303)338-7521

Health Images At South Potomac
1300 S Potomac St Ste 104
Aurora, CO 80012-4526
(303)750-8400
FAX: (303)751-0360

Kaiser Permanente Smoky Hill Medical Office
16290 E Quincy Ave
Aurora, CO 80015-1594
(303)338-3456
FAX: (303)239-7553

Smi Imaging , Llc - Aurora
14301 E Cedar Ave, Unit E
Aurora, CO 80012-1433
(720)492-1985
FAX: (602)714-6126

The Breast Care Center At Parker Adventist At Southlands
6069 S Southlands Pkwy
Aurora, CO 80016-5316
(303)269-4150
FAX: (303)269-4151

University Of Colorado Hospital Breast Imaging Center
1635 Aurora Ct, Box F-724 Third Fl
Aurora, CO 80045-2541
(720)848-1604
FAX: (720)848-1650

Boulder

Boulder Community Health Foothills Hospital
4747 Arapahoe Ave
Boulder, CO 80303-1131
(303)440-2170
FAX: (303)415-7555

Kaiser Permanente Baseline Medical Offices
580 Mohawk Dr
Boulder, CO 80303-3712
(303)338-3456
FAX: (303)764-4823

Brighton

Kaiser Permanente Brighton Medical Offices
859 S 4th Ave
Brighton, CO 80601-3205
(303)338-3456
FAX: (303)764-4823

Platte Valley Medical Center
1600 Prairie Center Pkwy
Brighton, CO 80601-4006
(303)498-1700
FAX: (303)498-1788

Spectrum Medical Imaging
1610 Prairie Center Pkwy, Ste 2100
Brighton, CO 80601-4001
(303)558-1755
FAX: (720)523-0176

Brush

East Morgan County Hospital
2400 Edison St
Brush, CO 80723-1640
(970)842-6288
FAX: (970)842-6294

Burlington

Kit Carson County Memorial Hospital
286 16th St
Burlington, CO 80807-1697
(719)346-4752
FAX: (719)346-4755

Canon City

St. Thomas More Hospital
1338 Phay Ave
Canon City, CO 81212-2399
(719)285-2255
FAX: (719)285-2316

Castle Rock

Castle Rock Adventist Hospital
2350 Meadows Blvd
Castle Rock, CO 80109-8405
(720)455-2506
FAX: (720)455-0601

Centennial

Colorado Breast Care At Cmp
14200 E Arapahoe Rd
Centennial, CO 80112-4065
(303)269-3241
FAX: (303)269-3242

Kaiser Permanente Arapahoe Medical Office
5555 E Arapahoe Rd
Centennial, CO 80122-2300
(303)338-3456
FAX: (303)850-2176

Cheyenne Wells

Keefe Memorial Hospital
602 N 6th St W, Radiology Department
Cheyenne Wells, CO 80810-5125
(719)767-5662
FAX: (719)767-8042

Colorado Springs

Kaiser Permanente Premier Medical Offices
3920 N Union Blvd Ste 130
Colorado Springs, CO 80907-4907
(303)338-3456
FAX: (303)360-1339

Optum Medical Group - Colorado - Briargate Facility
2405 Research Pkwy
Colorado Springs, CO 80920-1044
(719)667-4139
FAX: (719)473-8843

Optum Medical Group Colorado, Llc
1633 Medical Center Pt
Colorado Springs, CO 80907-5700
(719)463-5775
FAX: (719)473-8843

Penrad Imaging
3050 N Circle Dr
Colorado Springs, CO 80909-1175
(719)785-9000
FAX: (719)867-7900

Penrad Imaging At Broadmoor
1263 Lake Plaza Dr, Ste 100
Colorado Springs, CO 80906-3510
(719)785-9000
FAX: (719)867-7900

Penrad Imaging At Sisters Grove Pavilion
6011 E Woodmen Rd Ste 10
Colorado Springs, CO 80923-2603
(719)785-9000
FAX: (719)867-6900

The Center For Women's Imaging At Penrose Hospital
2312 N Nevada Ave Ste 220
Colorado Springs, CO 80907-5311
(719)776-8010
FAX: (719)776-2307

Uchealth Mlbbcc Briargate
8890 N Union Blvd Ste 100
Colorado Springs, CO 80920-2700
(719)365-2900
FAX: (719)365-2510

Uchealth Mlbbcc Ppmp
175 S Union Blvd Ste 340
Colorado Springs, CO 80910-3143
(719)365-2900
FAX: (719)365-5529

Women's Center At Colorado Springs Imaging
6005 Delmonico Dr Ste 170
Colorado Springs, CO 80919-2264
(719)260-6500
FAX: (719)260-7750

Cortez

Southwest Health System, Inc.
1311 N Mildred Rd
Cortez, CO 81321-2231
(970)564-2050
FAX: (970)564-2069

Craig

The Memorial Hospital
750 Hospital Loop
Craig, CO 81625-8750
(970)826-2231
FAX: (970)826-2239

Delta

Delta County Memorial Hospital
1501 E 3rd St
Delta, CO 81416-2815
(970)874-2214
FAX: (970)874-2407

Denver

Colorado Breast Care At Green Valley Ranch Imaging
4809 Argonne St, Ste 120
Denver, CO 80249-6835
(303)563-2770
FAX: (303)563-2771

Denver Health Medical Center - Mobile Mammography
777 Bannock St
Denver, CO 80204-4507
(303)602-4122
FAX: (303)602-4163

Denver Health Medical Center Department Of Mammography
660 Bannock St
Denver, CO 80204-4506
(303)602-4140
FAX: (303)602-4163

Health Images Breast Center At Diamond Hill
2490 W 26th Ave, Ste 50A
Denver, CO 80211-5346
(303)964-1444
FAX: (303)500-1485

Invision Sally Jobe At Psl
2055 N High St Ste 180
Denver, CO 80205-5552
(720)493-3700
FAX: (720)874-4410

Kaiser Permanente East Denver Medical Office
10400 E Alameda Ave
Denver, CO 80247-5199
(303)338-3456
FAX: (303)360-1339

Kaiser Permanente Franklin Med Office
2045 Franklin St
Denver, CO 80205-5494
(303)338-3456
FAX: (303)764-5222

Porter Breast Care
2525 S Downing St, Porter Breast Center
Denver, CO 80210-5817
(303)765-3705
FAX: (303)778-5268

Saint Joseph Hospital Breast Care Center
1825 N Marion St, Breast Care Center
Denver, CO 80218-1122
(303)318-3400
FAX: (303)318-3439

Saint Joseph Hospital Mobile Mammo Unit-Mobile
1825 N Marion St
Denver, CO 80218-1122
(303)318-1326
FAX: (303)318-3433

Solis Mammography Of Central Park, Llc
10405 Martin Luther King Blvd, Ste 130
Denver, CO 80238-2399
(303)329-7511
FAX: (303)320-2565

Solis Mammography, A Dept. Of Rose Medical Center
4700 Hale Pkwy Ste 450
Denver, CO 80220-4052
(303)329-7511
FAX: (303)320-2565

The Women's Imaging Center
3773 E Cherry Creek North Dr Ste 101
Denver, CO 80209-3821
(303)321-2273
FAX: (303)321-3641

Uchealth Imaging Services, Llc
100 Cook St, Ste 212
Denver, CO 80206-5328
(720)516-9211
FAX: (720)516-9211

Durango

Mercy Regional Medical Center
1010 Three Springs Blvd, Breast Care Center
Durango, CO 81301-8296
(970)764-2525
FAX: (970)764-2520

Edwards

Vail Health The Sonnenalp Breast Center
322 Beard Creek Rd
Edwards, CO 81632-6433
(970)569-7690
FAX: (970)470-1141

Erie

Boulder Community Health - Erie Medical Center
101 Erie Pkwy
Erie, CO 80516-4070
(303)415-5170
FAX: (303)440-2168

Estes Park

Estes Park Health
555 Prospect Ave
Estes Park, CO 80517-6312
(970)577-4545
FAX: (970)577-4338

Fort Carson

Evans U.S. Army Community Hospital
1650 Cochrane Cir
Fort Carson, CO 80913-4604
(719)526-7301
FAX: (719)526-7978

Fort Collins

Banner Fort Collins Medical Center
4700 Lady Moon Dr
Fort Collins, CO 80528-4426
(970)810-6070
FAX: (970)821-4079

Fort Collins Mammography Center
3519 Richmond Dr, Ste A
Fort Collins, CO 80526-5993
(970)495-6255
FAX: (970)495-6254

Miramont Family Medicine
4674 Snow Mesa Dr Ste 140
Fort Collins, CO 80528-8614
(970)225-5023
FAX: (970)482-9646

Poudre Valley Hospital - Breast Diagnostic Center
2127 E Harmony Rd Ste 100
Fort Collins, CO 80528-3406
(970)207-4700
FAX: (970)207-4755

The Women's Clinic Of Northern Colorado
1107 S Lemay Ave Ste 300
Fort Collins, CO 80524-3955
(970)493-7442
FAX: (970)493-2990

Fort Morgan

Colorado Plains Medical Center
1000 Lincoln St
Fort Morgan, CO 80701-3290
(970)542-3351
FAX: (970)542-3368

Frisco

St Anthony's Summit Medical Center
340 Peak One Dr.
Frisco, CO 80443
(970)668-9595
FAX: (970)668-4789

Vail Health The Shaw Breast Center
323 W Main St, Ste 101
Frisco, CO 80443-5966
(970)569-7690
FAX: (970)470-6681

Fruita

Colorado Canyons Hospital And Medical Center
300 W Ottley Ave
Fruita, CO 81521-2118
(970)858-2503
FAX: (970)858-2200

Glenwood Springs

Valley View Hospital
1906 Blake Ave
Glenwood Springs, CO 81601-4259
(970)384-7640
FAX: (970)384-8165

Golden

Invision Sally Jobe Golden Lakewood
400 Indiana St, Ste 130
Golden, CO 80401-5043
(720)493-3687
FAX: (720)874-4410

Granby

Middle Park Health - Granby
1000 Granby Park Dr S
Granby, CO 80446
(970)887-5886
FAX: (970)887-5804

Grand Junction

Community Hospital
2373 G Rd Ste 140
Grand Junction, CO 81505-1003
(970)644-3157
FAX: (970)644-4379

Grand Junction Diagnostics
3150 N 12th St
Grand Junction, CO 81506-2863
(970)241-6014
FAX: (970)242-0497

Pavilion Imaging St Marys Hospital
750 Wellington Ave
Grand Junction, CO 81501-6132
(970)298-6900
FAX: (970)298-7900

Greeley

Banner Imaging Services Colorado
2001 70th Ave Ste 102, Summit View Medical Commons
Greeley, CO 80634-4628
(970)810-6070
FAX: (970)810-2621

Uchealth Breast Diagnostic Center- Greeley
6767 29th St
Greeley, CO 80634-5474
(970)207-4700
FAX: (970)207-4705

Greenwood Village

Invision Sally Jobe At The Centrum Dtc
8200 E Belleview Ave Ste 200E
Greenwood Village, CO 80111-2857
(720)493-3700
FAX: (720)874-4410

Gunnison

Gunnison Valley Hospital
711 N Taylor St
Gunnison, CO 81230-2296
(970)648-7126
FAX: (970)641-7299

Highlands Ranch

The Womens Imaging Center At Highlands Ranch
1265 Sgt Jon Stiles Dr, Unit H
Highlands Ranch, CO 80129-2266
(303)321-2273
FAX: (303)321-3641

Uchealth Imaging Services Llc
1500 Park Central Dr, Uchealth Highlands Ranch Hospital
Highlands Ranch, CO 80129-6688
(720)516-1002
FAX: (720)516-0230

Holyoke

Melissa Memorial Hospital
1001 E Johnson St
Holyoke, CO 80734-1854
(970)854-2241
FAX: (970)854-4370

Hugo

Lincoln Community Hospital
PO Box 248, 111 6th St
Hugo, CO 80821-0248
(719)743-2421
FAX: (719)743-2167

La Junta

Arkansas Valley Regional Medical Center
1100 Carson Ave
La Junta, CO 81050-2799
(719)383-6169
FAX: (719)383-6493

Lafayette

Boulder Community Health - Community Medical Center
1000 W South Boulder Rd
Lafayette, CO 80026-2752
(303)415-5170
FAX: (303)440-2168

Kaiser Permanente Rock Creek Medical Offices
280 Exempla Cir
Lafayette, CO 80026-3370
(303)338-3456
FAX: (303)764-4823

Scl Health Good Samaritan Medical Center
200 Exempla Cir
Lafayette, CO 80026-3370
(303)689-4180
FAX: (303)689-4187

Lakewood

Kaiser Permanente Lakewood Medical Office
8383 W Alameda Ave
Lakewood, CO 80226-3007
(303)338-3456
FAX: (303)239-7553

St Anthony Breast Center
11700 W 2nd Pl, Ste 210
Lakewood, CO 80228-1716
(720)321-0400
FAX: (720)321-8231

The Women's Imaging Center-Lakewood
215 Union Blvd Ste 100
Lakewood, CO 80228-1840
(303)321-2273
FAX: (303)321-3641

Lamar

Prowers Medical Center
401 Kendall Dr
Lamar, CO 81052-3993
(719)336-7042
FAX: (719)336-6794

Littleton

Centura Health Littleton Adventist Hospital
7700 S Broadway
Littleton, CO 80122-2602
(303)738-2767
FAX: (303)738-2600

Invision Sally Jobe At Littleton
8200 Southpark Ter
Littleton, CO 80120-5614
(720)493-3700
FAX: (720)874-4410

Invision Sally Jobe At Southwest Healthpark
6169 S Balsam Way Ste 170
Littleton, CO 80123-3086
(720)493-3700
FAX: (720)874-4410

Kaiser Permanente South West Medical Office
5257 S Wadsworth Blvd
Littleton, CO 80123-2228
(303)338-3456
FAX: (303)972-5404

The Breast Care Center-West Littleton Adventist Hospital
9670 W Coal Mine Ave
Littleton, CO 80123-4004
(303)738-2767
FAX: (303)738-2763

Lone Tree

Invision Sally Jobe At Sky Ridge
10107 Ridgegate Pkwy, Ste 110
Lone Tree, CO 80124-5638
(720)493-3700
FAX: (720)874-4410

Kaiser Permanente Lone Tree Medical Office
10240 Park Meadows Dr
Lone Tree, CO 80124-5425
(303)338-3456
FAX: (303)764-4823

University Of Colorado Hospital Lone Tree Breast Center
9544 Park Meadows Drive, Suite 100
Lone Tree, CO 80134
(720)553-1200
FAX: (720)553-1201

Longmont

Kaiser Permanente Longmont Medical Offices
2345 Bent Way
Longmont, CO 80503-7614
(303)338-3456
FAX: (303)239-7313

Poudrevalley Medical Group Llc Dba Colo Health Medical Group
1925 Mountain View Ave
Longmont, CO 80501-3128
(303)684-7888
FAX: (303)684-7889

Women's Imaging Center Longmont United Hospital Centura
1380 Tulip St Ste B
Longmont, CO 80501-3157
(303)651-5161
FAX: (303)651-5173

Louisville

Centura Health Avista Adventist Hospital
100 Health Park Dr
Louisville, CO 80027-9583
(303)673-1233
FAX: (303)673-1113

Loveland

Banner Imaging Services Colorado
1900 Boise Ave Ste 110
Loveland, CO 80538-5004
(970)820-6191
FAX: (970)820-6745

Breast Diagnostic Ctr. At Medical Center Of The Rockies
2500 Rocky Mountain Ave
Loveland, CO 80538-9004
(970)207-4700
FAX: (970)207-4755

Kaiser Permanente Loveland Medical Office
4901 Thompson Pkwy
Loveland, CO 80534-6426
(303)338-3456
FAX: (970)613-2395

The Women's Clinic Of Northern Colorado
2500 Rocky Mountain Ave Ste 150, N Medical Office Bldg
Loveland, CO 80538-9004
(970)493-7442
FAX: (970)493-2990

Meeker

Eastern Rio Blanco Cty Hlth Svc Dist Dba Pioneers Med Ctr
100 Pioneers Medical Center Dr
Meeker, CO 81641-3181
(970)878-9269
FAX: (970)878-3754

Montrose

Montrose Memorial Hospital
800 S 3rd St
Montrose, CO 81401-4212
(970)252-2540
FAX: (970)252-2541

Monument

Penrad Imaging At Tri-Lakes Pavilion
17230 Jackson Creek Pkwy Ste 160
Monument, CO 80132-7302
(719)785-9000
FAX: (719)867-7900

Pagosa Springs

Pagosa Springs Medical Center
95 S Pagosa Blvd
Pagosa Springs, CO 81147-8329
(970)507-3755
FAX: (970)731-0504

Parker

Breast Care Center At Parker Adventist Hospital
9399 Crown Crest Blvd, Ste 100
Parker, CO 80138-8507
(303)269-4150
FAX: (303)269-4151

Invision Sally Jobe Parker
12219 Pine Bluffs Way, Ste 111
Parker, CO 80134-4486
(720)493-3700
FAX: (720)874-4410

Miramont Family Medicine
9251 Twenty Mile Rd
Parker, CO 80134-4980
(303)805-5528
FAX: (678)905-0947

Smi Imaging, Llc
11960 Lioness Way, Ste 140
Parker, CO 80134-5643
(303)643-0200
FAX: (303)643-0201

Peterson Afb

Peterson Afb 21 Mdg Mdss/Sgsar
559 Vincent St
Peterson Afb, CO 80914-1541
(719)556-1121
FAX: (719)556-1122

Pueblo

Park West Imaging
3676 Parker Blvd Ste 165
Pueblo, CO 81008-2212
(719)595-7600
FAX: (719)595-7661

Parkview Medical Center
400 W 16th St
Pueblo, CO 81003-2781
(719)584-1300
FAX: (719)584-4016

St.Mary Corwin Medical Center Breast Center Of Excellence
1008 Minnequa Ave, Breast Screening And Diagnostic Center
Pueblo, CO 81004-3733
(719)557-4000
FAX: (719)557-4095

Rangely

Rangely District Hospital
225 Eagle Crest Dr
Rangely, CO 81648-2104
(970)675-5011
FAX: (970)675-2163

Rifle

Grand River Hospital District
501 Airport Rd
Rifle, CO 81650-8510
(970)625-6442
FAX: (970)625-6443

Salida

Heart Of The Rockies Regional Medical Center
PO Box 429
Salida, CO 81201-0429
(719)530-2241
FAX: (719)530-2203

Steamboat Springs

Uchealth Gloria Gossard Breast Care Center
1100 Central Park Dr, Ste 1100
Steamboat Springs, CO 80487-8818
(970)871-2399
FAX: (970)871-2570

Sterling

Sterling Regional Medcenter
615 Fairhurst St
Sterling, CO 80751-4523
(970)521-3147
FAX: (970)521-5383

Thornton

North Suburban Medical Center
9195 Grant St Ste 304
Thornton, CO 80229-4386
(303)450-3344
FAX: (303)453-2271

Trinidad

Mt. San Rafael Hospital
410 Benedicta Ave
Trinidad, CO 81082-2093
(719)846-8081
FAX: (719)846-8082

Usaf Academy

USAF Academy Mammography Department
4102 Pinion Dr, 10MDG/MSGS/SGCR
Usaf Academy, CO 80840-2502
(719)333-5171
FAX: (719)333-0507

Walsenburg

Spanish Peaks Regional Health Center
23500 US Highway 160
Walsenburg, CO 81089-9524
(719)738-5152
FAX: (719)738-4504

Westminster

Kaiser Permanente Westminster Medical Office
11245 Huron St
Westminster, CO 80234-2866
(303)338-3456
FAX: (303)457-6587

St Anthony North Health Campus
14300 Orchard Pkwy
Westminster, CO 80023-9206
(303)426-2400
FAX: (720)627-3297

The Women's Imaging Center - North Office
9035 Wadsworth Pkwy, Ste 2800
Westminster, CO 80021-8683
(303)321-2273
FAX: (303)321-3641

Wheat Ridge

Kaiser Permanente Wheat Ridge Med Office
4803 Ward Rd
Wheat Ridge, CO 80033-1902
(303)338-3456
FAX: (303)467-5178

Lutheran Breast Care Ctr - Diagnostic Suite
3655 Lutheran Pkwy, Ste 108
Wheat Ridge, CO 80033-6009
(303)425-2285
FAX: (303)403-3007

Touchstone Imaging Wheat Ridge
7615 W 38th Ave, Unit B107
Wheat Ridge, CO 80033-6138
(720)683-3005
FAX: (303)632-2730

Woodland Park

Uchealth Pikes Peak Regional Hospital
16420 West Hwy 24
Woodland Park, CO 80863
(719)374-6095
FAX: (719)686-5882

Wray

Wray Community District Hospital
1017 W 7th St
Wray, CO 80758-1420
(970)332-2233
FAX: (970)332-2312

Yuma

Yuma District Hospital
1000 W 8th Ave
Yuma, CO 80759-2641
(970)848-4642
FAX: (970)848-3144

CONNECTICUT

Avon

Connecticut Imaging Partners
100 Simsbury Rd Ste 101
Avon, CT 06001-3793
(860)289-3375
FAX: (860)783-5750

J Gershon Breast Imaging
21 Arch Rd
Avon, CT 06001-4202
(860)673-8379
FAX: (860)271-8025

Radiology Associates Of Hartford, P. C. - Avon, Ct
35 Nod Rd, Ste 101
Avon, CT 06001-3826
(860)409-1952
FAX: (860)409-1942

Womens Health Connecticut-Avon
20 W Avon Rd, Ste 205
Avon, CT 06001-3677
(860)561-7222
FAX: (860)561-7228

Bloomfield

Connecticut Imaging Partners
6 Northwestern Dr
Bloomfield, CT 06002-3463
(860)289-3375
FAX: (860)783-5750

Radiology Associates Of Hartford P.C
673 Cottage Grove Rd
Bloomfield, CT 06002-3033
(860)969-6400
FAX: (860)969-6392

Branford

Radiology Group, P.C.
6 Business Park Dr, Ste 103
Branford, CT 06405-2988
(203)481-5397
FAX: (203)483-8322

Bridgeport

Bridgeport Hospital
267 Grant St
Bridgeport, CT 06610-2870
(203)384-3177
FAX: (203)384-3224

Bridgeport Hospital Outpatient Radiology
4699 Main St, Ste 108
Bridgeport, CT 06606-1830
(203)447-5581
FAX: (203)378-4788

St. Vincent's Medical Center
2800 Main St
Bridgeport, CT 06606-4292
(475)210-7042
FAX: (475)210-6592

Women's Health Connecticut Obstetrics And Gynecology
3180 Main St, Suite 202 And 204
Bridgeport, CT 06606-4237
(203)374-0404
FAX: (203)372-4167

Bristol

Bristol Radiology Center
25 Collins Rd
Bristol, CT 06010-3867
(860)589-2642
FAX: (860)584-9998

Womens Health Resource At Bristol Hospital
41 Brewster Rd
Bristol, CT 06010-5161
(860)585-3020
FAX: (860)585-3665

Cheshire

Cheshire Imaging Center
280 S Main St
Cheshire, CT 06410-3112
(203)250-4030
FAX: (203)272-3995

Colchester

Colchester Backus Health Center
163 Broadway St
Colchester, CT 06415-1022
(860)823-6304
FAX: (860)537-8957

Danbury

Danbury Radiological Assoc Dba Connecticut Women's Imaging
103 Newtown Rd Ste 1B
Danbury, CT 06810-4195
(203)743-5356
FAX: (203)791-8693

Danbury Radiological Assoc Dba Connecticut Women's Imaging
90 Locust Ave Ste 1B
Danbury, CT 06810-6034
(203)792-5005
FAX: (203)792-0273

Danbury Radiological Assoc. Dba Connecticut Women's Imaging
2 Riverview Dr
Danbury, CT 06810-6268
(203)791-9011
FAX: (203)426-6411

Northeast Radiology
67 Sand Pit Rd, Ste 101
Danbury, CT 06810-4032
(203)797-1770
FAX: (203)797-2071

Western Ct Breast Imaging Center
20 Germantown Rd
Danbury, CT 06810-5023
(203)739-4999
FAX: (203)739-8811

Darien

Stamford Health Breast Imaging Center - Darien
6 Thorndal Cir
Darien, CT 06820-5415
(203)276-6134
FAX: (203)276-4007

Derby

The Hewitt Center For Breast Wellness At Griffin Hospital
350 Seymour Ave Ste 102
Derby, CT 06418-1336
(203)732-7101
FAX: (203)732-1559

Enfield

Baystate Radiology And Imaging, Inc.
113 Elm St Ste 206
Enfield, CT 06082-3738
(866)209-7271
FAX: (860)745-6995

Connecticut Imaging Partners Llc
100 Hazard Ave
Enfield, CT 06082-5446
(860)289-3375
FAX: (860)783-5750

Johnson Memorial Hospital, Inc
148 Hazard Ave, Johnson Surgery Center
Enfield, CT 06082-4520
(860)684-8555
FAX: (860)272-2910

North Central Imaging Llc
139 Hazard Ave, Ste 6
Enfield, CT 06082-4597
(860)749-0221
FAX: (860)749-1602

Radiology Associates Of Hartford P.C.
9 Cranbrook Blvd Ste 102
Enfield, CT 06082-3868
(860)714-9410
FAX: (860)714-9409

Fairfield

Advanced Radiology Consultants - Fairfield
1055 Post Rd
Fairfield, CT 06824-6019
(203)337-9729
FAX: (203)459-0116

Bridgeport Hospital Outpatient Radiology
425 Post Rd
Fairfield, CT 06824-6232
(203)673-0167
FAX: (203)378-4788

Farmington

Connecticut Imaging Partners-Farmington
399 Farmington Ave
Farmington, CT 06032-1936
(860)289-3375
FAX: (860)783-5750

Uconn Health - John Dempsey Hosp.
135 Dowling Way
Farmington, CT 06030-2803
(860)679-4798
FAX: (860)679-1352

Glastonbury

Connecticut Imaging Partners-Glastonbury
704 Hebron Ave Ste 100
Glastonbury, CT 06033-5020
(860)289-3375
FAX: (860)783-5750

Radiology Associates Of Hartford P.C.
31 Sycamore St Ste 101
Glastonbury, CT 06033-4540
(860)714-9710
FAX: (860)714-8185

Womens Health Connecticut-Glastonbury
330 Western Blvd, Ste 102
Glastonbury, CT 06033-4383
(860)291-1361
FAX: (860)561-7228

Granby

Connecticut Imaging Partners, Granby
18 E Granby Rd
Granby, CT 06035-2201
(860)289-3375
FAX: (860)783-5750

Greenwich

Greenwich Hospital Breast Center
77 Lafayette Pl
Greenwich, CT 06830-5426
(203)863-3031
FAX: (203)863-4603

Stamford Health Breast Imaging Center-Greenwich
75 Holly Hill Ln, Ste 200
Greenwich, CT 06830-2911
(203)276-8595
FAX: (203)276-4084

Westmed Medical Group
644 W Putnam Ave, Ste 4
Greenwich, CT 06830-2910
(914)682-6430
FAX: (914)719-5769

Groton

Pequot Health Center
52 Hazelnut Hill Rd
Groton, CT 06340-3268
(860)444-3778
FAX: (860)444-4785

Guilford

Guilford Radiology
1591 Boston Post Rd Ste 106
Guilford, CT 06437-4335
(203)453-5123
FAX: (203)458-0427

Yale New Haven Hospital - Shoreline Medical Center
111 Goose Ln
Guilford, CT 06437-5101
(203)688-1010
FAX: (203)688-9258

Hamden

Radiology Group, P.C.
2447 Whitney Ave, Ste 104
Hamden, CT 06518-3211
(203)288-7975
FAX: (203)288-1012

Hartford

Connecticut Imaging Partners, Hartford
85 Seymour St Ste 200
Hartford, CT 06106-5509
(860)289-3375
FAX: (860)783-5750

Hartford Hospital
PO Box 5037, 80 Seymour St
Hartford, CT 06102-5037
(860)972-2813
FAX: (860)696-3030

The Comprehensive Women's Health Center At Saint Francis
114 Woodland St
Hartford, CT 06105-1208
(860)714-9729
FAX: (860)714-8313

Madison

Madison Radiology, P.C.
2A Samson Rock Dr
Madison, CT 06443-3005
(203)245-7351
FAX: (203)245-8838

Manchester

Manchester Ob/Gyn Associates
388 W Center St
Manchester, CT 06040-4735
(860)291-1361
FAX: (860)649-7328

Prospect Manchester Memorial Hospital
71 Haynes St
Manchester, CT 06040-4188
(860)872-5150
FAX: (860)474-1700

Mansfield

Windham Hospital Center For Women's Health At Mansfield
7A Ledgebrook Dr
Mansfield, CT 06250-1664
(860)456-7237
FAX: (860)423-3225

Marlborough

Middlesex Hospital Marlborough Medical Center
12 Jones Hollow Rd, Middlesex Health Marlborough Medical Cen
Marlborough, CT 06447-1139
(860)358-2600
FAX: (860)358-2626

Meriden

Midstate Medical Center
435 Lewis Ave
Meriden, CT 06451-2101
(203)694-8405
FAX: (203)694-7652

Middletown

Middlesex Hospital Outpatient Center Radiology
534 Saybrook Rd, Middlesex Health- Out Patient Center
Middletown, CT 06457-4754
(860)358-2600
FAX: (860)358-2626

Milford

Diagnostic Imaging Of Milford
30 Commerce Park, Ste 1
Milford, CT 06460-3551
(203)878-2341
FAX: (203)878-3429

Mystic

Mystic Imaging
100 Perkins Farm Dr Ste 101
Mystic, CT 06355-4041
(860)572-2670
FAX: (860)245-0027

New Britain

Hospital Of Central Connecticut
100 Grand St, New Britain General Hospital/Dept Of Rad
New Britain, CT 06052-2016
(860)224-5244
FAX: (860)224-5907

Starling Radiology
300 Kensington Ave
New Britain, CT 06051-3916
(860)224-6222
FAX: (860)826-6986

New Haven

Yale New Haven Hospital Dept Of Diagnostic Imaging
35 Park St
New Haven, CT 06519-1110
(203)688-1010
FAX: (203)688-9258

Yale New Haven Radiology At Long Wharf
150 Sargent Dr
New Haven, CT 06511-6100
(203)688-1010
FAX: (203)688-9258

Yale-New Haven Hospital - Mobile
20 York St, Department Of Diagnostic Imaging
New Haven, CT 06510-3202
(203)200-1550
FAX: (203)200-5264

New London

Lawrence & Memorial Hospital
365 Montauk Ave
New London, CT 06320-4769
(860)444-3778
FAX: (860)444-4785

New Milford

New Milford Hospital
21 Elm St
New Milford, CT 06776-2993
(860)210-5555
FAX: (860)210-5252

North Haven

Breast Imaging North Haven Devine At Yale New Haven Hospital
6 Devine St, Mammography 1st Floor
North Haven, CT 06473-2195
(203)688-1010
FAX: (203)688-9258

Norwalk

Norwalk Radiology & Mammography Center
148 East Ave Ste 1M
Norwalk, CT 06851-5721
(203)838-4886
FAX: (203)855-4169

Norwalk Radiology Consultants
148 East Ave, Second Floor, Suite 2L
Norwalk, CT 06851-5700
(203)276-4311
FAX: (203)899-3160

Norwich

Backus Outpatient Care Center
111 Salem Tpke
Norwich, CT 06360-7403
(860)823-6304
FAX: (860)425-0847

William W. Backus Hospital
326 Washington St
Norwich, CT 06360-2714
(860)889-8331
FAX: (860)892-6965

Plainfield

Day Kimball Healthcare Plainfield Diagnostic Center
12 Lathrop Rd
Plainfield, CT 06374-2061
(860)963-6356
FAX: (860)963-6335

Plainfield Backus Emergency Care Center
582 Norwich Rd
Plainfield, CT 06374-1727
(860)823-6304
FAX: (860)892-6965

Plainville

Comprehensive Breast Health Center
201 N Mountain Rd
Plainville, CT 06062-1848
(860)827-4171
FAX: (860)832-8694

Prospect

Prospect Diagnostic Imaging
166 Waterbury Rd Ste 105
Prospect, CT 06712-1247
(203)758-7700
FAX: (203)758-7877

Putnam

Day Kimball Hospital
320 Pomfret St
Putnam, CT 06260-1869
(860)928-6541
FAX: (860)963-6335

Ridgefield

Western Connecticut Imaging
901 Ethan Allen Hwy Ste 104
Ridgefield, CT 06877-2838
(203)894-1444
FAX: (203)749-9149

Rockville

Prospect Rockville General Hospital
31 Union St
Rockville, CT 06066-3160
(860)872-5150
FAX: (860)872-5352

Sharon

Sharon Hospital
50 Hospital Hill Rd
Sharon, CT 06069-2092
(860)364-4070
FAX: (860)364-4224

South Windsor

Prospect Rockville Hosp Inc D/B/A Womens Center For Wellness
2600 Tamarack Ave Ste 100
South Windsor, CT 06074-5560
(860)533-4646
FAX: (860)533-2946

Southbury

Diagnostic Imaging Of Southbury
385 Main St S, Bldg 2
Southbury, CT 06488-4243
(203)267-5800
FAX: (203)267-5801

Women's Imaging Center / Dra Of Southbury
32 Poverty Rd Ste B
Southbury, CT 06488-2386
(203)262-6797
FAX: (203)262-6006

Southington

Hospital Of Central Connecticut Breast Imaging
55 Meriden Ave Ste 2E
Southington, CT 06489-3237
(860)276-5299
FAX: (860)276-5297

Physicians For Women's Health Dba Central Ct Ob/Gyn
1131 West St Ste 2
Southington, CT 06489-6006
(860)276-6800
FAX: (860)276-6801

Stamford

Advanced Radiology Consultants - Stamford
1259 E Main St
Stamford, CT 06902-3538
(203)337-9729
FAX: (203)459-0116

Greenwich Hospital Diagnostic Center
2015 W Main St, Fl 3
Stamford, CT 06902-4536
(203)863-2870
FAX: (203)863-2879

Obstetrics & Gynecology Associates
29 Hospital Plz, Ste 400
Stamford, CT 06902-3602
(203)325-4321
FAX: (203)975-7515

Stamford Health Breast Imaging Center - Tully
32 Strawberry Hill Ct, Ste 41052
Stamford, CT 06902-2777
(203)276-8595
FAX: (203)276-4084

Stratford

Advanced Radiology Consultants Stratford
2876 Main St
Stratford, CT 06614-4984
(203)337-9729
FAX: (203)459-0116

Bridgeport Hospital Outpatient Radiology
2909 Main St
Stratford, CT 06614-4960
(203)673-0167
FAX: (203)378-4788

Tolland

Tic, Llc
6 Fieldstone Cmns Ste E
Tolland, CT 06084-3419
(860)896-4848
FAX: (860)896-4849

Torrington

Charlotte Hungerford Hospital Hungerford Diagnostic Center
220 Kennedy Dr
Torrington, CT 06790-7204
(860)496-6860
FAX: (860)496-0834

Trumbull

Advanced Womens Imaging Center
15 Corporate Dr
Trumbull, CT 06611-1351
(203)337-9794
FAX: (203)459-0116

Bridgeport Hospital Outpatient Radiology
5520 Park Ave, Level 1 Suite 400
Trumbull, CT 06611-3463
(203)673-0153
FAX: (203)378-4788

Women's Choice Mammography
115 Technology Dr, Unit B301
Trumbull, CT 06611-6347
(203)445-0101
FAX: (203)445-0022

Vernon

Vernon Imaging
35 Talcottville Rd, Ste 4
Vernon, CT 06066-5261
(203)694-8405
FAX: (203)694-7756

Wallingford

Meriden Imaging Center/Dba Wallingford Imaging
863 N Main Street Ext
Wallingford, CT 06492-2434
(203)694-8405
FAX: (203)694-7652

Waterbury

Diagnostic Radiology Associates
134 Grandview Ave
Waterbury, CT 06708-2571
(203)756-8911
FAX: (203)574-3298

Naugatuck Valley Radiology Associates
1389 W Main St Ste 107
Waterbury, CT 06708-3115
(203)574-1311
FAX: (203)573-1062

Prospect Ct Medical Foundation
140 Grandview Ave Ste 202
Waterbury, CT 06708-2518
(203)755-2344
FAX: (203)573-8166

Pwh, Llc D/B/A Women's Health Breast Imaging Of Waterbury
134 Grandview Ave, Ste 201
Waterbury, CT 06708-2507
(203)754-2535
FAX: (203)591-9135

Saint Mary's Hospital
56 Franklin St
Waterbury, CT 06706-1281
(203)709-6020
FAX: (203)709-7788

Valley Imaging Partners,Llc
140 Grandview Ave, Ste 204
Waterbury, CT 06708-2518
(203)756-8911
FAX: (203)574-3298

Waterbury Hospital
64 Robbins St, Radiology Department
Waterbury, CT 06708-2600
(203)573-7124
FAX: (203)573-6731

Westwood Womens Health
60 Westwood Ave, Ste 250
Waterbury, CT 06708-2470
(203)574-5501
FAX: (877)436-2310

Waterford

L & M Diagnostic Imaging At Crossroads
196 Pky. South, Ste. 102
Waterford, CT 06385
(860)444-3778
FAX: (860)444-4785

West Hartford

Connecticut Imaging Partners-West Hartford
941 Farmington Ave
West Hartford, CT 06107-2203
(860)289-3375
FAX: (860)783-5750

Meriden Imaging Center, Inc Dba West Hartford Imaging
65 Memorial Rd Ste 510
West Hartford, CT 06107-4233
(860)236-6517
FAX: (860)233-4823

Womens Health Connecticut-West Hartford
345 N Main St, Ste 201
West Hartford, CT 06117-2508
(860)561-7222
FAX: (860)561-7228

West Haven

Diagnostic Imaging Of West Haven
687 Campbell Ave Ste 1
West Haven, CT 06516-3774
(203)934-4482
FAX: (203)934-8803

Westbrook

Middlesex Hospital, Shoreline Medical Center
250 Flat Rock Pl, Middlesex Health- Shoreline Medical Cent
Westbrook, CT 06498-3585
(860)358-2600
FAX: (860)358-2626

Westport

Avery Center Ob-Gyn
12 Avery Pl
Westport, CT 06880-3223
(203)227-5125
FAX: (203)222-7180

Wethersfield

Connecticut Imaging Partners
1260 Silas Deane Hwy, Ste 104
Wethersfield, CT 06109-4363
(860)289-3375
FAX: (860)783-5733

Willimantic

Windham Community Memorial Hospital
112 Mansfield Ave
Willimantic, CT 06226-2045
(860)456-9116
FAX: (860)456-6975

Wilton

Advanced Radiology-Wilton
30 Danbury Rd
Wilton, CT 06897-4457
(203)337-9729
FAX: (203)459-0116

Stamford Health Breast Imaging Center - Wilton
372 Danbury Rd, Ste 181
Wilton, CT 06897-2523
(203)276-8595
FAX: (203)276-4084

Winsted

Harford Healthcare Health Center At Winsted
80 S Main St, Ste 100
Winsted, CT 06098-4013
(860)738-6664
FAX: (860)738-6663

DELAWARE

Dover

Bayhealth Medical Center, Kent General Hospital
640 S State St
Dover, DE 19901-3530
(302)744-7400
FAX: (302)735-3210

Mid-Delaware Imaging
710 S Queen St
Dover, DE 19904-3567
(302)734-9888
FAX: (302)734-1024

Women's Imaging Center At Bayhealth, Kent Campus
540 S Governors Ave Ste 200
Dover, DE 19904-3530
(302)744-7400
FAX: (302)735-3210

Georgetown

Beebe Imaging Georgetown
21635 Biden Ave
Georgetown, DE 19947-4574
(302)645-3278
FAX: (302)856-6020

Lewes

Beebe Healthcare, Inc.
424 Savannah Rd
Lewes, DE 19958-1462
(302)645-3642
FAX: (302)645-3133

Middletown

Delaware Imaging Network
120 Sandhill Dr Ste 2
Middletown, DE 19709-5864
(302)999-9729
FAX: (302)357-3384

Middletown Diagnostic Center
209 E Main St
Middletown, DE 19709-1449
(302)378-1199
FAX: (302)376-1590

Milford

Bayhealth Hospital - Sussex Campus
100 Wellness Way
Milford, DE 19963-4364
(302)430-5707
FAX: (302)430-5050

Bayhealth Outpatient Center - Sussex
1020 Mattlind Way
Milford, DE 19963-5300
(302)430-5707
FAX: (302)430-5050

Millsboro

Beebe Imaging Millsboro
28538 Dupont Blvd Unit 2
Millsboro, DE 19966-4791
(302)645-3278
FAX: (302)645-3011

Millville

Beebe Imaging - Millville
32566 Docs Pl, Unit 10
Millville, DE 19967-6959
(302)539-8749
FAX: (302)541-8056

Milton

Ocean Medical Imaging Of Delaware Inc
611 Federal St Ste 4
Milton, DE 19968-1157
(302)684-5151
FAX: (302)684-1977

Newark

Christiana Care Breast Ctr - Helen F. Graham Cancer Ctr
4701 Ogletown Stanton Rd Ste 1400, West Entrance
Newark, DE 19713-7012
(302)623-4231
FAX: (302)623-4204

Christiana Care Imaging Svcs Springside Plaza
300 Biddle Ave, Suite 100 Connor Building
Newark, DE 19702-3969
(302)838-3001
FAX: (302)838-3004

Delaware Imaging Network
40 Polly Drummond Hill Rd
Newark, DE 19711-5703
(302)999-9729
FAX: (302)738-9176

Delaware Imaging Network
2600 Glasgow Ave, Ste 122
Newark, DE 19702-4777
(302)999-9729
FAX: (302)738-9176

Delaware Imaging Network
J-24 Omega Dr.
Newark, DE 19713
(302)738-9100
FAX: (302)738-9176

Rehoboth

Beebe Health Campus
18941 John J Williams Hwy
Rehoboth, DE 19971-4404
(302)645-3278
FAX: (302)645-3011

Seaford

Nanticoke Diagnostic At Mears Center
Tidalhealth Nanticoke
100 Rawlins Dr
Seaford, DE 19973-5881
(302)628-1507
FAX: (302)629-0286

Smyrna

Christiana Care Imaging Services Smyrna
100 S Main St Ste 100
Smyrna, DE 19977-1478
(302)562-6451
FAX: (302)838-3004

Smyrna Medical Center
401 Carter Road
Smyrna, DE 19977
(302)653-2010
FAX: (302)653-2697

Wilmington

Christiana Care Health Services - Wilmington Hospital
501 W 14th St, Wilmington Hosptial
Wilmington, DE 19801-1038
(302)320-4901
FAX: (302)320-4901

Christiana Care Imaging Svcs. Foulkstone Plaza- North
1401 Foulk Rd Ste 100C
Wilmington, DE 19803-2764
(302)838-3001
FAX: (302)838-3004

Delaware Diagnostic Imaging, Pa
2055 Limestone Rd Ste 104
Wilmington, DE 19808-5536
(302)633-6200
FAX: (302)575-9322

Delaware Imaging Network
3105 Limestone Rd, Ste 106
Wilmington, DE 19808-2147
(302)999-9729
FAX: (302)738-9176

Delaware Imaging Network
3206 Concord Pike
Wilmington, DE 19803-5015
(302)999-9729
FAX: (302)738-9176

N. Wilmington Women's Ctr/St. Francis Healthcare Svcs
2002 Foulk Rd Ste A
Wilmington, DE 19810-3643
(302)421-4141
FAX: (302)529-7955

St Francis-The Women's Center- Greenhill
532 Greenhill Ave
Wilmington, DE 19805-1851
(302)421-4141
FAX: (302)421-4974

St. Francis Hospital
701 N Clayton St
Wilmington, DE 19805-3155
(302)421-4141
FAX: (302)421-4974

Virginia B. Clemmer, M.D.- Clinical Breast Imaging
2401 Pennsylvania Ave Ste 115, The Devon
Wilmington, DE 19806-1432
(302)658-4800
FAX: (302)658-4844

DISTRICT OF COLUMBIA

Washington

Breast Care For Washington
4 Atlantic St SW
Washington, DC 20032-2350
(202)465-7164
FAX: (202)905-0159

Breast Care For Washington - Mobile Mammography
4 Atlantic St SW
Washington, DC 20032-2350
(202)745-7164
FAX: (202)905-0159

George Washington Hospital
2300 M St NW, Ste 910 8th Fl
Washington, DC 20037-1434
(202)741-3038
FAX: (202)741-3011

George Washington Imaging Center At 19th Street
1145 19th St NW, Ste 205
Washington, DC 20036-3719
(202)715-5679
FAX: (202)715-4007

Howard University Faculty Practice Plan
4414 Benning Rd NE, Ste 2400
Washington, DC 20019-4555
(202)865-2120
FAX: (202)617-2998

Howard University Hospital
2041 Georgia Ave NW
Washington, DC 20060-0002
(202)865-3610
FAX: (202)865-6636

Kaiser Permanente - Northwest
2301 M St NW
Washington, DC 20037-1427
(877)390-0033
FAX: (301)548-5849

Kaiser Permanente Capitol Hill
700 2nd St NE
Washington, DC 20002-8100
(877)390-0033
FAX: (301)548-5849

Medstar Georgetown University Hospital
3800 Reservoir Rd NW, Radiology Department
Washington, DC 20007-2196
(202)444-3315
FAX: (202)444-7081

Medstar Radiology Network At Foxhall
3301 New Mexico Ave NW, Ste 324
Washington, DC 20016-3613
(202)686-1316
FAX: (202)244-1391

Medstar Radiology Network At Lafayette
1133 21st St NW, Ste 800
Washington, DC 20036-3371
(202)748-8840
FAX: (202)650-8830

Not For Profit Hospital Corp. Dba United Medical Center
1310 Southern Ave SE
Washington, DC 20032-4623
(202)574-7169
FAX: (202)274-7499

Providence Hospital
1150 Varnum St NE, 3rd Floor Wellness Suite
Washington, DC 20017-2104
(202)854-7560
FAX: (202)854-7951

The Sullivan Center For Breast Health
5255 Loughboro Rd NW
Washington, DC 20016-2633
(202)537-4545
FAX: (202)537-4505

Washington Hospital Center
110 Irving St NW Ste 1300, Center For Breast Health
Washington, DC 20010-3017
(202)877-9729
FAX: (202)877-9338

Washington Radiology Associates P.C.
2141 K St NW Ste 200
Washington, DC 20037-1876
(703)280-9800
FAX: (202)223-0021

FLORIDA

Altamonte Springs

Adventhealth Imaging Altamonte Springs
661 E Altamonte Dr Ste 130
Altamonte Springs, FL 32701-5102
(407)303-2273
FAX: (407)303-2259

Ohri, Llc Dba Orlando Health Imaging Centers
398 E Altamonte Dr
Altamonte Springs, FL 32701-4402
(407)331-9355
FAX: (407)331-9481

Simonmed Imaging Florida, Llc - Altamonte III
745 Orienta Ave, Ste 1161
Altamonte Springs, FL 32701-6609
(321)207-4474
FAX: (407)475-6801

Amelia Island

Ackerman Cancer Center
1340 S 18th St Ste 103, Medical Office Bldg A
Amelia Island, FL 32034-4733
(904)277-2700
FAX: (904)277-2220

Apopka

Adventhealth Apopka
2100 Ocoee Apopka Rd, Womens Center
Apopka, FL 32703-9210
(407)200-0538
FAX: (407)609-7287

Adventhealth Imaging Center Apopka
1480 W Orange Blossom Trl
Apopka, FL 32712-2637
(407)303-2273
FAX: (407)598-9266

Emery Medical Solutions, Inc.
840 E Semoran Blvd
Apopka, FL 32703-5517
(407)628-9100
FAX: (407)628-0748

Arcadia

Desoto Memorial Hospital
900 N Robert Ave, Ofc
Arcadia, FL 34266-8713
(863)494-8440
FAX: (863)993-7755

Manatee Diagnostic Center Arcadia
833 N Robert Ave
Arcadia, FL 34266-9578
(863)491-9970
FAX: (863)491-9971

Aventura

Alfa Diagnostic, Llc
21355 E Dixie Hwy, Ste 101
Aventura, FL 33180-1239
(305)705-4775
FAX: (786)955-2700

Aventura Breast Diagnostic Center
20950 NE 27th Ct Ste 101
Aventura, FL 33180-1232
(877)341-7017
FAX: (305)792-5829

Comprehensive Breast Care Center
20601 E Dixie Hwy Ste 310
Aventura, FL 33180-1542
(305)931-1344
FAX: (305)931-1346

Mt Sinai Aventura Womens Imaging Center
2845 Aventura Blvd Ste 145
Aventura, FL 33180-3120
(305)535-3434
FAX: (305)535-3380

Vilma B Biaggi MD Breast Diagnostics
21355 E Dixie Hwy Ste 117
Aventura, FL 33180-1244
(305)932-0282
FAX: (877)635-1453

Bayonet Point

Tower Radiology Center - Bayonet Point
7525 State Road 52
Bayonet Point, FL 34667-6716
(727)847-5122
FAX: (727)819-1549

Belle Glade

Lakeside Medical Ctr-Hlth Care District Palm Bch Co
39200 Hooker Hwy
Belle Glade, FL 33430-5368
(561)996-6571
FAX: (561)996-2423

Boca Raton

Akumin- Boca Raton
1590 NW 10th Ave Ste 202
Boca Raton, FL 33486-1323
(561)368-7956
FAX: (561)447-9373

Boca Raton Mammography
880 NW 13th St, Ste 2C
Boca Raton, FL 33486-2342
(561)300-0220
FAX: (561)334-2147

Care Diagnostics Llc
8903 Glades Rd, Ste H1
Boca Raton, FL 33434-4023
(561)361-7872
FAX: (561)361-7873

Center For Breast Care - Boca Clinic
1601 Clint Moore Rd, Ste 140
Boca Raton, FL 33487-5714
(561)955-4700
FAX: (561)955-4444

Center For Breast Care - Boca Raton Regional Hospital
690 Meadows Rd
Boca Raton, FL 33486-2344
(561)955-4700
FAX: (561)955-2107

Diagnostic Centers Of America
23071 State Road 7
Boca Raton, FL 33428-5433
(561)496-6935
FAX: (561)496-6936

Diagnostic Centers Of America
8142 Glades Rd
Boca Raton, FL 33434-4064
(561)314-2500
FAX: (561)314-2501

Mammovan At Boca Raton Regional Hosp. - Mobile
690 Meadows Rd
Boca Raton, FL 33486-2344
(561)955-4700
FAX: (561)955-4444

Rm Imaging, Inc.
2499 Glades Rd, Ste 206
Boca Raton, FL 33431-7201
(561)361-8090
FAX: (561)361-8033

University Mri & Diagnostic Imaging Centers
3848 Fau Blvd Ste 200
Boca Raton, FL 33431-6437
(561)362-9191
FAX: (561)394-5674

West Boca Diagnostic Imaging Center
7070 W Palmetto Park Rd
Boca Raton, FL 33433-3411
(561)417-7920
FAX: (561)417-7425

Bonifay

Doctors Memorial Hospital
2600 Hospital Dr
Bonifay, FL 32425-4264
(850)547-8166
FAX: (850)547-8175

Bonita Springs

Bonita Community Health Center
3501 Health Center Blvd
Bonita Springs, FL 34135-8127
(239)949-6112
FAX: (239)949-6125

Nch Healthcare Bonita
24040 S Tamiami Trl
Bonita Springs, FL 34134-7040
(239)624-6630
FAX: (239)513-2316

Radiology Regional Center
9776 Bonita Beach Rd SE, Ste 101A
Bonita Springs, FL 34135-4773
(239)936-2316
FAX: (239)936-0611

Boynton Beach

Bethesda Women's Health Center
10301 Hagen Ranch Rd, Ste A920
Boynton Beach, FL 33437-3732
(561)374-5300
FAX: (561)374-5310

Diagnostic Centers Of America
1425 Gateway Blvd Ste 100
Boynton Beach, FL 33426-8313
(561)900-9600
FAX: (561)900-9660

Diagnostic Centers Of America
6080 Boynton Beach Blvd Ste 140
Boynton Beach, FL 33437-3586
(561)736-3227
FAX: (561)424-0888

Bradenton

Blake Medical Center - Center For Breast Health
2020 59th St W
Bradenton, FL 34209-4604
(866)463-7004
FAX: (941)761-0260

Bowes Imaging Center
6207 Cortez Rd W
Bradenton, FL 34210-2602
(941)782-0490
FAX: (941)782-0496

Intercoastal Medical Group Lwr Radiology
11505 Rangeland Pkwy
Bradenton, FL 34211-4041
(941)365-1102
FAX: (941)362-8634

Lakewood Ranch Breast Health Center
8340 Lakewood Ranch Blvd, Ste 160
Bradenton, FL 34202-5184
(941)782-2264
FAX: (941)782-2556

Manatee Diagnostic Center
300 Riverside Dr E Ste 3000
Bradenton, FL 34208-1024
(941)747-3034
FAX: (941)748-5819

Manatee Gynecology
2310 60th Street Ct W
Bradenton, FL 34209-6609
(941)792-4993
FAX: (941)795-2905

Mdc Pointe West Women's Center And Mri
2301 60th Street Ct W Ste C
Bradenton, FL 34209-5512
(941)747-3034
FAX: (941)748-5819

Obgyn Women's Centre Of Lakewood Ranch
8340 Lakewood Ranch Blvd, Ste 240
Bradenton, FL 34202-5185
(941)254-2717
FAX: (941)907-3036

Partners Imaging Center Of Bradenton
5101 4th Avenue Cir E
Bradenton, FL 34208-5630
(941)782-0414
FAX: (941)782-0418

Sarasota Memorial Hlth Care Ctr At Heritage Harbour
1040 River Heritage Blvd
Bradenton, FL 34212-6348
(941)917-7069
FAX: (941)917-4366

Women's Health Services Of Bradenton Dba In A Woman's Image
5323 4th Avenue Cir E
Bradenton, FL 34208-5623
(941)567-2090
FAX: (941)567-2091

Brandon

Brandon Regional Hospital
119 Oakfield Dr
Brandon, FL 33511-5779
(813)681-0555
FAX: (813)916-2942

Mri Associates Of Brandon Llc D/B/A Brandon Mri
403 S Kings Ave
Brandon, FL 33511-5905
(813)210-8995
FAX: (813)409-2914

Mri Associates Of Winter Haven Dba Winter Haven Mri
PO Box 2570
Brandon, FL 33509-2570
(863)294-0999
FAX: (863)294-5025

Simonmed Imaging Florida, Llc - Brandon
613 Oakfield Dr
Brandon, FL 33511-5714
(813)703-8027
FAX: (407)865-6091

Tower Radiology Center Bloomingdale
3350 Bell Shoals Rd
Brandon, FL 33511-7637
(813)654-4883
FAX: (813)676-0346

Tower Radiology Center Parsons
427 S Parsons Ave Ste 100
Brandon, FL 33511-5252
(813)874-3177
FAX: (813)315-2091

Tower Radiology Robertson
414 W Robertson St
Brandon, FL 33511-5007
(813)657-6767
FAX: (813)654-7014

Womens Care Florida
515 S Kings Ave
Brandon, FL 33511-6060
(813)378-8575
FAX: (813)564-0518

Brooksville

Advanced Imaging Concepts Pl
13470 Taft St
Brooksville, FL 34613-6820
(352)597-0016
FAX: (352)597-0089

Bayfront Health Brooksville
17240 Cortez Blvd
Brooksville, FL 34601-8921
(352)796-5111
FAX: (352)544-6149

Oak Hill Hospital
11375 Cortez Blvd
Brooksville, FL 34613-5409
(352)606-7028
FAX: (352)597-6052

Summit Imaging
12037 Cortez Blvd
Brooksville, FL 34613-7349
(352)597-8880
FAX: (352)597-1008

Cape Coral

Lee Health Breast Health Center At Surfside
2441 Surfside Blvd
Cape Coral, FL 33914-3861
(239)424-1499
FAX: (239)343-9428

Millennium Physician Group
1528 Del Prado Blvd S
Cape Coral, FL 33990-3798
(855)674-4624
FAX: (941)249-4170

Premier Womens Care
1265 Viscaya Pkwy
Cape Coral, FL 33990-3237
(239)574-2229
FAX: (877)219-1575

Radiology Regional Center
805 Del Prado Blvd S
Cape Coral, FL 33990-2666
(239)936-4068
FAX: (239)936-0611

Radiology Regional Center
1708 Cape Coral Pkwy W, Suites 3 & 13
Cape Coral, FL 33914-6985
(239)936-2316
FAX: (239)425-4796

Radiology Regional Center
428 Del Prado Blvd N Ste 106B
Cape Coral, FL 33909-2218
(239)936-2316
FAX: (239)425-4796

Celebration

Adventhealth Imaging Celebration
380 Celebration Pl
Celebration, FL 34747-4606
(407)303-4111
FAX: (407)303-4309

Chipley

Northwest Florida Community Hospital
1360 Brickyard Rd
Chipley, FL 32428-6303
(850)415-8111
FAX: (850)415-8108

Clearwater

Akumin-Clearwater
501 S Lincoln Ave
Clearwater, FL 33756-5945
(727)771-2795
FAX: (727)683-9507

Diagnostic Clinic Medical
3131 N McMullen Booth Rd
Clearwater, FL 33761-2008
(727)726-8871
FAX: (727)669-3241

Susan Cheek Needler Breast Center
400 Pinellas St Ste 100
Clearwater, FL 33756-3312
(727)298-6673
FAX: (727)462-7742

Clermont

Clermont Radiology
871 Oakley Seaver Dr
Clermont, FL 34711-1968
(352)241-6100
FAX: (352)241-6101

Clermont Radiology - Kings Ridge
3725 S Highway 27, Ste 104
Clermont, FL 34711-7600
(352)241-6100
FAX: (352)241-6101

Simonmed Imaging Florida Llc - Clermont
265 Citrus Tower Blvd, Ste 100
Clermont, FL 34711-1908
(352)241-7440
FAX: (407)865-6080

South Lake Hospital - Centre For Women's Health
1900 Don Wickham Dr
Clermont, FL 34711-1979
(352)394-4071
FAX: (352)241-7245

Clewiston

Hendry Regional Medical Center
524 W Sagamore Ave
Clewiston, FL 33440-3514
(863)902-3061
FAX: (863)983-1696

Cocoa

North Brevard County Hospital District Dba Parrish Medical C
5005 Port St John Pkwy
Cocoa, FL 32927-4305
(321)268-6150
FAX: (321)268-6681

Cocoa Beach

Cape Canaveral Hospital Breast Center
699 W Cocoa Beach Cswy, Ste 602
Cocoa Beach, FL 32931-3562
(321)868-7217
FAX: (321)868-7239

Coconut Creek

Ultracare Imaging Serv Inc.
4310 W Hillsboro Blvd
Coconut Creek, FL 33073-3214
(954)428-4833
FAX: (954)481-2019

Cooper City

Pom Mri & Imaging Center Of Cooper City
11011 Sheridan St Ste 101
Cooper City, FL 33026-1501
(954)239-7466
FAX: (954)239-7489

Coral Gables

Ambulatory Diagnostic Center
747 Ponce De Leon Blvd, 1st Fl
Coral Gables, FL 33134-2049
(305)446-7893
FAX: (305)442-1183

Baptist Medical Plaza At Coral Gables
10 Giralda Ave Ste 120
Coral Gables, FL 33134-5303
(786)467-5052
FAX: (786)467-5051

Coral Gables Hospital
3100 S Douglas Rd
Coral Gables, FL 33134-6923
(305)441-6810
FAX: (305)529-6797

De La Pedraja Radiology Associates, Inc
4776 SW 8th St
Coral Gables, FL 33134-2564
(305)447-1415
FAX: (305)446-2435

Solis Mammography Of Miami, Llc.
1545 San Remo Ave
Coral Gables, FL 33146-3008
(305)403-4930
FAX: (305)403-4940

University Of Miami Hospital & Clinics-Lennar
5555 Ponce De Leon Blvd, Ste 455B
Coral Gables, FL 33146-2513
(305)689-0431
FAX: (305)689-0790

Coral Springs

Akumin - Coral Springs Women's Center
2232A N University Dr
Coral Springs, FL 33071-6184
(954)753-3800
FAX: (954)753-1645

Akumin Royal Palm
8110 Royal Palm Blvd Ste 100
Coral Springs, FL 33065-5742
(954)341-4200
FAX: (954)341-5360

Baptist Medical Plaza At Coral Springs
6264 W Sample Rd Ste 120
Coral Springs, FL 33067-3273
(954)837-1000
FAX: (954)837-1021

Broward Health Coral Springs Women's Center
2901 Coral Hills Dr, Ste 270
Coral Springs, FL 33065-4176
(954)759-7500
FAX: (954)346-5474

Cleveland Clinic Florida Coral Springs
5701 N University Dr
Coral Springs, FL 33067-1703
(954)689-5980
FAX: (954)689-5118

Comprehensive Breast Center Of Coral Springs
1311 N University Dr
Coral Springs, FL 33071-6622
(954)345-2718
FAX: (954)753-2683

Gentle Touch Breast Diagnostics, Inc
1505 N University Dr, Ste 100
Coral Springs, FL 33071-8975
(754)702-7267
FAX: (866)663-1071

Palms Mri Diagnostic Imaging Center Inc
3111 N University Dr, Ste 115
Coral Springs, FL 33065-5049
(954)688-7256
FAX: (954)688-7750

Crestview

North Okaloosa Medical Center
550 Redstone Ave W Ste 100, Mammography Department
Crestview, FL 32536-6429
(850)682-2475
FAX: (850)683-5198

Crystal River

Bayfront Health Seven Rivers
6201 N Suncoast Blvd
Crystal River, FL 34428-6712
(352)795-8365
FAX: (352)795-8369

Citrus Diagnostic Center
922 N Citrus Ave
Crystal River, FL 34428-3421
(352)795-9200
FAX: (352)795-6460

Cutler Bay

La Colonia Diagnostic Center
20407 Old Cutler Rd
Cutler Bay, FL 33189-1833
(786)438-2348
FAX: (305)602-4891

Davenport

Advance Technological Radiology, P.A.
2235 North Blvd W
Davenport, FL 33837-8990
(863)421-8674
FAX: (863)421-2615

Advent Health Heart Of Florida
40100 Highway 27
Davenport, FL 33837-5906
(863)419-2270
FAX: (863)419-2478

Adventhealth Breast Surgery At Davenport
40124 Highway 27, Ste 207
Davenport, FL 33837-5905
(863)421-7276
FAX: (863)421-7109

Daytona Beach

Twin Lakes Imaging Center
1890 Lpga Blvd Ste 110
Daytona Beach, FL 32117-7131
(386)274-6000
FAX: (386)274-7260

Deerfield Beach

Broward Health North
201 E Sample Rd, Radiology Department
Deerfield Beach, FL 33064-3502
(954)786-6450
FAX: (954)786-6487

Cntr For Breast Care Boca Raton Regional Hospital-Deerfield
3313 W Hillsboro Blvd
Deerfield Beach, FL 33442-9423
(954)420-0100
FAX: (954)420-0992

University Of Miami Hospital & Clinics - Deerfield
1192 E Newport Center Dr Ste 100
Deerfield Beach, FL 33442-7749
(954)571-0169
FAX: (954)698-3646

Deland

Adventhealth Imaging Womens Center Deland
151 Victoria Commons Blvd Ste 101
Deland, FL 32724-7722
(386)943-4610
FAX: (386)734-4781

Delray Beach

Diagnostic Centers Of America
15340 S Jog Rd Ste 160
Delray Beach, FL 33446-2170
(561)496-6935
FAX: (561)496-6936

Dmc Imaging At Palm Court
5130 Linton Blvd, Ste I1
Delray Beach, FL 33484-6597
(561)637-5400
FAX: (561)637-5343

Deltona

Adventhealth Imaging Deltona
1745 Sterling Silver Blvd, Ste 101
Deltona, FL 32725-4332
(386)917-5428
FAX: (386)917-7501

Akumin- Deltona
1555 Saxon Blvd Ste 401
Deltona, FL 32725-5845
(386)860-9336
FAX: (386)860-2225

Radiology Associates Imaging Deltona
3400 E Halifax Crossing Blvd Ste 170
Deltona, FL 32725-2914
(386)259-5959
FAX: (386)259-5999

Doral

Doral Medical Imaging
8181 NW 36th St Ste 3
Doral, FL 33166-6628
(305)471-4581
FAX: (305)471-4593

Idaca Llc
8353 NW 36th St, Ste B
Doral, FL 33166-6615
(305)557-0330
FAX: (786)534-8420

Life Radiology, Llc
3470 NW 82nd Ave Ste 119, One Park Square
Doral, FL 33122-1026
(786)446-8541
FAX: (786)446-8542

Sanitas
2000 NW 87th Ave, Ste 102
Doral, FL 33172-2656
(844)665-4827
FAX: (305)718-9191

Vital Imaging Diagnostic Centers Llc.
3155 NW 82nd Ave Ste 201
Doral, FL 33122-1056
(305)596-9992
FAX: (305)596-0942

Dunedin

Mease Dunedin Hospital
601 Main St
Dunedin, FL 34698-5848
(727)298-6045
FAX: (727)734-6462

Eglin Afb

Eglin Air Force Base - 96 Medical Group
307 Boatner Rd Ste 114, 96 Mdg/Sgcs/Sgcr
Eglin Afb, FL 32542-1302
(850)883-8335
FAX: (850)883-8290

Englewood

Radiology Associates Of Venice & Englewood
900 Pine St Ste 116
Englewood, FL 34223-4457
(941)475-5471
FAX: (941)475-4264

The Women's Center At Englewood Community Hospital
700 Medical Blvd
Englewood, FL 34223-3964
(941)473-5023
FAX: (941)473-5038

Estero

Lee Health Coconut Point
23450 Via Coconut Pt
Estero, FL 34135-1877
(239)343-1999
FAX: (239)343-9428

Radiology Regional Center
10201 Arcos Ave Ste 101, Estero Medical Center
Estero, FL 33928-9460
(239)936-4068
FAX: (239)936-0611

Fernandina Beach

Baptist Medical Center Nassau
1250 S 18th St
Fernandina Beach, FL 32034-3098
(904)202-2222
FAX: (904)321-3715

Fleming Island

Akumin-Fleming Island
4565 US Highway 17, Ste 150
Fleming Island, FL 32003-4823
(904)592-4700
FAX: (904)592-4701

Baptist Diagnostic Imaging At Clay
1771 Baptist Clay Dr
Fleming Island, FL 32003-8501
(904)202-2901
FAX: (904)516-1536

Precision Imaging Centers
1540 Business Center Dr, Ste B
Fleming Island, FL 32003-4419
(904)996-8100
FAX: (904)996-8101

Precision Imaging Centers
1540 Business Center Dr Ste B
Fleming Island, FL 32003-4419
(904)996-8100
FAX: (904)996-8101

Fort Lauderdale

Broward Health Imaging
1601 S Andrews Ave, 1st Floor, Suite 136
Fort Lauderdale, FL 33316-2509
(954)320-2603
FAX: (954)767-8347

Broward Health-Imperial Point
6401 N Federal Hwy
Fort Lauderdale, FL 33308-1427
(954)776-8750
FAX: (954)776-8569

Lillian S Wells Women's Health Center
1600 S Andrews Ave
Fort Lauderdale, FL 33316-2510
(954)355-4353
FAX: (954)712-8305

Pom Mri & Radiology Center Of Fort Lauderdale
4331 N Federal Hwy Ste 200
Fort Lauderdale, FL 33308-5252
(954)900-2020
FAX: (954)380-8039

Fort Myers

Lee Health Breast Health Center Healthpark Commons
16281 Bass Rd Ste 204, Healthpark Commons
Fort Myers, FL 33908-9687
(239)343-1999
FAX: (239)343-9428

Lee Health Breast Health Center Sanctuary
8960 Colonial Center Dr Ste 100
Fort Myers, FL 33905-7810
(239)424-1499
FAX: (239)343-9428

Premier Womens Care
9021 Park Royal Dr
Fort Myers, FL 33908-9617
(239)432-5858
FAX: (877)633-1520

Radiology Regional Center
3680 Broadway
Fort Myers, FL 33901-8005
(239)936-2316
FAX: (239)425-4796

Radiology Regional Center
6140 Winkler Rd Ste A
Fort Myers, FL 33919-8188
(239)936-4068
FAX: (239)936-0611

Radiology Regional Center - Mobile Unit
3660 Broadway
Fort Myers, FL 33901-8005
(239)936-2316
FAX: (239)425-4796

Fort Pierce

Diagnostic Radiology Center Of The Treasure Coast, Inc.
2011 S 25th St Ste 106
Fort Pierce, FL 34947-4795
(772)468-7020
FAX: (772)801-2900

Radiology Imaging Associates
2306 Nebraska Ave
Fort Pierce, FL 34950-4892
(772)464-1650
FAX: (772)464-4898

Windsor Imaging
1000 Virginia Ave
Fort Pierce, FL 34982-3522
(772)466-5050
FAX: (772)467-1003

Fort Walton Beach

Fort Walton Beach Medical Center
1032 Mar Walt Dr, Unit 150
Fort Walton Beach, FL 32547-6662
(888)894-2114
FAX: (850)315-7844

Institute Of Diagnostic Imaging
424 Racetrack Rd NW
Fort Walton Beach, FL 32547-1556
(850)314-7575
FAX: (850)314-7494

White-Wilson Medical Center
1005 Mar Walt Dr
Fort Walton Beach, FL 32547-6796
(850)863-8110
FAX: (850)862-3839

Ft Lauderdale

Akumin
2000 NE 45th St
Ft Lauderdale, FL 33308-5122
(954)492-8151
FAX: (954)772-7753

Dorothy Mangurian Cwc At Holy Cross Healthplex
1000 NE 56th St
Ft Lauderdale, FL 33334-4149
(954)771-8000
FAX: (954)229-8697

Florida Medical Center A Campus Of North Shore
5000 W Oakland Park Blvd
Ft Lauderdale, FL 33313-1503
(954)735-6000
FAX: (954)677-2675

Ft Myers

Advanced Radiology Imaging Associates, Llc
13731 Metropolis Ave
Ft Myers, FL 33912-7150
(239)333-2742
FAX: (239)333-4329

Millennium Physician Group
13813 Metro Pkwy
Ft Myers, FL 33912-4343
(855)674-4624
FAX: (941)249-4190

Gainesville

Arlene M. Weinshelbaum, M.D. P.A.
6820 NW 11th Pl
Gainesville, FL 32605-4217
(352)331-0115
FAX: (352)331-2044

Comprehensive Women's Health
724 NW 43rd St
Gainesville, FL 32607-6110
(352)332-7222
FAX: (352)332-7222

Doctors Imaging Group
6716 NW 11th Pl Ste 200
Gainesville, FL 32605-4201
(352)331-9729
FAX: (352)331-8692

Mammography & Ultrasound Imaging Center, Pllc
7550 W University Ave Ste A
Gainesville, FL 32607-7608
(352)727-4911
FAX: (352)505-5211

North Florida Regional Medical Center
6440 W Newberry Rd
Gainesville, FL 32605-4381
(352)333-5415
FAX: (352)333-5416

Simedhealth Llc
4343 Newberry Rd Ste 5
Gainesville, FL 32607-2824
(352)224-2263
FAX: (352)224-2476

Uf Health Women's And Diagnostic Imaging — Springhill
4037 NW 86th Ter
Gainesville, FL 32606-9277
(352)265-0000
FAX: (352)265-8123

Geneva

Women's Mobile Medical Services, Llc-Mobile
760 Valley Stream Dr
Geneva, FL 32732-9231
(407)349-2007
FAX: (407)349-2006

Gulf Breeze

Optimal Imaging Sacred Heart
4033 Gulf Breeze Pkwy
Gulf Breeze, FL 32563-3506
(850)416-1894
FAX: (850)416-1895

Women's Imaging/Gulf Breeze Hospital
1110 Gulf Breeze Pkwy
Gulf Breeze, FL 32561-4897
(850)934-7500
FAX: (850)934-2394

Hialeah

B & G Diagnostic Services
444 W 51st Pl
Hialeah, FL 33012-3620
(305)818-2006
FAX: (305)818-2009

Diagnostic Medical Imaging
2170 W 68th St Ste 101
Hialeah, FL 33016-1876
(305)398-4220
FAX: (305)398-4225

Hialeah Hospital
651 E 25th St
Hialeah, FL 33013-3878
(305)835-4619
FAX: (305)835-4556

Idaca, Llc
21 W 49th St
Hialeah, FL 33012-3709
(305)557-0330
FAX: (786)534-8420

Just For Women Diag. Ctr. At Palmetto Gen. Hospital
7160 W 20th Ave Ste M121
Hialeah, FL 33016-5535
(786)639-1800
FAX: (786)819-1349

La Colonia Diagnostic Center
395 W 10th St
Hialeah, FL 33010-3810
(305)608-1082
FAX: (305)823-3312

Leon Medical Centers
590 E 25th St
Hialeah, FL 33013-3841
(305)646-3764
FAX: (305)646-3763

Medical City Llc
3595 W 20th Ave Ste 145
Hialeah, FL 33012-4537
(305)557-4424
FAX: (305)557-4426

Millennium Diagnostic Imaging Center
900 E 9th St
Hialeah, FL 33010-4650
(305)885-3232
FAX: (305)889-2040

Rivero Diagnostic Center, Inc
285 W 49th St
Hialeah, FL 33012-3713
(305)826-6040
FAX: (305)698-0470

Unlimited Diagnostic Center
2360 W 68th St Ste 128
Hialeah, FL 33016-5502
(786)431-5876
FAX: (786)431-5704

Vital Imaging Diagnostic Centers Llc.
3333 Palm Ave, Unit 1
Hialeah, FL 33012-5212
(305)596-9992
FAX: (786)527-3216

Hollywood

Akumin Hollywood
3800 Johnson St Ste B
Hollywood, FL 33021-6030
(954)964-3800
FAX: (954)986-8153

Diagnostic Medical Imaging Of Hollywood, Llc
6517 Taft St Ste 103
Hollywood, FL 33024-4063
(954)780-5566
FAX: (954)780-5567

Hollywood Diagnostics Center
4224 Hollywood Blvd
Hollywood, FL 33021-6633
(954)966-3600
FAX: (954)967-1962

Memorial Regional Hospital
3501 Johnson St
Hollywood, FL 33021-5421
(954)265-3259
FAX: (954)986-8484

Memorial Regional Hospital South Women's Imaging Ctr
3600 Washington St
Hollywood, FL 33021-8216
(954)276-5500
FAX: (954)518-2250

Radiology Consultants
210 S Federal Hwy Ste 200 - Fl 2nd
Hollywood, FL 33020-6811
(954)927-1776
FAX: (954)920-5657

Total Mri And Diagnostic Center
4440 Sheridan St Ste B
Hollywood, FL 33021-3535
(786)756-3038
FAX: (786)756-3039

Homestead

Homestead Diagnostic Center
650 NE 22nd Ter, Ste 100
Homestead, FL 33033-4710
(305)246-5600
FAX: (305)246-1320

Homestead Hospital
975 Baptist Way
Homestead, FL 33033-7600
(786)243-8520
FAX: (786)243-8562

Vital Imaging Diagnostic Centers Llc.
610 Washington Ave
Homestead, FL 33030-6038
(305)596-9992
FAX: (305)847-2355

Homosassa

Sugar Mill Diagnostic Imaging
8303 S Suncoast Blvd
Homosassa, FL 34446-5028
(352)628-9900
FAX: (352)628-9700

Hudson

Pasco Imaging And Open Mri
7615 Jacque Rd
Hudson, FL 34667-7132
(727)697-0100
FAX: (727)697-1240

Inverness

Citrus Memorial Hospital - Medical Office Building
131 S Citrus Ave
Inverness, FL 34452-4701
(877)351-7012
FAX: (352)344-6908

Citrus Open Mri Center
2687 E Gulf To Lake Hwy
Inverness, FL 34453-3216
(352)637-4466
FAX: (352)637-4482

Inverness Medical Imaging
2105 Highway 44 W
Inverness, FL 34453-3805
(352)637-6100
FAX: (352)637-6900

Jacksonville

Ackerman Cancer Center
10881 San Jose Blvd
Jacksonville, FL 32223-6612
(904)880-5522
FAX: (904)880-5533

Akumin
6500 Fort Caroline Rd Ste B
Jacksonville, FL 32277-2084
(904)745-5900
FAX: (904)745-3737

Akumin
1215 Dunn Ave Ste 4
Jacksonville, FL 32218-4897
(904)696-8400
FAX: (904)696-8499

Akumin
4171 Roosevelt Blvd
Jacksonville, FL 32210-1837
(813)467-6109
FAX: (855)855-0050

Ascension St. Vincent's Mobile Mammography
1 Shircliff Way
Jacksonville, FL 32204-4748
(904)308-7428
FAX: (904)308-5457

Ascension St. Vincent's Riverside
1 Shircliff Way
Jacksonville, FL 32204-4748
(904)308-7428
FAX: (904)308-8093

Ascension St. Vincent's Southside
4201 Belfort Rd
Jacksonville, FL 32216-1431
(904)308-7428
FAX: (904)308-8093

Baptist Medical Center South
14550 Old Saint Augustine Rd
Jacksonville, FL 32258-2460
(904)202-2222
FAX: (904)271-6286

Baptist North Medical Campus
11250 Baptist Health Dr
Jacksonville, FL 32218-2978
(904)202-6926
FAX: (904)391-5411

Innovative Imaging Jacksonville
10696 Old Saint Augustine Rd
Jacksonville, FL 32257-1000
(904)268-1080
FAX: (904)268-3060

Mayo Clinic Florida
4500 San Pablo Rd S
Jacksonville, FL 32224-3899
(904)953-0323
FAX: (904)953-2966

Mayo Clinic Primary Care, Gate Parkway
7826 Ozark Dr
Jacksonville, FL 32256-5839
(904)956-8000
FAX: (904)956-8020

Memorial Hospital Healthcare Plaza-Breast Imaging
3901 University Blvd S
Jacksonville, FL 32216-4312
(888)887-1979
FAX: (904)702-6369

Monument 9-A Imaging & Diagnostic Center
1201 Monument Rd Ste 101
Jacksonville, FL 32225-6445
(904)855-0700
FAX: (904)855-0739

North Florida Obgyn, Llc
3 Shircliff Way, Ste 200B
Jacksonville, FL 32204-4785
(904)365-5685
FAX: (888)316-2547

Optimal Imaging St Vincent's Healthcare-Town Center
6699 Gate Pkwy Ste C
Jacksonville, FL 32256-8079
(904)381-9994
FAX: (904)389-6866

Optimal Imaging St. Vincent's Healthcare - Southside
4203 Belfort Rd, Ste 103
Jacksonville, FL 32216-1411
(904)733-7770
FAX: (904)733-7778

Optimal Imaging St. Vincent's Healthcare-Mandarin
10503 San Jose Blvd
Jacksonville, FL 32257-6295
(904)450-6680
FAX: (904)384-5733

Optimal Imaging St. Vincent's Healthcare-Westside
6488 103rd St, Ste C
Jacksonville, FL 32210-7161
(904)450-6980
FAX: (904)450-6981

Optimal Imaging St.Vincent's Healthcare - Forbes
2345 Forbes St
Jacksonville, FL 32204-4311
(904)381-9994
FAX: (904)389-6866

Precision Imaging Centers- Beach
14444 Beach Blvd, Ste 23
Jacksonville, FL 32250-2079
(904)996-8100
FAX: (904)996-8101

Sekine, Rasner, And Brock Md, Pa - Ob/Gyn
11945 San Jose Blvd Ste 400
Jacksonville, FL 32223-1627
(904)262-5333
FAX: (904)262-5337

Shands Jacksonville Advanced Breast Ctr At Emerson
4549 Emerson St Ste 200
Jacksonville, FL 32207-4961
(904)383-1024
FAX: (904)244-0822

Shands Jacksonville Womens Center
580 W 8th St, Plaza 2, 4th Flr
Jacksonville, FL 32209-6599
(904)383-1024
FAX: (904)244-9441

The Hill Breast Ctr At Baptist Medical Ctr
1235 San Marco Blvd, 3rd & 4th Flrs
Jacksonville, FL 32207-8554
(904)202-2222
FAX: (904)202-3489

U.S. Naval Hospital - Jacksonville
2080 Child St, Naval Air Station
Jacksonville, FL 32214-5000
(904)542-9360
FAX: (904)542-7357

Uf Health Imaging Center - Baymeadows
8060 Philips Hwy, Unit 201
Jacksonville, FL 32256-7477
(904)427-8431
FAX: (904)427-8444

Uf Health Jacksonville North
15255 Max Leggett Pkwy
Jacksonville, FL 32218-7273
(904)383-1024
FAX: (904)244-0822

Jacksonville Beach

Baptist Medical Center - Beaches
1577 Roberts Dr, Ste 102
Jacksonville Beach, FL 32250-3264
(904)202-2222
FAX: (904)202-4090

Jay

Jay Hospital
14114 Alabama St
Jay, FL 32565-1219
(850)675-8053
FAX: (850)675-8172

Jensen Beach

Women's Health Specialists
3498 NW Federal Hwy
Jensen Beach, FL 34957-4441
(772)219-1081
FAX: (772)219-1078

Jupiter

Jupiter Medical Center - Margaret W. Niedland Breast Ctr.
2111 Military Trl, Ste 100
Jupiter, FL 33458-8098
(561)263-4414
FAX: (561)263-5024

Ob/Gyn Specialists Of The Palm Beaches Ii, Llc
345 Jupiter Lakes Blvd Ste 200
Jupiter, FL 33458-7100
(561)275-7666
FAX: (561)275-1143

Key West

Mammography Of Key West
2503 Flagler Ave
Key West, FL 33040-3934
(305)395-1292
FAX: (305)602-7662

Women's Imaging Center
1111 12th St, Ste 414
Key West, FL 33040-3002
(305)294-5535
FAX: (305)292-1519

Kissimmee

Adventhealth Imaging Partin Settlement
2488 E Irlo Bronson Memorial Hwy, Ste 101
Kissimmee, FL 34744-4948
(407)303-2273
FAX: (407)861-3337

Adventhealth Kissimmee
2450 N Orange Blossom Trl
Kissimmee, FL 34744-2316
(407)303-7500
FAX: (407)933-6646

Akumin-Kissimmee West
1503 W Oak St
Kissimmee, FL 34741-4065
(407)847-8864
FAX: (407)847-5137

Obstetrics & Gynecology Associates Of Central Florida, Llc
2400 N Orange Blossom Trl Ste 300
Kissimmee, FL 34744-2308
(407)846-7200
FAX: (407)846-3989

Osceola Imaging Center
730 W Oak St
Kissimmee, FL 34741-4938
(407)518-3257
FAX: (407)518-3760

Poinciana Medical Center
325 Cypress Pkwy
Kissimmee, FL 34759-3326
(407)530-2350
FAX: (407)530-2310

Professional Imaging Centers
911 E Oak St
Kissimmee, FL 34744-5836
(407)657-7979
FAX: (407)678-9938

Simonmed Imaging Florida, Llc - Hunters Creek
1125 Miranda Ln
Kissimmee, FL 34741-0763
(689)204-0153
FAX: (407)865-6098

Simonmed Imaging Florida, Llc - Kissimmee
208 W Oak St
Kissimmee, FL 34741-4420
(407)846-8700
FAX: (407)846-0868

Labelle

Hendry Regional Convenient Care Center
450 S Main St
Labelle, FL 33935-4629
(863)675-2356
FAX: (863)675-2407

Lady Lake

Sand Lake Imaging
809 County Road 466 Unit 400
Lady Lake, FL 32159
(352)753-2660
FAX: (352)753-2259

Lake City

Invision
3140 NW Medical Center Ln, Ste 100
Lake City, FL 32055-4735
(386)755-0101
FAX: (386)755-0690

Physicians Imaging-Lake City, Llc
404 NW Hall Of Fame Dr
Lake City, FL 32055-4833
(386)487-3970
FAX: (386)487-3972

Lake Mary

Adventhealth Imaging Lake Mary
775 Primera Blvd
Lake Mary, FL 32746-2190
(407)333-9766
FAX: (407)829-7915

Cyrus Diagnostic Imaging
165 Waymont Ct
Lake Mary, FL 32746-6093
(407)321-3012
FAX: (407)321-9006

Ohri, Llc Dba Orlando Health Imaging Centers
392 Rinehart Rd Ste 1040
Lake Mary, FL 32746-2577
(407)331-9355
FAX: (407)704-8437

Simonmed Imaging Florida Llc - Lake Mary II
917 Rinehart Rd, Ste 1051
Lake Mary, FL 32746-4853
(407)708-0475
FAX: (407)865-6077

Lake Wales

Advance Technological Radiology Pa
24040 Hwy 27
Lake Wales, FL 33859-7813
(863)419-8832
FAX: (863)508-6314

Adventhealth Lake Wales
410 S 11th St
Lake Wales, FL 33853-4203
(863)679-6858
FAX: (863)678-3931

Lake Worth

Akumin Lake Worth
5051 S Congress Ave
Lake Worth, FL 33461-4704
(561)795-5558
FAX: (561)965-5827

Breast Institute At Jfk Medical Center
4685 S Congress Ave Ste 200
Lake Worth, FL 33461-4761
(561)548-3530
FAX: (561)548-3832

Good Samaritan Medical Center Outpatient Imaging Lake Worth
3713 S Congress Ave
Lake Worth, FL 33461-3753
(561)697-3001
FAX: (561)697-3284

Womens Care Florida - Palm Beach Obgyn
4671 S Congress Ave, Ste 100B
Lake Worth, FL 33461-4783
(561)434-0111
FAX: (561)440-2748

Lakeland

Radiology And Imaging Specialists
2125 Crystal Grove Dr
Lakeland, FL 33801-6875
(407)847-9674
FAX: (407)847-6344

Ris & Lrh Pablo Campus
130 Pablo St
Lakeland, FL 33803-3818
(863)688-2334
FAX: (863)577-0301

Watson Clinic Llp Highlands
2300 E County Road 540A
Lakeland, FL 33813-3825
(863)680-7755
FAX: (863)616-2478

Watson Clinic Llp Women's Center
1400 Lakeland Hills Blvd
Lakeland, FL 33805-3202
(863)680-7755
FAX: (863)616-2478

Women's Care Florida - Lakeland Ob/Gyn
1733 Lakeland Hills Blvd
Lakeland, FL 33805-3016
(863)688-1528
FAX: (863)777-2937

Women's Imaging Center
2120 Lakeland Hills Blvd
Lakeland, FL 33805-2906
(863)688-2334
FAX: (863)577-0288

Largo

Akumin Largo
13787 Belcher Rd S Ste 300
Largo, FL 33771-4065
(727)531-5444
FAX: (727)531-1122

Baycare Outpatient Imaging
8787 Bryan Dairy Rd
Largo, FL 33777-1251
(727)461-8555
FAX: (727)461-8760

Diagnostic Clinic
1301 2nd Ave SW
Largo, FL 33770-2298
(727)584-7706
FAX: (727)559-0594

Largo Medical Center
201 14th St SW
Largo, FL 33770-3199
(727)588-5291
FAX: (727)588-5670

Women's Care Florida Contemporary Women's Care
1301 2nd Ave SW 6th Fl
Largo, FL 33770-3120
(727)462-2229
FAX: (727)314-7520

Lauderdale Lakes

Broward Pet Imaging Center Llc
4850 W Oakland Park Blvd Ste 1A
Lauderdale Lakes, FL 33313-7265
(954)735-6330
FAX: (954)739-1924

Sanitas Lauderdale Lakes
4850 W Oakland Park Blvd Ste 136
Lauderdale Lakes, FL 33313-7277
(305)470-2929
FAX: (305)675-2430

Leesburg

Lake Medical Imaging And Vascular Institute Leesburg
801 E Dixie Ave Ste 104
Leesburg, FL 34748-7601
(352)365-0777
FAX: (352)787-4655

Simonmed Imaging Florida, Llc
211 N 1st St
Leesburg, FL 34748-5150
(352)241-7446
FAX: (407)865-6089

Uf Leesburg Hospital
600 E Dixie Ave
Leesburg, FL 34748-5925
(352)751-8888
FAX: (352)751-8880

Lehigh Acres

Radiology Regional Center
5220 Lee Blvd Unit 1
Lehigh Acres, FL 33971-1038
(239)936-4068
FAX: (239)936-0611

Radiology Regional Center
1110 Lee Blvd
Lehigh Acres, FL 33936-4844
(239)936-2316
FAX: (239)936-0611

Longwood

Simonmed Imaging Florida, Llc - Longwood
225 W State Road 434, Ste 104
Longwood, FL 32750-4980
(407)304-1000
FAX: (407)682-0746

Loxahatchee

Palms West Breast Center
12989 Southern Blvd Ste 101
Loxahatchee, FL 33470-9205
(877)331-7023
FAX: (561)792-1012

Lutz

Baycare OP Imaging - Van Dyke
4091 Van Dyke Rd
Lutz, FL 33558-8007
(813)265-6300
FAX: (813)265-6319

St Josephs Hospital North
4211 Van Dyke Rd, Imaging Center
Lutz, FL 33558-8005
(813)443-7447
FAX: (813)443-7535

Tower Radiology - North Dale Mabry
17503 N Dale Mabry Hwy
Lutz, FL 33548-4521
(813)874-3177
FAX: (813)968-4502

Macclenny

Ed Fraser Memorial Hospital
159 N 3rd St
Macclenny, FL 32063-2103
(904)259-3151
FAX: (904)653-1808

Madison

Madison County Memorial Hospital
224 NW Crane Ave
Madison, FL 32340-1400
(850)253-1958
FAX: (850)253-3696

Maitland

Sand Lake Imaging- Maitland
1640 N Maitland Ave
Maitland, FL 32751-3320
(407)363-2772
FAX: (407)477-9966

Marathon

Fishermen's Community Hospital
3301 Overseas Hwy
Marathon, FL 33050-2398
(305)434-1601
FAX: (786)260-0533

Margate

Northwest Medical Center
2801 N State Road 7
Margate, FL 33063-5727
(877)331-7031
FAX: (866)205-9556

Marianna

Jackson Hospital
4230 Hospital Dr, Ste 110
Marianna, FL 32446-1927
(850)718-2580
FAX: (850)718-2573

Melbourne

Health First Breast Center
1223 Gateway Dr
Melbourne, FL 32901-2607
(321)728-6006
FAX: (321)728-6014

Health First Diagnostic Ctr - Viera Medical Plaza
8725 N Wickham Rd, Ste 101
Melbourne, FL 32940-2240
(321)434-6100
FAX: (321)434-9259

Omni Healthcare - Atlantis Diagnostics
1344 S Apollo Blvd, Ste 102
Melbourne, FL 32901-3180
(321)777-7888
FAX: (321)773-7738

Steward Melbourne Hospital, Inc.
250 N Wickham Rd
Melbourne, FL 32935-8625
(321)637-3030
FAX: (321)242-5872

Tepas Breast Center
1140 Broadband Dr
Melbourne, FL 32901-2609
(321)312-4178
FAX: (321)733-0211

University Center Imaging
1800 W Hibiscus Blvd Ste 100
Melbourne, FL 32901-2624
(321)726-3800
FAX: (321)726-3842

University Center Imaging - Suntree
6300 N Wickham Rd Ste 100
Melbourne, FL 32940-2030
(321)775-7100
FAX: (321)775-7101

Viera Diagnostic Center
6609 N Wickham Rd, Ste 101
Melbourne, FL 32940-2043
(321)254-7880
FAX: (321)254-7707

Merritt Island

Health First Diagnostic Center Merritt Island
255 Borman Dr 2nd Fl
Merritt Island, FL 32953-3486
(321)434-5842
FAX: (321)434-5841

Miami

Advance Cardiovascular Imaging Inc
10260 SW 56th St, Ste 102
Miami, FL 33165-7021
(305)270-7855
FAX: (305)270-7857

Ambulatory Diagnostic Center
9090 SW 87th Ct
Miami, FL 33176-2315
(305)446-7893
FAX: (305)442-1183

Baptist Diagnostic Ctr At West Kendall Hosp
15955 SW 96th St Ste 101
Miami, FL 33196-1272
(786)573-6000
FAX: (786)533-9686

Baptist Mammography Center In Macy's, The Falls
9100 SW 136th St
Miami, FL 33176-5881
(786)573-6000
FAX: (786)533-9724

Baptist Medical Plaza At Brickell
2660 Brickell Ave
Miami, FL 33129-2800
(786)467-5351
FAX: (786)533-9568

Baptist Medical Plaza At Doral
9915 NW 41st St Ste 120
Miami, FL 33178-2445
(786)573-6000
FAX: (786)596-3821

Baptist Medical Plaza At Palmetto Bay
8750 SW 144th St Ste 120
Miami, FL 33176-7229
(786)573-6000
FAX: (756)596-3839

Baptist Medical Plaza At Tamiami Trail
14660 SW 8th St, Ste 120
Miami, FL 33184-3135
(786)573-6000
FAX: (786)596-4201

Baptist Medical Plaza At Westchester
8840 SW 40th St Ste 300
Miami, FL 33165-5482
(786)573-3882
FAX: (786)573-3881

Baptist Outpatient Center
8950 N Kendall Dr, Ste 200 2nd Fl
Miami, FL 33176-2131
(786)596-3886
FAX: (786)533-9724

Cms Diagnostic Services, Inc.
9200 SW 72nd St, Bldg 4
Miami, FL 33173-3240
(305)227-2500
FAX: (305)220-7133

Community Health Of South Florida, Inc.
10300 SW 216th St
Miami, FL 33190-1099
(305)252-4818
FAX: (305)254-4971

Comprehensive Breast Care Center
10300 SW 72nd St, Ste 400
Miami, FL 33173-3013
(305)602-0692
FAX: (305)602-0693

Diagnostic Center For Women
7500 SW 87th Ave Ste 100
Miami, FL 33173-5426
(305)740-5100
FAX: (305)596-0606

Fiu Herbert Wertheim College Of Medicine
11200 SW 8th St Ahc II Rom 559
Miami, FL 33199-2516
(305)348-2940
FAX: (305)348-1494

G & G Medical Center.
8000 W Flagler St, Ste 206
Miami, FL 33144-2153
(786)703-9779
FAX: (786)703-9784

Healthcare Imaging Of Kendall
11410 N Kendall Dr Ste 101
Miami, FL 33176-1031
(305)398-3575
FAX: (305)398-3579

Jackson Memorial Hospital - Mobile
1611 NW 12th Ave, Dtc 1st Floor Breast Health Center
Miami, FL 33136-1096
(305)585-0311
FAX: (305)585-0040

Jackson Memorial Hospital Breast Health Center
1611 NW 12th Ave, Breast Health Center
Miami, FL 33136-1096
(305)585-6000
FAX: (305)585-0040

Kendall Regional Medical Center
11750 SW 40th St
Miami, FL 33175-3530
(877)341-7019
FAX: (786)315-4197

Leon Medical Centers
12515 SW 88th St
Miami, FL 33186-1829
(305)646-3764
FAX: (305)646-3763

Mercy Hospital A Campus Of Plantation General Hospital
3641 S Miami Ave, Radiology Dept.
Miami, FL 33133-4204
(305)854-4400
FAX: (305)285-2946

Miami Cancer Institute Baptist Hospital
8900 N Kendall Dr 2nd Fl
Miami, FL 33176-2118
(786)662-4778
FAX: (786)662-4806

Midtown Women's Center
2751 N Miami Ave, Ste 4
Miami, FL 33127-4439
(786)375-6600
FAX: (305)573-0186

Millennium Diagnostic Imaging Center Inc
8900 SW 24th St Ste 100
Miami, FL 33165-2075
(305)229-9511
FAX: (305)229-9112

North Shore Medical Center
1100 NW 95th St
Miami, FL 33150-2038
(305)835-6105
FAX: (305)694-3402

Palmetto Bay Medical Center
9765 SW 184th St
Miami, FL 33157-6932
(305)255-3950
FAX: (305)233-2503

Pet-Ct & Mri Of Miami Llc
12905 SW 42nd St Ste 106
Miami, FL 33175-2910
(305)229-2020
FAX: (305)229-2218

Pinnacle Imaging Center
2390 NW 7th St Ste 103
Miami, FL 33125-3227
(305)642-7388
FAX: (305)642-4988

Precision Health Center
2975 Coral Way
Miami, FL 33145-3205
(786)615-2027
FAX: (305)982-8323

Sanitas Miami Lakes
Suite 101
Miami, FL 33015
(844)665-4827
FAX: (305)675-2430

South Florida Diagnostic Imaging
11801 SW 90th St Ste 102
Miami, FL 33186-2182
(305)270-6001
FAX: (305)270-6955

South Miami Hospital
6200 SW 73rd St, Imaging Services
Miami, FL 33143-4679
(786)662-0656
FAX: (786)662-5350

Sunset Radiology, Inc.
7000 SW 97th Ave Ste 117
Miami, FL 33173-1474
(305)273-6602
FAX: (305)273-6603

University Of Miami Hospital And Clinics-Sccc
1475 NW 12th Ave Ste 3301, Mammography Dept.
Miami, FL 33136-1002
(305)243-4954
FAX: (305)243-4955

Vital Imaging Diagnostic Centers Llc.
7101 SW 99th Ave Ste 106
Miami, FL 33173-4661
(305)596-9992
FAX: (305)596-0942

Vital Imaging Diagnostic Centers Llc.
3150 Coral Way
Miami, FL 33145
(305)596-9992
FAX: (786)527-3216

West Kendall Obgyn
8200 SW 117th Ave, Ste 304
Miami, FL 33183-4826
(305)203-1446
FAX: (561)423-0675

Westchester General Hospital, Inc.
2500 SW 75th Ave
Miami, FL 33155-2895
(305)264-5252
FAX: (305)267-6920

Miami Beach

Baptist Medical Hub At Miami Beach
709 Alton Rd Ste 100, Imaging Mammography Department
Miami Beach, FL 33139-5520
(786)573-6000
FAX: (786)533-9741

Mt. Sinai Comprehensive Breast Center
4306 Alton Rd 2nd Fl
Miami Beach, FL 33140-2840
(305)535-3379
FAX: (305)535-3380

Miami Lakes

Baptist Outpatient Services, Inc. Med. Plaza At Miami Lakes
14701 NW 77th Ave Ste 120
Miami Lakes, FL 33014-2500
(786)573-6000
FAX: (786)596-2352

Cms Diagnostic Services.
15100 NW 67th Ave Ste 103
Miami Lakes, FL 33014-2103
(305)227-2500
FAX: (305)220-7133

Lakes Radiology
14575 NW 77th Ave Ste 100/200
Miami Lakes, FL 33014-2547
(305)231-1115
FAX: (305)231-1116

Universal Imaging & Radiology Llc
14462 Commerce Way
Miami Lakes, FL 33016-1508
(305)821-8585
FAX: (305)821-8586

Middleburg

Ascension St. Vincent's Clay County
1670 St Vincents Way
Middleburg, FL 32068-8447
(904)602-2600
FAX: (904)602-2828

Optimal Imaging St. Vincent's Healthcare-Clay
1786 Blanding Blvd, Ste 11
Middleburg, FL 32068-3806
(904)450-6940
FAX: (904)384-5733

Milton

Santa Rosa Medical Center Medical Office Building
5992 Berryhill Rd, Ste 302
Milton, FL 32570-1017
(850)626-5129
FAX: (850)626-5292

Miramar

Memorial Hospital Miramar
1901 SW 172nd Ave
Miramar, FL 33029-5592
(954)276-5595
FAX: (954)538-5058

Mount Dora

Akumin- Mount Dora
3615 Lake Center Dr
Mount Dora, FL 32757-2364
(352)405-4545
FAX: (352)388-9464

N Miami Beach

Comprehensive Breast Care Center
1380 NE Miami Gardens Dr Ste 105
N Miami Beach, FL 33179-4708
(305)944-3132
FAX: (305)944-3437

Naples

A Womans Place Naples, Llc
1660 Medical Blvd, Ste 100
Naples, FL 34110-1415
(239)513-0053
FAX: (239)596-0900

Breast Center Of Naples, Pllc
3555 Kraft Rd Ste 350
Naples, FL 34105-5037
(239)238-1210
FAX: (239)238-1212

Millennium Physician Group
88 12th St N, Unit 110
Naples, FL 34102-6250
(855)674-4624
FAX: (941)883-8386

Nch Imaging 9th Street
311 Tamiami Trl N, Ste 104
Naples, FL 34102-5886
(239)624-4443
FAX: (239)513-2316

Nch Imaging Southeast
7717 Collier Blvd
Naples, FL 34114-2768
(239)624-6630
FAX: (239)624-8331

Nch Imaging- Medical Blvd
1715 Medical Blvd
Naples, FL 34110-1402
(239)624-6630
FAX: (239)513-2316

Nchmd, Inc Radiology Commons
800 Goodlette-Frank Rd N Ste 230
Naples, FL 34102-5461
(239)624-4443
FAX: (239)624-0751

Physicians Regional Healthcare System
6101 Pine Ridge Rd
Naples, FL 34119-3900
(239)304-4888
FAX: (239)304-5126

Physicians Regional Medical Center Collier Blvd.
8300 Collier Blvd
Naples, FL 34114-3549
(239)354-6442
FAX: (239)354-6134

Proscan Imaging
1020 Crosspointe Dr, Ste 103
Naples, FL 34110-0918
(239)598-0035
FAX: (239)598-0038

Radiology Regional Center
1875 Veterans Park Dr Ste 2101
Naples, FL 34109-0596
(239)936-2316
FAX: (239)425-4796

Radiology Regional Center
700 Goodlette-Frank Rd N
Naples, FL 34102-5644
(239)936-4068
FAX: (239)425-4796

Navarre

Baptist Medical Park Navarre-Diagnostic Center
8888 Navarre Pkwy
Navarre, FL 32566-3615
(850)939-4888
FAX: (850)939-4620

New Port Richey

Excel Medical Imaging
5626 Gulf Dr
New Port Richey, FL 34652-4020
(727)841-8212
FAX: (727)841-9589

Tower Radiology Center New Port Richey
5539 Marine Pkwy
New Port Richey, FL 34652-4329
(727)847-5122
FAX: (727)843-8832

New Smyrna Beach

Adventhealth Imaging-New Smyrna Health Park
125 Florida Memorial Pkwy, Imaging
New Smyrna Beach, FL 32168-9311
(386)409-6827
FAX: (386)409-6904

Adventhealth New Smyrna Beach
401 Palmetto St
New Smyrna Beach, FL 32168-7322
(386)424-5046
FAX: (386)424-5077

Niceville

Women's Health & Imaging
552 Twin Cities Blvd Ste B
Niceville, FL 32578-1059
(888)894-2115
FAX: (850)729-8900

North Miami

Lakes Radiology Ii, Inc
2085 NE 120th Rd
North Miami, FL 33181-3321
(954)634-5272
FAX: (954)634-5274

North Miami Beach

Jackson North Medical Center
160 NW 170th St
North Miami Beach, FL 33169-5576
(305)654-5010
FAX: (305)654-5256

North Palm Beach

Palm Beach Radiology
733 US Highway 1, Ste A Ste B
North Palm Beach, FL 33408-4513
(561)841-8588
FAX: (561)841-8533

North Port

Sarasota Memorial Health Care Center & Er At North Port
2345 Bobcat Village Center Rd
North Port, FL 34288-8999
(941)917-7069
FAX: (941)917-6443

Ocala

Invision Diagnostics Of Florida, Llc
3233 SW 33rd Rd Ste 301
Ocala, FL 34474-8425
(877)318-1349
FAX: (772)263-8887

Ocala Gynecology
1500 SE 17th St, Ste 200
Ocala, FL 34471-4649
(352)351-0060
FAX: (352)351-4130

Ocala Health Imaging Srv Llc Dba Advanced Imaging Ctrs-Main
2300 SE 17th St Ste 800
Ocala, FL 34471-9142
(352)867-9606
FAX: (352)620-1494

Project Health Inc Dba Langley Health Services Ocala
7205 SE Maricamp Rd
Ocala, FL 34472-2105
(352)680-0324
FAX: (352)687-3413

Radiology Imaging Specialists Llc
1714 SW 17th St, Ste 300
Ocala, FL 34471-1227
(352)274-9565
FAX: (888)978-5541

The Women's Imaging Center
1901 SE 18th Ave Ste 200
Ocala, FL 34471-8214
(352)671-4300
FAX: (352)671-4292

Timberridge Imaging Center
9521 SW Highway 200
Ocala, FL 34481-7719
(352)671-4300
FAX: (352)671-4393

Ocoee

Health Central Hospital
10000 W Colonial Dr
Ocoee, FL 34761-3499
(407)296-1190
FAX: (407)253-1677

Ohri, Llc Dba Orlando Health Imaging Centers
10885 W Colonial Dr
Ocoee, FL 34761-2939
(407)656-6040
FAX: (407)680-0436

Simonmed Imaging Florida Llc - Ocoee II
10125 W Colonial Dr, Ste 114
Ocoee, FL 34761-4212
(407)531-9853
FAX: (407)865-6075

Okeechobee

Raulerson Hospital
1796 US Highway 441 N
Okeechobee, FL 34972-1918
(877)331-7027
FAX: (863)824-2315

Oldsmar

Tower Radiology Center - Oldsmar
3870 Tampa Rd
Oldsmar, FL 34677-3133
(813)874-3177
FAX: (813)814-1615

Orange Park

Akumin
2020 Professional Center Dr
Orange Park, FL 32073-4461
(904)696-8400
FAX: (904)696-8447

North Florida Ob-Gyn
1680 Eagle Harbor Pkwy, Ste A
Orange Park, FL 32003-4821
(904)264-9555
FAX: (904)215-7960

Optimal Imaging St Vincent's Healthcare-Orange Park
2300 Park Ave, Ste 104
Orange Park, FL 32073-5571
(904)381-9994
FAX: (904)389-6866

Orange Park Medical Center
2001 Kingsley Ave, Breast Care Center
Orange Park, FL 32073-5156
(888)887-6675
FAX: (904)639-8617

Park Avenue Imaging
2128 Park Ave
Orange Park, FL 32073-5584
(904)375-8884
FAX: (904)644-7308

Orlando

Adventhealth Imaging East Orlando
7975 Lake Underhill Rd Ste 100
Orlando, FL 32822-8203
(407)303-2273
FAX: (407)303-6555

Adventhealth Imaging Lake Nona
9975 Tavistock Lakes Blvd, Ste 120
Orlando, FL 32827-7665
(407)834-8722
FAX: (407)303-0887

Adventhealth Imaging Princeton
235 E Princeton St
Orlando, FL 32804-5553
(407)834-8722
FAX: (407)303-1420

Adventhealth Imaging Waterford Lakes
12301 Lake Underhill Rd Ste 113
Orlando, FL 32828-4509
(407)834-8722
FAX: (407)277-4911

Ohri, Llc D/B/A Orlando Health Imaging Centers
7243 Della Dr, Ste C
Orlando, FL 32819-5106
(407)331-9355
FAX: (407)637-8356

Ohri,Llc Dba Orlando Health Imaging Centers
1800 S Orange Ave
Orlando, FL 32806-2925
(407)839-3800
FAX: (407)434-0644

Ormc Ambulatory Care Center Women's Imaging
22 W Underwood St
Orlando, FL 32806-1110
(321)841-5274
FAX: (407)843-6010

Professional Imaging Centers
7806 Lake Underhill Rd Ste 101
Orlando, FL 32822-8232
(407)608-6800
FAX: (407)608-6747

Sand Lake Imaging
9350 Turkey Lake Rd
Orlando, FL 32819-7319
(407)363-2772
FAX: (407)447-9966

Simonmed Imaging Florida, Llc - Waterford Lakes
775 N Alafaya Trl
Orlando, FL 32828-7047
(321)235-8700
FAX: (321)235-8777

Simonmed Imaging Florida, Llc- Kaley II
2121 S Orange Ave
Orlando, FL 32806-3067
(407)514-1870
FAX: (407)865-6092

Smi Imaging Florida , Llc - Sand Lake
6000 Turkey Lake Rd, Ste 102
Orlando, FL 32819-4205
(407)514-1840
FAX: (407)865-6016

The Women's Center Of Orlando
3000 Hunters Creek Blvd, Ste 3
Orlando, FL 32837-6901
(407)857-2502
FAX: (407)857-1855

Ucf Lake Nona Medical Center
6700 Lake Nona Blvd
Orlando, FL 32827-7729
(954)328-8362
FAX: (689)216-8036

Women's Center For Radiology
1621 N Mills Ave
Orlando, FL 32803-1849
(407)841-0822
FAX: (407)841-0411

Women's Center For Radiology
1718 S Orange Ave
Orlando, FL 32806-2923
(407)841-0822
FAX: (407)841-0411

Womencare Of Baldwin Park
930 Lake Baldwin Ln
Orlando, FL 32814-6651
(407)898-1500
FAX: (407)898-3022

Ormond Beach

Adventhealth Imaging Ormond Beach
335 Clyde Morris Blvd Ste 250
Ormond Beach, FL 32174-3196
(386)671-4785
FAX: (386)898-0257

Osprey

Sarasota Memorial Health Care Center At Blackburn Point
929 S Tamiami Trl Ste 100
Osprey, FL 34229-9241
(941)917-7069
FAX: (941)917-4366

Oviedo

Adventhealth Imaging Oviedo
8000 Red Bug Lake Rd Ste 120
Oviedo, FL 32765-9226
(407)303-2273
FAX: (407)977-7431

Oviedo Medical Center
8300 Red Bug Lake Rd
Oviedo, FL 32765-6801
(888)454-7974
FAX: (407)890-2121

Simonmed Imaging Florida, Llc - Oviedo
7424 Red Bug Lake Rd
Oviedo, FL 32765-7154
(407)971-6344
FAX: (407)971-6343

Pace

Ann Baroco Center At Pace Of Optimal Imaging
3754 Highway 90 Ste 110, Sacred Heart Medical Park At Pace - Mamm
Pace, FL 32571-1097
(850)746-0694
FAX: (850)746-0688

Palatka

Express Medical Imaging
6300 Saint Johns Ave
Palatka, FL 32177-3884
(386)280-0080
FAX: (386)280-0081

Putnam Diagnostic Imaging Center
611 Zeagler Dr
Palatka, FL 32177-3810
(386)328-4225
FAX: (386)328-4599

Putnam Radiology Group
6121 Saint Johns Ave
Palatka, FL 32177-3889
(386)326-0077
FAX: (386)326-0188

Palm Bay

Florida Diagnostic Imaging
5201 Babcock St NE Ste 5
Palm Bay, FL 32905-4697
(321)676-5323
FAX: (321)951-9253

Health First Palm Bay Hospital
1425 Malabar Rd NE
Palm Bay, FL 32907-2506
(321)434-6100
FAX: (321)434-6040

Palm Beach Gardens

Midtown Imaging
2529 Burns Rd
Palm Beach Gardens, FL 33410-5204
(561)697-3001
FAX: (561)697-3284

Obgyn Specialists Of The Palm Beaches Ii, Llc
2979 Pga Blvd Ste 100
Palm Beach Gardens, FL 33410-3002
(561)275-7666
FAX: (561)275-1143

Palm Beach Gardens Medical Center
3360 Burns Rd
Palm Beach Gardens, FL 33410-4384
(561)694-7163
FAX: (561)625-5060

Palm City

Invision Diagnostics Of Florida, Llc
1025 SW Martin Downs Blvd Ste 201
Palm City, FL 34990-2868
(919)606-2856
FAX: (704)966-2407

Palm Coast

Adventhealth Imaging Palm Coast
120 Cypress Edge Dr Ste 103
Palm Coast, FL 32164-8454
(386)586-1650
FAX: (386)586-1690

Adventhealth Palm Coast
60 Memorial Medical Pkwy
Palm Coast, FL 32164-5980
(386)586-4402
FAX: (386)586-4618

Palm Coast Imaging Center
3 Pine Cone Dr Ste 101
Palm Coast, FL 32137-8684
(386)446-5200
FAX: (386)446-9437

Town Center Imaging
21 Hospital Dr Ste 130
Palm Coast, FL 32164-2453
(386)446-5200
FAX: (386)597-5675

Palm Harbor

Akumin Boot Ranch
4133 Woodlands Pkwy
Palm Harbor, FL 34685-3462
(727)781-3888
FAX: (727)781-3881

Akumin- Palm Harbor
36463 US Highway 19 N
Palm Harbor, FL 34684-1329
(727)771-2795
FAX: (727)786-7265

Mri Assoc Of Palm Harbor Inc Dba Palm Harbor Mri Inc
32615 US Highway 19 N Ste 4
Palm Harbor, FL 34684-3176
(727)787-6900
FAX: (727)787-1892

Panama City

Bay Radiology Women's Imaging Center, Llc
330 W 23rd St Ste A
Panama City, FL 32405-4540
(850)747-4900
FAX: (850)215-0408

Emerald Coast Obgyn Of The Panhandle
103 E 23rd St
Panama City, FL 32405-4501
(850)769-0338
FAX: (850)785-6088

Medical Evaluators Inc. Dba Gulf Imaging
406 W 19th St
Panama City, FL 32405-4602
(850)784-0545
FAX: (850)215-4045

The Diagnostic Center At Gulf Coast Medical Center
2024 State Ave
Panama City, FL 32405-4558
(850)747-7775
FAX: (877)304-4525

Parrish

Manatee Diagnostic Center- Parrish
11255 US Highway 301 N Unit 105
Parrish, FL 34219-8706
(941)747-3034
FAX: (941)748-5819

Pembroke Pines

Akumin Pines
701 NW 179th Ave Ste 102
Pembroke Pines, FL 33029-2820
(954)538-0050
FAX: (954)538-0036

Akumin, Pembroke Pines East
10950 Pines Blvd
Pembroke Pines, FL 33026-5208
(954)430-2044
FAX: (954)430-2055

Baptist Medical Plaza At Pembroke Pines
15885 Pines Blvd
Pembroke Pines, FL 33027-1220
(954)837-1352
FAX: (954)837-1351

Diagnostic Medical Imaging Of Pembroke Pines
330 S Flamingo Rd
Pembroke Pines, FL 33027-1770
(954)780-5566
FAX: (954)780-5567

La Colonia Diagnostic Center
8399 Pines Blvd
Pembroke Pines, FL 33024-6607
(305)608-1082
FAX: (305)823-3312

Memorial Hospital West
703 N Flamingo Rd
Pembroke Pines, FL 33028-1014
(954)844-5056
FAX: (954)450-4416

Pembroke Pink Imaging
15735 Pines Blvd
Pembroke Pines, FL 33027-1207
(954)517-1725
FAX: (954)517-1729

Qualcare Medical Group
9050 Pines Blvd Ste 170
Pembroke Pines, FL 33024-6400
(954)431-7627
FAX: (954)431-7733

Pensacola

Angel Williamson Imaging Center
5120 Bayou Blvd, Ste 9
Pensacola, FL 32503-2135
(850)476-1161
FAX: (850)476-3575

Ann L. Baroco Center At Optimal Imaging
1890 Summit Blvd Ste 110
Pensacola, FL 32503-3357
(850)746-0694
FAX: (850)746-0688

Baptist Hospital Women's Imaging
1717 N E St Ste 104
Pensacola, FL 32501-6339
(850)469-7500
FAX: (850)469-2309

Community Health Northwest Florida
2315 W Jackson St
Pensacola, FL 32505-7552
(850)436-4630
FAX: (850)436-2095

Naval Hospital Pensacola
6000 W Highway 98, Naval Hospital, Code 39
Pensacola, FL 32512-0003
(850)505-6719
FAX: (850)505-6527

Optimal Imaging Sacred Heart
13137 Sorrento Rd
Pensacola, FL 32507-8777
(850)416-0020
FAX: (850)416-1893

Optimal Imaging Sacred Heart
2156 W Nine Mile Rd Ste A
Pensacola, FL 32534-9464
(850)416-1830
FAX: (850)416-1831

The Women's Group Llc
2114 Airport Blvd Ste 1000
Pensacola, FL 32504-8926
(850)476-3696
FAX: (850)476-0955

West Florida Hospital
8383 N Davis Hwy
Pensacola, FL 32514-6088
(888)894-2113
FAX: (850)494-5359

Women's Services At Baptist Medical Park
9400 University Pkwy
Pensacola, FL 32514-5752
(850)469-7500
FAX: (850)208-6049

Woodlands Medical Specialists
4724 N Davis Hwy, 1st Floor Imaging
Pensacola, FL 32503-2339
(850)696-4200
FAX: (850)607-7553

Perry

Doctors' Memorial Hospital
333 N Byron Butler Pkwy
Perry, FL 32347-2300
(850)584-0877
FAX: (850)584-0642

Pinellas Park

Gateway Radiology Consultants P.A.
4800 Park Blvd N
Pinellas Park, FL 33781-3534
(727)522-1061
FAX: (727)528-7916

Plant City

Plant City Imaging
206 W Alexander St Ste 1
Plant City, FL 33563-7100
(813)750-1724
FAX: (813)750-1971

South Florida Baptist Hospital Breast Center
301 N Alexander St, South Florida Baptist Hospital
Plant City, FL 33563-4303
(813)757-8350
FAX: (813)757-8001

Plantation

Akumin Plantation
8300 W Sunrise Blvd
Plantation, FL 33322-5406
(954)577-6000
FAX: (954)577-5910

Akumin, Plantation East
7301 NW 4th St
Plantation, FL 33317-2234
(954)449-7023
FAX: (954)449-7027

Baptist Health Diagnostic Imaging At Plantation
1228 S Pine Island Rd, Ste 120
Plantation, FL 33324-4580
(954)837-1420
FAX: (954)837-1061

Diagnostic Medical Imaging Of Plantation, Llc
7050 NW 4th St Ste 202
Plantation, FL 33317-2247
(954)780-5566
FAX: (954)780-5567

Pom Mri & Imaging Center Of Plantation
4373 W Sunrise Blvd
Plantation, FL 33313-6749
(954)318-0551
FAX: (954)343-1855

Sanitas Plantation
180 SW 84th Ave
Plantation, FL 33324-2731
(786)860-4741
FAX: (305)675-2430

University Of Miami Hospital & Clinics - Plantation
8100 SW 10th St Ste 1901, Crossroads Office Park Building 3
Plantation, FL 33324-3279
(954)210-1156
FAX: (954)210-1291

Westside Regional Medical Center
8201 W Broward Blvd
Plantation, FL 33324-2798
(954)476-3918
FAX: (954)476-3983

Poinciana

Simonmed Imaging Florida, Llc - Poinciana
875 Cypress Pkwy
Poinciana, FL 34759-3408
(407)944-2220
FAX: (407)865-6086

Ponte Vedra

Flagler Health Plus Imaging
351 Town Plaza Ave Ste 101
Ponte Vedra, FL 32081-5178
(904)819-4707
FAX: (904)819-4948

Ponte Vedra Beach

Baptist Healthplace At Nocatee
400 Colonnade Dr
Ponte Vedra Beach, FL 32081-6235
(904)271-7574
FAX: (904)271-7527

Port Charlotte

Akumin- Port Charlotte
2625 Tamiami Trl Ste 1
Port Charlotte, FL 33952-6403
(813)467-6109
FAX: (941)235-4660

American Imaging Of Southwest Florida
23081 Harborview Rd
Port Charlotte, FL 33980-2153
(941)235-8762
FAX: (941)237-5691

Bayfront Health Port Charlotte
2500 Harbor Blvd
Port Charlotte, FL 33952-5000
(941)766-4810
FAX: (941)766-4708

Fawcett Memorial Hospital
21298 Olean Blvd
Port Charlotte, FL 33952-6765
(866)463-7103
FAX: (866)402-7296

Millennium Physician Group Womens Center
19621 Cochran Blvd, Ste 1
Port Charlotte, FL 33948-2070
(855)674-4624
FAX: (941)255-8671

Radiology Regional Center
18300 Murdock Cir Unit 101 Bldg 15
Port Charlotte, FL 33948-1116
(239)936-2316
FAX: (239)425-4799

Simonmed Imaging Fl, Llc Dba Simonmed Imaging Port Charlotte
4161 Tamiami Trl, Bldg 2 Unit 202/204
Port Charlotte, FL 33952-9204
(941)235-3280
FAX: (407)865-6097

Port Orange

Port Orange Imaging Center
1195 Dunlawton Ave
Port Orange, FL 32127-4745
(386)763-5300
FAX: (386)322-5330

Port Saint Lucie

Radiology Imaging Associates
1825 SE Tiffany Ave Ste 104
Port Saint Lucie, FL 34952-7554
(772)398-2233
FAX: (772)398-2244

Women's Health Specialists
10771 SW Trade St
Port Saint Lucie, FL 34987-2119
(772)219-1081
FAX: (772)219-1078

Port St Joe

Sacred Heart Hospital On The Gulf
3801 E Highway 98
Port St Joe, FL 32456-5318
(850)229-5802
FAX: (850)229-5688

Port St Lucie

Cleveland Clinic Imaging
1095 NW Saint Lucie West Blvd
Port St Lucie, FL 34986-1719
(772)785-5566
FAX: (772)785-5539

Diagnostic Radiology Center Of The Treasure Coast Inc.
1501 SE Lennard Rd, Drctc-St. Lucie
Port St Lucie, FL 34952-6542
(772)468-7020
FAX: (772)924-3231

Physicians To Women Pa
1949 SE Port St Lucie Blvd
Port St Lucie, FL 34952-5535
(772)288-2992
FAX: (772)236-4816

St. Lucie Medical Center
1700 SE Hillmoor Dr, Ste 400
Port St Lucie, FL 34952-7559
(772)335-4000
FAX: (772)398-3687

Punta Gorda

Millennium Physician Group
315 E Olympia Ave
Punta Gorda, FL 33950-3831
(855)674-4624
FAX: (941)249-4190

Riverview

Akumin Riverview
7329 Highway 301 S
Riverview, FL 33578
(813)677-2020
FAX: (813)677-3888

Baycare Outpatient Imaging - Big Bend
10141 Big Bend Rd Ste 102
Riverview, FL 33578-7419
(813)302-8925
FAX: (813)302-8929

Shimberg Breast Center At St. Joseph's Hospital-South
6901 Simmons Loop
Riverview, FL 33578-9498
(813)302-8016
FAX: (813)302-8032

Tower Radiology Center Riverview
10621 Big Bend Rd
Riverview, FL 33579-7176
(813)672-0608
FAX: (813)672-0612

Women's Care Florida-Div 4400 Ob/Gyn Assoc., Riverview
13149 Elk Mountain Dr
Riverview, FL 33579-7184
(813)675-8335
FAX: (813)675-8338

Rockledge

Rockledge Mri & Pet Center
1910 US Highway 1 Ste 102
Rockledge, FL 32955-3751
(321)636-6599
FAX: (321)636-6614

Steward Rockledge Hospital, Inc
110 Longwood Ave MS 70
Rockledge, FL 32955-2828
(321)637-3030
FAX: (321)690-6677

Royal Palm Beach

Midtown Imaging - Good Samaritan Medical Center
440 N State Road 7, Ste 104
Royal Palm Beach, FL 33411-3504
(561)697-3001
FAX: (561)697-3284

Safety Harbor

Baycare Outpatient Imaging-Countryside
1840 Mease Dr Ste 103
Safety Harbor, FL 34695-6603
(727)461-8555
FAX: (727)725-6384

Saint Augustine

Flagler Health Plus Imaging
70 Turin Ter Ste 120
Saint Augustine, FL 32092-0849
(904)819-4707
FAX: (904)819-4948

Saint Cloud

Orlando Health St Cloud Hospital
2900 17th St, Ste 5
Saint Cloud, FL 34769-6098
(407)498-3486
FAX: (407)891-2980

Saint Johns

Optimal Imaging St. Vincent's Healthcare-St. John's
2001 County Road 210 W
Saint Johns, FL 32259-2063
(904)450-6270
FAX: (904)450-6279

Saint Petersburg

Simonmed Imaging Florida, Llc - St. Petersburg
840 Dr Martin Luther King Jr St N, Ste 100
Saint Petersburg, FL 33705-1214
(727)440-8250
FAX: (407)865-6090

Sanford

Central Florida Regional Hospital
1401 W Seminole Blvd
Sanford, FL 32771-6764
(407)302-7372
FAX: (407)302-7311

Simonmed Imaging Florida, Llc Dba Simonmed Imaging-Sanford
303 W 1st St
Sanford, FL 32771-1205
(321)275-3132
FAX: (407)865-6094

Santa Rosa Beach

Ascension Sacred Heart Emerald Coast
179 Mack Bayou Loop, Suite 102
Santa Rosa Beach, FL 32459
(850)278-3063
FAX: (850)278-3989

Sarasota

Akumin Sarasota
4917 Clark Rd
Sarasota, FL 34233-3252
(941)927-7711
FAX: (941)927-7710

Breast Care Ctr At Doctors Hospital
5741 Bee Ridge Rd Ste 130
Sarasota, FL 34233-5060
(800)921-7184
FAX: (866)385-0589

Breast Health Center
1921 Waldemere St Ste 110
Sarasota, FL 34239-2941
(941)917-7322
FAX: (941)917-1400

Choice Diagnostic Imaging
5831 Bee Ridge Rd Ste 102
Sarasota, FL 34233-5089
(941)954-1900
FAX: (941)371-8284

Gulf Coast Obstetrics And Gynecology Of Sarasota
1950 Arlington St, Ste 203
Sarasota, FL 34239-3516
(941)379-6331
FAX: (941)379-5443

Intercoastal Medical Group Inc.
3333 Cattlemen Rd Ste 102
Sarasota, FL 34232-6057
(941)371-3871
FAX: (941)371-5727

Partners Imaging Center Of Sarasota
1250 S Tamiami Trl Ste 101
Sarasota, FL 34239-2221
(941)951-2100
FAX: (941)487-5800

Radiology Associates Of Venice & Englewood
3501 Cattlemen Rd, Ste C
Sarasota, FL 34232-6054
(941)488-7781
FAX: (941)342-8283

Sarasota Memorial Ambulatory Ctr At University Pkwy
5350 University Pkwy Ste 100
Sarasota, FL 34243-5813
(941)917-7069
FAX: (941)917-4366

Sarasota Memorial Health Care Center At Clark Road
5880 Rand Blvd, Ste 100
Sarasota, FL 34238-5118
(941)917-7069
FAX: (941)917-4366

Sebastian

Sebastian River Medical Center
13695 US Highway 1
Sebastian, FL 32958-3230
(772)589-3186
FAX: (772)388-1864

Sebring

Adventhealth Imaging Sebring
2950 Alt. 27 South, Ste C
Sebring, FL 33870
(863)402-3383
FAX: (863)402-5379

Adventhealth Sebring
4200 Sun N Lake Blvd
Sebring, FL 33872-1986
(863)402-7575
FAX: (863)402-3449

Highlands Breast And Imaging Center
114 Medical Center Ave 115
Sebring, FL 33870-5422
(863)385-6655
FAX: (863)385-2282

Highlands Regional Medical Center
3600 S Highlands Ave
Sebring, FL 33870-5495
(863)471-5813
FAX: (863)314-3164

South Miami

South Miami Open Mri, Llc
6161 Sunset Dr, Ste A
South Miami, FL 33143-5045
(305)665-4674
FAX: (305)669-4674

Spring Hill

Bayfront Health Spring Hill
10461 Quality Dr
Spring Hill, FL 34609-9634
(352)684-7555
FAX: (352)684-7577

Mri Associates Of Spring Hill, Inc. D/B/A Spring Hill Mri
6451 Toucan Trl
Spring Hill, FL 34607-2642
(352)684-2811
FAX: (352)684-0212

West Hernando Diagnostic Center
3315 Commercial Way
Spring Hill, FL 34606-2699
(352)688-5860
FAX: (352)688-4347

West Hernando Womens Imaging Center
3389 Mariner Blvd
Spring Hill, FL 34609-2461
(352)610-4394
FAX: (352)610-4397

St Augustine

Flagler Health Plus Imaging
101 Health Park Blvd
St Augustine, FL 32086-5777
(904)819-4707
FAX: (904)819-4901

Maven Mammography - Mobile
521 Costa Del Sol Dr
St Augustine, FL 32095-4868
(904)562-4884
FAX: (904)600-4581

Precision Imaging Centers - St. Augustine
1000 Plantation Island Dr S Ste 1
St Augustine, FL 32080-3106
(904)996-8100
FAX: (904)996-8101

St. Augustine Imaging Center
190 Southpark Blvd Ste 101
St Augustine, FL 32086-4209
(904)827-9191
FAX: (904)829-2221

St Petersburg

Akumin- St Petersburg
3451 66th St N Ste B
St Petersburg, FL 33710-1568
(813)467-6109
FAX: (727)781-1310

Baycare Outpatient Imaging Carillon
900 Carillon Pkwy, Ste 105
St Petersburg, FL 33716-1117
(727)734-6442
FAX: (727)561-2341

Baycare Outpatient Imaging St. Anthony's
620 10th St N No S-100
St Petersburg, FL 33705-1407
(727)502-4200
FAX: (727)502-4201

Gateway Radiology Consultants, Pa
2100 1st Ave S
St Petersburg, FL 33712-1212
(727)525-2121
FAX: (727)528-7916

Ohi West, Inc D/B/A Bayfront Health St Petersburg
603 7th St S
St Petersburg, FL 33701-4719
(727)893-6044
FAX: (727)553-7802

Palms Of Pasadena Hospital
1501 Pasadena Ave S
St Petersburg, FL 33707-3798
(727)341-7533
FAX: (727)341-7674

Price, Hoffman, Stone And Associates, M.D.'s, P.A.
747 6th Ave S
St Petersburg, FL 33701-4595
(727)898-3647
FAX: (727)823-3080

St. Petersburg General Hospital - Breast Center
6500 38th Ave N
St Petersburg, FL 33710-1629
(800)617-7095
FAX: (727)341-4944

Susan Shepard McGillicuddy Breast Center At St. Anthony's
1201 5th Ave N Ste 105
St Petersburg, FL 33705-1410
(727)461-8555
FAX: (727)825-1411

Women's Care Florida Center For Breast Health
2191 9th Ave N, Ste 120
St Petersburg, FL 33713-7147
(727)954-6519
FAX: (727)954-6524

Starke

North Florida Regional Medical Center Starke Campus
922 E Call St
Starke, FL 32091-3616
(904)452-2200
FAX: (904)452-2233

Stuart

Cleveland Clinic Imaging
3801 S Kanner Hwy
Stuart, FL 34994-4801
(772)288-5817
FAX: (772)223-2877

Physicians To Women Pa
1815 S Kanner Hwy
Stuart, FL 34994-7204
(772)288-2992
FAX: (772)288-2999

Radiology Imaging Associates
835 SE Osceola St
Stuart, FL 34994-2431
(772)283-3331
FAX: (772)283-9484

Sumterville

Project Health, Inc.
1389 S US 301 Ste B
Sumterville, FL 33585-5143
(352)568-1966
FAX: (352)568-0551

Sun City Center

Sun City Hospital Inc, Dba South Bay Hospital
4016 Sun City Blvd
Sun City Center, FL 33573
(813)634-0366
FAX: (813)634-0452

Tower Radiology Center Sun City
3862 Sun City Center Blvd
Sun City Center, FL 33573-6806
(813)642-9299
FAX: (813)633-3565

Sun City Ctr

Simonmed Imaging Florida, Llc
4051 Upper Creek Dr, Ste 103A
Sun City Ctr, FL 33573-6848
(813)634-0010
FAX: (813)634-0011

Tower Radiology Sun City 301
16521 S US Hwy 301
Sun City Ctr, FL 33573
(813)874-3177
FAX: (813)879-1809

Sunrise

Wiinhealth Women's Imaging And Interventions
8397 W Oakland Park Blvd
Sunrise, FL 33351-7307
(954)998-1887
FAX: (251)235-8378

Tallahassee

Capital Regional Comprehensive Breast Center
2626 Care Dr Ste 100
Tallahassee, FL 32308-4489
(888)702-2152
FAX: (877)304-4526

Mammography Center Of Capital Health Plan
1491 Governors Square Blvd
Tallahassee, FL 32301-3049
(850)523-7246
FAX: (850)523-7316

Tallahassee Primary Care Associates
1803 Miccosukee Commons Dr
Tallahassee, FL 32308-7403
(850)942-6624
FAX: (850)219-1044

Tech Care X - Ray Llc Mobile
106 W 5th Ave
Tallahassee, FL 32303-6125
(850)562-1656
FAX: (850)562-7209

The Women's Imaging Center
1600 Phillips Rd
Tallahassee, FL 32308-5304
(850)878-6104
FAX: (850)309-0650

Tmh Inc Dba Sharon E. Walker Breast Health Center
1300 Miccosukee Rd Ste 700
Tallahassee, FL 32308-5054
(850)431-5433
FAX: (850)431-7439

Tamarac

University Hospital And Medical Center
7201 N University Dr, Radiology Department
Tamarac, FL 33321-2996
(877)331-7030
FAX: (954)724-6564

Tampa

Advent Health Tampa- Kay Meyer Breast Care Center
3000 Medical Park Dr, Ste 100
Tampa, FL 33613-4691
(813)615-7107
FAX: (813)615-8110

Advent Health West Florida Imaging Inc.
14055 Riveredge Dr, Ste 250
Tampa, FL 33637-2141
(813)601-1925
FAX: (813)436-8437

Adventhealth Carrollwood
7171 N Dale Mabry Hwy
Tampa, FL 33614-2665
(813)558-8025
FAX: (813)558-8021

Adventhealth Imaging Center-Westchase
10987 Sheldon Rd
Tampa, FL 33626-4702
(813)467-4850
FAX: (813)467-4898

Akumin Tampa
5107 N Armenia Ave Bldg B
Tampa, FL 33603-1405
(813)874-2999
FAX: (813)874-7673

Baycare Outpatient Imaging South Tampa
711 S Mabry Hwy, Suite 101
Tampa, FL 33609
(813)259-1900
FAX: (813)259-1999

Baycare Outpatient Imaging-Hampton Lakes
12780 Race Track Rd Ste 100
Tampa, FL 33626-1395
(813)749-7810
FAX: (813)749-7815

Bayview Radiology
10010 N Dale Mabry Hwy Ste 150
Tampa, FL 33618-4469
(813)964-8439
FAX: (813)964-0908

Breast Diagnostic Center - Habana
4719 N Habana Ave
Tampa, FL 33614-7105
(813)874-7000
FAX: (813)877-1854

Insignia Care For Women
3268 Cove Bend Dr
Tampa, FL 33613-2752
(813)971-4555
FAX: (813)463-0258

Macdill Air Force Base Hq 6th Medical Group
3250 Zemke Ave Bldg 1078
Tampa, FL 33621-5023
(813)827-9630
FAX: (813)828-4404

Memorial Hospital Of Tampa
2901 W Swann Ave
Tampa, FL 33609-4057
(855)865-5380
FAX: (813)466-7191

Moffitt Cancer Center At International Plaza
4104 Jim Walter Blvd.
Tampa, FL 33607
(813)745-1600
FAX: (813)449-8548

Moffitt McKinley Outpatient Center
10920 McKinley Dr
Tampa, FL 33612-6471
(813)745-8410
FAX: (813)745-4718

Sabal Park Clinic
9208 King Palm Dr
Tampa, FL 33619-1328
(813)827-9734
FAX: (813)828-4404

Simonmed Imaging Florida, Llc
14302 Bruce B Downs Blvd
Tampa, FL 33613-2601
(813)979-7580
FAX: (813)979-7581

Simonmed Imaging Florida, Llc - Macdill
110 S Macdill Ave, Ste 203
Tampa, FL 33609-3589
(813)499-0541
FAX: (407)865-6099

St. Joseph's Womens Hospital - Shimberg Breast Ctr
3030 W Dr Martin Luther King Jr Blvd
Tampa, FL 33607-6308
(813)872-3949
FAX: (813)872-3930

Tampa General Hospital
1 Tampa General Cir
Tampa, FL 33606-3571
(813)844-8288
FAX: (813)844-8063

Tower Breast Diagnostic Center Northside
2716 University Square Dr
Tampa, FL 33612-5513
(813)971-2050
FAX: (813)775-3410

Tower Radiology Center Carrollwood
14499 N Dale Mabry Hwy, Ste 152 Ste 150
Tampa, FL 33618-2049
(813)968-6998
FAX: (813)960-5147

Tower Radiology Center New Tampa
17416 Brookside Trace Ct
Tampa, FL 33647-6200
(813)874-3177
FAX: (813)660-6632

Tower Radiology Center South Tampa
2106 S Lois Ave
Tampa, FL 33629-5659
(813)874-3177
FAX: (813)288-8849

University Medical Service Association
2A Tampa General Circle, 1st Floor
Tampa, FL 33606
(813)259-8845
FAX: (813)259-8846

University Medical Service Association Morsani
13330 Usf Laurel Dr
Tampa, FL 33612-6601
(813)396-2372
FAX: (813)905-9959

Women's Care Florida Division 1100 Partners In Ob/Gyn
2818 W Virginia Ave
Tampa, FL 33607-6330
(813)872-8551
FAX: (813)999-4066

Tarpon Springs

Advent Health North Pinellas
1395 S Pinellas Ave
Tarpon Springs, FL 34689-3790
(727)942-5180
FAX: (727)943-3498

Tavares

Advent Health Waterman
1000 Waterman Way
Tavares, FL 32778-5266
(352)253-3333
FAX: (352)253-3231

Serene Diagnostic Imaging Corp
1751 David Walker Dr
Tavares, FL 32778-5745
(352)800-6500
FAX: (352)800-6501

Tavernier

Mariners Hospital Tassell Medical Arts Building
91550 Overseas Hwy
Tavernier, FL 33070-2506
(305)434-3688
FAX: (305)434-1587

The Villages

Lake Med Imag & Breast Ctr At The Villages Mulberry Grove
8801 SE 165th Mulberry Ln
The Villages, FL 32162-5887
(352)365-0777
FAX: (352)787-4655

Lake Medical Imaging & Breast Center At Colony Plaza
340 Heald Way
The Villages, FL 32163-6087
(352)365-0777
FAX: (352)315-6329

Lake Medical Imaging & Breast Center At The Villages Llc
910 Old Camp Rd Ste 120
The Villages, FL 32162-5605
(352)365-0777
FAX: (352)391-9165

Lake Medical Imaging And Breast Ctr
1400 N US Highway 441, Ste 511
The Villages, FL 32159-8983
(352)365-0777
FAX: (352)315-6329

Lake Medical Imaging At Cahb
2955 Brownwood Blvd, Ste 112
The Villages, FL 32163-2036
(352)787-5858
FAX: (352)315-6329

Simonmed Imaging Florida, Llc
13940 N US Highway 441 Ste 201
The Villages, FL 32159-8909
(352)241-7448
FAX: (407)865-6088

Titusville

North Brevard County Hospital District Dba Parrish Medical C
951 N Washington Ave, Radiology Dept.
Titusville, FL 32796-2163
(321)268-6140
FAX: (321)268-6681

Parrish Medical Group
250 Harrison St
Titusville, FL 32780-5094
(321)268-6674
FAX: (321)268-6820

Trinity

Akumin Trinity
2144 Duck Slough Blvd, Ste 102
Trinity, FL 34655-5009
(727)375-8880
FAX: (727)375-8887

Baycare Outpatient Imaging Trinity
2102 Trinity Oaks Blvd
Trinity, FL 34655-4409
(727)372-4047
FAX: (727)372-4135

New Port Richey Hospital Inc Dba The Medical Ctr Of Trinity
9330 State Road 54
Trinity, FL 34655-1808
(727)816-2662
FAX: (727)372-7205

Tower Radiology Center Trinity
2115 Little Rd
Trinity, FL 34655-4410
(727)847-5122
FAX: (727)569-0499

Tyndall Afb

325th Medical Group /Diagnostic Imaging Dept
340 Magnolia Cir
Tyndall Afb, FL 32403-5612
(850)283-7541
FAX: (850)283-7634

Valrico

Baycare Outpatient Imaging Bloomingdale
2470 Bloomingdale Ave
Valrico, FL 33596-6403
(813)586-8500
FAX: (813)586-8516

Venice

Radiology Associates Of Venice & Englewood
512 - 516 Nokomis Ave S.
Venice, FL 34285
(941)488-7781
FAX: (941)488-0791

Sarasota Memorial Urgent Care Center At Venice
997 US Highway 41 Byp N
Venice, FL 34285-6046
(941)917-7069
FAX: (941)917-4366

Venice Health Park
1201 Jacaranda Blvd
Venice, FL 34292-4535
(941)483-7205
FAX: (941)483-7697

Vero Beach

Indian River Mri, Inc.
1850 37th St, Ste A
Vero Beach, FL 32960-4856
(772)562-3030
FAX: (772)778-0766

Vero Radiology Associates
3725 11th Cir
Vero Beach, FL 32960-4804
(772)562-0163
FAX: (772)410-0302

Viera

Viera Diagnostic Center
7000 Spyglass Ct, Ste 260
Viera, FL 32940-8291
(321)254-7880
FAX: (321)254-7707

Wauchula

Adventhealth Wauchula
735 S 5th Ave
Wauchula, FL 33873-3158
(863)402-3383
FAX: (863)402-5379

Wellington

Akumin Wellington
3347 S State Road 7 Ste 100
Wellington, FL 33449-8148
(561)795-5558
FAX: (561)792-7300

Bethesda Womens Health At Wellington
10520 Forest Hill Blvd, Ste 300
Wellington, FL 33414-3179
(561)336-7164
FAX: (561)795-7888

Diagnostic Centers Of America
2565 S State Road 7, Ste 100
Wellington, FL 33414-9368
(561)727-2300
FAX: (561)727-2333

Ob/Gyn Specialists Of The Palm Beaches Ii, Llc
1447 Medical Park Blvd, Ste 300
Wellington, FL 33414-3183
(561)276-7666
FAX: (561)275-1143

The Comprehensive Womens Imaging Center At Wellington
1395 S State Road 7 Ste 200
Wellington, FL 33414-9326
(561)798-8513
FAX: (561)753-2615

Wesley Chapel

Akumin Wesley Chapel
27662 Cashford Cir
Wesley Chapel, FL 33544-6912
(813)788-2500
FAX: (813)788-2922

Florida Hospital Wesley Chapel
2600 Bruce B Downs Blvd
Wesley Chapel, FL 33544-9207
(813)929-5327
FAX: (813)929-5556

Florida Medical Clinic
2352 Bruce B Downs Blvd, Ste 106
Wesley Chapel, FL 33544-9203
(813)751-3371
FAX: (813)377-1671

Tower Radiology Center Wesley Chapel
2324 Oak Myrtle Ln
Wesley Chapel, FL 33544-6319
(813)874-3177
FAX: (813)751-0423

West Palm Beach

Cleveland Clinic Florida Health And Wellness Ctr
525 Okeechobee Blvd
West Palm Beach, FL 33401-6349
(561)804-0227
FAX: (561)804-0229

Diagnostic Centers Of America
1572 Palm Beach Lakes Blvd Ste 2
West Palm Beach, FL 33401-2338
(561)496-6935
FAX: (561)496-6936

Foundcare, Inc
2330 S Congress Ave
West Palm Beach, FL 33406-7608
(561)660-5468
FAX: (561)283-0677

Good Samaritan Medical Center
1309 N Flagler Dr
West Palm Beach, FL 33401-3499
(561)650-6441
FAX: (561)671-7441

Ob-Gyn Specialists Of The Palm Beaches Ii, Llc
770 Northpoint Pkwy Ste 200
West Palm Beach, FL 33407-1901
(561)275-7666
FAX: (561)275-1143

Outpatient Imaging Wpb Dba Good Samaritan Medical Center
5405 Okeechobee Blvd, Ste 101
West Palm Beach, FL 33417-4544
(561)697-3001
FAX: (561)687-0754

St. Mary's Medical Center
901 45th St
West Palm Beach, FL 33407-2495
(561)881-2828
FAX: (561)882-1085

The Breast Institute At Jfk Medical Center North Campus
4631 N Congress Ave Ste 100
West Palm Beach, FL 33407-3209
(877)331-7024
FAX: (877)600-9829

Ultrasound And Mammography Associates
603 Village Blvd, Ste 202
West Palm Beach, FL 33409-1972
(561)687-9633
FAX: (561)684-5969

Weston

Bhw Women's Diagnostics
2300 N Commerce Pkwy Ste 110
Weston, FL 33326-3255
(954)217-3200
FAX: (954)217-3201

Cleveland Clinic Florida Health System Nonprofit Corporation
3100 Weston Rd
Weston, FL 33331-3602
(954)689-5125
FAX: (954)689-5651

Windermere

Ohri,Llc Dba Orlando Health Imaging Centers
5151 Winter Garden Vineland Rd
Windermere, FL 34786-6098
(407)331-9355
FAX: (407)331-9481

Winter Garden

Adventhealth Imaging Winter Garden
2200 Fowler Grove Blvd, Ste 060
Winter Garden, FL 34787-5597
(407)614-0565
FAX: (407)614-0563

Winter Haven

Advance Technological Radiology, P.A.
315 E Central Ave
Winter Haven, FL 33880-3047
(863)421-9393
FAX: (863)295-5719

Akumin-Winter Haven
7524 Cypress Gardens Blvd
Winter Haven, FL 33884-3200
(813)467-6109
FAX: (863)271-9892

Bond Clinic Women's Diagnostic Center
199 Avenue B NW
Winter Haven, FL 33881-4546
(863)293-1191
FAX: (863)837-5326

Gessler Clinic, P. A.
635 1st St N
Winter Haven, FL 33881-4191
(863)294-0670
FAX: (863)298-3513

Winter Haven Women's Hospital
101 Avenue O SE, Breast And Imaging Center
Winter Haven, FL 33880-4333
(863)297-1885
FAX: (863)291-5901

Winter Park

Adventhealth Women's Center Winter Park
100 N Edinburgh Dr Ste 101
Winter Park, FL 32792-4125
(407)646-7798
FAX: (407)646-7880

Central Florida Breast Center, P.A.
2200 Glenwood Dr Ste 201
Winter Park, FL 32792-3315
(407)740-5127
FAX: (407)740-0827

Ohri, Llc Dba Orlando Health Imaging Centers
1111 W Fairbanks Ave, Ste 140
Winter Park, FL 32789-4777
(407)794-6350
FAX: (407)794-1915

Simonmed Imaging Florida, Llc - Winter Park
1110 W Fairbanks Ave
Winter Park, FL 32789-4721
(407)629-7474
FAX: (407)629-7475

Simonmed Imaging Florida, Llc - Winter Park III
1350 W Fairbanks Ave
Winter Park, FL 32789-4804
(321)203-5731
FAX: (602)708-7706

University Diagnostic Institute Winter Park Pllc
111 N Lakemont Ave
Winter Park, FL 32792-3213
(407)975-3315
FAX: (407)622-1035

Women's Care Florida Ob &Gyn Specialists
1551 Clay St
Winter Park, FL 32789-5499
(407)644-5371
FAX: (863)271-7811

Women's Care Florida Winter Park Ob-Gyn
100 N Edinburgh Dr, Ste 200
Winter Park, FL 32792-4125
(407)645-5565
FAX: (407)919-6412

Winter Springs

Vinmed Medical Services
5732 Canton Cv
Winter Springs, FL 32708-5079
(407)699-7787
FAX: (407)699-7963

Yulee

Uf Health Imaging Services - Wildlight
76011 William Burgess Rd
Yulee, FL 32097-5428
(904)427-8488
FAX: (904)427-8593

Zephyrhills

Adventhealth Zephyrhills
7050 Gall Blvd
Zephyrhills, FL 33541-1347
(813)779-6278
FAX: (813)779-6279

Akumin Zephyrhills
6900 Gall Blvd
Zephyrhills, FL 33542-2513
(813)783-6736
FAX: (813)788-4299

Florida Medical Clinic
38135 Market Sq
Zephyrhills, FL 33542-7539
(813)782-8829
FAX: (813)355-5099

GEORGIA

Acworth

Northside Acworth Imaging
4791 S Main St Ste 140
Acworth, GA 30101-5324
(678)701-6868
FAX: (770)529-0042

Wellstar Acworth Health Park Mammography - Kennestone
4550 Cobb Parkway North NW Ste 109
Acworth, GA 30101-4181
(678)581-5900
FAX: (770)529-1374

Adel

Tift Regional Health System, Inc. D/B/A Southwell Medical, A
260 Mj Taylor Rd
Adel, GA 31620-3485
(229)896-8066
FAX: (229)896-8194

Albany

Carlton Breast Health Center
427 W 3rd Ave Ste 400
Albany, GA 31701-1975
(229)312-4800
FAX: (229)312-4015

One Meredyth Pl-Carlton Breast Hlth Ctr Outpatient Diag
2709 Meredyth Dr Ste 260
Albany, GA 31707-0218
(229)312-4800
FAX: (229)312-4015

The Veranda, P.C.
2701 Meredyth Dr
Albany, GA 31707-2267
(229)883-7010
FAX: (229)883-4475

Alma

Bacon County Hospital
302 S Wayne St
Alma, GA 31510-2922
(912)632-8961
FAX: (912)632-8414

Alpharetta

Breast Care Specialists Llc Alpharetta
3180 North Point Pkwy Ste 203
Alpharetta, GA 30005-4381
(404)255-8086
FAX: (404)255-5592

Kaiser Permanente - Alpharetta Medical Office
3550 Preston Ridge Rd
Alpharetta, GA 30005-3821
(404)365-0966
FAX: (855)232-0488

Northside / North Crescent
11975 Morris Rd Ste 120
Alpharetta, GA 30005-4444
(770)667-4370
FAX: (770)667-4373

Northside Alpharetta Breast Care Center
3400C Old Milton Pkwy Ste 145
Alpharetta, GA 30005-4438
(770)667-4280
FAX: (770)667-4281

Northside Screen Atlanta - Mobile
3400 Old Milton Pkwy Bldg C Ste 145
Alpharetta, GA 30005-3707
(770)667-4400
FAX: (770)667-4441

Wellstar North Fulton Avalon Health Park Imaging Center
2450 Old Milton Pkwy Ste 101
Alpharetta, GA 30009-2520
(470)267-0295
FAX: (770)999-2701

Americus

Phoebe Sumter Medical Center
126 US Highway 280 W
Americus, GA 31719-8645
(229)931-1375
FAX: (229)931-1214

Athens

Athens Ob-Gyn L.L.C.
740 Prince Ave Ste 3
Athens, GA 30606-5903
(706)548-4272
FAX: (706)548-9181

Piedmont Athens Regional Medical Center Inc.
1199 Prince Ave
Athens, GA 30606-2767
(706)475-4960
FAX: (706)475-5979

St. Mary's Diagnostic Imaging Ctr.
2470 Daniels Bridge Rd Ste 300
Athens, GA 30606-6192
(706)389-2075
FAX: (706)389-2061

St. Mary's Health Care System
1230 Baxter St
Athens, GA 30606-3712
(706)389-2300
FAX: (706)389-2346

Women's Healthcare Associates
355 Hawthorne Ln
Athens, GA 30606-2153
(706)369-0019
FAX: (706)369-1989

Atlanta

Atlanta Women's Healthcare Specialists
275 Collier Rd NW Ste 280
Atlanta, GA 30309-1701
(678)500-7120
FAX: (678)500-7121

Breast Care Specialists, Llc
975 Johnson Ferry Rd, Ste 500
Atlanta, GA 30342-4737
(404)255-8086
FAX: (404)255-5592

Diagnostic Radiology, Ultrasound & Breast Center, Pc
755 Mount Vernon Hwy NE, Ste 310
Atlanta, GA 30328-4288
(404)252-3430
FAX: (404)843-9398

Doris Shaheen Breast Health Center Piedmont Hospital
1968 Peachtree Rd NW, Bldg 77 Floor 3rd
Atlanta, GA 30309-1281
(404)605-4427
FAX: (404)609-6725

Emory University Hospital - Midtown
550 Peachtree St NE
Atlanta, GA 30308-2247
(404)778-7465
FAX: (404)778-4947

Emory University Hospital Breast Imaging Center
1701 Upper Gate Dr NE, Wci Bldg, Ste C1104,1st Fl
Atlanta, GA 30322-1023
(404)778-3416
FAX: (404)778-1901

Grady Comprehensive Care Center At Camp Creek
3896 Princeton Lakes Way SW
Atlanta, GA 30331-5510
(404)561-6059
FAX: (404)616-2178

Grady Health System Breast Imaging
PO Box 26278, 80 Jesse Hill Jr Dr SE
Atlanta, GA 30303-0005
(404)561-6059
FAX: (404)616-5910

Kaiser Permanente - Cumberland Medical Office
2525 Cumberland Pkwy SE
Atlanta, GA 30339-3915
(404)365-0966
FAX: (855)232-0488

Kaiser Permanente - Glenlake Medical Office
20 Glenlake Pkwy
Atlanta, GA 30328-3473
(404)365-0966
FAX: (855)232-0488

Kaiser Permanente Cascade Medical Office
1175 Cascade Pkwy SW
Atlanta, GA 30311-3090
(404)365-0966
FAX: (855)232-0488

Northside Hospital Breast Care Center Imaging
1000 Johnson Ferry Rd, Breast Care Center Imaging
Atlanta, GA 30342-1606
(404)845-5700
FAX: (404)845-5732

Northside Hospital Outpatient Center At Meridian Mark
5445 Meridian Mark Rd Ste 450
Atlanta, GA 30342-4766
(404)303-3688
FAX: (404)459-1880

Northside Interchange Mammography
5780 Peachtree Dunwoody Rd, Ste 100
Atlanta, GA 30342-1513
(404)459-1810
FAX: (404)459-1650

Northside Midtown Imaging
1110 W Peachtree St NW, Ste 900
Atlanta, GA 30309-3609
(404)875-2640
FAX: (404)874-6752

Out Patient Imaging
2284 Peachtree Rd NW
Atlanta, GA 30309-1147
(404)225-5674
FAX: (678)623-5610

Peachtree Women's Clinic
5780 Peachtree Dunwoody Rd Ste 200
Atlanta, GA 30342-1558
(404)255-8022
FAX: (404)255-7248

Piedmont Imaging Brookhaven
3925 Peachtree Rd NE, Ste 210
Atlanta, GA 30319-5256
(404)605-4427
FAX: (404)609-6725

Piedmont West Mammography Center
1800 Howell Mill Rd NW Ste 100
Atlanta, GA 30318-0916
(404)605-4427
FAX: (404)609-6725

The Awhg Breast Center, Llc
5780 Peachtree Dunwoody Rd, Ste 175
Atlanta, GA 30342-1558
(678)651-2840
FAX: (404)506-9440

The Ed & Dora Voyles Breast Health Center At Saint Josephs
5673 Peachtree Dunwoody Rd Ste 175
Atlanta, GA 30342-1797
(678)843-7472
FAX: (678)843-7461

Wellstar Atlanta Medical Center
320 Parkway Dr NE, Health Pavilion, 1st Floor
Atlanta, GA 30312-1213
(404)265-3828
FAX: (404)265-4477

Wellstar Outpatient Imaging And Specialty Care At Campcreek
3890 Redwine Rd SW Ste 104
Atlanta, GA 30331-5583
(404)629-4700
FAX: (404)629-4727

Wellstar Primary Care Imaging Services
670 Dekalb Avenue, NE, Suite 105
Atlanta, GA 30312
(404)265-3828
FAX: (770)999-2723

Augusta

Au Health Imaging
3722 Wheeler Rd
Augusta, GA 30909-6648
(706)723-8860
FAX: (706)723-8861

Au Medical Center, Inc.
1120 15th St
Augusta, GA 30912-0004
(706)721-9729
FAX: (706)721-7319

Obgyn Partners Of Augusta, Pc
1348 Walton Way Ste 4100
Augusta, GA 30901-5107
(706)722-1381
FAX: (706)823-6871

Univ Health Srv Inc Mobile Mammography
818 Saint Sebastian Way Ste 100, Professional Center 2
Augusta, GA 30901-2652
(706)774-2482
FAX: (706)774-2582

University Breast Health Imaging
818 Saint Sebastian Way Ste 100
Augusta, GA 30901-2652
(706)722-3574
FAX: (706)774-2582

West Augusta Ob/Gyn
1126 Medical Center Dr
Augusta, GA 30909-1810
(706)863-5082
FAX: (706)863-4082

Women's Diagnostic Center - Doctors Hospital Augusta
3624 J Dewey Gray Cir Ste 100
Augusta, GA 30909-6585
(877)357-0159
FAX: (706)651-2240

Women's Health Of Augusta, P.C.
1303 Dantignac St Ste 2500
Augusta, GA 30901-2792
(888)233-6121
FAX: (520)572-7138

Austell

Kaiser Permanente- West Cobb Medical Center
3640 Tramore Pointe Pkwy
Austell, GA 30106-6825
(404)365-0966
FAX: (770)931-6399

Wellstar Cobb Hospital Mammography
3950 Austell Rd
Austell, GA 30106-1121
(678)581-5900
FAX: (770)732-7288

Bainbridge

Memorial Hospital And Manor
1500 E Shotwell St
Bainbridge, GA 39819-4294
(229)246-3500
FAX: (229)243-3325

Baxley

Appling Healthcare System
163 E Tollison St
Baxley, GA 31513-0144
(912)367-9841
FAX: (912)367-6001

Blairsville

Union General Hospital
35 Hospital St.
Blairsville, GA 30512
(706)439-6450
FAX: (706)439-6408

Blue Ridge

Fannin Regional Hospital
2855 Old Highway 5, Ste 107
Blue Ridge, GA 30513-6239
(706)632-3711
FAX: (706)632-4209

Braselton

Imaging Center Braselton
1515 River Pl Ste 190
Braselton, GA 30517-5604
(770)219-7666
FAX: (770)219-3823

Bremen

Higgins General Hospital
200 Allen Memorial Dr
Bremen, GA 30110-2012
(770)836-9721
FAX: (770)824-2375

Brunswick

Sghs, Inc. Dba Southeast Georgia Health System - Brunswick
3025 Shrine Rd Ste 160
Brunswick, GA 31520-4784
(912)466-1240
FAX: (912)466-1213

Sghs, Inc. Dba Southeast Georgia Health System - Brunswick
2415 Parkwood Dr
Brunswick, GA 31520-4722
(912)466-1240
FAX: (912)466-5214

Sghs, Inc. Dba Southeast Georgia Health System - Brunswick
2500 Starling St Ste 202
Brunswick, GA 31520-4267
(912)466-5235
FAX: (912)466-5214

Buford

Northside Sugar Hill Imaging
4700 Nelson Brogdon Blvd Ste 100
Buford, GA 30518-5403
(404)851-6577
FAX: (770)844-4031

Byron

Medical Center Of Peach County Navicent Health
1960 Ga Highway 247 Connector
Byron, GA 31008-5663
(478)654-2162
FAX: (478)654-2168

Cairo

Grady General Hospital
1155 5th St SE
Cairo, GA 39828-3162
(229)377-0481
FAX: (229)584-5926

Calhoun

Adventhealth Gordon
1035 Red Bud Rd NE
Calhoun, GA 30701-6010
(706)602-7800
FAX: (706)629-8785

Camilla

Mitchell County Hospital
90 E Stephens St
Camilla, GA 31730-1899
(229)336-4653
FAX: (229)336-4681

Canton

Northside Canton Breast Care Center
470 Northside Cherokee Blvd, Ste T70
Canton, GA 30115-8032
(770)721-9700
FAX: (770)721-9701

Northside Riverstone Imaging
720 Transit Ave Ste 201
Canton, GA 30114-2544
(770)479-3722
FAX: (770)479-4211

Outpatient Imaging- Canton
2000 Village Professional Dr, Ste 100
Canton, GA 30114-8499
(678)324-1306
FAX: (700)800-2424

Piedmont Mountainside Hospital Outpt Imaging Ctr Canton
15 Reinhardt College Pkwy, Parkway Ste 105
Canton, GA 30114-5257
(706)301-5404
FAX: (706)301-5405

Carrollton

Tanner Breast Health
706 Dixie St Ste 110
Carrollton, GA 30117-3858
(770)836-9721
FAX: (770)838-8286

Cartersville

Cartersville Medical Women's Center
100 Market Place Blvd Ste 107
Cartersville, GA 30121-8715
(855)828-5136
FAX: (470)490-1980

Harbin Clinic Cartersville Imaging Center
150 Gentilly Blvd
Cartersville, GA 30120-8522
(706)378-8144
FAX: (706)236-6454

Cedartown

Polk Medical Center
2360 Rockmart Hwy, Radiology Department
Cedartown, GA 30125-6029
(770)749-4060
FAX: (770)749-4061

Chatsworth

Adventhealth Murray
707 Old Dalton Ellijay Rd
Chatsworth, GA 30705-2029
(706)517-2064
FAX: (706)517-3714

Claxton

Evans Memorial Hospital
200 N River St
Claxton, GA 30417-1659
(912)739-5010
FAX: (912)739-5011

Colquitt

Miller County Hospital
PO Box 7, 209 N Cuthbert St
Colquitt, GA 39837-0007
(229)758-4268
FAX: (229)758-5919

Columbus

Brookstone Comprehensive Breast Care Center, Llc
1000 Centre Brook Ct
Columbus, GA 31904-4573
(706)507-7055
FAX: (706)507-7056

Columbus Diagnostic Center
2040 10th Ave
Columbus, GA 31901-1491
(706)322-3000
FAX: (706)596-2038

Elena Diaz-Verson Amos Center For Breast Health St. Francis
2300 Manchester Expy Ste A001, Butler Pavillon
Columbus, GA 31904-6805
(706)257-7700
FAX: (706)257-7701

Pink Monarch Breast Center
1538 13th Ave Ste B200
Columbus, GA 31901-2562
(706)507-7465
FAX: (706)221-5212

Pink Monarch Breast Center North
3081 Williams Rd, Unit B200
Columbus, GA 31909-5717
(706)507-7465
FAX: (706)221-5212

St Francis Columbus Clinic
610 19th St
Columbus, GA 31901-1534
(706)660-2112
FAX: (706)660-2189

The Breast Care Center
1831 5th Ave
Columbus, GA 31904-8915
(706)571-1234
FAX: (706)660-6438

Conyers

Advanced Southern Imaging Llc
1390 Business Center Dr SW Ste 700
Conyers, GA 30094-6600
(844)337-2837
FAX: (706)608-8296

Advanced Southern Imaging- Conyers
1415 Milstead Rd NE, Ste D
Conyers, GA 30012-3807
(844)337-2837
FAX: (706)608-8296

Digital Mammography Specialists - Conyers, Llc.
3242 Avalon Blvd
Conyers, GA 30013-6320
(678)904-6823
FAX: (770)679-1425

Piedmont Rockdale Hospital
1412 Milstead Ave NE
Conyers, GA 30012-3899
(770)918-3707
FAX: (770)918-3738

Cordele

Crisp Regional Hospital, Inc.
902 N 7th St
Cordele, GA 31015-3270
(229)276-3345
FAX: (229)276-3382

Covington

Piedmont Newton Hospital
4181 Hospital Dr NE Ste 301, Physicians Pavilion
Covington, GA 30014-2541
(770)385-7800
FAX: (770)385-7858

Cumming

Breast Care Center At Northside Forsyth
1800 Northside Forsyth Dr, Ste 160
Cumming, GA 30041-8485
(404)851-6577
FAX: (770)844-4031

Peachtree Women's Clinic
1800 Northside Forsyth Dr, Ste 250
Cumming, GA 30041-8482
(470)533-1466
FAX: (770)888-3358

Women's Imaging Specialists - Cumming, Llc
3970 Deputy Bill Cantrell Mem, Ste 204
Cumming, GA 30040-3069
(866)300-8512
FAX: (800)613-8386

Dacula

Northside Hamilton Mill
2078 Teron Trce Ste 200
Dacula, GA 30019-1606
(678)312-3444
FAX: (678)312-9736

Dalton

Dalton Imaging
1502 N Thornton Ave
Dalton, GA 30720-3064
(762)226-8048
FAX: (762)226-8049

Peeples Cancer Institute
1215 Memorial Dr
Dalton, GA 30720-2530
(706)272-6599
FAX: (706)272-6046

Dawsonville

Imaging Center Dawsonville
108 Prominence Ct
Dawsonville, GA 30534-6339
(770)219-7666
FAX: (770)219-7665

Northside Dawson Imaging
81 Northside Dawson Dr, Ste 150
Dawsonville, GA 30534-7165
(404)851-6577
FAX: (706)344-3333

Decatur

Emory Decatur Hospital
2665 N Decatur Rd Ste 120
Decatur, GA 30033-6136
(404)501-2660
FAX: (404)501-7279

First Medical Care
2536 Lawrenceville Hwy
Decatur, GA 30033-3227
(770)934-6832
FAX: (770)934-6337

Demorest

Habersham County Medical Center
Hwy. 441
Demorest, GA 30577
(706)754-2161
FAX: (706)754-5345

Donalsonville

Donalsonville Hospital, Inc.
102 Hospital Cir
Donalsonville, GA 39845-1199
(229)524-5217
FAX: (229)524-2979

Douglas

Crmc Outpatient Imaging
190 Westside Dr Ste D
Douglas, GA 31533-3534
(912)383-6918
FAX: (912)383-5675

Douglasville

Wellstar Douglas Hospital
8954 Hospital Dr, Frnt
Douglasville, GA 30134-5604
(470)644-6601
FAX: (470)644-6610

Dublin

The Imaging Center, A Department Of Fairview Park Hospital
104 Fairview Park Dr Ste 100 Hospital
Dublin, GA 31021-2567
(478)274-3919
FAX: (478)274-3906

Women's Imaging Specialists - Dublin, Llc
1000 Hillcrest Pkwy
Dublin, GA 31021-4208
(478)241-0241
FAX: (800)613-8386

Duluth

Kaiser Permanente - Gwinnett Medical Office
3650 Steve Reynolds Blvd
Duluth, GA 30096-4506
(404)365-0966
FAX: (855)232-0488

Northside Duluth Breast Center
3805 Pleasant Hill Rd
Duluth, GA 30096-4808
(678)584-7741
FAX: (678)312-7616

Northside Duluth Hudgens Professional Building
3855 Pleasant Hill Rd Ste 340
Duluth, GA 30096-8030
(678)312-3444
FAX: (770)623-8793

East Ellijay

Piedmont Mountainside Hospital OP Diagnostic Center
309 Highland Pkwy Ste 100
East Ellijay, GA 30540-7093
(706)301-5404
FAX: (706)635-1682

East Point

Wellstar Atlanta Medical Center South, Breast Center
1170 Cleveland Ave
East Point, GA 30344-3615
(404)629-4700
FAX: (404)466-1588

Eastman

Dodge County Hospital
901 Griffin Ave
Eastman, GA 31023-6784
(478)448-4047
FAX: (478)374-9797

Eatonton

Putnam General Hospital
101 Greensboro Rd
Eatonton, GA 31024-8512
(706)485-2711
FAX: (706)485-2849

Elberton

Elbert Memorial Hospital
4 Medical Dr
Elberton, GA 30635-1897
(706)213-2569
FAX: (706)213-2577

Evans

Brown And Radiology Associates
4350 Towne Centre Dr, The Evans Imaging Center Ste. 1000
Evans, GA 30809-3301
(706)868-3940
FAX: (706)750-8397

Ob/Gyn Partners Of Augusta
465 N Belair Rd, Ste 1B
Evans, GA 30809-3189
(706)855-6244
FAX: (706)786-6364

Fayetteville

Piedmont Fayette Women's Imaging
1279 Highway 54 W Ste 120
Fayetteville, GA 30214-4551
(770)719-7007
FAX: (770)719-6611

Fitzgerald

Dorminy Medical Center
PO Box 1447, 200 Perry House Rd
Fitzgerald, GA 31750-1447
(229)424-1409
FAX: (229)424-7283

Forsyth

Diagnostics Monroe Navicent Health
120 N Lee St
Forsyth, GA 31029-2122
(478)633-7020
FAX: (478)633-8998

Monroe County Hospital
88 Martin Luther King Jr Dr
Forsyth, GA 31029-1605
(478)394-6285
FAX: (478)974-0854

Fort Benning

Martin Army Community Hospital
6600 Van Aalst Blvd
Fort Benning, GA 31905-2102
(762)408-2079
FAX: (762)408-2054

Fort Gordon

Eisenhower Army Medical Center
Bldg. 300, E Hospital Rd.
Fort Gordon, GA 30905
(706)787-2171
FAX: (706)787-0553

Fort Stewart

Winn Army Community Hospital
1061 Harmon Ave Ste 1D03
Fort Stewart, GA 31314-5641
(912)435-6056
FAX: (912)435-5636

Gainesville

Northeast Georgia Diagnostic Associates And Clinic, Llc
1240 Jesse Jewell Pkwy SE Ste 500
Gainesville, GA 30501-3861
(770)536-9864
FAX: (770)297-5016

The Imaging Center Of Northeast Georgia Medical Center
1315 Jessie Jewell Pkwy
Gainesville, GA 30501
(770)219-7666
FAX: (770)219-7665

The Longstreet Clinic, P.C.
705 Jesse Jewell Pkwy SE Ste 295, The Longstreet Clinic, P.C.
Gainesville, GA 30501-3869
(770)539-9391
FAX: (770)718-1281

Grayson

Northside Grayson Imaging Center
1132 Athens Hwy Ste 207
Grayson, GA 30017-1760
(678)442-4782
FAX: (770)312-2036

Greensboro

Diagnostic Cowles Clinic Navicent Health Baldwin
1000 Cowles Clinc Way, Pine Building
Greensboro, GA 30642-5285
(706)454-4266
FAX: (706)454-2658

Good Samaritan Hospital
5401 Lake Oconee Pkwy
Greensboro, GA 30642-4232
(706)453-5040
FAX: (706)453-7324

Griffin

Griffin Obgyn Clinic
517 S 8th St
Griffin, GA 30224-4211
(770)227-0167
FAX: (678)692-0002

Wellstar Spalding Regional Medical Center
601 S 8th St, Mammography Department
Griffin, GA 30224-4213
(678)688-5969
FAX: (678)688-2404

Hawkinsville

Taylor Regional Hospital
222 Perry Hwy
Hawkinsville, GA 31036-6748
(478)783-0288
FAX: (478)783-0345

Hazlehurst

Jeff Davis Hospital
163 S Tallahassee St
Hazlehurst, GA 31539-6465
(912)375-7781
FAX: (912)379-5190

Hinesville

Liberty Regional Medical Center
462 Elma G Miles Pkwy
Hinesville, GA 31313-4000
(912)369-9488
FAX: (912)369-3658

Hiram

Wellstar Paulding Imaging Center
144 Bill Carruth Pkwy
Hiram, GA 30141-3818
(678)581-5900
FAX: (770)443-7717

Holly Springs

Northside Imaging At Holly Springs
684 Sixes Rd Ste 100
Holly Springs, GA 30115-8720
(404)851-6577
FAX: (678)388-5461

Wellstar Cherokee Health Park
1120 Wellstar Way, Ste 104
Holly Springs, GA 30114-8952
(678)581-5900
FAX: (678)494-2628

Homerville

Clinch Memorial Hospital
1050 Valdosta Hwy
Homerville, GA 31634-9701
(912)487-5211
FAX: (912)487-4339

Jasper

Northside Imaging Jasper
134 Mountainside Village Pkwy, Bldg 400 Suite 110
Jasper, GA 30143-8694
(404)851-6577
FAX: (706)692-3990

Piedmont Mountainside Hospital
1266 Highway 515 S
Jasper, GA 30143-4872
(706)301-5402
FAX: (706)301-5405

Jesup

Wayne Memorial Hospital
865 S 1st St
Jesup, GA 31545-0210
(912)530-3197
FAX: (912)530-3160

Johns Creek

Emory Johns Creek Hospital
6335 Hospital Pkwy, Ste 106
Johns Creek, GA 30097-1550
(678)474-5602
FAX: (678)474-7908

North Atlanta Women's Specialists- Johns Creek
11459 Johns Creek Pkwy
Johns Creek, GA 30097-3515
(770)623-0910
FAX: (770)622-8144

Northside Medlock Medical Imaging
11459 Johns Creek Pkwy, Ste 120
Johns Creek, GA 30097-3518
(678)584-2210
FAX: (678)584-2211

Jonesboro

Kaiser Permanente - Southwood Medical Office
2400 Mount Zion Pkwy
Jonesboro, GA 30236-2500
(404)365-0966
FAX: (855)232-0488

Prime Healthcare Women's Center At Spivey Station
7823 Spivey Station Blvd Ste 250
Jonesboro, GA 30236-0001
(770)991-8144
FAX: (770)991-8448

Kennesaw

Kaiser Permanente - Townpark Medical Facility
750 Townpark Ln NW
Kennesaw, GA 30144-5579
(404)365-0966
FAX: (855)232-0488

Piedmont Imaging At Kennesaw
3525 Busbee Dr NW Ste 150
Kennesaw, GA 30144-5685
(404)605-4427
FAX: (404)609-6725

Lagrange

Emory Clark-Holder Clinic
303 Smith St
Lagrange, GA 30240-2784
(706)812-4249
FAX: (706)812-4097

La Grange Internal Medicine
1602 Vernon Rd Ste 400
Lagrange, GA 30240-4129
(706)882-9341
FAX: (706)884-0131

Wellstar West Georgia Medical Center Women's Health Center
1420 Vernon Rd
Lagrange, GA 30240-2942
(706)845-3000
FAX: (706)884-5183

Lavonia

St Mary's Sacred Heart Hospital
PO Box 788, 367 Clear Creek Pkwy
Lavonia, GA 30553-0788
(706)356-7420
FAX: (706)356-7422

Lawrenceville

Gwinette's Progressive Healthcare For Women
601-A Professional Blvd., Suite 260
Lawrenceville, GA 30046
(770)339-4000
FAX: (770)339-9037

Gwinnett Clinic Ltd
475 Philip Blvd, Ste 300
Lawrenceville, GA 30046-8736
(770)995-3300
FAX: (770)682-8024

Maternal Gynerations Of Georgia, Llc
600 Professional Dr, Ste 200
Lawrenceville, GA 30046-7651
(404)444-5046
FAX: (877)617-2267

Northside Gwinnett Breast Center
631 Professional Dr Ste 250
Lawrenceville, GA 30046-3370
(678)312-3444
FAX: (678)312-0950

Northside Lawrenceville Imaging
555 Old Norcross Rd Ste 115
Lawrenceville, GA 30046-8703
(770)277-0501
FAX: (770)277-4324

Reagan Medical Center, L.L.C., Dba/Georgia Diagnostic Center
2878 Five Forks Trickum Rd, Ste 1A
Lawrenceville, GA 30044-5896
(678)344-8700
FAX: (678)344-8600

Women's Imaging Specialists - Gwinnett, Llc
601A Professional Dr., Suite 160
Lawrenceville, GA 30046
(866)300-8512
FAX: (800)613-8386

Women's Imaging Specialists-Lawrenceville, Llc
1730 Lawrenceville Suwanee Rd Ste B
Lawrenceville, GA 30043-3507
(706)438-8777
FAX: (770)234-5311

Lithonia

Emory Hillandale Hospital
2801 Dekalb Medical Pkwy
Lithonia, GA 30058-4996
(404)501-2660
FAX: (404)501-8138

Kaiser Permanente - Panola Medical Office
5440 Hillandale Dr
Lithonia, GA 30058-4865
(404)365-0966
FAX: (855)232-0488

Sisters By Choice-Mobile
5910 Hillandale Dr Ste 104
Lithonia, GA 30058-1877
(678)418-3990
FAX: (678)418-3995

Loganville

Eastside Medical Center- Loganville
3445 Highway 81
Loganville, GA 30052-9138
(678)628-1230
FAX: (678)639-1601

Louisville

Jefferson Hospital
1067 Peachtree St
Louisville, GA 30434-1599
(478)625-7000
FAX: (478)625-9110

Macon

Breast Center Navicent Health
800 1st St, Ste 310
Macon, GA 31201-8399
(478)633-4066
FAX: (478)633-8199

Coliseum Medical Centers - Women's Center
350 Hospital Dr
Macon, GA 31217-3838
(478)765-4889
FAX: (478)765-4428

Coliseum Northside Hospital
400 Charter Blvd
Macon, GA 31210-4853
(478)757-6030
FAX: (478)757-6037

Diagnostics Hardeman Navicent Health
1650 Hardeman Ave
Macon, GA 31201-1418
(478)633-4066
FAX: (478)633-2637

Internal Medicine Associates, Pc
330 Hospital Dr, Ste 200 Ste 200
Macon, GA 31217-8034
(478)745-1191
FAX: (478)752-3867

Navicent Health Diagnostics Zebulon
5925 Zebulon Rd
Macon, GA 31210-1917
(478)757-7877
FAX: (478)757-7876

Obgyn Specialists, Llp
380 Hospital Dr, Ste 100 Suite 100
Macon, GA 31217-8005
(478)743-4646
FAX: (877)590-2158

Madison

Morgan Medical Center
1740 Lions Club Rd
Madison, GA 30650-4762
(706)752-2169
FAX: (706)342-1718

Marietta

Cqv Dba Quantum Radiology
790 Church St NE, Ste 400
Marietta, GA 30060-8957
(678)626-0745
FAX: (800)311-6482

North Atlanta Women's Specialists-East Cobb
4800 Olde Towne Pkwy Ste 350
Marietta, GA 30068-4396
(770)977-1510
FAX: (770)508-8858

Northside Marietta Imaging
780 Canton Rd NE Ste 230
Marietta, GA 30060-8928
(770)792-1234
FAX: (770)424-1194

Northside/East Cobb Imaging
4800 Olde Towne Pkwy Ste 100
Marietta, GA 30068-4357
(770)973-9702
FAX: (770)973-9775

Obgyn Of Atlanta
4800 Olde Towne Pkwy, Ste 200
Marietta, GA 30068-4391
(770)565-5604
FAX: (770)578-9712

Surgical Oncology Of North Georgia Dba Advanced Breast Care
790 Church St NE Ste 570
Marietta, GA 30060-8967
(404)841-6262
FAX: (888)343-1740

Wellstar East Cobb Health Park Mammography
3747 Roswell Rd, Ste 102
Marietta, GA 30062-6227
(470)956-8770
FAX: (678)560-5936

Wellstar Kennestone OP Womens Imaging Ctr
699 Church St NE Ste 100
Marietta, GA 30060-1116
(678)581-5900
FAX: (470)793-0083

Wellstar Mammography At The Breast Center
702 Canton Rd NE
Marietta, GA 30060-7271
(470)793-0060
FAX: (770)427-0618

Wellstar Windy Hill Hospital
2540 Windy Hill Rd SE
Marietta, GA 30067-8632
(770)644-1173
FAX: (770)644-1175

McDonough

Kaiser Permanente - Henry Towne Centre
1125 Town Center Village Dr
McDonough, GA 30253-5970
(404)365-0966
FAX: (855)232-0488

Metter

Candler County Hospital
400 Cedar St
Metter, GA 30439-3338
(912)685-1779
FAX: (912)685-1789

Milledgeville

Milledgeville Ob-Gyn
750 N Cobb St, Ste 240
Milledgeville, GA 31061-7163
(478)453-8511
FAX: (478)295-3560

Navicent Health Oconee, Llc, D/B/A Navicent Health Baldwin
821 N Cobb St
Milledgeville, GA 31061-2343
(478)776-4802
FAX: (478)776-4803

Monroe

Piedmont Walton Hospital
2151 W Spring St
Monroe, GA 30655-3202
(770)267-1720
FAX: (770)267-1713

Women's Imaging Specialists - Monroe, Llc
500 Great Oaks Dr, Ste 13
Monroe, GA 30655-8228
(706)785-0500
FAX: (678)635-0818

Monticello

Jasper Health Services
898 College St
Monticello, GA 31064-1258
(706)468-4509
FAX: (706)468-9880

Moultrie

Colquitt Regional Medical Center
3 Sweet Bay Ct
Moultrie, GA 31768-6784
(229)891-9287
FAX: (229)890-4089

Nashville

Sgmc Berrien Campus
1221 E McPherson Ave
Nashville, GA 31639-2326
(229)433-8750
FAX: (229)433-8782

Newnan

Outpatient Imaging Llc
60 Oak Hill Blvd Ste 101
Newnan, GA 30265-2314
(770)502-9883
FAX: (770)251-2130

Piedmont Newnan Faye Hendrix-Ware Breast Health Center
775 Poplar Rd Ste 110
Newnan, GA 30265-8301
(770)400-4305
FAX: (770)400-4310

Piedmont Outpatient Center
1755 Highway 34 E Ste 1200
Newnan, GA 30265-3185
(770)254-3252
FAX: (770)254-3266

Southeastern Regional Medical Center, Llc
600 Celebrate Life Pkwy
Newnan, GA 30265-8001
(770)400-6482
FAX: (770)400-6941

Norcross

Mri Imaging Specialist
6760 Jimmy Carter Blvd Ste 165
Norcross, GA 30071-1256
(678)969-0904
FAX: (678)969-0908

Ocilla

Irwin County Hospital
710 N Irwin Ave
Ocilla, GA 31774-5098
(229)468-3836
FAX: (229)468-3841

Peachtree City

Lifeboat Medical Associates
1201 Georgian Park
Peachtree City, GA 30269-6972
(770)631-4873
FAX: (770)631-0684

Outpatient Imaging
10 Eastbrook Bnd, Ste 100
Peachtree City, GA 30269-1545
(770)305-4674
FAX: (770)305-4682

Peachtree City Obstetrics And Gynecology, Pc
210 Clover Reach
Peachtree City, GA 30269-1657
(770)487-9604
FAX: (770)631-0540

Peachtree Corners

Northside Peachtree Corners
5277 Peachtree Pkwy
Peachtree Corners, GA 30092-2552
(678)312-3444
FAX: (678)442-9736

Perry

Perry Hospital
1120 Morningside Dr
Perry, GA 31069-2953
(478)218-1659
FAX: (478)218-1787

Pooler

St. Joseph's/Candler Pooler Campus
101 Saint Josephs Candler Dr
Pooler, GA 31322-9584
(912)819-6800
FAX: (912)330-0097

Quitman

Brooks County Hospital
903 N Court St
Quitman, GA 31643-1315
(229)263-6314
FAX: (229)263-6305

Rincon

Effingham Health System Imaging Center
110 Goshen Rd
Rincon, GA 31326-5744
(912)826-1427
FAX: (912)826-1490

Ringgold

Chi Memorial Parkway Imaging Center
4700 Battlefield Pkwy Ste 100
Ringgold, GA 30736-5167
(706)858-2166
FAX: (423)495-5048

Prime Imaging Battlefield
4632 Battlefield Pkwy
Ringgold, GA 30736-8004
(706)806-1100
FAX: (706)806-0200

Riverdale

South Atlanta Radiology Associates, P.C.
119 Upper Riverdale Rd SW
Riverdale, GA 30274-2540
(770)991-1010
FAX: (770)997-8242

Southern Regional Medical Center
11 Upper Riverdale Rd SW
Riverdale, GA 30274-2600
(770)991-8144
FAX: (770)991-8211

Rome

Northwest Georgia Medical Clinic
15 Riverbend Dr SW, Ste 200
Rome, GA 30161-6005
(706)291-0884
FAX: (706)378-8267

Redmond Regional Medical Center
501 Redmond Rd NW
Rome, GA 30165-1415
(706)802-3890
FAX: (706)802-3561

The Breast Center At Floyd Medical Center
255 West 5th St. Ste. 300
Rome, GA 30161
(706)509-6840
FAX: (706)509-6841

Roswell

Roswell Imaging Center - Wellstar North Fulton Hospital
4500 Hospital Blvd Ste 100
Roswell, GA 30076-0001
(770)751-2531
FAX: (770)751-2731

Royston

Piedmont Royston Health Campus
930 Franklin Springs St
Royston, GA 30662-3908
(706)745-5896
FAX: (706)475-5979

Saint Marys

Sghs, Inc.Dba Southeast Georgia Health System-Camden
2000 Dan Proctor Dr
Saint Marys, GA 31558-3810
(912)576-6177
FAX: (912)576-6163

Sandersville

Washington County Regional Medical Center
610 Sparta Rd
Sandersville, GA 31082-1893
(478)240-2135
FAX: (478)240-2387

Sandy Springs

Obstetrics And Gynecology Of Atlanta, P.C.
1100 Johnson Ferry Rd Ste 800, Bldg 2
Sandy Springs, GA 30342-1708
(404)252-1137
FAX: (866)912-2454

Savannah

Curtis V. Cooper Primary Health Care
106 E Broad St
Savannah, GA 31401-2917
(912)527-1122
FAX: (912)527-1123

Savannah Health Services, Llc D/B/A Memorial Health Umc
4700 Waters Ave
Savannah, GA 31404-6220
(912)350-2766
FAX: (912)350-7920

Southcoast Imaging Center
1326-B Eisenhower Dr Bldg 1
Savannah, GA 31406
(912)691-4266
FAX: (912)691-4209

St. Joseph's Candler - Mobile Mammography
5353 Reynolds St
Savannah, GA 31405-6015
(912)819-6140
FAX: (912)691-9321

St. Joseph's Hospital
11705 Mercy Blvd
Savannah, GA 31419-1791
(912)819-4114
FAX: (912)819-2517

Telfair Breast Imaging-Eisenhower
527 Eisenhower Dr
Savannah, GA 31406-2668
(912)691-1460
FAX: (912)691-1462

Telfair Pavilion
5353 Reynolds St
Savannah, GA 31405-6015
(912)819-8488
FAX: (912)691-9010

Tuttle Army Health Clinic
230 Duncan Dr
Savannah, GA 31409-5107
(912)315-6464
FAX: (912)315-2486

Smyrna

Innovative Women's Healthcare & Diagnostics Center
3200 Highlands Pkwy SE, Ste 420
Smyrna, GA 30082-5192
(678)424-1123
FAX: (678)424-1127

Wellstar -Vinings Health Park-Imaging
4441 Atlanta Rd SE
Smyrna, GA 30080-6406
(470)956-0378
FAX: (678)842-5518

Snellville

Eastside Medical Ctr - Breast And Diagnostic Ctr
1700 Tree Ln Ste 100
Snellville, GA 30078-6749
(770)736-2551
FAX: (770)736-2336

Springfield

Effingham Hospital
459 Ga Highway 119 S, Radiology Department
Springfield, GA 31329-3085
(912)754-0419
FAX: (912)754-0303

Statesboro

Out Patient Imaging
1601 Fair Rd Ste 100
Statesboro, GA 30458-0801
(912)800-4674
FAX: (912)357-6352

Statesboro Imaging Center
8 Coach Lee Hill Blvd
Statesboro, GA 30458-4786
(912)764-5656
FAX: (855)753-7307

Stockbridge

Eagle's Landing Health
1100 Hospital Dr
Stockbridge, GA 30281-6381
(404)907-6118
FAX: (678)432-3677

Eagle's Landing Ob-Gyn
350 Country Club Dr Ste D
Stockbridge, GA 30281-9084
(770)474-1919
FAX: (770)389-8090

Northside Stockbridge Women's Imaging
239 Village Center Pkwy Ste 160
Stockbridge, GA 30281-5090
(678)565-6937
FAX: (678)565-6940

Piedmont Henry Breast Health Center
1240 Eagles Landing Pkwy Ste 200
Stockbridge, GA 30281-5173
(678)289-7605
FAX: (678)289-9706

Piedmont Henry Hospital
1133 Eagles Landing Pkwy
Stockbridge, GA 30281-5085
(678)604-1055
FAX: (678)289-9706

South Atlanta Radiology Associates,P.C.
130 Eagle Spring Ct Ste D
Stockbridge, GA 30281-7252
(770)991-1010
FAX: (770)997-8242

Women's Imaging Specialists - Eagles Landing, Llc.
115 Eagle Spring Dr, Ste 100 - Lower Level
Stockbridge, GA 30281-6486
(678)904-7209
FAX: (770)507-5199

Suwanee

Obstetrics And Gynecology Of Atlanta, P.C
3890 Johns Creek Pkwy Ste 300
Suwanee, GA 30024-1286
(678)775-2300
FAX: (678)775-2359

Women's Imaging Specialists - Johns Creek, Llc
3855 Johns Creek Pkwy, Ste B
Suwanee, GA 30024-1293
(678)960-8555
FAX: (800)889-0010

Swainsboro

Emanuel Medical Center
PO Box 879, 117 Kite Rd
Swainsboro, GA 30401-0879
(478)289-1285
FAX: (478)289-1289

Thomaston

Upson Regional Medical Center
801 W Gordon St
Thomaston, GA 30286-3474
(706)647-8111
FAX: (706)647-9370

Thomasville

Archbold Women's Center
947 S Broad St
Thomasville, GA 31792-6161
(229)228-3710
FAX: (229)228-3790

Shaw Center For Women's Health, Pa
918 S Broad St, Ste 1
Thomasville, GA 31792-6166
(229)226-8800
FAX: (229)226-8232

Thomson

University Hospital McDuffie
2460 Washington Rd
Thomson, GA 30824-6600
(706)597-5359
FAX: (706)597-9512

Tifton

Tift Regional Medical Center
901 18th St E, Women's Imaging
Tifton, GA 31794-3699
(229)382-7120
FAX: (229)353-6594

Toccoa

Stephens County Hospital
163 Hospital Dr
Toccoa, GA 30577-6820
(706)282-4270
FAX: (706)282-4470

Tucker

Kaiser Permanente - Crescent Center Medical Office
200 Crescent Center Pkwy
Tucker, GA 30084-7047
(404)365-0966
FAX: (855)232-0488

Valdosta

South Georgia Medical Ctr - Imaging Ctr
2409 N Patterson St, Dept Of Radiology
Valdosta, GA 31602-2512
(229)293-3600
FAX: (229)293-3645

Southern Ob-Gyn Associates, P.C.
220 Northside Dr
Valdosta, GA 31602-1858
(229)241-2800
FAX: (229)245-0888

Southwell Ob/Gyn
814 Northwood Park Dr
Valdosta, GA 31602-1398
(229)262-6810
FAX: (229)219-1634

Vidalia

Memorial Health Meadows Hospital
1 Meadows Pkwy
Vidalia, GA 30474-8759
(912)535-5783
FAX: (912)535-5058

Memorial Health Meadows Hospital - Imaging Center
1707 Meadows Ln
Vidalia, GA 30474-7200
(912)535-7100
FAX: (912)535-7120

Villa Rica

Tanner Breast Health / Villa Rica
705 Dallas Hwy Ste 102
Villa Rica, GA 30180-1243
(770)456-3402
FAX: (770)456-3404

Warm Springs

Warm Springs Medical Center
5995 Spring St
Warm Springs, GA 31830-2149
(706)655-9204
FAX: (706)655-9217

Warner Robins

Houston Health Pavilion Diagnostic Center
233 N Houston Rd, Ste 140I Ste 140 - I
Warner Robins, GA 31093-3023
(478)329-3200
FAX: (478)975-6774

The Imaging Center
2706 Watson Blvd Ste D
Warner Robins, GA 31093-8034
(478)953-6033
FAX: (478)953-6047

Women's Imaging Specialists - Warner Robins, Llc
101 Willie Lee Pkwy, Ste 400
Warner Robins, GA 31088-9245
(478)242-3880
FAX: (800)889-0010

Watkinsville

Piedmont Oconee Health Campus
1305 Jennings Mill Rd, Ste 280
Watkinsville, GA 30677-7203
(706)475-4960
FAX: (706)475-5979

Women's Imaging Specialists - Athens, Llc.
1360 Caduceus Way, Bldg 400 Suite 101
Watkinsville, GA 30677-7300
(678)801-9862
FAX: (800)613-8386

Waycross

Memorial Satilla Health
1900 Tebeau St
Waycross, GA 31501-6357
(912)287-2650
FAX: (912)287-2653

Waynesboro

Burke Medical Center
351 S Liberty St
Waynesboro, GA 30830-9686
(706)554-4435
FAX: (706)437-8685

Winder

Northeast Georgia Medical Center Barrow
316 N Broad St, Ste 230
Winder, GA 30680-2150
(770)868-5173
FAX: (770)307-5438

Woodstock

Northside Cherokee Towne Lake Imaging
900 Towne Lake Pkwy Ste 100
Woodstock, GA 30189-1603
(404)851-6577
FAX: (770)591-1647

Wellstar Kennestone At Towne Lake Medical Imaging
120 Stonebridge Pkwy Ste 300
Woodstock, GA 30189-3769
(470)956-0895
FAX: (678)494-3542

HAWAII

Aiea

Pali Momi Women's Center
98-1005 Moanalua Rd Unit Fs2
Aiea, HI 96701-4703
(808)485-4500
FAX: (808)485-3171

Ewa Beach

The Queen's Medical Center-West Oahu
91-2141 Fort Weaver Rd
Ewa Beach, HI 96706-1993
(808)691-3663
FAX: (808)691-3804

Hilo

Kaiser Permanente Hilo Clinic
1292 Waianuenue Ave, Kaiser Permanente Hilo Clinic
Hilo, HI 96720-1228
(808)432-5100
FAX: (808)432-7340

Women's Imaging Center - Hawaii Radiologic Associates, Ltd.
82 Puuhonu Pl Ste 102
Hilo, HI 96720-2010
(808)961-4745
FAX: (808)933-2532

Honolulu

Frank J. Voralik, M.D.
1441 Kapiolani Blvd Ste 403
Honolulu, HI 96814-4497
(808)944-9144
FAX: (808)944-9444

Kaiser Moanalua Medical Center - Kaiser Permanente
3288 Moanalua Rd, Kaiser Permanente Medical Center
Honolulu, HI 96819-1469
(808)432-5100
FAX: (808)432-7340

Kaiser Permanente - Honolulu Clinic
1010 Pensacola St
Honolulu, HI 96814-2120
(808)432-5100
FAX: (808)432-7340

Kapiolani Women's Center
1907 S Beretania St
Honolulu, HI 96826-1301
(808)535-7000
FAX: (808)973-4762

Kuakini Medical Center
347 N Kuakini St
Honolulu, HI 96817-2381
(808)547-9545
FAX: (808)547-9585

Queens Physicians Office Bldg., III
550 S Beretania St, Bsmt
Honolulu, HI 96813-2414
(808)691-7171
FAX: (808)691-7079

Straub Medical Center
888 S King St
Honolulu, HI 96813-3097
(808)522-4221
FAX: (808)522-4241

Straub Medical Center - Hawaii Kai Clinic
7192 Kalanianaole Hwy Ste A200, Koko Marina Shopping Center
Honolulu, HI 96825-1845
(808)396-6321
FAX: (808)395-7160

The Queen's Medical Center
1301 Punchbowl St
Honolulu, HI 96813-2499
(808)691-7171
FAX: (808)691-7007

Kahuku

Kahuku Medical Center
56-117 Pualalea St
Kahuku, HI 96731-2052
(808)380-1426
FAX: (808)293-5584

Kahului

Maui Diagnostic Imaging
425 Koloa St Ste 102
Kahului, HI 96732-2486
(808)877-6402
FAX: (808)873-8762

Kailua

Adventist Health Castle
640 Ulukahiki St
Kailua, HI 96734-4454
(808)263-5191
FAX: (808)263-5411

Kailua Kona

Hawaii Radiologic Associates, Ltd.
75-5653 Kuakini Hwy Ste 110
Kailua Kona, HI 96740-1620
(808)329-7314
FAX: (808)329-5510

Kaiser Kona Clinic
74-517 Honokohau St
Kailua Kona, HI 96740-2715
(808)432-5100
FAX: (808)432-7340

Kamuela

North Hawaii Community Hospital, Inc.
67-1125 Mamalahoa Hwy
Kamuela, HI 96743-8496
(808)881-4881
FAX: (808)881-4841

Kaneohe

Kaiser Permanente Koolau Clinic
45-602 Kamehameha Hwy
Kaneohe, HI 96744-2098
(808)432-5100
FAX: (808)432-7340

Straub Clinic & Hospital
46-056 Kamehameha Hwy, Ste 221
Kaneohe, HI 96744-6706
(808)233-6200
FAX: (808)522-4241

Kapolei

Kaiser Permanente West Oahu Medical Office
401 Kamokila Blvd
Kapolei, HI 96707-5607
(808)432-5100
FAX: (808)432-3144

Kaunakakai

Molokai General Hospital
280 Homeolu St
Kaunakakai, HI 96748
(808)553-3132
FAX: (808)553-3135

Lihue

Wilcox Medical Center
3-3420 Kuhio Hwy, Ste B
Lihue, HI 96766-1098
(808)245-1030
FAX: (808)245-1116

Mililani

Straub Clinic & Hospital - Mililani Clinic
95-1249 Meheula Pkwy, Ste 187 Ste C2
Mililani, HI 96789-1791
(808)625-6444
FAX: (808)522-4241

Pearl Harbor

Naval Health Clinic Hawaii
480 Central Ave Bldg 1750, Mammography/Radiology Dept.
Pearl Harbor, HI 96860-4908
(808)473-1880
FAX: (808)473-0857

Schofield Barracks

Schofield Barracks Health Clinic
Bldg 685 Radiology
Schofield Barracks, HI 96857
(808)433-8355
FAX: (808)433-8505

Tripler Amc

Women's Imaging Center Tripler Army Medical Center
1 Jarrett White Rd, Dept Of Radiology McHk-Dr
Tripler Amc, HI 96859-5001
(808)433-2778
FAX: (808)433-4688

Wahiawa

Wahiawa General Hospital
128 Lehua St
Wahiawa, HI 96786-2099
(808)621-4177
FAX: (808)621-4106

Waianae

Waianae Coast Comprehensive Health Center
86-260 Farrington Hwy
Waianae, HI 96792-3199
(808)697-3327
FAX: (808)697-3454

Wailuku

Kaiser Permanente - Wailuku Clinic
80 Mahalani St
Wailuku, HI 96793-2531
(808)243-6500
FAX: (808)432-7340

Maui Health System
221 Mahalani St
Wailuku, HI 96793-2526
(808)242-3012
FAX: (808)242-1940

Maui Medical Group
2180 Main St
Wailuku, HI 96793-1625
(808)243-2390
FAX: (808)243-2352

Waimea

Kauai Veterans Memorial Hospital
PO Box 337, 4643 Waimea Canyon Rd
Waimea, HI 96796-0337
(808)338-9435
FAX: (808)338-9480

Waipahu

Hawaii Diagnostic Radiology Services, Llc
94-229 Waipahu Depot St Ste 308
Waipahu, HI 96797-3033
(808)949-0091
FAX: (808)957-0005

Kaiser Permanente Waipio Clinic
94-1480 Moaniani St, X-Ray Department
Waipahu, HI 96797-4632
(808)432-5100
FAX: (808)432-7340

IDAHO

Blackfoot

Bingham Memorial Hospital
98 Poplar St, Radiology Department
Blackfoot, ID 83221-1799
(208)785-3807
FAX: (208)785-3811

Blackfoot Medical Center- An Affiliate Of Mountain View Hosp
1441 Parkway Dr
Blackfoot, ID 83221-1667
(208)785-8145
FAX: (208)785-1762

Boise

Saint Alphonsus R.M.C. Breast Care Center
6200 W Emerald St, Breast Care Center
Boise, ID 83704-8730
(208)367-8787
FAX: (208)367-3390

Saint Alphonsus Rmc Mobile Health Screening Unit - Mobile
6200 W Emerald St, Saint Alphonsus Breast Care Center
Boise, ID 83704-8730
(208)367-8787
FAX: (208)367-3390

St. Lukes Breast Cancer Detection Center - Rifleman
8050 W Rifleman St Ste 300
Boise, ID 83704-9012
(208)706-2055
FAX: (208)381-2165

St. Lukes Breast Cancer Detection Center- East Office
247 W Washington St
Boise, ID 83702-5941
(208)706-2055
FAX: (208)381-2165

St. Lukes Regional Medical Center For Breast Imaging
190 E Bannock St
Boise, ID 83712-6241
(208)706-2055
FAX: (208)381-2165

Womens Health Associates Pllc
333 N 1st St, Ste 240
Boise, ID 83702-6132
(208)338-8900
FAX: (877)207-1070

Bonners Ferry

Boundary Community Hospital
6640 Kaniksu St
Bonners Ferry, ID 83805-7532
(208)267-3141
FAX: (208)267-7167

Burley

Cassia Regional Medical Center
1501 Hiland Ave, Ste Frnt
Burley, ID 83318-2682
(208)677-6515
FAX: (208)677-6313

Caldwell

Imaging Center Of Idaho
4519 Enterprise Way, Ste 101
Caldwell, ID 83605-8060
(208)455-7482
FAX: (208)455-7538

West Valley Medical Center
1717 Arlington Ave
Caldwell, ID 83605-4800
(208)455-3905
FAX: (208)455-3945

Coeur D Alene

N. Idaho Imaging Ctr Llc Dba Kootenai Outpatient Imaging
700 W Ironwood Dr Ste 175
Coeur D Alene, ID 83814-4401
(208)625-6300
FAX: (208)625-6301

Driggs

Teton Valley Health Care, Inc.
120 E Howard St
Driggs, ID 83422-5112
(208)354-6313
FAX: (208)354-6308

Eagle

Breast Care Ctr At Eagle Health Plaza
323 E Riverside Dr Ste 132
Eagle, ID 83616-6864
(208)367-8787
FAX: (208)367-3390

St. Luke's Breast Cancer Detection Center - Eagle
3101 E State St Ste 2101
Eagle, ID 83616-6232
(208)706-2055
FAX: (208)381-2165

Fruitland

St. Luke's Breast Cancer Detection Center - Fruitland
909 NW 16th St Ste C
Fruitland, ID 83619-2274
(208)706-2055
FAX: (208)381-2165

Gooding

North Canyon Medical Center
267 N Canyon Dr
Gooding, ID 83330-5500
(208)934-4433
FAX: (208)934-9662

Idaho Falls

Eastern Idaho Women's Imaging
2860 Channing Way Ste 121
Idaho Falls, ID 83404-7532
(208)227-2612
FAX: (208)535-4547

Mountain View Hospital
2325 Coronado St
Idaho Falls, ID 83404-7407
(208)557-2864
FAX: (208)542-7336

Teton Radiology Diagnostics, Llc Dba Teton Radiology
2001 S Woodruff Ave Ste 17
Idaho Falls, ID 83404-6372
(208)524-7237
FAX: (208)522-3017

Jerome

St. Luke's Jerome
709 N Lincoln Ave
Jerome, ID 83338-1851
(208)814-9733
FAX: (208)814-9592

Kellogg

Shoshone Medical Center
25 Jacobs Gulch Rd
Kellogg, ID 83837-2023
(208)784-1384
FAX: (208)784-8761

Ketchum

St. Luke's Wood River Women's Imaging Center
PO Box 1 100 Hospital Dr Pob Ste 202
Ketchum, ID 83340-0001
(208)727-8190
FAX: (208)727-8195

Lewiston

Catalyst Medical Group,Pllc
2315 8th St
Lewiston, ID 83501-7301
(208)746-1383
FAX: (208)298-4531

St. Joseph Breast Imaging Center
1630 23rd Ave Ste 601
Lewiston, ID 83501-6358
(208)799-6505
FAX: (208)799-0673

St. Joseph Regional Medical Center
415 6th St
Lewiston, ID 83501-2434
(208)799-5335
FAX: (208)798-0673

McCall

St. Luke's McCall Medical Center
1000 State St
McCall, ID 83638-3704
(208)630-2260
FAX: (208)634-3218

Meridian

St Luke's Breast Cancer Detection Ctr-Meadowlake
3525 E Louise Dr Ste 320
Meridian, ID 83642-6303
(208)706-2055
FAX: (208)381-2165

St. Luke's Meridian Med Ctr For Breast Imaging
520 S Eagle Rd
Meridian, ID 83642-6351
(208)706-2055
FAX: (208)706-5673

Montpelier

Bear Lake Memorial Hospital
164 S 5th St
Montpelier, ID 83254-1597
(208)847-1630
FAX: (208)847-2201

Moscow

Women's Imaging Center
700 S Main St
Moscow, ID 83843-3056
(208)882-5377
FAX: (208)883-6583

Mountain Home

St. Luke's Breast Cancer Detection Ctr At Elmore Medical Ctr
895 N 6th E
Mountain Home, ID 83647-2207
(208)706-2055
FAX: (208)381-2165

Mountain Home Afb

366 Medical Treatment Facility/Diagnostic Imaging
90 Hope Dr Bldg 6000, 366 Medical Group Acc /Rad Dept Sgsq
Mountain Home Afb, ID 83648-1062
(208)828-7810
FAX: (208)828-3793

Nampa

Saint Alphonsus Nampa Breast Care Center
4400 E Flamingo Ave
Nampa, ID 83687-9203
(208)367-8787
FAX: (208)205-0635

St. Luke's Nampa Breast Care Services
9850 W St Lukes Dr
Nampa, ID 83687-7912
(208)706-2055
FAX: (208)381-2165

Pocatello

Idaho Medical Imaging Portneuf Medical Center
1151 Hospital Way Bldg B
Pocatello, ID 83201-5091
(208)239-1500
FAX: (208)239-2750

Portneuf Medical Center
777 Hospital Way, Ste 300
Pocatello, ID 83201-5176
(208)239-1560
FAX: (208)239-3718

Post Falls

Kootenai Outpatient Imaging Center
1300 E Mullan Ave Ste 700, Kmc Health Park
Post Falls, ID 83854-6054
(208)625-6307
FAX: (208)625-6307

Preston

Franklin County Medical Center
44 N 1st E
Preston, ID 83263-1326
(208)852-4123
FAX: (208)852-3240

Rexburg

Teton Radiology Madison
425 E 4th N
Rexburg, ID 83440-5390
(208)524-7237
FAX: (208)522-3017

Rupert

Minidoka Memorial Hospital
1224 8th St, Radiology Dept.
Rupert, ID 83350-1599
(208)436-8143
FAX: (208)436-8015

Salmon

Steele Memorial Medical Center
203 S Daisy St
Salmon, ID 83467-4709
(208)756-5641
FAX: (208)756-5743

Sandpoint

Bonner General Health
423 N Third Ave
Sandpoint, ID 83864-1511
(208)265-3349
FAX: (208)265-3348

St Maries

Benewah Community Hospital
229 S 7th St
St Maries, ID 83861-1894
(208)245-7631
FAX: (208)245-2471

Twin Falls

St Luke's Magic Valley Womens Imaging
762 N College Rd
Twin Falls, ID 83301-5392
(208)814-7210
FAX: (208)814-7222

ILLINOIS

Addison

Alexian Bros. Immediate Care Center
1339 W Lake St
Addison, IL 60101-1836
(877)717-7700
FAX: (847)590-2634

Elmhurst Memorial Addison Center For Health
303 W Lake St
Addison, IL 60101-2586
(331)221-3511
FAX: (331)221-3701

Aledo

Genesis Medical Center - Aledo
409 NW 9th Ave
Aledo, IL 61231-1258
(309)582-9140
FAX: (309)582-9149

Algonquin

Advocate Sherman Outpatient Center - Algonquin
600 S Randall Rd
Algonquin, IL 60102-5935
(224)783-8972
FAX: (224)783-2960

Alton

Alton Memorial Hospital
1 Memorial Dr
Alton, IL 62002-6755
(618)463-7426
FAX: (618)463-7420

Alton Multispecialists Physicians
1 Professional Dr
Alton, IL 62002-5068
(618)463-8530
FAX: (618)463-8536

Brightway Imaging
3 Professional Dr Ste A
Alton, IL 62002-5011
(618)465-4674
FAX: (618)465-4676

OSF Saint Anthony's Health Center
1 Saint Anthonys Way, Saint Anthony's Way
Alton, IL 62002-4579
(618)465-4520
FAX: (618)465-4529

Anna

Anna Hospital Corp Dba Union County Hospital
517 N Main St
Anna, IL 62906-1668
(618)833-4511
FAX: (618)833-5106

Arlington Heights

Arlington Heights Health Center
3250 N Arlington Heights Rd
Arlington Heights, IL 60004-1563
(847)506-4010
FAX: (847)934-9243

Nch Breast Center At Arlington Heights Road
1410 N Arlington Heights Rd
Arlington Heights, IL 60004-4822
(847)618-2760
FAX: (847)618-2769

Northwest Community Hospital
800 W Central Rd, Radiology Department
Arlington Heights, IL 60005-2349
(847)618-3700
FAX: (847)618-5888

Aurora

Dreyer Clinic, Inc
1221 N Highland Ave
Aurora, IL 60506-1404
(630)859-6777
FAX: (630)264-8522

Presence Mercy Medical Center
1325 N Highland Ave
Aurora, IL 60506-1449
(630)801-2505
FAX: (630)801-5669

Vna Health Care
400 N Highland Ave
Aurora, IL 60506-3814
(630)978-2532
FAX: (630)801-8933

Barrington

Good Shepherd Hospital Breast Care Center
450 W Il Route 22, Breast Care Center
Barrington, IL 60010-1999
(847)842-4130
FAX: (847)842-4804

Bartlett

St. Alexius Breast Care Center At Bartlett
1041 W Stearns Rd
Bartlett, IL 60103-4509
(877)717-7700
FAX: (847)252-8804

Bedford Park

Bright Light Medcial Imaging
7456 S State Rd Ste 100
Bedford Park, IL 60638-6625
(708)930-1420
FAX: (708)924-1214

Belleville

Hshs Imaging Center, Belleville
180 S 3rd St, Ste 101
Belleville, IL 62220-1952
(618)222-4639
FAX: (618)222-4626

Memorial Hospital
4500 Memorial Dr
Belleville, IL 62226-5399
(618)257-4949
FAX: (618)624-4862

Belvidere

Samc - Belvidere
1625 S State St
Belvidere, IL 61008-5907
(779)696-7676
FAX: (779)696-5561

Benton

Franklin Hospital
201 Bailey Ln
Benton, IL 62812-1999
(618)439-3161
FAX: (618)435-3999

Berwyn

Gottlieb Community Health Services Corporation D/B/A Macneal
3249 Oak Park Ave
Berwyn, IL 60402-3429
(708)216-1065
FAX: (708)783-0769

Bloomingdale

Dupage Medical Group At Stratford
220 Springfield Dr, Ste 110
Bloomingdale, IL 60108-2215
(630)545-7880
FAX: (630)539-6067

Nm Cdh Diagnostic Imaging-Bloomingdale
235 S Gary Ave
Bloomingdale, IL 60108-2213
(630)933-5000
FAX: (630)933-5800

Bloomington

Carle Bromenn Med Ctr/Carle Bromenn OP Ctr
3024 E Empire St
Bloomington, IL 61704-5402
(309)268-5705
FAX: (309)268-5915

OSF - Sjmc College Ave Imaging Services
1701 E College Ave
Bloomington, IL 61704-2100
(309)664-3272
FAX: (309)664-3496

OSF St. Joseph Medical Center
2200 E Washington St
Bloomington, IL 61701-4364
(309)665-5160
FAX: (309)662-5512

Blue Island

Blue Island Medical Clinic
12757 Western Ave
Blue Island, IL 60406-2155
(312)864-0413
FAX: (708)864-9512

Dupage Medical Group Blue Island
2320 High St
Blue Island, IL 60406-2426
(708)388-5500
FAX: (708)293-3086

Bolingbrook

Edward Hospital Radiology Bolingbrook
130 N Weber Rd
Bolingbrook, IL 60440-1518
(630)527-3200
FAX: (630)548-1884

Womens Imaging Ctr Amita Health Adventist Medical Center Bol
396 Remington Blvd, Ste 235
Bolingbrook, IL 60440-4304
(630)312-5464
FAX: (630)312-6856

Bourbonnais

Amita Health Medical Imaging Bourbonnais
100 Provena Way Ste 104
Bourbonnais, IL 60914-4797
(815)937-3089
FAX: (815)929-5801

Riverside Medical Center Bourbonnais Plaza
300 Riverside Dr
Bourbonnais, IL 60914-4996
(815)935-7525
FAX: (815)928-6265

Breese

St. Joseph's Hospital
9515 Holy Cross Ln
Breese, IL 62230-3618
(618)526-4511
FAX: (618)526-0556

Buffalo Grove

Northwest Community Healthcare - Treatment Center
15 S McHenry Rd
Buffalo Grove, IL 60089-6705
(847)618-3700
FAX: (847)618-3709

Burr Ridge

Loyola Center For Health At Burr Ridge
6800 N Frontage Rd
Burr Ridge, IL 60527-7819
(708)216-8563
FAX: (708)216-6207

Cairo

Cairo Diagnostic Center
13289 Kessler Rd
Cairo, IL 62914-3101
(618)734-1500
FAX: (618)731-4258

Calumet City

Ingalls Family Care Center
1600 Torrence Ave
Calumet City, IL 60409-5435
(708)915-8442
FAX: (708)915-2755

Canton

Graham Hospital
210 W Walnut St
Canton, IL 61520-2497
(309)649-5140
FAX: (309)649-5121

Carbondale

The Breast Center
1237 E Main St, Ste C1
Carbondale, IL 62901-3148
(618)457-2281
FAX: (618)529-0572

Carlinville

Carlinville Area Hospital
20733 N Broad St, Radiology Department
Carlinville, IL 62626-1499
(217)854-3141
FAX: (217)854-3804

Carol Stream

Molecular Imaging Chicago
640 E Saint Charles Rd, Ste 106
Carol Stream, IL 60188-2600
(630)462-0793
FAX: (630)462-1376

Carrollton

Thomas H. Boyd Memorial Hospital
800 School St
Carrollton, IL 62016-1498
(217)942-6946
FAX: (217)942-5021

Carthage

Memorial Hospital
PO Box 160, 1454 Ncr 2050
Carthage, IL 62321-0160
(217)357-8660
FAX: (217)357-8663

Centralia

Ssm Health St. Mary's Hospital
400 N Pleasant Ave
Centralia, IL 62801-3098
(618)436-7003
FAX: (618)436-8020

Centreville

Touchette Regional Hospital
5900 Bond Ave
Centreville, IL 62207-2397
(618)332-5462
FAX: (618)332-5409

Champaign

Christie Clinic
101 W University Ave
Champaign, IL 61820-3981
(217)366-1285
FAX: (217)366-5645

Christie Clinic
1801 W Windsor Rd, Ste A
Champaign, IL 61822-6218
(217)366-1285
FAX: (217)366-6129

Channahon

Morris Hospital Ridge Rd Campus
27240 W Saxony Dr
Channahon, IL 60410-1416
(815)942-2932
FAX: (815)941-1568

Chester

Memorial Hospital
1900 State St, Radiology Department
Chester, IL 62233-1116
(618)826-4581
FAX: (618)826-3361

Chicago

Advocate Illinois Masonic Medical Center
3000 N Halsted St Ste 220 - Moc
Chicago, IL 60657-5190
(773)296-3000
FAX: (773)296-3020

Advocate Medical Group - Irving And Western
4025 N Western Ave
Chicago, IL 60618-3726
(773)279-6535
FAX: (773)279-6791

Advocate Medical Group - Sykes
2535 S. Martin Luther King Dr.
Chicago, IL 60616
(312)674-5094
FAX: (312)842-1948

Advocate Medical Group-Beverly
9831 S Western Ave
Chicago, IL 60643-1740
(773)445-3500
FAX: (773)298-2865

Advocate Trinity Hospital
2320 E 93rd St
Chicago, IL 60617-3982
(773)967-1000
FAX: (773)967-3954

Amita Health Saints Mary And Elizabeth Medical Center
2233 W Division St, Radiology Department - Mammography
Chicago, IL 60622-8151
(312)770-3006
FAX: (312)770-2161

Community First Medical Center
5645 W Addison St, Radiology Department
Chicago, IL 60634-2881
(773)794-7678
FAX: (773)794-7694

Diagnostic Imaging Specialists Of Chicago
60 E Delaware Pl Ste 1410
Chicago, IL 60611-6559
(312)867-9000
FAX: (312)867-9127

Dr. Jorge Prieto Family Health Center
2424 S Pulaski Rd
Chicago, IL 60623-3718
(312)864-0413
FAX: (312)864-9512

Edgebrook Radiology Management Services Inc.
5320 W Devon Ave
Chicago, IL 60646-4108
(773)774-6440
FAX: (773)774-4372

Holy Cross Hospital
2701 W 68th St
Chicago, IL 60629-1882
(773)257-4040
FAX: (773)884-8061

Humboldt Park Health
1044 N Francisco Ave, Radiology Department
Chicago, IL 60622-2743
(773)292-8200
FAX: (773)278-8871

Jackson Park Hospital And Medical Center
7531 S Stony Island Ave
Chicago, IL 60649-3993
(773)947-7990
FAX: (773)947-7895

John H. Stroger Jr. Hospital Of Cook County
1901 W Harrison St, Radiology Dept.
Chicago, IL 60612-3714
(312)864-3809
FAX: (312)864-9889

Lavillita Clinic Radiology
3303 W 26th St
Chicago, IL 60623-4036
(773)257-2407
FAX: (773)257-5726

Loretto Hospital
645 S Central Ave, Department Of Radiology
Chicago, IL 60644-5059
(773)854-5225
FAX: (773)626-1309

Mercy Family Health Center At Oakwood Shores
3753 S Cottage Grove Ave
Chicago, IL 60653-1662
(312)567-2273
FAX: (312)567-6157

Mercy Hospital And Medical Center
2525 S Michigan Ave, 12th Fl. Breast Center
Chicago, IL 60616-2332
(312)567-2273
FAX: (312)567-6157

Mount Sinai Hospital
1500 S Fairfield Ave
Chicago, IL 60608-1782
(773)257-4040
FAX: (773)257-2666

Northshore At 680
680 N Lake Shore Dr Ste 115
Chicago, IL 60611-4495
(847)926-5070
FAX: (847)926-5320

Northwestern Mem Hosp Lynn Sage Comprehensive Ctr.
250 E Superior St, Prentice 4th Fl
Chicago, IL 60611-2914
(312)926-5522
FAX: (312)472-0498

Northwestern Memorial Hospital Bucktown Radiology
1776 N Milwaukee Ave
Chicago, IL 60647-5453
(312)926-0026
FAX: (312)926-8326

Northwestern Memorial Hospital Lakeview Imaging
1333 W Belmont Ave
Chicago, IL 60657-5785
(312)926-0026
FAX: (312)472-0498

Provident Hospital Of Cook County
500 E 51st St
Chicago, IL 60615-2494
(312)864-3809
FAX: (312)864-9889

Regenstein Breast Imaging Center
1725 W Harrison St, Professional Building I - Suite 717
Chicago, IL 60612-3841
(312)942-2027
FAX: (312)563-3272

Resurrection Medical Center Women's Imaging Center
7435 W Talcott Ave
Chicago, IL 60631-3707
(773)792-5556
FAX: (773)792-5124

Roseland Community Hospital
45 W 111th St
Chicago, IL 60628-4294
(773)995-3052
FAX: (773)995-6710

Rush Breast Imaging-South Loop
1411 S Michigan Ave, 4th Floor-Mammography Dept
Chicago, IL 60605-2810
(312)942-2027
FAX: (312)563-3272

Saint Joseph Hospital Amita Health - Chicago
2900 N Lake Shore Dr
Chicago, IL 60657-6274
(773)665-3827
FAX: (773)665-6228

Solis Mammography
355 E Grand Ave, Ste 202
Chicago, IL 60611-5389
(773)786-1811
FAX: (773)786-1811

South Shore Hospital
8012 S Crandon Ave
Chicago, IL 60617-1175
(773)356-5399
FAX: (773)768-8690

St. Anthony Hospital
2875 W 19th St
Chicago, IL 60623-3596
(773)484-4100
FAX: (773)521-1632

St. Bernard Ambulatory Care Center
6307 S Stewart Ave
Chicago, IL 60621-3116
(773)962-4030
FAX: (773)962-4399

Swedish Covenant Hospital
5145 N California Ave, Dept. Of Radiology
Chicago, IL 60625-3687
(773)878-8200
FAX: (773)878-5884

Thorek Hospital & Medical Center
850 W Irving Park Rd
Chicago, IL 60613-3099
(773)975-6775
FAX: (773)975-6741

Union Health Service, Inc.
1634 W Polk St
Chicago, IL 60612-4352
(312)423-4223
FAX: (312)423-4324

University Of Chicago Medicine
5758 S Maryland Ave, Duchossois Ctr For Advanced Medicine
Chicago, IL 60637-1426
(773)834-3443
FAX: (773)834-3443

University Of Illinois Hospital & Health Sciences System
1801 W Taylor St Ste 2-C, Mammography
Chicago, IL 60612-4795
(312)996-0267
FAX: (312)413-3328

University Of Illinois Hospital And Health Sciences System
1220 S Wood St
Chicago, IL 60608-1202
(312)996-0267
FAX: (312)413-3328

Weiss Memorial Hospital
4646 N Marine Dr
Chicago, IL 60640-5759
(773)564-7777
FAX: (773)564-5152

Clinton

Warner Hospital & Health Services
422 W White St
Clinton, IL 61727-2272
(217)937-5246
FAX: (217)937-5292

Coal City

Riverside Medical Center West Campus
5775 E State Route 113
Coal City, IL 60416-7111
(815)935-7525
FAX: (815)928-6265

Crystal Lake

Advocate Good Shepherd OP Ctr - Crystal Lake
525 E Congress Pkwy
Crystal Lake, IL 60014-6245
(815)479-7380
FAX: (815)479-7390

Northwestern Medicine Gavers Breast Center
360 N Terra Cotta Rd
Crystal Lake, IL 60012-3749
(815)334-5566
FAX: (815)356-7124

Danville

OSF Sacred Heart Medical Center
812 N Logan Ave
Danville, IL 61832-3752
(217)443-5273
FAX: (217)431-5594

The Carle Foundation Hospital
311 W Fairchild St
Danville, IL 61832-3876
(217)431-7730
FAX: (217)554-1890

Darien

Bright Light Medical Imaging, Darien
7372 Route 83
Darien, IL 60561-4283
(630)455-5552
FAX: (630)455-1090

Decatur

Decatur Memorial Hospital
2300 N Edward St, Radiology Department
Decatur, IL 62526-4192
(217)876-1111
FAX: (217)876-2335

South Shores Imaging Center
1689 S Franklin Street Rd
Decatur, IL 62521-4018
(217)876-1111
FAX: (217)876-5065

St Marys Health Center
2965 N Main
Decatur, IL 62521
(217)464-2984
FAX: (217)464-1631

St. Mary's Hospital
1800 E Lake Shore Dr, Radiology Department
Decatur, IL 62521-3883
(217)464-2976
FAX: (217)464-1631

Dekalb

Northwestern Medicine Kish Hospital Breast Health Center
5 Kish Hospital Dr, Ste 102
Dekalb, IL 60115-9602
(815)766-7521
FAX: (815)766-9754

Des Plaines

Advocate Outpatient Center
77 Rand Rd
Des Plaines, IL 60016-1005
(847)460-7412
FAX: (847)460-7344

Amita Health Holy Family Medical Center Des Plaines
100 N River Rd, Women's Imaging Center
Des Plaines, IL 60016-1209
(847)813-3200
FAX: (847)813-3201

Midwest Advanced Radiology Center
9680 Golf Rd
Des Plaines, IL 60016-1522
(847)296-5366
FAX: (847)296-0067

Diamond

Morris Hospital Diamond Coal City Campus
1450 E Division St
Diamond, IL 60416-6050
(815)705-7131
FAX: (815)941-1568

Dixon

Katherine Shaw Bethea Hospital
403 E 1st St
Dixon, IL 61021-3187
(815)284-5700
FAX: (815)285-5623

Downers Grove

Advocate Good Samaritan OP Ctr Downers Grove
6840 Main St, Ste 202
Downers Grove, IL 60516-3451
(630)275-5562
FAX: (630)275-5770

Good Samaritan Hospital-Advocate
3815 Highland Ave
Downers Grove, IL 60515-1590
(630)275-5562
FAX: (630)275-5770

Du Quoin

Marshall Browning Hospital
900 N Washington St
Du Quoin, IL 62832-1233
(618)542-2146
FAX: (618)542-4790

Edwardsville

Edwardsville Imaging Center
1261 University Dr
Edwardsville, IL 62025-5586
(618)659-9520
FAX: (618)307-3411

Effingham

Hshs St.Anthony's Womens Wellness Center
900 W Temple Ave, Ste 108 Ste 2100
Effingham, IL 62401-2186
(217)347-1540
FAX: (217)347-1792

St. Anthony's Mammography At Effingham Ob/Gyn
912 N Henrietta St
Effingham, IL 62401-1788
(217)347-1540
FAX: (217)347-1792

Eldorado

Ferrell Hospital
1201 Pine St
Eldorado, IL 62930-1634
(618)273-3361
FAX: (618)273-3602

Elgin

Advocate Sherman Hospital
1425 N Randall Rd
Elgin, IL 60123-2300
(224)783-8972
FAX: (224)783-2960

Advocate Sherman Imaging Center - Randall
1710 N Randall Rd, Ste 180
Elgin, IL 60123-9403
(224)783-8972
FAX: (224)783-2960

Amita Health St. Joseph Hospital Elgin
77 N Airlite St
Elgin, IL 60123-4912
(847)695-3200
FAX: (847)608-5187

Elk Grove Village

Alexian Brothers Medical Center - Women's Ctr
800 Biesterfield Rd
Elk Grove Village, IL 60007-3396
(877)717-7700
FAX: (847)590-2634

Bright Light Medical Imaging
31 Arlington Heights Rd
Elk Grove Village, IL 60007-1405
(847)439-2315
FAX: (847)439-3935

Elmhurst

Elmhurst Memorial Center For Health
1200 S York St, Ste 1250
Elmhurst, IL 60126-5627
(331)221-0005
FAX: (331)221-3701

Eureka

Carle Eureka Hospital
101 S Major St
Eureka, IL 61530-1278
(309)467-2371
FAX: (309)467-4831

Evanston

Breast Center Of St. Francis Hospital
800 Austin St Ste 551, East Tower
Evanston, IL 60202-3456
(847)316-3011
FAX: (847)316-2445

Northshore Evanston Hospital
2650 Ridge Ave Ste 1155
Evanston, IL 60201-1797
(547)570-2325
FAX: (847)570-2942

Evergreen Park

OSF Healthcare Little Company Of Mary Medical Center
2800 W 95th St
Evergreen Park, IL 60805-2701
(708)229-5621
FAX: (708)422-9659

Fairfield

Fairfield Memorial Hospital
303 NW 11th St
Fairfield, IL 62837-1206
(618)847-8249
FAX: (618)847-8375

Flora

Clay County Hospital
911 Stacey Burk Dr
Flora, IL 62839-3241
(618)844-3059
FAX: (618)662-1489

Flossmoor

Ingalls Family Care Center Flossmoor
19550 Governors Hwy
Flossmoor, IL 60422-2125
(708)915-8442
FAX: (708)915-2752

Forsyth

Forsyth Imaging Center
389 W Weaver Rd, Ste 1
Forsyth, IL 62535-9803
(217)876-1111
FAX: (217)876-5345

Freeport

Fhn Memorial Hospital
1045 W Stephenson St
Freeport, IL 61032-4899
(815)599-6363
FAX: (815)599-6141

Monroe Clinic Highland Womens Care
3103 W Kunkle Blvd
Freeport, IL 61032-6922
(815)233-0999
FAX: (815)233-7255

Galena

Midwest Medical Center
1 Medical Center Dr
Galena, IL 61036-8118
(815)777-6135
FAX: (815)777-1565

Galesburg

Galesburg Cottage Hospital
695 N Kellogg St
Galesburg, IL 61401-2885
(309)345-4219
FAX: (309)345-4523

OSF St. Mary Medical Ctr
3333 N Seminary St
Galesburg, IL 61401-1299
(309)344-3161
FAX: (309)344-9750

Geneseo

Hammond Henry Hospital
600 N College Ave
Geneseo, IL 61254-1099
(309)944-9135
FAX: (309)944-9286

Geneva

Center For Diagnostic Imaging
1416C S Randall Rd., Ste. C1
Geneva, IL 60134
(630)208-9325
FAX: (630)208-9326

The Delnor Center For Breast Health
300 Randall Rd
Geneva, IL 60134-4200
(630)933-5000
FAX: (630)933-5800

Gibson City

Gibson Area Hospital & Health Services
1120 N Melvin St
Gibson City, IL 60936-1477
(217)784-2682
FAX: (217)784-2676

Glen Ellyn

Dupage Medical Group- Glen Ellyn
430 Pennsylvania Ave, Ste 110
Glen Ellyn, IL 60137-4464
(630)545-7880
FAX: (630)545-7841

Nm Cdh Diagnostic Imaging - Glen Ellyn
885 Roosevelt Rd
Glen Ellyn, IL 60137-6141
(630)933-5000
FAX: (630)384-6230

Glendale Heights

Amita Health Adventist Medical Center, Glenoaks
701 Winthrop Ave
Glendale Heights, IL 60139-1405
(630)545-8200
FAX: (630)545-8240

Glenview

Northshore Glenbrook Hospital
2050 Pfingsten Rd, Ste 330 Ste 130
Glenview, IL 60026-1300
(847)926-5070
FAX: (847)926-5320

Northwestern Medicine Imaging Center At Glenview
2701 Patriot Blvd Ste 175
Glenview, IL 60026-8039
(847)535-7796
FAX: (847)998-9882

Granite City

Gateway Regional Medical Center
2100 Madison Ave
Granite City, IL 62040-4713
(618)876-2255
FAX: (618)798-3744

Grayslake

Northwestern Grayslake
1475 E Belvidere Rd Dept 1069
Grayslake, IL 60030-2085
(847)535-8000
FAX: (847)535-8001

Northwestern Lake Forest Hospital
1475 E Belvidere Rd Ste 284
Grayslake, IL 60030-2015
(847)535-8000
FAX: (847)535-8001

Greenville

Hshs Holy Family Hospital, Inc.
200 Health Care Dr, Diagnostic Imaging Department
Greenville, IL 62246-1154
(618)664-1230
FAX: (618)664-9678

Gurnee

Advocate Condell Medical Center
1435 N Hunt Club Rd
Gurnee, IL 60031-2656
(847)990-6000
FAX: (847)599-7372

Northshore - Gurnee - Rollins Rd
7900 Rollins Rd
Gurnee, IL 60031-1512
(847)926-5070
FAX: (847)926-5320

Northwestern Medicine Lake Forest Hospital Gurnee Imaging
6155 Grand Ave, Ste 101
Gurnee, IL 60031-1651
(847)535-8000
FAX: (847)535-8415

Vista Imaging Ctr - Gurnee A Dept Of Vista Medical Ctr E.
95 N Greenleaf St
Gurnee, IL 60031-3309
(847)360-4187
FAX: (847)782-3895

Harrisburg

Harrisburg Medical Center, Inc.
100 Dr Warren Tuttle Dr
Harrisburg, IL 62946-2718
(618)253-0222
FAX: (618)253-0468

Harvey

Ingalls Hospital
1 Ingalls Dr Ste 100, Professional Office Building
Harvey, IL 60426-3591
(708)915-5987
FAX: (708)915-2755

Havana

Mason District Hospital
615 N Promenade St, Ste 1
Havana, IL 62644-1274
(309)543-8596
FAX: (309)543-8539

Hazel Crest

Advocate South Suburban Hospital
17800 Kedzie Ave
Hazel Crest, IL 60429-0989
(708)213-1000
FAX: (708)213-0108

Highland

St. Joseph Hospital
12866 Troxler Ave
Highland, IL 62249-1698
(618)651-2790
FAX: (618)651-2795

Highland Park

Northshore Highland Park Hospital
777 Park Ave W Ste B400
Highland Park, IL 60035-2497
(847)570-2325
FAX: (847)926-5320

Hillsboro

Hillsboro Area Hospital
1200 E Tremont St
Hillsboro, IL 62049-1900
(217)532-4196
FAX: (217)532-4428

Hinsdale

Amita Health Cancer Institute & Outpatient Center
1 Salt Creek Ln
Hinsdale, IL 60521-2936
(630)286-5719
FAX: (630)286-5974

Dupage Medical Group Hinsdale
40 S Clay St, Suite Ll10, West Building
Hinsdale, IL 60521-3257
(630)545-7880
FAX: (630)348-3018

Edward-Elmhurst Health Center/Hinsdale
8 Salt Creek Ln
Hinsdale, IL 60521-2903
(331)221-0005
FAX: (331)221-3701

Hoffman Estates

The Breast Care Center At St. Alexius Medical Center
1555 Barrington Rd, Dob 3 Ste 1600
Hoffman Estates, IL 60169-1099
(877)717-7700
FAX: (847)252-8804

Hoopeston

Hoopeston Community Memorial Hospital
701 E Orange St
Hoopeston, IL 60942-1801
(217)383-3270
FAX: (217)383-4015

Hopedale

Hopedale Medical Complex
107 Tremont St
Hopedale, IL 61747-7525
(309)449-4230
FAX: (309)449-6014

Huntley

Advocate Outpatient Center Radiology
13900 Quality Dr
Huntley, IL 60142-8098
(847)961-7800
FAX: (847)961-7811

Northwestern Medicine Huntley Medical Office Building 1
10350 Haligus Rd
Huntley, IL 60142-9545
(815)334-5566
FAX: (847)802-7113

Jacksonville

Passavant Memorial Area Hospital
1600 W Walnut St
Jacksonville, IL 62650-1199
(217)479-2996
FAX: (217)479-5751

Jerseyville

Jersey Community Hospital
400 Maple Summit Rd
Jerseyville, IL 62052-2028
(618)498-8383
FAX: (618)498-8315

Joliet

Amita St. Joseph Medical Center
333 Madison St
Joliet, IL 60435-8200
(815)725-7133
FAX: (815)773-7759

Dupage Medical Group Joliet
2100 Glenwood Ave, Frnt
Joliet, IL 60435-5488
(630)545-7880
FAX: (815)730-6391

Future Diagnostics Group
254 Republic Ave
Joliet, IL 60435-6518
(815)730-3344
FAX: (815)730-3888

Primary Care Physicians Of Joliet Sc
2025 S Chicago St
Joliet, IL 60436-3172
(815)726-2200
FAX: (815)727-5815

Kankakee

Presence St. Mary's Hospital
500 W Court St
Kankakee, IL 60901-3691
(815)937-3475
FAX: (815)937-2468

Riverside Healthcare
350 N Wall St
Kankakee, IL 60901-2991
(815)935-7531
FAX: (815)928-6265

Kewanee

OSF Saint Luke Medical Center
1051 W South St
Kewanee, IL 61443-8354
(309)852-7550
FAX: (309)852-7836

Kildeer

Northwest Community Hospital
21481 N Rand Rd
Kildeer, IL 60047-3061
(847)618-2750
FAX: (847)618-2759

Lake Zurich

Advocate Good Shepherd OP Ctr-Lake Zurich
350 Surryse Rd Ste 140
Lake Zurich, IL 60047-3217
(847)842-4380
FAX: (847)842-4804

Lawrenceville

Lawrence County Memorial Hospital
2200 State St
Lawrenceville, IL 62439-1899
(618)943-7221
FAX: (618)943-7240

Libertyville

Advocate Condell Medical Center
801 S Milwaukee Ave
Libertyville, IL 60048-3204
(847)990-2844
FAX: (847)573-4237

Lincoln

Abraham Lincoln Memorial Hospital
200 Stahlhut Dr
Lincoln, IL 62656-5066
(217)605-5108
FAX: (217)735-2869

Lindenhurst

Vista Ambulatory Care Centtesting Dept Of Vista Med Ctr East
1050 Red Oak Ln
Lindenhurst, IL 60046-4998
(847)360-4187
FAX: (847)782-3895

Lisle

Dupage Medical Group - Lisle
430 Warrenville Rd Ste 110
Lisle, IL 60532-1348
(630)545-7880
FAX: (630)241-1385

Litchfield

St. Francis Hospital
1215 Franciscan Dr
Litchfield, IL 62056-1799
(217)324-8555
FAX: (217)324-8705

Lombard

Andrew A. Roth, M.D., S.C.
500 E 22nd St Ste A
Lombard, IL 60148-6102
(630)932-2055
FAX: (630)932-2059

Dupage Medical Group At Lombard
1801 S Highland Ave
Lombard, IL 60148-4932
(630)545-7880
FAX: (630)873-8801

Elmhurst Memorial Lombard Health Care
130 S Main St
Lombard, IL 60148-2670
(331)221-0005
FAX: (331)221-3701

Loves Park

OSF Center For Health- Rock Cut
9951 Rock Cut Xing
Loves Park, IL 61111-1999
(815)395-5444
FAX: (815)395-4674

Macomb

McDonough District Hospital
525 E Grant St
Macomb, IL 61455-3318
(309)833-1550
FAX: (309)836-1552

Marion

Heartland Regional Medical Center
3333 W Deyoung St
Marion, IL 62959-5884
(618)998-7001
FAX: (618)998-7623

The Breast Center
3117 Williamson County Pkwy
Marion, IL 62959-5235
(800)360-6902
FAX: (618)997-3107

Maryville

Maryville Imaging, Llc
2023 Vadalabene Dr, Ste 100
Maryville, IL 62062-5636
(618)288-4929
FAX: (618)288-4531

The Friends Of Hope Breast Diagnostic Center
2227 Vadalabene Dr
Maryville, IL 62062-5823
(618)391-6820
FAX: (618)288-4586

Mattoon

Chci - Mattoon
2512 Hurst Dr
Mattoon, IL 61938-9200
(217)383-5920
FAX: (217)383-4980

Hshs St. Anthony's Diagnostic Center- Mattoon
101, Coles Centre Pkwy Suite B
Mattoon, IL 61938
(217)347-1540
FAX: (217)347-1377

Sarah Bush Lincoln Health Center
1000 Health Center Dr
Mattoon, IL 61938-4644
(217)258-2588
FAX: (217)258-2336

Maywood

Loyola University Medical Center Loyola Outpatient Ctr
2160 S 1st Ave, Bldg 150
Maywood, IL 60153-3328
(708)216-8474
FAX: (708)327-2010

McHenry

Northwestern Medicine McHenry Hospital
4201 W Medical Center Dr
McHenry, IL 60050-8409
(815)344-5566
FAX: (815)759-4319

McLeansboro

Hamilton Memorial Hospital
PO Box 429 611 S Marshall Ave, Radiology Dept.
McLeansboro, IL 62859-0429
(618)643-2361
FAX: (618)643-2087

Melrose Park

Bright Light Medical Imaging
8319 W North Ave
Melrose Park, IL 60160-1605
(708)450-9800
FAX: (708)450-9975

Gottlieb Memorial Hospital
701 W North Ave, Medical Imaging Dept.
Melrose Park, IL 60160-1699
(708)538-4917
FAX: (708)538-5333

Mendota

Mendota Community Hospital Dba OSF Saint Paul Medical Center
1401 E 12th St, Radiology Department
Mendota, IL 61342-9216
(815)539-1403
FAX: (815)539-1463

Metropolis

Massac Memorial Hospital
28 Chick St
Metropolis, IL 62960-2467
(618)524-2176
FAX: (618)524-1056

Mokena

Prime Medical Imaging
10260 191st St, Ste 106
Mokena, IL 60448-8803
(708)215-3800
FAX: (708)215-3801

Moline

Advanced Imaging Center, Llc
615 Valley View Dr Ste 101
Moline, IL 61265-6150
(309)743-0445
FAX: (309)764-4712

Genesis Imaging Center, Moline
3900 28th Avenue Dr, Ste 110
Moline, IL 61265-5536
(563)421-9729
FAX: (563)441-0617

Medical Arts Associates, Ltd.
600 John Deere Rd Ste 200
Moline, IL 61265-6897
(309)779-4295
FAX: (309)779-4307

Unitypoint Health- Trinity Moline
500 John Deere Rd
Moline, IL 61265-6892
(309)779-5114
FAX: (309)779-5113

Monmouth

OSF Holy Family Medical Center
1000 W Harlem Ave
Monmouth, IL 61462-1007
(309)734-1407
FAX: (309)734-1697

Monticello

Kirby Medical Center
1000 Medical Center Dr, Radiology Department
Monticello, IL 61856-2116
(217)762-1811
FAX: (217)762-1812

Morris

Morris Hospital And Health Care Centers
150 W High St
Morris, IL 60450-1463
(815)942-4105
FAX: (815)941-1568

Morton

OSF St. Francis Center For Breast Health Morton
435 Maxine Dr
Morton, IL 61550-2498
(309)683-5522
FAX: (309)683-5588

Morton Grove

3t Imaging Of Morton Grove
9000 Waukegan Rd Ste 110
Morton Grove, IL 60053-2128
(847)213-2700
FAX: (847)213-2709

Mount Vernon

Crossroads Community Hospital
8 Doctors Park Rd
Mount Vernon, IL 62864-6224
(618)244-5500
FAX: (618)242-2436

Ssm Health Good Samaritan Hospital
2 Good Samaritan Way, Mammography Dept.
Mount Vernon, IL 62864-2408
(618)899-1234
FAX: (618)899-4751

Mt Carmell

Wabash General Hospital - Mobile
1418 College Dr
Mt Carmell, IL 62863-2638
(618)263-6362
FAX: (618)263-6462

Naperville

Dupage Medical Group Naperville Breast Center
808 Rickert Dr Ste 101
Naperville, IL 60540-0907
(630)961-4177
FAX: (630)946-2520

Dupage Medical Group On Rolling Ridge Road
2940 Rollingridge Rd Ste 202
Naperville, IL 60564-4217
(630)545-7880
FAX: (630)545-7841

Edward Hospital
801 S Washington St
Naperville, IL 60540-7499
(630)527-3200
FAX: (630)548-1884

Edward Hospital - Book Road
2007 95th St
Naperville, IL 60564-8459
(630)527-3200
FAX: (630)527-3099

Edward Hospital Radiology - Hobson
1220 Hobson Rd Ste 124
Naperville, IL 60540-8137
(630)527-3200
FAX: (630)548-1884

Naperville Medical Imaging
1888 Bay Scott Cir
Naperville, IL 60540-1106
(630)717-3700
FAX: (630)717-3701

Nm Cdh Diagnostic Imaging- Naperville
636 Raymond Dr Ste 106
Naperville, IL 60563-9790
(630)315-1770
FAX: (630)778-8499

Rush Copley Medical Center Dba Midwest Ctr For Advanced Img.
4355 Montgomery Road
Naperville, IL 60564
(630)236-8300
FAX: (630)236-9860

Nashville

Washington County Hospital
705 S Grand St
Nashville, IL 62263-1534
(618)327-2323
FAX: (618)327-2331

New Lenox

Amita Healing Arts Pavilion
410 E Lincoln Hwy
New Lenox, IL 60451-1975
(815)462-5566
FAX: (815)741-7389

Silver Cross Center For Women's Health
1870 Silver Cross Blvd, Ste 150
New Lenox, IL 60451-8648
(815)300-6350
FAX: (815)300-6374

Normal

Carle Bromenn Medical Center
1304 Franklin Ave
Normal, IL 61761-3558
(309)268-5223
FAX: (309)268-2157

Fort Jesse Imaging Center
2200 Fort Jesse Rd, Ste 130
Normal, IL 61761-6289
(309)452-9001
FAX: (309)452-9299

North Riverside

Loyola Family Health Center At North Riverside
1950 Harlem Ave
North Riverside, IL 60546-1470
(708)354-9936
FAX: (708)354-8765

Northbrook

Northshore At Northbrook Court
1182 Northbrook Ct
Northbrook, IL 60062-1435
(847)926-5070
FAX: (847)926-5320

O Fallon

St. Elizabeth's Hospital
1 Saint Elizabeth Blvd
O Fallon, IL 62269-1099
(618)222-4639
FAX: (618)222-4626

St. Elizabeth's Medical Park
1512 N Green Mount Rd
O Fallon, IL 62269-2083
(618)624-3750
FAX: (618)624-5421

Oak Brook

Rush Breast Imaging - Oak Brook
2011 York Rd 2nd Fl
Oak Brook, IL 60523-1992
(312)942-2027
FAX: (630)724-1760

Oak Lawn

Advocate Aurora Health
9555 S 52nd Ave
Oak Lawn, IL 60453-3054
(708)634-0921
FAX: (708)634-0934

Advocate Christ Center For Breast Care
4545 W 103rd St
Oak Lawn, IL 60453-4860
(708)684-1000
FAX: (708)684-4369

Dupage Medical Group Oak Lawn
4061 W 95th St Ste 10
Oak Lawn, IL 60453-2611
(630)545-7880
FAX: (630)946-2520

OSF Healthcare Center For Health
6700 W 95th St
Oak Lawn, IL 60453-2199
(708)499-8550
FAX: (708)422-9659

Oak Park

Edward Elmhurst Health Center Oak Park
940 Lake St, Rm 315
Oak Park, IL 60301-1204
(331)221-0005
FAX: (331)331-3701

Rush Oak Park Hospital
520 S Maple Ave
Oak Park, IL 60304-1097
(708)660-6268
FAX: (708)660-6366

Oakbrook Terrace

Loyola Oakbrook Terrace Primary Care Center
1S260 Summit Ave
Oakbrook Terrace, IL 60181-3941
(630)953-6900
FAX: (630)953-6901

Olney

Richland Memorial Hospital, Inc.
800 E Locust St
Olney, IL 62450-2598
(618)395-6048
FAX: (618)392-1136

Olympia Fields

Franciscan Health Olympia Fields
3900 W 203rd St
Olympia Fields, IL 60461-1183
(708)747-4000
FAX: (708)679-2339

Orland Park

Advocate Medical Group Orland Park
9550 W 167th St
Orland Park, IL 60467-5561
(708)873-4500
FAX: (708)873-4533

Palos Diagnostic & Women's Health Center
15300 West Ave Ste 120
Orland Park, IL 60462-4508
(708)923-5588
FAX: (708)923-8584

Solis Mammography
14290 S La Grange Rd, 14290 S. Lagrange Road
Orland Park, IL 60462-2023
(773)778-1811
FAX: (312)584-0990

Oswego

Edward Oswego Center
6701 US Highway 34
Oswego, IL 60543-9129
(630)527-3200
FAX: (630)548-1884

Ottawa

Morris Hospital Ob And Gynegology Specialists
1300 Starfire Dr
Ottawa, IL 61350-1619
(815)942-4105
FAX: (815)942-0713

OSF Saint Elizabeth Medical Center
1614 E Norris Dr
Ottawa, IL 61350-3681
(815)431-3151
FAX: (815)431-8231

OSF Saint Elizabeth Medical Center
1100 E Norris Dr
Ottawa, IL 61350-1604
(815)431-5773
FAX: (815)433-3212

Palos Heights

High Tech Medical Park
11800 Southwest Hwy
Palos Heights, IL 60463-1065
(708)923-3074
FAX: (708)923-3269

Palos Community Hospital
12251 S 80th Ave
Palos Heights, IL 60463-0930
(708)923-5588
FAX: (708)923-8584

Pana

Pana Community Hospital
101 E 9th St
Pana, IL 62557-1785
(217)562-6368
FAX: (217)562-6251

Paris

Paris Community Hospital
721 E Court St
Paris, IL 61944-2420
(217)465-4141
FAX: (217)466-4702

Park Ridge

Advocate Medical Nesset Radiology
1775 Ballard Rd
Park Ridge, IL 60068-1005
(847)318-2796
FAX: (847)318-2933

Lutheran General Hospital- Center For Advanced Care
1700 Luther Ln, Caldwell Breast Center
Park Ridge, IL 60068-1270
(847)723-3100
FAX: (847)723-2236

Women's Health Specialists
1875 Dempster St Ste 245
Park Ridge, IL 60068-1126
(847)692-9234
FAX: (847)692-5267

Pekin

Women's Diagnostic Center Of Unitypoint Health-Pekin
600 S 13th St
Pekin, IL 61554-4969
(309)353-0931
FAX: (309)353-0708

Peoria

OSF Saint Francis Center For Breast Health
8800 State Route 91, Osf St. Francis Center For Health
Peoria, IL 61615-9473
(309)683-5536
FAX: (309)683-5588

OSF St. Francis Center For Breast Health, Main
530 NE Glen Oak Ave
Peoria, IL 61637-0001
(309)683-5536
FAX: (309)683-5588

Unitypoint Health Proctor
5409 N Knoxville Ave, Ste 1
Peoria, IL 61614-5071
(309)691-1071
FAX: (309)689-8307

Unitypoint Health-Methodist
2338 W Van Winkle Way
Peoria, IL 61615-7483
(309)671-8282
FAX: (309)672-4575

Unitypoint Health-Methodist
112 NE Crescent Ave
Peoria, IL 61606-1901
(309)671-8282
FAX: (309)672-4229

Peru

St Margaret's Health-Peru
925 West St
Peru, IL 61354-2757
(815)780-3199
FAX: (815)780-3198

Pinckneyville

Pinckneyville Community Hospital
5383 State Route 154
Pinckneyville, IL 62274-3342
(618)357-5909
FAX: (618)357-8882

Pittsfield

Blessing Care Corp. Dba Illini Community Hospital
640 W Washington St
Pittsfield, IL 62363-1350
(217)285-2113
FAX: (217)285-5062

Quincy Medical Group
320 N Madison St
Pittsfield, IL 62363-1412
(217)285-9661
FAX: (217)285-4641

Plainfield

Adventist Plainfield Imaging And Outpatient Center
15720 S Route 59
Plainfield, IL 60544-2693
(630)312-3300
FAX: (815)436-7748

Amita Plainfield Healing Arts Pavilion
16615 S Route 59
Plainfield, IL 60586-2941
(815)725-7133
FAX: (815)773-7759

Edward Hospital - South Plainfield
16519 S Route 59
Plainfield, IL 60586-2607
(630)527-3200
FAX: (630)548-1884

Edward Hospital Plainfield
24600 W 127th St
Plainfield, IL 60585-9507
(630)527-3142
FAX: (630)548-1884

Pontiac

OSF Saint James John W. Albrecht Medical Center
2500 W Reynolds St
Pontiac, IL 61764-9774
(815)842-6859
FAX: (815)842-4994

Princeton

Perry Memorial Hospital
530 Park Ave E
Princeton, IL 61356-2598
(815)876-2050
FAX: (815)876-2033

Quincy

Blessing Hospital
927 Broadway St Ste 320, Breast Center
Quincy, IL 62301-2726
(217)223-8400
FAX: (217)223-3906

Quincy Medical Group
1118 Hampshire St
Quincy, IL 62301-3027
(217)222-6550
FAX: (217)277-2341

Red Bud

Red Bud Regional Hospital
325 Spring St
Red Bud, IL 62278-1105
(618)282-5144
FAX: (618)282-5658

River Forest

River Forest Breast Care Center
420 William St 2nd Fl
River Forest, IL 60305-1970
(708)488-2300
FAX: (708)763-2782

Robinson

Crawford Memorial Hospital
1000 N Allen St
Robinson, IL 62454-1114
(618)546-2536
FAX: (618)546-2620

Rochelle

Rochelle Community Hospital
900 N 2nd St
Rochelle, IL 61068-1717
(815)562-2181
FAX: (815)561-3135

Rockford

Forest City Diagnostic Imaging, Llc
3849 N Perryville Rd
Rockford, IL 61114-8080
(815)654-2486
FAX: (815)654-2680

Mercyhealth Rockton Avenue
2300 N Rockton Ave
Rockford, IL 61103-3619
(815)971-2299
FAX: (815)971-9753

Mercyhealth Women's Center
7180 Spring Brook Rd Ste B
Rockford, IL 61114-6700
(815)971-2299
FAX: (815)971-9959

OSF Saint Anthony Medical Center
5666 E State St
Rockford, IL 61108-2472
(815)395-5444
FAX: (815)395-5427

Swedish American Center For Women
1340 Charles St Ste 201
Rockford, IL 61104-2200
(779)696-7676
FAX: (779)696-5522

Romeoville

Presence Healing Arts Pavilion Romeoville
500 S Weber Rd
Romeoville, IL 60446-6528
(815)725-7133
FAX: (815)773-7759

Roscoe

Mercy Health Roscoe
5000 Prairie Rose Dr
Roscoe, IL 61073-7792
(815)971-2299
FAX: (815)971-9753

Northpointe Health And Wellness Campus
5605 E Rockton Rd
Roscoe, IL 61073-7601
(815)525-4210
FAX: (815)525-4205

Samg/Stateline Clinic
4282 E Rockton Rd
Roscoe, IL 61073-7420
(779)696-9000
FAX: (779)696-8170

Rosiclare

Hardin County General Hospital
PO Box 2467, 6 Ferrel Rd
Rosiclare, IL 62982-2467
(618)285-6634
FAX: (618)285-6651

Rushville

Culbertson Memorial Hospital
238 S Congress St
Rushville, IL 62681-1472
(217)322-4321
FAX: (217)322-2008

Salem

Salem Township Hospital
1201 Ricker Rd
Salem, IL 62881-4263
(618)548-3194
FAX: (618)548-4177

Sandwich

Valley West Hospital
1302 N Main St
Sandwich, IL 60548-2587
(815)981-7130
FAX: (815)981-7375

Schaumburg

Northwest Community Hospital-Schaumburg Imaging Ctr
519 S Roselle Rd
Schaumburg, IL 60193-2925
(847)618-3700
FAX: (847)352-2450

St. Alexius Outpatient Center
347 W Golf Rd
Schaumburg, IL 60195-3607
(877)717-7700
FAX: (847)590-2634

Scott Afb

375th Medical Group
310 W Losey St
Scott Afb, IL 62225-5252
(618)256-1494
FAX: (618)256-7253

Shelbyville

Hshs Good Shepherd Hospital
200 S Cedar St
Shelbyville, IL 62565-1838
(217)774-3961
FAX: (217)774-6414

Shiloh

Memorial Hospital East
1404 Cross St
Shiloh, IL 62269-2988
(618)607-1203
FAX: (618)624-4862

Memorial Hospital East M.O.B. A
1414 Cross St, Medical Office Buliding A Suite 220
Shiloh, IL 62269-2988
(618)257-4949
FAX: (618)624-4862

Silvis

Genesis Health System Dba Genesis Medical Ctr Silvis Campus
801 Illini Dr
Silvis, IL 61282-1804
(309)281-4140
FAX: (309)281-4149

Skokie

Midwest Center For Women's Healthcare
4905 Old Orchard Ctr, Ste 200
Skokie, IL 60077-1462
(847)673-3130
FAX: (847)673-3183

Northshore Nordstrom
4937 Old Orchard Ctr
Skokie, IL 60077-1439
(847)570-2325
FAX: (847)570-2942

Northshore Skokie Hospital
9650 Gross Point Rd, 3rd Fl
Skokie, IL 60076-5080
(847)570-2325
FAX: (224)251-3365

South Elgin

Advocate Sherman Outpatient Center - South Elgin
2000 McDonald Rd
South Elgin, IL 60177-3323
(224)783-8972
FAX: (224)783-2960

Sparta

Sparta Community Hospital
818 E Broadway St
Sparta, IL 62286-1820
(618)443-1396
FAX: (618)443-1373

Spring Valley

St. Margaret's Health - Spring Valley
600 E 1st St
Spring Valley, IL 61362-1512
(815)664-1365
FAX: (815)664-1159

Springfield

Memorial Breast Diagnostic Services At Baylis
747 N. Rutledge
Springfield, IL 62781-0001
(217)788-4042
FAX: (217)788-5596

Springfield Clinic
1025 S 6th St
Springfield, IL 62703-2499
(217)528-7541
FAX: (217)527-3848

Springfield Clinic 1st
800 N 1st St
Springfield, IL 62702-3778
(217)528-7541
FAX: (217)527-1709

St. John's Health Center - Mammography
1100 Lincolnshire Blvd
Springfield, IL 62701
(217)757-6400
FAX: (217)757-6517

Women's And Children's Clinic
400 North Ninth Street
Springfield, IL 62769-0001
(217)993-0480
FAX: (217)757-6517

St Charles

Dreyer Clinic, Inc.
3310 W Main St, Ste 200
St Charles, IL 60175-1024
(630)859-6777
FAX: (630)264-8522

Staunton

Community Hospital Of Staunton
400 N Caldwell St
Staunton, IL 62088-1499
(618)635-4323
FAX: (618)635-4346

Sterling

Cgh Medical Center
100 E Le Fevre Rd
Sterling, IL 61081-1279
(815)625-0400
FAX: (815)625-4960

Streator

OSF Healthcare Center For Health-Streator
111 Spring St
Streator, IL 61364-3332
(815)673-4641
FAX: (815)673-5624

Taylorville

Taylorville Memorial Hospital
201 E Pleasant St
Taylorville, IL 62568-1597
(217)707-5555
FAX: (217)707-5241

Tinley Park

Dupage Medical Group Tinley Park
17495 La Grange Rd
Tinley Park, IL 60487-7581
(708)226-7000
FAX: (708)226-7159

High Tech Medical Park
18210 La Grange Rd Ste 106
Tinley Park, IL 60487-7723
(708)361-0220
FAX: (708)923-3269

Ingalls Family Care Center R. K. Desser, M.D. Breast Ctr
6701 159th St
Tinley Park, IL 60477-1758
(708)915-8442
FAX: (708)915-2755

Urbana

Carle Foundation Hospital
509 W University Ave
Urbana, IL 61801-1645
(217)383-5920
FAX: (217)388-4980

OSF Heart Of Mary Medical Center
1400 W Park St
Urbana, IL 61801-2334
(217)337-2621
FAX: (217)337-2526

Vandalia

Fayette County Hospital
650 W Taylor St
Vandalia, IL 62471-1296
(618)283-5466
FAX: (618)283-4849

Vernon Hills

Northshore Vernon Hills
225 N Milwaukee Ave
Vernon Hills, IL 60061-4304
(847)926-5070
FAX: (847)926-5320

Northwestern Vernon Hills Diagnostic Imaging Center
870 N Milwaukee Ave
Vernon Hills, IL 60061-1521
(847)535-7796
FAX: (847)535-8415

Washington

OSF St. Francis Ctr. For Breast Hlth-Washington St Clare
10 Saint Clare Ct
Washington, IL 61571-9239
(309)683-5536
FAX: (309)683-5588

Waterloo

Gateway Imaging Of Waterloo
509 Hamacher St Ste 300
Waterloo, IL 62298-1592
(618)798-3704
FAX: (618)798-3744

Watseka

Iroquois Memorial Hospital
200 E Fairman Ave
Watseka, IL 60970-1644
(815)432-7727
FAX: (815)432-7827

Waukegan

Vista Medical Center East Diagnostic Imaging
1324 N Sheridan Rd, Diagnostic Imaging
Waukegan, IL 60085-2161
(847)360-4187
FAX: (847)782-3895

Westmont

Amita Health - Westmont Imaging Center
6311 S Cass Ave
Westmont, IL 60559-3206
(630)856-4060
FAX: (630)856-4067

Dupage Medical Group Westmont
303 W Ogden Ave, Ste 13
Westmont, IL 60559-1419
(630)545-7880
FAX: (630)946-2520

Willowbrook

Amita Health Willowbrook Mammography Center
545 Plainfield Rd
Willowbrook, IL 60527-7600
(630)286-5719
FAX: (630)286-5975

Winfield

Nm Central Dupage Hospital
25 N Winfield Rd
Winfield, IL 60190-1379
(630)933-5000
FAX: (630)933-2872

Woodridge

Amita Healthcare Woodridge Ambulatory Center
2363 63rd St
Woodridge, IL 60517-1300
(630)856-7070
FAX: (630)856-7060

Woodstock

Mercy Woodstock Medical Center
2000 Lake Ave
Woodstock, IL 60098-7401
(877)976-3729
FAX: (815)337-4298

Northwestern Medicine Woodstock Hospital
3701 Doty Rd
Woodstock, IL 60098-7509
(815)338-2500
FAX: (815)334-3974

Yorkville

Edward Hospital - Yorkville
76 W Countryside Pkwy
Yorkville, IL 60560-1967
(630)527-3200
FAX: (630)548-1884

Rush Copley Health Center Diagnostic Imaging
1100 W Veterans Pkwy
Yorkville, IL 60560-4728
(630)236-8300
FAX: (630)236-9860

Zion

Midwestern Regional Medical Center, Llc
2520 Elisha Ave
Zion, IL 60099-2587
(800)458-1975
FAX: (847)872-3353

INDIANA

Anderson

Ascension St. Vincent Anderson Women's Center
2020 Meridian St Ste 150
Anderson, IN 46016-4343
(765)683-3234
FAX: (765)683-3278

Community Hospital Anderson Women's Center
1515 N Madison Ave
Anderson, IN 46011-3453
(765)298-5386
FAX: (765)298-5823

Angola

Cameron Memorial Community Hospital
416 E Maumee St
Angola, IN 46703-2015
(260)665-2141
FAX: (260)665-7805

Auburn

Parkview Dekalb Hospital
PO Box 542, 1316 E Seventh St
Auburn, IN 46706-0542
(260)920-2513
FAX: (260)925-7648

Avon

Center For Diagnostic Imaging
8607 E US Highway 36
Avon, IN 46123-7960
(317)846-0717
FAX: (317)846-0557

Iu Health West Hospital
1111 Ronald Reagan Pkwy
Avon, IN 46123-7085
(317)217-3171
FAX: (317)217-3268

Batesville

Margaret Mary Health
321 Mitchell Ave
Batesville, IN 47006-8890
(812)933-5434
FAX: (812)933-5305

Bedford

Ascension St.Vincent Dunn
1600 23rd St
Bedford, IN 47421-4704
(812)276-1300
FAX: (812)276-1297

Indiana University Health Bedford, Inc.
2900 16th St
Bedford, IN 47421-3510
(812)275-1270
FAX: (812)275-1238

Bloomington

Monroe Women's Center
4011 S Monroe Medical Park Blvd, Monroe Hospital
Bloomington, IN 47403-8000
(812)825-0818
FAX: (812)825-0787

Sira Imaging Center, Llc
500 S Landmark Ave
Bloomington, IN 47403-3239
(812)333-7676
FAX: (812)333-7689

Bluffton

Bluffton Hlth Systems Llc Dba Bluffton Regional Med Ctr
303 S Main St, Radiology Department
Bluffton, IN 46714-2503
(260)919-3830
FAX: (260)824-7059

Brazil

Ascension St. Vincent Clay
1206 E National Ave
Brazil, IN 47834-2718
(812)442-2560
FAX: (812)442-2565

Bremen

Community Hospital Of Bremen
PO Box 8, 1020 High Rd
Bremen, IN 46506-0008
(574)546-8081
FAX: (574)546-4055

Brownsburg

Ascension Medical Group St. Vincent - Brownsburg Imaging
590 Pit Rd, Ste 200
Brownsburg, IN 46112-7830
(317)456-1159
FAX: (317)456-1111

Hendricks Regional Health Brownsburg Hospital
5492 N Ronald Reagan Pkwy, Sandy Kelly
Brownsburg, IN 46112-5618
(317)745-3404
FAX: (317)718-4340

Iu Health Brownsburg
1375 N Green St
Brownsburg, IN 46112-8705
(317)948-9729
FAX: (317)852-6536

Carmel

Ascension St Vincent Carmel Breast Center
13420 N Meridian St Ste 100
Carmel, IN 46032-1581
(317)582-7474
FAX: (317)582-7476

Community Breast Screening Carmel
11911 N Meridian St Ste 175
Carmel, IN 46032-6944
(317)806-8265
FAX: (317)806-8291

Indiana University Health North Hospital
11700 N Meridian St, Women's Diagnostic Breast Center
Carmel, IN 46032-4656
(317)688-2955
FAX: (317)688-2874

Moon And Associates Llc
12400 N Meridian St, Ste 100
Carmel, IN 46032-4601
(317)559-3320
FAX: (317)559-3321

Chesterton

Fsah - Chesterton Health And Er Center
770 Indian Boundary Rd
Chesterton, IN 46304-1519
(219)921-2040
FAX: (219)395-8280

Clarksville

Community Medical Associates
2051 Clevidence Blvd
Clarksville, IN 47129-2278
(812)280-9145
FAX: (812)280-6628

Clinton

Union Hospital Clinton
801 S Main St
Clinton, IN 47842-2261
(765)832-1317
FAX: (765)832-1315

Columbia City

Parkview Whitley Hospital Breast Diagnostic Center
1260 E State Road 205
Columbia City, IN 46725-9492
(260)248-9504
FAX: (260)248-9178

Columbus

The Breast Health Center At Columbus Regional Hospital
2326 18th St Ste 110
Columbus, IN 47201-5362
(812)376-5150
FAX: (812)376-5989

Connersville

Reid Health-Connersville
1941 Virginia Ave
Connersville, IN 47331-2879
(765)827-7703
FAX: (765)827-7781

Corydon

Baptist Health Imaging
313 Federal Dr NW Ste 20, Northfield Plaza
Corydon, IN 47112-3080
(812)734-3920
FAX: (812)734-3940

Harrison County Hospital
1141 Hospital Dr NW
Corydon, IN 47112-1774
(812)738-4251
FAX: (812)738-7825

Crawfordsville

Ascension Medical Group St. Vincent - Crawfordsville Imaging
1684 Bush Ln, Ste 100
Crawfordsville, IN 47933-3364
(765)365-9650
FAX: (765)365-9556

Franciscan Health Crawfordsville
1710 Lafayette Rd
Crawfordsville, IN 47933-1033
(765)364-8597
FAX: (765)361-3010

Crown Point

Community Stroke And Rehabilitation Center
10215 Broadway
Crown Point, IN 46307-8001
(219)661-6143
FAX: (219)703-6818

Franciscan Alliance Inc Dba Franciscan Health Crown Point
1201 S Main St
Crown Point, IN 46307-8483
(219)757-6010
FAX: (219)681-6770

Pinnacle Hospital
9301 Connecticut Dr
Crown Point, IN 46307-7486
(219)756-2100
FAX: (219)756-0413

Danville

Hendricks Regional Health
1000 E Main St
Danville, IN 46122-1948
(317)745-3404
FAX: (317)718-4340

Decatur

Adams Memorial Hospital
1100 Mercer Ave
Decatur, IN 46733-2303
(260)724-2145
FAX: (260)728-3856

Dyer

Franciscan Health - Dyer
24 Joliet St
Dyer, IN 46311-1705
(219)922-4070
FAX: (219)864-2609

East Chicago

St. Catherine Hospital
4321 Fir St
East Chicago, IN 46312-3097
(219)392-7321
FAX: (219)392-7325

Elkhart

Elkhart General Hospital
600 East Blvd
Elkhart, IN 46514-2499
(574)523-3444
FAX: (574)523-3435

Elwood

Ascension St. Vincent Mercy
1331 S A St
Elwood, IN 46036-1942
(765)552-4698
FAX: (765)552-4750

Evansville

Ascension St. Vincent Westside Crossing
100 S Rosenberger Ave Ste A320
Evansville, IN 47712-6504
(812)485-5722
FAX: (812)485-6890

Deaconess Breast Center
520 Mary St Ste 140
Evansville, IN 47710-1669
(812)450-6614
FAX: (812)424-4163

Fishers

Ascension St Vincent Fishers Breast Center
13914 Southeastern Pkwy, Ste 101
Fishers, IN 46037-7124
(317)582-8070
FAX: (317)415-9012

Community Breast Screening Saxony
13121 Olio Rd Ste 120
Fishers, IN 46037-7240
(317)806-8265
FAX: (317)621-3070

Iu Health Saxony Hospital Women's Services
13000 E 136th St
Fishers, IN 46037-9478
(317)962-3580
FAX: (317)678-1704

Fort Wayne

Anthony Breast Center - St Joseph Hospital
5717 S Anthony Blvd Ste 900
Fort Wayne, IN 46806-3393
(260)425-2685
FAX: (260)425-2698

Breast Diagnostic Center
1818 Carew St, Ste 40
Fort Wayne, IN 46805-4764
(260)266-8120
FAX: (260)266-8130

Breast Diagnostic Center
3707 New Vision Dr
Fort Wayne, IN 46845-1702
(260)266-8120
FAX: (260)266-8130

Breast Diagnostic Center- Mobile
3707 New Vision Dr
Fort Wayne, IN 46845-1702
(260)266-8120
FAX: (260)266-8130

Dupont Hospital Center For Breast Health
2510 E Dupont Rd Ste 207
Fort Wayne, IN 46825-1602
(260)416-3006
FAX: (260)416-3310

Indiana University Health Fort Wayne Physicians, Llc
7411 Hope Dr Ste B
Fort Wayne, IN 46815-5687
(260)234-5390
FAX: (260)234-5396

Lutheran MD Imaging
7900 W Jefferson Blvd Ste 103
Fort Wayne, IN 46804-4128
(260)435-7956
FAX: (260)435-7749

Parkview Cancer Institute
11050 Parkview Circle Dr
Fort Wayne, IN 46845-1739
(260)266-6216
FAX: (260)266-6945

St. Joseph Hospital
700 Broadway, Mob Suite 220
Fort Wayne, IN 46802-1493
(260)425-3983
FAX: (260)425-3040

The Imaging Center
7631 W Jefferson Blvd
Fort Wayne, IN 46804-4133
(260)436-7770
FAX: (260)436-3570

Women's Health Advantage
7988 W Jefferson Blvd
Fort Wayne, IN 46804-4140
(260)432-4400
FAX: (260)969-6834

Frankfort

Ascension Medical Group St. Vincent Frankfort
2485 E Wabash St
Frankfort, IN 46041-9400
(765)656-3900
FAX: (765)656-3921

Iu Health Frankfort Hospital
1300 S Jackson St
Frankfort, IN 46041-3313
(765)656-3650
FAX: (765)656-3595

Franklin

The Breast Care Center Of Johnson Memorial Health
1125 W Jefferson St
Franklin, IN 46131-2140
(317)346-3800
FAX: (317)346-3801

Ft Wayne

Women's Health Advantage
2518 E Dupont Rd
Ft Wayne, IN 46825-1675
(260)432-4400
FAX: (260)969-6826

Gary

Methodist Hospital Northlake
600 Grant St
Gary, IN 46402-6099
(219)981-5440
FAX: (219)738-6685

Goshen

Goshen Health The Retreat Women's Health Center
1135 Professional Dr
Goshen, IN 46526-3800
(574)364-4604
FAX: (574)364-4630

Granger

Granger Family Medicine
52500 Fir Rd
Granger, IN 46530-8579
(574)237-9203
FAX: (574)237-9311

Memorial Lighthouse Medical Imaging
6901 N Main St Ste 100
Granger, IN 46530-8022
(574)647-2901
FAX: (574)647-2910

Greencastle

Putnam County Hospital
1542 S Bloomington St
Greencastle, IN 46135-2297
(765)301-7310
FAX: (765)301-7328

Greenfield

James T. Anderson MD Center For Women's Health
801 N State St
Greenfield, IN 46140-1270
(317)468-4600
FAX: (317)468-4629

Parkway Imaging Center
300 E Boyd Ave Ste 130
Greenfield, IN 46140-2818
(317)468-4600
FAX: (317)477-6577

Greensburg

Decatur County Memorial Hospital
720 N Lincoln St
Greensburg, IN 47240-1398
(812)663-1157
FAX: (812)663-1198

Greenwood

Community Imaging Center South
333 E County Line Rd Ste A
Greenwood, IN 46143-1080
(317)497-2842
FAX: (317)497-6301

Franciscan Stones Crossing
1703 W Stones Crossing Rd Ste 350
Greenwood, IN 46143-8552
(317)528-5129
FAX: (317)528-2229

Northwest Radiology Network, Pc
853 N Emerson Ave, Ste A
Greenwood, IN 46143-5676
(317)328-5050
FAX: (317)489-5176

Stones Crossing Health Pavilion
3000 S State Road 135, Ste 120
Greenwood, IN 46143-9829
(317)355-4680
FAX: (317)351-2024

Hammond

Northshore Health Center
1828 165th St
Hammond, IN 46320-2823
(219)763-8112
FAX: (219)962-1646

Hartford City

Indiana University Health Blackford Hospital, Inc.
410 Pilgrim Blvd
Hartford City, IN 47348-1382
(765)331-2150
FAX: (765)331-2158

Hobart

Women's Diagnostic Center Of St. Mary
300 W 61st Ave
Hobart, IN 46342-6490
(219)947-6830
FAX: (219)947-6837

Huntington

Parkview Huntington Hospital
2001 Stults Rd
Huntington, IN 46750-1291
(260)355-3400
FAX: (260)355-3404

Indianapolis

Ascension St Vincent Indianapolis Breast Center And Mobile
8550 Naab Rd Ste 300
Indianapolis, IN 46260-2086
(317)338-9595
FAX: (317)583-2626

Barrington Radiologic Services
3403 E Raymond St
Indianapolis, IN 46203-4744
(317)957-2110
FAX: (317)957-2111

Breast Diagnostic Center East
1400 N Ritter Ave Ste 170
Indianapolis, IN 46219-3060
(317)806-8265
FAX: (317)355-1575

Breast Diagnostic Center North
7120 Clearvista Dr Ste 3100
Indianapolis, IN 46256-0030
(317)806-8265
FAX: (317)621-2320

Center For Diagnostic Imaging
7151 Marsh Rd, Ste 100
Indianapolis, IN 46278-1631
(317)846-0717
FAX: (317)846-0557

Community Breast Screening West
3660 Guion Rd Ste 102
Indianapolis, IN 46222-1691
(317)920-7528
FAX: (317)920-7229

Community Breast Screening/X-Ray Washington
10122 E 10th St Ste 101
Indianapolis, IN 46229-3046
(317)806-8265
FAX: (317)355-1712

Community Imaging Center South Campus
1440 E County Line Rd, Ste 3100
Indianapolis, IN 46227-0963
(317)497-6900
FAX: (317)497-6928

Franciscan Health Indianapolis
8111 S Emerson Ave
Indianapolis, IN 46237-8601
(317)528-5129
FAX: (317)528-2229

Iu Health Methodist Hospital Breast Center
1801 Senate Blvd
Indianapolis, IN 46202-1228
(317)962-3580
FAX: (317)962-7564

Iu Health Radiology Methodist Medical Plaza East
9660 E Washington St
Indianapolis, IN 46229-3032
(317)962-3580
FAX: (317)890-5429

Iu Health University Hospital
550 University Blvd
Indianapolis, IN 46202-5149
(317)962-3580
FAX: (317)948-8773

Iuhealth-Methodist Medical Plaza Eagle Highlands
6850 Parkdale Pl, X-Ray Department
Indianapolis, IN 46254-4670
(317)962-3580
FAX: (317)329-7299

Methodist Medical Plaza South - Indiana University Hlth
8830 S Meridian St
Indianapolis, IN 46217-5029
(317)865-6788
FAX: (317)865-6672

Northwest Radiology Network
10603 N Meridian St
Indianapolis, IN 46290-1055
(317)844-2511
FAX: (317)846-3658

Obstetrics & Gynecology Of Indiana, Llc
8360 S Emerson Ave Ste 100
Indianapolis, IN 46237-8746
(317)859-2535
FAX: (463)777-5735

Obstetrics & Gynecology Of Indiana, Llc
8091 Township Line Rd, Fl 2 Suite 206
Indianapolis, IN 46260-2494
(317)415-1000
FAX: (317)415-1010

St. Margaret's Hospital Guild Diagnostic Breast Center
720 Eskenazi Ave, St. Margaret's Guild Diagnostic Breast C
Indianapolis, IN 46202-5187
(317)880-7258
FAX: (317)880-4890

St. Margaret's Hospital Guild Diagnostic Breast Center
5515 W 38th St, Eskenazi Health
Indianapolis, IN 46254-2919
(317)880-7280
FAX: (317)880-4890

Jasper

Memorial Hospital & Health Care Center
800 W 9th St, The Women's Center
Jasper, IN 47546-2516
(812)996-8550
FAX: (812)996-0103

Jeffersonville

Clark Memorial Hospital Women's Imaging Center
1220 Missouri Ave
Jeffersonville, IN 47130-3743
(812)283-2405
FAX: (812)283-2951

Kendallville

Parkview Noble Hospital
PO Box 728, 401 Sawyer Rd
Kendallville, IN 46755-0728
(260)347-8611
FAX: (260)347-8256

Knox

Knox Hospital Company Llc
102 E Culver Rd
Knox, IN 46534-2216
(574)772-1177
FAX: (574)772-1233

Kokomo

Advanced Medical Imaging
2008 W Boulevard
Kokomo, IN 46902-6079
(765)454-9729
FAX: (765)454-9766

Ascension St. Vincent Women's Center Kokomo
305 S Berkley Rd Ste 120
Kokomo, IN 46901-5114
(765)456-5000
FAX: (765)456-5110

Community Howard Regional Health Women's Center
2201 W Boulevard
Kokomo, IN 46902-6070
(765)776-8929
FAX: (765)455-1711

Lafayette

Franciscan Health Lafayette Breast Center
1345 Unity Pl Ste 220
Lafayette, IN 47905-5761
(765)423-6170
FAX: (765)446-5475

Franciscan Health Lafayette Screening Breast Center
3920 St Francis Way Ste 215
Lafayette, IN 47905-4917
(765)423-6170
FAX: (765)428-5887

Lagrange

Parkview Lagrange Hospital
207 N Townline Rd
Lagrange, IN 46761-1325
(877)225-5747
FAX: (877)747-3291

Lake Station

Northshore Health Centers
2490 Central Ave
Lake Station, IN 46405-2122
(219)763-8112
FAX: (219)962-1646

Laporte

Franciscan Beacon Hospital
1010 Sr 2
Laporte, IN 46350
(219)575-6701
FAX: (219)575-6699

Northwest Health - Laporte
1331 State St
Laporte, IN 46350-3112
(219)326-2444
FAX: (219)325-5464

Lawrenceburg

St. Elizabeth Dearborn
606 Wilson Creek Rd Ste 120, Professional Bldg
Lawrenceburg, IN 47025-1035
(812)532-7500
FAX: (812)537-8464

Lebanon

Witham Memorial Hospital Women's Center
2705 N Lebanon St Ste 110
Lebanon, IN 46052-8621
(765)485-8370
FAX: (765)485-8379

Linton

Greene County General Hospital
1185 N 1000 W
Linton, IN 47441-5282
(812)847-5204
FAX: (812)847-5218

Logansport

Logansport Memorial Hospital
1101 Michigan Ave
Logansport, IN 46947-1596
(574)753-1488
FAX: (574)753-1584

Madison

King's Daughters' Health
1373 N Sr 62
Madison, IN 47250-7328
(812)801-8080
FAX: (812)801-8063

Marion

Marion General Hospital South Marion Diagnostics
1410 W Bella Dr
Marion, IN 46953-5229
(765)660-6222
FAX: (765)674-7023

Martinsville

Indiana University Health Morgan
2209 John R Wooden Dr
Martinsville, IN 46151-1840
(765)349-6440
FAX: (765)349-5415

McCordsville

McCordsville Medical Office
8535 N Clearview Dr
McCordsville, IN 46055-6240
(317)468-4600
FAX: (317)335-5033

Merrillville

Indiana Regional Imaging Center
7891 Broadway Ste A
Merrillville, IN 46410-5556
(219)793-9655
FAX: (219)793-9692

Northwest Indiana Breast Care Ctr At Methodist Hospitals
101 E 87th Ave, Pavilion A. 2nd Fl
Merrillville, IN 46410-7335
(219)981-5440
FAX: (219)738-6685

Michigan City

Franciscan Health Mc Breast Center
3500 Franciscan Way
Michigan City, IN 46360-0021
(219)877-1987
FAX: (219)877-1069

Northwest Health - Lifeworks - Women's Imaging
3777 N Frontage Rd Ste 700
Michigan City, IN 46360-7698
(844)865-7459
FAX: (219)326-2493

Mishawaka

Saint Joseph Regional Medical Ctr-South Bend Campus, Inc
611 E Douglas Rd Ste 123
Mishawaka, IN 46545-1464
(574)335-4500
FAX: (574)335-6217

The South Bend Clinic Day Road
301 E Day Rd
Mishawaka, IN 46545-3455
(574)237-9203
FAX: (574)237-9311

Monticello

Indiana University Health White Memorial Hospital
720 S 6th St
Monticello, IN 47960-8182
(574)583-1714
FAX: (574)583-1753

Mooresville

Franciscan Health Mooresville
1201 Hadley Rd
Mooresville, IN 46158-1737
(317)528-5129
FAX: (317)528-2229

Muncie

Center For Diagnostic Imaging
3631 N Morrison Rd
Muncie, IN 47304-5547
(317)846-0717
FAX: (317)846-0557

Iu Health Ball Memorial Breast Center
2598 W White River Blvd
Muncie, IN 47303-5251
(765)751-2727
FAX: (765)282-7356

Munster

Community Diagnostic Center
10020 Don S Powers Dr
Munster, IN 46321-4054
(219)934-8869
FAX: (219)934-8870

Franciscan Health Munster
701 Superior Ave
Munster, IN 46321-4037
(219)922-4070
FAX: (219)934-4009

New Albany

Baptist Health Floyd
1850 State St
New Albany, IN 47150-4990
(812)949-5570
FAX: (812)949-5712

Northgate Medical Imaging Llc Dba Priority Radiology
807 Northgate Blvd
New Albany, IN 47150-6419
(812)949-0807
FAX: (812)949-0806

New Castle

Henry County Hospital
1000 N 16th St
New Castle, IN 47362-4395
(765)521-1415
FAX: (765)521-1433

New Palestine

Healthway Park
4055 Roy Wilson Way
New Palestine, IN 46163-8032
(317)468-4600
FAX: (317)861-5325

Newburgh

Ascension St. Vincent Evansville Breast Center
100 St Marys Epworth Xing Ste A500
Newburgh, IN 47630-9497
(812)485-4437
FAX: (812)485-6890

Ascension St.Vincent Evansville Breast Center - Mobile
100 St Marys Epworth Xing Ste A5
Newburgh, IN 47630-9497
(812)485-4437
FAX: (812)485-6890

The Breast Center At The Women's Hospital
4199 Gateway Blvd Ste 3200
Newburgh, IN 47630-8976
(812)842-4995
FAX: (812)858-4615

Noblesville

Riverview Women's Center
395 Westfield Rd
Noblesville, IN 46060-1425
(317)776-7495
FAX: (317)776-7208

North Vernon

Ascension St. Vincent Jennings
301 Henry St
North Vernon, IN 47265-1030
(812)352-4310
FAX: (812)352-4380

Paoli

Iu Health Paoli, Inc.
642 W Hospital Rd
Paoli, IN 47454-9672
(812)723-7966
FAX: (812)723-7501

Peru

Dukes Memorial Hospital
275 W 12th St
Peru, IN 46970-1655
(765)472-8001
FAX: (765)472-9062

Plainfield

Ascension Medical Group St. Vincent - Plainfield Imaging
2155 E Main St, Ste 150
Plainfield, IN 46168-1816
(317)204-6850
FAX: (317)204-6824

Franciscan Plainfield Health Center
315 N Dan Jones Rd
Plainfield, IN 46168-2817
(317)528-5129
FAX: (317)528-2229

Hendricks Regional Health-Plainfield
1100 Southfield Dr Ste 1130
Plainfield, IN 46168-4499
(317)745-3404
FAX: (317)718-4340

Plymouth

Saint Joseph Regional Medical Center
1915 Lake Ave
Plymouth, IN 46563-9393
(574)335-4500
FAX: (574)367-7634

Portage

Northshore Health Centers Portage
6050 Sterling Creek Rd, Mammography Department
Portage, IN 46368-7752
(219)763-8112
FAX: (219)962-1646

Northwest Health - Portage
3630 Willowcreek Rd
Portage, IN 46368-5075
(219)364-3301
FAX: (219)364-3305

Portland

Iu Health Jay
500 W Votaw St
Portland, IN 47371-1322
(260)726-1821
FAX: (260)726-1921

Princeton

Gibson General Hospital, Inc.
1808 Sherman Dr
Princeton, IN 47670-1000
(812)385-9248
FAX: (812)385-9367

Rensselaer

Franciscan Health Rensselaer
1104 E Grace St
Rensselaer, IN 47978-3211
(219)866-2051
FAX: (219)866-2050

Richmond

Reid Health Mammography
1100 Reid Pkwy, Occ Bldg.
Richmond, IN 47374-1157
(765)935-8728
FAX: (765)935-8701

Rochester

Woodlawn Hospital
1400 E 9th St
Rochester, IN 46975-8937
(574)224-1151
FAX: (574)224-1276

Rushville

Rush Memorial Hospital
PO Box 608, 1300 N Main St
Rushville, IN 46173-0608
(765)932-7556
FAX: (765)932-7552

Salem

Ascension St. Vincent Salem
911 N Shelby St
Salem, IN 47167-2304
(812)883-5881
FAX: (812)883-8590

Schererville

Schererville Imaging Center
7860 Burr St
Schererville, IN 46375-3402
(219)981-5440
FAX: (219)864-2910

Scottsburg

Scott Memorial Health
1451 N Gardner St
Scottsburg, IN 47170-7751
(812)752-8597
FAX: (812)752-8563

Seymour

Schneck Medical Center
411 W Tipton St, Radiology Department
Seymour, IN 47274-2363
(812)523-4874
FAX: (812)524-3366

Shelbyville

Major Hospital
2451 Intelliplex Dr, Ste 100
Shelbyville, IN 46176-8581
(317)421-5678
FAX: (317)398-1812

South Bend

Memorial Regional Breast Care Center
100 Navarre Pl, Ste 6655
South Bend, IN 46601-1174
(574)647-7519
FAX: (574)647-1818

The South Bend Clinic
211 N Eddy St
South Bend, IN 46617-3096
(574)237-9203
FAX: (574)237-9311

The South Bend Clinic Portage
4400 Portage Ave
South Bend, IN 46628-9570
(574)204-6200
FAX: (574)239-1520

St John

Community Hospital Outpatient Centre
9660 Wicker Ave
St John, IN 46373-9487
(219)226-2291
FAX: (219)226-2293

Sullivan

Sullivan County Community Hospital
2200 N Section St
Sullivan, IN 47882-7523
(812)268-4311
FAX: (812)268-2662

Tell City

Perry County Memorial Hospital
8885 State Road 237
Tell City, IN 47586-8567
(812)547-0185
FAX: (812)547-0188

Terre Haute

Clara Fairbanks Center For Women
1711 N 6th 1/2 St, Ste 301
Terre Haute, IN 47804-2770
(812)238-7766
FAX: (812)238-4511

Terre Haute Regional Hospital
3901 S 7th St
Terre Haute, IN 47802-4299
(812)237-1237
FAX: (812)237-9520

Union Hospital - Clara Fairbanks Thomas Plaza
5500 S US Highway 41 Ste 106
Terre Haute, IN 47802-4745
(812)238-7766
FAX: (812)238-4511

Tipton

Indiana University Health Tipton Hospital
1000 S Main St, Women's Center
Tipton, IN 46072-9753
(765)675-8538
FAX: (765)675-8178

Valparaiso

Northwest Health - Porter
85 E US Highway 6, Ste 120
Valparaiso, IN 46383-8948
(219)983-6120
FAX: (219)983-6020

Northwest Health - Valparaiso
1900 Roosevelt Rd
Valparaiso, IN 46383-2780
(219)263-4925
FAX: (219)263-7226

Women's Diagnostic Center Of St. Mary's
3800 Saint Mary Rd
Valparaiso, IN 46383-3986
(219)286-3711
FAX: (219)286-3712

Vincennes

Good Samaritan Breast Care Center
520 S 7th St 1st Fl
Vincennes, IN 47591-1038
(812)885-3353
FAX: (812)885-3626

Wabash

Parkview Wabash Hospital
10 John Kissinger Dr
Wabash, IN 46992-1648
(260)569-2117
FAX: (260)569-2398

Warsaw

Parkview Warsaw Medical Complex
1355 Mariners Dr
Warsaw, IN 46582-7145
(574)372-0080
FAX: (574)372-0089

Warsaw Health System Llc Dba Kosciusko Community Hospital
2101 Dubois Dr
Warsaw, IN 46580-3210
(574)372-7601
FAX: (574)372-5879

Warsaw Women's Center, P.C.
1275 Provident Dr
Warsaw, IN 46580-3265
(574)269-4026
FAX: (574)269-7444

Washington

Daviess Community Hospital
1314 E Walnut St
Washington, IN 47501-2132
(812)444-9020
FAX: (812)254-8890

West Lafayette

Iu Health Arnett West Mob
253 Sagamore Pkwy W
West Lafayette, IN 47906-1501
(765)448-8100
FAX: (765)838-4078

Westfield

Riverview Health Westfield Hospital
17600 Shamrock Blvd
Westfield, IN 46074-7002
(317)776-7247
FAX: (317)776-7208

Williamsport

Ascension St. Vincent Williamsport
412 N Monroe St
Williamsport, IN 47993-1049
(765)762-4080
FAX: (765)762-4075

Winamac

Pulaski Memorial Hospital
616 E 13th St
Winamac, IN 46996-1117
(574)946-2136
FAX: (574)946-2139

Winchester

Ascension St. Vincent Randolph
473 SE Greenville Ave
Winchester, IN 47394-9436
(765)584-0296
FAX: (765)584-0312

Zionsville

Witham Health Services At Anson
6085 Heartland Dr Ste 105
Zionsville, IN 46077-4433
(765)485-8080
FAX: (765)485-8088

IOWA

Albia

Monroe County Hospital
6580 165th St
Albia, IA 52531-8893
(641)932-2134
FAX: (641)932-1662

Algona

Kossuth Regional Health Center
1515 S Phillips St
Algona, IA 50511-3649
(515)295-4460
FAX: (515)295-4467

Ames

Mary Greeley Medical Center
1111 Duff Ave
Ames, IA 50010-5792
(515)239-2131
FAX: (515)239-2492

McFarland Clinic Ames
1215 Duff Ave
Ames, IA 50010-5469
(515)239-4436
FAX: (515)239-4761

Anamosa

Jones Regional Medical Center
1795 Highway 64 E
Anamosa, IA 52205-2112
(319)481-6369
FAX: (319)481-6125

Ankeny

Iowa Diagnostic Imaging And Procedure Center Dba - Ankeny
3625 N Ankeny Blvd Ste H
Ankeny, IA 50023-4611
(515)226-7468
FAX: (515)963-7619

Mercyone Ankeny Mammography
800 E 1st St, Ste 1100
Ankeny, IA 50021-2078
(515)247-4444
FAX: (515)643-8867

The Iowa Clinic
1410 SW Tradition Dr Ste 180
Ankeny, IA 50023-9188
(515)875-9500
FAX: (515)875-9672

Atlantic

Cass County Memorial Hospital
1501 E 10th St
Atlantic, IA 50022-1997
(712)243-7451
FAX: (712)243-7560

Audubon

Audubon County Memorial Hospital
515 Pacific Ave, Ste 1
Audubon, IA 50025-1056
(712)563-5265
FAX: (712)563-5282

Belmond

Iowa Specialty Hospital Belmond
403 1st St SE
Belmond, IA 50421-1201
(515)532-9258
FAX: (641)444-5691

Bettendorf

Genesis Imaging Center Bettendorf
2140 53rd Ave
Bettendorf, IA 52722-6279
(563)421-5641
FAX: (563)441-0617

Trinity Medical Center-Bettendorf
4500 Utica Ridge Rd
Bettendorf, IA 52722-1626
(309)779-5870
FAX: (309)779-5113

Bloomfield

Davis County Hospital
509 N Madison St
Bloomfield, IA 52537-1299
(641)664-7139
FAX: (641)664-3847

Boone

Boone County Hospital
1015 Union St
Boone, IA 50036-4898
(515)433-8160
FAX: (515)433-8916

Britt

Hancock County Memorial Hospital
532 1st St NW, Radiology Department
Britt, IA 50423-1227
(641)843-5190
FAX: (641)843-5008

Carroll

McFarland Clinic Carroll
1214 S Grant Rd
Carroll, IA 51401-3102
(712)792-1500
FAX: (712)792-7597

St. Anthony Regional Hospital And Nursing Home
311 S Clark St
Carroll, IA 51401-3038
(712)794-5201
FAX: (712)794-5488

Cedar Falls

Mercyone Cedar Falls Medical Center
515 College St
Cedar Falls, IA 50613-2500
(319)268-3060
FAX: (319)268-3326

Prairie Parkway Imaging
5100 Prairie Pkwy
Cedar Falls, IA 50613-8155
(319)222-2902
FAX: (319)222-2992

Cedar Rapids

Mercy Medical Center/Mercy Women's Center
701 10th St SE
Cedar Rapids, IA 52403-1251
(319)398-6359
FAX: (319)398-6959

Ob-Gyn Associates
855 A Ave NE
Cedar Rapids, IA 52402-5050
(319)368-5500
FAX: (319)368-5512

Radiology Consultants Of Iowa, Plc
1948 1st Ave NE
Cedar Rapids, IA 52402-5377
(319)364-0121
FAX: (319)364-5684

Unity Point St. Luke's Breast And Bone Health - Pci
202 10th St SE, Ste 265
Cedar Rapids, IA 52403-2420
(319)369-7216
FAX: (319)369-7808

Unity Point St. Luke's Breast And Bone Health - Westdale
4325 Williams Blvd SW 2nd Fl
Cedar Rapids, IA 52404-3436
(319)369-8255
FAX: (319)861-6750

Centerville

Mercyone Centerville Medical Center
1 Saint Joseph Dr
Centerville, IA 52544-9017
(641)437-3462
FAX: (641)437-3497

Chariton

Lucas County Health Center
1200 N 7th St
Chariton, IA 50049-1258
(641)774-3000
FAX: (641)774-3312

Charles City

Floyd County Medical Center
800 11th St, Radiology Department
Charles City, IA 50616-3468
(641)257-4325
FAX: (641)228-8012

Cherokee

Cherokee Regional Medical Center
300 Sioux Valley Dr
Cherokee, IA 51012-1205
(712)225-1501
FAX: (712)225-6880

Clarinda

Clarinda Regional Health Center
220 Essie Davison Dr
Clarinda, IA 51632-2915
(712)542-8278
FAX: (712)542-8262

Clarion

Iowa Specialty Hospital
1316 S Main St
Clarion, IA 50525-2019
(515)532-2811
FAX: (515)532-9243

Clinton

Mercyone Clinton Medical Center
1410 N 4th St
Clinton, IA 52732-2999
(563)244-5642
FAX: (563)244-5957

Mercyone Clinton North Health Plaza
915 13th Ave N
Clinton, IA 52732-5067
(563)243-2511
FAX: (563)243-6270

Clive

Iowa Radiology
12368 Stratford Dr, Ste 300
Clive, IA 50325-8149
(515)226-7437
FAX: (515)369-7437

Mercyone Clive Mammography
1601 NW 114th St, Ste 128
Clive, IA 50325-7036
(515)247-4444
FAX: (515)643-8867

Coralville

Corridor Radiology
2769 Heartland Dr Ste 105
Coralville, IA 52241-2732
(319)545-7300
FAX: (319)545-7309

Iowa River Landing
105 E 9th St
Coralville, IA 52241-2209
(319)356-3444
FAX: (319)467-2085

Corning

Chi Mercy Corning
603 Rosary Dr
Corning, IA 50841-1683
(641)322-6230
FAX: (641)322-5104

Corydon

Wayne County Hospital
PO Box 305, 417 S East St
Corydon, IA 50060-0305
(641)872-5237
FAX: (641)872-3097

Council Bluffs

Chi Mercy Hospital
800 Mercy Dr
Council Bluffs, IA 51503-3192
(866)731-3267
FAX: (712)328-5115

Methodist Jennie Edmundson Hospital
933 E Pierce St, Breast Imaging Department
Council Bluffs, IA 51503-4652
(712)396-6224
FAX: (712)396-6286

Methodist Jennie Edmundson Medical Plaza
808 E Pierce St, Imaging Suite
Council Bluffs, IA 51503-4601
(712)396-7600
FAX: (712)396-6286

Cresco

Regional Health Services Of Howard County
235 8th Ave W
Cresco, IA 52136-1062
(563)547-6333
FAX: (563)547-6475

Creston

Greater Regional Medical Center
1700 W Townline St, Ste 3
Creston, IA 50801-1054
(641)782-3508
FAX: (641)782-3805

Davenport

Genesis - Kenneth H. McKay, M.D. Center For Breast Health
1228 E Rusholme St Ste 2100
Davenport, IA 52803-2467
(563)421-7625
FAX: (563)421-7659

Genesis Imaging Center 53rd St
1970 E 53rd St
Davenport, IA 52807-2710
(563)421-5641
FAX: (563)441-0617

Decorah

Gundersen Health System - Decorah
1830 State Highway 9
Decorah, IA 52101-7301
(608)775-2682
FAX: (608)775-6674

Winneshiek Medical Center
901 Montgomery St
Decorah, IA 52101-2325
(563)387-3018
FAX: (563)382-1539

Denison

Crawford County Memorial Hospital
100 Medical Pkwy, Radiology Department
Denison, IA 51442-2299
(712)265-2651
FAX: (712)263-1722

Des Moines

Broadlawns Medical Center
1801 Hickman Rd
Des Moines, IA 50314-1597
(515)282-2309
FAX: (515)282-5735

Iowa Radiology
1221 Pleasant St, Ste 350
Des Moines, IA 50309-1420
(515)226-9810
FAX: (515)226-7493

Mercyone Des Moines Mammography
411 Laurel St, Ste 1265
Des Moines, IA 50314-3017
(515)247-4444
FAX: (515)643-8867

The Iowa Clinic
1215 Pleasant St Ste 408
Des Moines, IA 50309-1418
(515)244-5109
FAX: (515)875-9672

Unitypoint Health Des Moines Lutheran Mammography
700 E University Ave Level A Mammogra
Des Moines, IA 50316-2302
(515)263-5726
FAX: (515)263-5719

Dewitt

Genesis Medical Center - Dewitt Campus
1118 11th St
Dewitt, IA 52742-1296
(309)281-4148
FAX: (309)281-4149

Dubuque

Finley Hospital
350 N Grandview Ave
Dubuque, IA 52001-6392
(563)589-2402
FAX: (563)589-2491

Grand River Medical Group
1515 Delhi St Ste 100
Dubuque, IA 52001-6320
(563)589-4051
FAX: (563)589-4052

Medical Associates Clinic, P.C.
1000 Langworthy St
Dubuque, IA 52001-7365
(563)584-3384
FAX: (563)584-3129

Mercyone Dubuque Medical Center
250 Mercy Dr
Dubuque, IA 52001-7360
(563)589-9040
FAX: (563)589-9079

Dyersville

Mercy One Dyersville Medical Center
1111 3rd St SW
Dyersville, IA 52040-1725
(563)875-2952
FAX: (563)875-2957

Elkader

Mercyone Elkader Medical Center
901 Davidson St NW
Elkader, IA 52043-9015
(563)245-7037
FAX: (563)245-7077

Emmetsburg

Palo Alto County Health System
3201 1st St
Emmetsburg, IA 50536-2599
(712)852-5416
FAX: (712)852-5478

Estherville

Avera Holy Family
826 N 8th St
Estherville, IA 51334-1528
(712)362-6137
FAX: (712)362-6283

Fairfield

Jefferson County Health Center
2000 S Main St
Fairfield, IA 52556-3793
(641)469-4325
FAX: (641)469-4340

Fort Dodge

Unitypoint Clinic Norma Schmoker Women's Center
625 L St
Fort Dodge, IA 50501-5706
(515)574-6015
FAX: (515)574-6016

Fort Madison

Fort Madison Community Hospital
5445 Avenue O
Fort Madison, IA 52627-9611
(319)376-2040
FAX: (319)376-2183

Greenfield

Adair County Memorial Hospital
609 SE Kent St
Greenfield, IA 50849-9494
(641)743-7211
FAX: (641)743-7218

Grinnell

Grinnell Regional Medical Center
210 4th Ave, Radiology Department
Grinnell, IA 50112-1898
(641)236-2355
FAX: (641)236-2521

Grundy Center

Grundy County Memorial Hospital
201 E J Ave
Grundy Center, IA 50638-2096
(319)824-5086
FAX: (319)824-6696

Guthrie Center

Guthrie County Hospital
710 N 12th St
Guthrie Center, IA 50115-1549
(641)332-3806
FAX: (641)332-3886

Guttenberg

Guttenberg Municipal Hospital
200 Main St
Guttenberg, IA 52052-9108
(563)252-5552
FAX: (563)252-5553

Hamburg

George C. Grape Community Hospital
2959 US Highway 275
Hamburg, IA 51640-5067
(712)382-1515
FAX: (712)382-2012

Hampton

Franklin General Hospital
1720 Central Ave E, Ste A
Hampton, IA 50441-1867
(641)456-5026
FAX: (641)456-5021

Harlan

Myrtue Medical Center
1213 Garfield Ave
Harlan, IA 51537-2057
(712)755-4373
FAX: (712)755-4263

Hawarden

Hawarden Regional Healthcare
1111 11th St
Hawarden, IA 51023-1903
(712)551-3109
FAX: (712)551-3177

Humboldt

Humboldt County Memorial Hospital
1000 15th St N
Humboldt, IA 50548-1075
(515)332-4200
FAX: (515)332-7687

Ida Grove

Horn Memorial Hospital
701 E 2nd St
Ida Grove, IA 51445-1699
(712)364-7237
FAX: (712)364-7249

Independence

Buchanan County Health Center
1600 1st St E, Radiology Department
Independence, IA 50644-3155
(319)332-0870
FAX: (319)332-0957

Indianola

Mercyone Clinics Imaging Indianola
2006 N 4th St, Ste 202B
Indianola, IA 50125-4500
(515)247-4444
FAX: (515)643-8867

Iowa City

Mercy Hospital Breast Imaging Center
500 E Market St
Iowa City, IA 52245-2633
(319)339-3948
FAX: (319)358-2679

University Of Iowa Hospital & Clinics
200 Hawkins Dr
Iowa City, IA 52242-1009
(319)356-4369
FAX: (319)356-8929

Iowa Falls

Ellsworth Municipal Hospital Dba Hansen Family Hospital
920 S Oak St
Iowa Falls, IA 50126-9507
(641)648-7024
FAX: (641)648-7023

Jefferson

Greene County Medical Center
1000 W Lincoln Way
Jefferson, IA 50129-1685
(515)386-0590
FAX: (515)386-2661

Keokuk

Blessing Health Keokuk
1600 Morgan St
Keokuk, IA 52632-3456
(319)526-8700
FAX: (319)524-1399

Keokuk Clinic
3285 Main St
Keokuk, IA 52632-2263
(319)524-6274
FAX: (319)524-9068

Keosauqua

Van Buren County Hospital And Clinics
304 Franklin St
Keosauqua, IA 52565-1164
(319)293-8721
FAX: (319)293-6281

Knoxville

Knoxville Hospital And Clinics
1002 S Lincoln St
Knoxville, IA 50138-3121
(641)842-1518
FAX: (641)842-1472

Lake City

Stewart Memorial Community Hospital
1301 W Main St
Lake City, IA 51449-1586
(712)464-3171
FAX: (712)464-4136

Lemars

Floyd Valley Healthcare
714 Lincoln St NE
Lemars, IA 51031-3341
(712)546-3382
FAX: (712)546-3483

Leon

Community Health Centers Of Southern Iowa
302 NE 14th St
Leon, IA 50144-1206
(641)446-2383
FAX: (641)446-2382

Manchester

Regional Medical Center
709 W Main St
Manchester, IA 52057-1526
(563)927-7338
FAX: (563)927-7407

Manning

Manning Regional Healthcare Center
1550 6th St
Manning, IA 51455-1004
(712)655-2072
FAX: (712)655-8173

Maquoketa

Jackson County Regional Health Center
PO Box 910
Maquoketa, IA 52060-0910
(563)652-4053
FAX: (563)652-4019

Marengo

Marengo Memorial Hospital Dba: Compass Memorial Healthcare
300 W May St
Marengo, IA 52301-1261
(319)642-8037
FAX: (319)642-5543

Marion

Unity Point St. Luke's Breast And Bone Health - Marion
2996 7th Ave
Marion, IA 52302-3713
(319)286-4376
FAX: (319)369-7808

Marshalltown

McFarland Clinic Marshalltown
312 E Main St
Marshalltown, IA 50158-1992
(641)844-2215
FAX: (641)844-2222

Unitypoint Health - Marshalltown
55 Central Iowa Dr
Marshalltown, IA 50158-4705
(641)754-5077
FAX: (641)753-2714

Mason City

Forest Park Imaging, Llc
1010 4th St SW, Ste 100
Mason City, IA 50401-2856
(641)428-7782
FAX: (641)428-5156

Missouri Valley

Chi Missouri Valley
631 N 8th St
Missouri Valley, IA 51555-1102
(712)642-9347
FAX: (712)642-9224

Mount Ayr

Ringgold County Hospital
504 N Cleveland St
Mount Ayr, IA 50854-2201
(641)464-4400
FAX: (641)464-4431

Mount Pleasant

Henry County Health Center Inc
106 N Jackson St Ste 103
Mount Pleasant, IA 52641-2063
(319)385-6158
FAX: (319)385-6719

Muscatine

Muscatine General Hospital
1518 Mulberry Ave, Radiology Dept
Muscatine, IA 52761-3433
(563)264-9205
FAX: (563)264-9298

Muscatine Radiology
2104 Cedarwood Dr Ste 100
Muscatine, IA 52761-2662
(563)263-3400
FAX: (563)263-3311

New Hampton

Mercyone New Hampton Medical Center
308 N Maple Ave, Radiology Department
New Hampton, IA 50659-1142
(515)394-4121
FAX: (515)394-1685

Newton

Mercyone Newton Medical Center
204 N 4th Ave E
Newton, IA 50208-3135
(641)791-4310
FAX: (641)791-4828

Oelwein

Bchc Family Medicine Oelwein
2405 Rock Island Rd
Oelwein, IA 50662-3102
(319)283-2651
FAX: (319)283-5635

Mercyone Oelwein Medical Center
201 8th Ave SE, Mammography Department
Oelwein, IA 50662-2447
(319)283-6055
FAX: (319)283-6269

Onawa

Burgess Health Center
1600 Diamond St
Onawa, IA 51040-1548
(712)423-9363
FAX: (712)423-9329

Orange City

Orange City Area Health System
1000 Lincoln Cir SE
Orange City, IA 51041-1862
(712)737-5322
FAX: (712)737-5371

Osage

Mitchell County Regional Health Center
616 N 8th St
Osage, IA 50461-1456
(641)732-6017
FAX: (641)732-6038

Osceola

Clarke County Hospital
800 S Fillmore St
Osceola, IA 50213-1694
(641)342-5410
FAX: (641)342-5368

Oskaloosa

Mahaska County Hospital
1229 C Ave E
Oskaloosa, IA 52577-4298
(641)672-3322
FAX: (641)672-3320

Ottumwa

Ottumwa Regional Health Center
1001 Pennsylvania Ave
Ottumwa, IA 52501-2186
(641)684-2430
FAX: (641)684-2433

Pella Regional Health Center - Ottumwa
920 N Quincy Ave
Ottumwa, IA 52501-3866
(641)455-5200
FAX: (641)455-5150

Pella

Pella Regional Health Center
404 Jefferson St
Pella, IA 50219-1257
(641)628-6620
FAX: (641)628-6672

Perry

Dallas County Hospital
610 10th St
Perry, IA 50220-2249
(515)465-7525
FAX: (515)465-7680

Pocahontas

Pocahontas Community Hospital
606 NW 7th St
Pocahontas, IA 50574-1099
(712)335-5227
FAX: (712)335-5223

Red Oak

Montgomery County Memorial Hospital
2301 Eastern Ave
Red Oak, IA 51566-1305
(712)623-7164
FAX: (712)623-6465

Rock Rapids

Avera Merrill Pioneer Hospital
1100 S 10th Ave
Rock Rapids, IA 51246-2020
(712)472-5401
FAX: (712)472-5505

Rock Valley

Hegg Health Center
1202 21st Ave
Rock Valley, IA 51247-1420
(712)476-8023
FAX: (712)476-8006

Sac City

Loring Hospital
211 Highland Ave
Sac City, IA 50583-2416
(712)662-6344
FAX: (712)662-6330

Sheldon

Sanford Sheldon Medical Center
PO Box 250, 118 N 7th Ave
Sheldon, IA 51201-0250
(712)324-6360
FAX: (712)324-6373

Shenandoah

Shenandoah Medical Center
300 Pershing Ave
Shenandoah, IA 51601-2355
(712)246-7288
FAX: (712)246-7309

Sibley

Osceola Community Hospital,Inc Dba Osceola Regional Hlth.Ctr
600 9th Ave N
Sibley, IA 51249-1012
(712)754-5360
FAX: (712)754-4494

Sigourney

Keokuk County Health Center
23019 Highway 149
Sigourney, IA 52591-1194
(641)622-2720
FAX: (641)243-8296

Sioux Center

Sioux Center Health
1101 9th St SE, Radiology Department
Sioux Center, IA 51250-2501
(712)722-8116
FAX: (712)722-8477

Sioux City

Mercyone Siouxland Medical Center
801 5th St
Sioux City, IA 51101-1326
(712)279-2046
FAX: (712)279-5619

Uph, St. Luke's Imaging & Breast Screening Services
5885 Sunnybrook Dr, Ste A100
Sioux City, IA 51106-4250
(712)266-2671
FAX: (712)277-8728

Spencer

Spencer Hospital
1200 1st Ave E
Spencer, IA 51301-4330
(712)264-6181
FAX: (712)264-6541

Spirit Lake

Lakes Regional Healthcare
2301 Highway 71
Spirit Lake, IA 51360-1185
(712)336-8777
FAX: (712)336-8636

Storm Lake

Buena Vista Regional Medical Center
1525 W 5th St
Storm Lake, IA 50588-3027
(712)213-8691
FAX: (712)732-8281

Sumner

Community Memorial Hospital
909 W 1st St
Sumner, IA 50674-1203
(563)578-3275
FAX: (563)578-2148

Vinton

Virginia Gay Hospital
502 N 9th Ave
Vinton, IA 52349-2299
(319)472-6288
FAX: (319)472-6484

W Burlington

Southeast Iowa Regional Medical Center
1221 S Gear Ave
W Burlington, IA 52655-1679
(319)768-3590
FAX: (319)768-4825

Washington

Washington County Hospital And Clinics
400 E Polk St
Washington, IA 52353-1254
(319)863-3964
FAX: (319)863-3978

Waterloo

Allen Memorial Hospital
Radiology Services, 1825 Logan Avenue
Waterloo, IA 50703
(319)235-3179
FAX: (319)235-5187

Mercyone Waterloo Breast Center
3421 W 9th St, Ste G4600
Waterloo, IA 50702-5401
(319)272-7039
FAX: (319)272-0045

Unity Point Health Allen At United Medical Park
1731 W Ridgeway Ave Ste 101
Waterloo, IA 50701-4595
(319)833-6001
FAX: (319)833-6003

Waukon

Veterans Memorial Hospital
40 1st St SE
Waukon, IA 52172-2099
(563)568-5500
FAX: (563)568-5573

Waverly

Waverly Health Center
312 9th St SW
Waverly, IA 50677-2999
(319)352-4926
FAX: (319)352-4828

Webster City

Hamilton County Hospital Dba Van Diest Family Health Clinic
2350 Hospital Dr
Webster City, IA 50595-6600
(515)832-7800
FAX: (515)832-1123

West Des Moines

The Iowa Clinic
5950 University Ave Ste 145
West Des Moines, IA 50266-8233
(515)244-5109
FAX: (515)875-9672

West Union

Gundersen Palmer Lutheran Hospital And Clinics
112 Jefferson St, Gundersen Palmer Lutheran Hospital And C
West Union, IA 52175-1022
(608)780-1839
FAX: (563)422-9793

Winterset

Madison County Memorial Hospital
300 W Hutchings St, Ste A
Winterset, IA 50273-2109
(515)462-5214
FAX: (515)462-5114

KANSAS

Abilene

Memorial Health System
511 NE 10th St
Abilene, KS 67410-2100
(785)263-2100
FAX: (785)263-6653

Anthony

Hospital District 6 Of Harper County Kansas
485 N Ks Hwy 2
Anthony, KS 67003-2526
(620)914-1200
FAX: (620)914-1254

Arkansas City

South Central Kansas Regional Medical Center
6401 Patterson Pkwy
Arkansas City, KS 67005-5701
(620)441-5758
FAX: (620)441-5962

Atchison

Atchison Hospital
800 Ravenhill Dr
Atchison, KS 66002-9204
(913)360-5542
FAX: (913)674-2014

Belleville

Republic County Hospital
2420 G St
Belleville, KS 66935-2400
(785)527-6064
FAX: (785)527-2602

Beloit

Mitchell County Hospital Health Systems
PO Box 399, 400 W 8th St
Beloit, KS 67420-0399
(785)738-9554
FAX: (785)738-9212

Burlington

Coffey County Hospital
801 N 4th St
Burlington, KS 66839-2602
(620)364-2121
FAX: (620)364-2208

Chanute

Neosho Memorial Regional Medical Center
629 S Plummer Ave
Chanute, KS 66720-1928
(620)432-5386
FAX: (620)432-5505

Clay Center

Clay County Medical Center
617 Liberty St
Clay Center, KS 67432-1564
(785)632-2144
FAX: (785)632-3196

Coffeyville

Coffeyville Regional Medical Center
1400 W 4th St
Coffeyville, KS 67337-3306
(620)252-1572
FAX: (620)252-1573

Colby

Citizens Medical Center
100 E College Dr
Colby, KS 67701-3799
(785)460-1250
FAX: (785)460-1235

Columbus

Mercy Hosp Columbus Dba Mercy Maude Norton Hosp - Mobile
220 N Pennsylvania Ave
Columbus, KS 66725-1110
(620)429-2545
FAX: (620)429-1984

Concordia

Cloud County Health Center
1100 Highland Dr
Concordia, KS 66901-3923
(785)243-8447
FAX: (785)243-8555

Council Grove

Morris County Hospital
600 N Washington St
Council Grove, KS 66846-1499
(620)767-6811
FAX: (620)767-5611

Derby

Family Medcenters Diagnostics
1101 N Rock Rd
Derby, KS 67037-3705
(316)789-1134
FAX: (316)789-1195

Dodge City

Dodge City Medical Center
2020 Central Ave
Dodge City, KS 67801-6411
(620)255-6326
FAX: (620)227-1234

Western Plains Medical Complex
3001 Avenue A
Dodge City, KS 67801-2270
(620)225-8487
FAX: (620)225-8482

El Dorado

Susan B. Allen Memorial Hospital
720 W Central Ave
El Dorado, KS 67042-2144
(316)322-4510
FAX: (316)322-4506

Emporia

Cotton O'Neil Emporia
1301 W 12th Ave, Ste 401
Emporia, KS 66801-2591
(620)343-2900
FAX: (620)342-1833

Newman Regional Health Ws & Ec Jones Breast Care Center
1201 W 12th Ave
Emporia, KS 66801-2504
(620)342-5222
FAX: (620)343-5919

Fort Leavenworth

Munson Army Health Center
550 Pope Ave, Radiology Dept.
Fort Leavenworth, KS 66027-2332
(913)684-6140
FAX: (913)684-6153

Fort Riley

Irwin Army Community Hospital
650 Huebner Rd
Fort Riley, KS 66442-4030
(785)239-7911
FAX: (785)239-7803

Fort Scott

Community Health Center Of Southeast Kansas - Fort Scott Pcc
PO Box 1104
Fort Scott, KS 66701-1104
(620)223-8484
FAX: (620)240-5674

Fredonia

Fredonia Regional Hospital
1527 Madison St
Fredonia, KS 66736-1751
(620)378-6209
FAX: (620)378-6211

Garden City

St. Catherine Hospital
401 E Spruce St
Garden City, KS 67846-5672
(620)272-2276
FAX: (620)272-2283

Garnett

Anderson County Hospital
421 S Maple St
Garnett, KS 66032-1334
(785)204-8000
FAX: (785)448-6381

Girard

Girard Medical Center
302 N Hospital Dr
Girard, KS 66743-2000
(620)724-5162
FAX: (620)724-8875

Goodland

Goodland Regional Medical Center
220 W 2nd St
Goodland, KS 67735-1602
(785)890-6033
FAX: (785)890-6082

Great Bend

University Of Kansas Health System Great Bend Campus
514 Cleveland St
Great Bend, KS 67530-3562
(620)792-7300
FAX: (620)792-7315

Hays

Hays Medical Center Inc.
2220 Canterbury Dr
Hays, KS 67601-2370
(785)623-6565
FAX: (785)261-6564

Herington

Herington Municipal Hospital
100 E Helen St
Herington, KS 67449-1697
(785)258-2207
FAX: (785)258-5127

Hiawatha

Amberwell Hiawatha
300 Utah St
Hiawatha, KS 66434-2314
(785)742-6270
FAX: (785)742-6506

Hoisington

Clara Barton Hospital
250 W 9th St
Hoisington, KS 67544-1799
(620)653-2114
FAX: (620)653-2673

Holton

Holton Community Hospital
1110 Columbine Dr
Holton, KS 66436-8824
(785)364-9677
FAX: (785)364-9616

Hutchinson

Hutchinson Clinic, P.A.
2101 N Waldron St
Hutchinson, KS 67502-1197
(620)669-2730
FAX: (620)694-4115

Junction City

Geary Community Hospital
1102 Saint Marys Rd
Junction City, KS 66441-4196
(785)210-3377
FAX: (785)210-3450

Kansas City

Diagnostic Imaging Centers P.A. Wyandotte
9201 Parallel Pkwy
Kansas City, KS 66112-1510
(913)344-9989
FAX: (913)696-0040

Providence Medical Center
8929 Parallel Pkwy
Kansas City, KS 66112-3607
(913)596-3352
FAX: (913)596-3890

Providence Medical Imaging Center
11011 Haskell Ave
Kansas City, KS 66109-8500
(913)667-5600
FAX: (913)667-5601

Kingman

Kingman Healthcare Center
750 Avenue D West
Kingman, KS 67068
(620)532-0114
FAX: (620)532-0169

Larned

Pawnee Valley Community Hospital
923 Carroll Ave
Larned, KS 67550-2429
(620)285-8607
FAX: (620)285-8885

Lawrence

Lmh Health West Campus
6265 Rock Chalk Dr Ste 2400
Lawrence, KS 66049-5232
(785)505-3300
FAX: (785)505-5262

Leavenworth

St. John Hospital
3550 S 4th St
Leavenworth, KS 66048-5071
(913)680-6297
FAX: (913)680-6408

Lenexa

Advent Health - Lenexa
23401 Prairie Star Pkwy
Lenexa, KS 66227-7268
(913)676-2505
FAX: (913)789-3212

Encompass Medical Group - Premier Imaging Lenexa
8550 Marshall Dr
Lenexa, KS 66214-1505
(913)495-2000
FAX: (913)495-2022

Liberal

Southwest Medical Center
315 W 15th St
Liberal, KS 67901-2455
(620)629-6329
FAX: (620)629-2435

Manhattan

Cotton O'Neil Manhattan
1133 College Ave Bldg E
Manhattan, KS 66502-2770
(785)537-2651
FAX: (785)354-5125

Via Christi Hospital Manhattan, Inc
1133 College Ave Bldg G Ste 130
Manhattan, KS 66502-2770
(785)565-4707
FAX: (785)532-9036

Marion

St. Luke Hospital
535 S Freeborn St
Marion, KS 66861-1256
(620)382-2177
FAX: (620)382-8926

Marysville

Community Memorial Healthcare Inc.
708 N 18th St
Marysville, KS 66508-1338
(785)562-2311
FAX: (785)562-4043

McPherson

McPherson Hospital, Inc.
1000 Hospital Dr
McPherson, KS 67460-2326
(620)241-2250
FAX: (620)241-8253

Meade

Meade District Hospital
510 E Carthage St
Meade, KS 67864-6401
(620)873-5589
FAX: (620)873-5521

Neodesha

Wilson Medical Center
PO Box 360, 2600 Ottawa Rd
Neodesha, KS 66757-0360
(620)325-8364
FAX: (620)325-8457

Newton

Breast Imaging Center At Nmc Health's Medical Center
600 Medical Center Dr
Newton, KS 67114-8780
(316)283-4744
FAX: (316)283-6867

Norton

Norton County Hospital
102 E Holme St
Norton, KS 67654-1406
(785)877-3351
FAX: (785)877-3029

Oberlin

Decatur Health Systems Inc.
810 W Columbia St
Oberlin, KS 67749-2450
(785)475-2208
FAX: (785)475-2401

Olathe

Diagnostic Imaging Centers Pa Olathe
13795 S Mur Len Rd
Olathe, KS 66062-1675
(913)397-7272
FAX: (913)397-7373

Olathe Medical Pavilion
21120 W 152nd St
Olathe, KS 66061-5307
(913)791-4395
FAX: (913)791-3532

Onaga

Community Healthcare System, Inc.
120 W 8th St
Onaga, KS 66521-9574
(785)889-4274
FAX: (785)889-4277

Osage City

Cotton O'Neil Clinic - Osage City
131 W Market St
Osage City, KS 66523-1000
(785)528-3161
FAX: (785)354-5125

Oskaloosa

Cotton-O'Neil Clinic - Oskaloosa
209 W Jefferson St
Oskaloosa, KS 66066-5359
(785)863-3417
FAX: (785)354-5125

Ottawa

Ransom Memorial Hospital
1301 S Main St
Ottawa, KS 66067-3598
(785)229-3340
FAX: (785)229-8289

Overland Park

Adventhealth South Overland Park Women's Imaging
7840 W 165th St, Ste 150
Overland Park, KS 66223-2994
(913)676-2505
FAX: (913)789-3889

Diagnostic Imaging Centers - Overland Park
6650 W 110th St, Ste 100
Overland Park, KS 66211-1544
(913)491-9299
FAX: (913)491-9363

Diagnostic Imaging Centers, P.A. Mobile 1
6650 W 110th St, Ste 110
Overland Park, KS 66211-1501
(913)319-8400
FAX: (816)554-9657

Goppert Center For Breast Care
12541 Foster St Ste 100
Overland Park, KS 66213-2305
(913)317-3100
FAX: (913)317-3124

Johnson County Imaging
11717 W 112th St
Overland Park, KS 66210-2761
(913)469-8998
FAX: (913)469-1698

Menorah Medical Center Breast Center
5721 W 119th St
Overland Park, KS 66209-3753
(913)498-6266
FAX: (913)498-7899

Overland Park Regional Medical Ctr
10550 Quivira Rd, Ste 130
Overland Park, KS 66215-2370
(913)541-5503
FAX: (913)541-5205

Overland Park Surgical Specialties, Llc
10600 Mastin St
Overland Park, KS 66212-5723
(913)956-4200
FAX: (913)825-2765

The University Of Kansas Dba Hosp. Indian Creek Campus
10710 Nall Ave
Overland Park, KS 66211-1206
(913)588-6804
FAX: (913)588-3440

Paola

Miami County Medical Center
2100 Baptiste Dr
Paola, KS 66071-1314
(913)294-6611
FAX: (913)294-6634

Parsons

Labette Health
PO Box 956, 1902 Hwy 59 S
Parsons, KS 67357-0956
(620)421-4880
FAX: (620)820-5189

Phillipsburg

Phillips County Hospital
1150 State St
Phillipsburg, KS 67661-1743
(785)540-4930
FAX: (785)543-8911

Pittsburg

Ascension Via Christi Hospital Pittsburg, Inc.
1 Mt Carmel Way
Pittsburg, KS 66762-7587
(620)232-0129
FAX: (620)235-7971

Plainville

Rooks County Health Center
1210 N Washington St Box 389
Plainville, KS 67663-1632
(785)688-4424
FAX: (785)434-2187

Pratt

Pratt Regional Medical Center
200 Commodore St
Pratt, KS 67124-3099
(620)450-1494
FAX: (620)450-1280

Roeland Park

Adventhealth Imaging Center Roeland Park
5675 Roe Blvd
Roeland Park, KS 66205-2515
(913)632-2634
FAX: (913)632-2635

Russell

Russell Regional Hospital
200 S Main St
Russell, KS 67665-2937
(785)483-0710
FAX: (785)483-0711

Sabetha

Sabetha Community Hospital
14th And Oregon St.
Sabetha, KS 66534
(785)284-1525
FAX: (785)284-1532

Salina

Mowery Clinic, Llc.
737 E Crawford St
Salina, KS 67401-5103
(785)822-0224
FAX: (785)833-5783

Salina Regional Breast Diagnostic Center
520 S Santa Fe Ave Ste 100
Salina, KS 67401-4190
(785)452-7000
FAX: (785)452-4995

Salina Regional Health Center Dba Comcare
2090 S Ohio St
Salina, KS 67401-6702
(785)515-5167
FAX: (785)309-2327

United Radiology Group, Mobile Imaging
119 W Iron Ave Fl 5
Salina, KS 67401-2600
(785)827-9526
FAX: (785)827-2854

Scott City

Scott County Hospital
201 Albert Ave
Scott City, KS 67871-6117
(620)872-7761
FAX: (620)872-5729

Seneca

Nemaha Valley Community Hospital
1600 Community Dr
Seneca, KS 66538-9758
(785)336-0455
FAX: (785)336-2764

Shawnee

Ku Med West
7405 Renner Rd
Shawnee, KS 66217-9414
(913)588-6804
FAX: (913)588-3440

Shawnee Mission

Adventhealth Shawnee Mission
9100 W 74th St
Shawnee Mission, KS 66204-4004
(913)632-9164
FAX: (913)789-3212

Smith Center

Smith County Memorial Hospital
921 E Highway 36
Smith Center, KS 66967-9582
(785)686-3140
FAX: (785)282-3327

Topeka

Cotton O'Neil Asbury Drive
2902 SW Asbury Dr
Topeka, KS 66614-4466
(785)354-6266
FAX: (785)354-5125

Stormont Vail Women's Center
823 SW Mulvane St Ste 102
Topeka, KS 66606-1679
(785)354-6266
FAX: (785)354-5125

The University Of Kansas Health System St. Francis
1700 SW 7th St
Topeka, KS 66606-2489
(785)295-8013
FAX: (785)231-5973

The University Of Kansas Health System St. Francis
601 SW Corporate Vw
Topeka, KS 66615-1244
(785)295-5470
FAX: (785)231-5973

Ulysses

Bob Wilson Memorial Grant Co Hospital
415 N Main St
Ulysses, KS 67880-2196
(620)356-6051
FAX: (620)424-2400

Wamego

Wamego Hospital Association Dba Wamego Health Center
711 Genn Dr
Wamego, KS 66547-1179
(785)456-7270
FAX: (785)458-7342

Washington

Washington County Hospital
304 E 3rd St
Washington, KS 66968-2098
(785)325-2211
FAX: (785)325-3149

Westwood

University Of Kansas Hospital
2650 Shawnee Mission Pkwy
Westwood, KS 66205-2003
(913)588-6804
FAX: (913)588-3440

Wichita

Amg Via Christi On Murdock
3311 E Murdock St
Wichita, KS 67208-3054
(316)274-8532
FAX: (316)274-8963

Ascension Medical Group- Founders Circle
1947 N Founders Cir
Wichita, KS 67206-3548
(316)858-0100
FAX: (316)691-6701

Ascension Via Christi Imaging L.L.C.
14700 W Saint Teresa St, Ste 150
Wichita, KS 67235-9611
(316)274-2020
FAX: (316)274-2030

Ascension Via Christi Imaging Wichita, Llc
928 N Saint Francis Ave
Wichita, KS 67214-3822
(316)274-8532
FAX: (316)691-6701

Ascension Via Christi St Joseph
3600 E Harry St
Wichita, KS 67218-3713
(316)858-4090
FAX: (316)689-6192

Cypress Women's Imaging
3232 E Murdock St
Wichita, KS 67208-3003
(316)681-1827
FAX: (316)219-5825

Cypress Women's Imaging - West
2131 N Ridge Rd Ste 105
Wichita, KS 67212-1571
(316)681-1827
FAX: (316)681-3224

Cypress Women's Imaging East
9300 E 29th St N Ste 202
Wichita, KS 67226-2183
(316)681-1827
FAX: (316)681-3224

Cypress Womens Imaging Cranbrook
10111 E 21st St N, Bldg 4 Suite 400
Wichita, KS 67206-3508
(316)779-8504
FAX: (316)681-3224

Wesley Medical Center
550 N Hillside St
Wichita, KS 67214-4976
(316)962-2900
FAX: (316)962-7814

West Wichita Family Physicians, P.A.
8200 W Central Ave, Ste 1 Ste One
Wichita, KS 67212-9501
(316)721-4544
FAX: (316)773-4563

Wichita Ob/Gyn Associates
551 N Hillside St, Ste 510
Wichita, KS 67214-4928
(316)685-0559
FAX: (877)334-2709

Winfield

William Newton Hospital
1300 E 5th Ave, Radiology Department
Winfield, KS 67156-2495
(620)221-2214
FAX: (620)222-6260

KENTUCKY

Albany

The Medical Center At Albany
723 Burkesville Rd
Albany, KY 42602-1654
(606)387-8000
FAX: (606)387-8550

Ashland

King's Daughters' Medical Center
2225 Central Ave
Ashland, KY 41101-7841
(606)408-2742
FAX: (606)408-6470

Barbourville

Barbourville Arh
80 Hospital Dr
Barbourville, KY 40906-7363
(606)545-5528
FAX: (606)545-5558

Bardstown

Baptist Health
3615 E John Rowan Blvd, Ste 101
Bardstown, KY 40004-3264
(502)350-3889
FAX: (502)350-3890

Flaget Memorial Hospital
4305 New Shepherdsville Rd, Hwy 245
Bardstown, KY 40004-1299
(502)350-5000
FAX: (502)350-5111

Benton

Marshall County Hospital
615 Old Symsonia Rd
Benton, KY 42025-1399
(270)527-4804
FAX: (270)527-4891

Berea

St. Joseph Berea
305 Estill St, Dept. Radiology
Berea, KY 40403-1909
(859)986-5563
FAX: (859)967-5617

Booneville

Owsley County Medical Clinic
Rt. 11 Beattyville Rd.
Booneville, KY 41314
(606)593-6395
FAX: (606)593-5916

Bowling Green

Graves Gilbert Clinic
201 Park St
Bowling Green, KY 42101-1708
(270)781-5111
FAX: (270)783-3779

Graves Gilbert Clinic Family Care Center
2724 Nashville Rd
Bowling Green, KY 42101-4000
(270)781-5111
FAX: (270)783-3779

Greenview Regional Hospital
1801 Ashley Cir
Bowling Green, KY 42104-3384
(270)793-2023
FAX: (270)793-2270

The Medical Center At Bowling Green
250 Park St
Bowling Green, KY 42101-1795
(270)745-1175
FAX: (270)745-1173

Western Kentucky Diagnostic Img - Dept Of The Med Ctr
1635 Scottsville Rd
Bowling Green, KY 42104-3244
(270)746-9500
FAX: (270)780-2739

Brandenburg

Baptist Health Diagnostics At Brandenburg
100 Commerce Dr
Brandenburg, KY 40108-9784
(270)422-1222
FAX: (270)422-1278

Cadiz

Trigg County Hospital
254 Main St
Cadiz, KY 42211-9153
(270)206-3638
FAX: (270)522-5438

Campbellsville

Taylor Regional Hospital
1700 Old Lebanon Rd, Radiology Department
Campbellsville, KY 42718-9600
(270)789-5832
FAX: (270)789-5835

Carrollton

Carroll County Memorial Hospital
309 11th St
Carrollton, KY 41008-1400
(502)732-3129
FAX: (502)732-3281

Corbin

Baptist Health Corbin
1 Trillium Way
Corbin, KY 40701-8426
(606)526-4268
FAX: (606)523-8738

Covington

St. Elizabeth Healthcare - Covington
1500 James Simpson Jr Way, Ste 302
Covington, KY 41011-0802
(859)655-7400
FAX: (859)655-7205

Crestwood

Baptist Crestwood
6580 Kenwood Crossing Rd
Crestwood, KY 40014-7614
(502)222-3304
FAX: (502)222-3629

Cynthiana

Harrison Memorial Hospital
1210 Ky Highway 36 E
Cynthiana, KY 41031-7498
(859)235-3559
FAX: (859)235-3688

Danville

Ephraim McDowell Diagnostic Center
101 Daniel Dr
Danville, KY 40422-2527
(859)936-8204
FAX: (859)239-6756

Edgewood

St. Elizabeth Healthcare - Edgewood
1 Medical Village Dr
Edgewood, KY 41017-3403
(859)655-7400
FAX: (859)301-6209

St. Elizabeth Healthcare-Women's Health Center
600 Medical Village Dr
Edgewood, KY 41017-3416
(859)655-7400
FAX: (859)301-6209

Elizabethtown

Baptist Health Hardin Diagnostic Main Campus
913 N Dixie Ave
Elizabethtown, KY 42701-2503
(270)706-5444
FAX: (270)706-5356

Baptist Health Hardin Elizabethtown
2409 Ring Rd Ste 114
Elizabethtown, KY 42701-5935
(270)982-3344
FAX: (270)982-2777

Flemingsburg

Fleming County Hospital
55 Foundation Dr, Radiology Department
Flemingsburg, KY 41041-9815
(606)849-5150
FAX: (606)849-5135

Florence

St. Elizabeth Healthcare-Florence
4900 Houston Rd
Florence, KY 41042-4824
(859)212-4830
FAX: (859)212-4324

Fort Campbell

Blanchfield Army Community Hospital
650 Joel Dr, Radiology Department
Fort Campbell, KY 42223-5318
(270)956-0033
FAX: (270)798-8243

Fort Knox

Ireland Army Health Clinic
200 Brule St, Bldg 872
Fort Knox, KY 40121-6100
(502)626-9941
FAX: (502)624-9343

Fort Thomas

St. Elizabeth Healthcare Ft. Thomas
85 N Grand Ave
Fort Thomas, KY 41075-1793
(859)572-3430
FAX: (859)572-2310

Frankfort

Capital Medical Group Imaging Services
1001 Leawood Dr Ste A
Frankfort, KY 40601-3375
(502)875-0882
FAX: (502)875-0872

Frankfort Regional Medical Center
299 Kings Daughters Dr
Frankfort, KY 40601-4186
(502)226-1665
FAX: (502)696-3472

Franklin

The Medical Center At Franklin
1100 Brookhaven Rd, Radiology Department
Franklin, KY 42134-2746
(270)598-4839
FAX: (270)598-4818

Ft Wright

The Christ Hospital Imaging Center - Ft Wright
1995 Dixie Hwy., Ste. E
Ft Wright, KY 41011
(513)585-2668
FAX: (513)564-1370

Georgetown

Baptist Health Lexington Breast Imag. Services At Georgetown
206 Bevins Ln
Georgetown, KY 40324-6130
(859)260-6050
FAX: (859)260-4151

Georgetown Community Hospital
1140 Lexington Rd
Georgetown, KY 40324-9330
(502)868-1270
FAX: (502)868-1107

Glasgow

Tj Health Pavilion
310 N L Rogers Wells Blvd
Glasgow, KY 42141-1300
(270)651-5591
FAX: (270)659-5858

Greensburg

Jane Todd Crawford Memorial Hospital
202 Milby St 206
Greensburg, KY 42743-1100
(270)932-4211
FAX: (270)932-3590

Hardinsburg

Breckinridge Memorial Hospital
1011 Old Highway 60
Hardinsburg, KY 40143-2597
(270)756-6546
FAX: (270)756-6584

Harlan

Harlan Appalachian Regional Hospital
81 Ball Park Rd
Harlan, KY 40831-1792
(606)573-8100
FAX: (606)573-8121

Harlan Medical Clinic
132 Village Center Rd
Harlan, KY 40831-1777
(606)573-7771
FAX: (606)573-2809

Harrodsburg

Ephraim McDowell James B. Haggin Hospital
464 Linden Ave
Harrodsburg, KY 40330-1882
(859)733-4810
FAX: (859)734-8334

Hartford

Ohio County Hospital
1211 Old Main St
Hartford, KY 42347-1619
(270)298-5450
FAX: (270)298-3407

Hazard

Hazard Arh Imaging Ctr. Llc - Med. Mall Imaging Ctr
210 Black Gold Blvd Ste 110
Hazard, KY 41701-2620
(606)487-7070
FAX: (606)487-7010

Primary Care Centers Of Eastern Kentucky
101 Town And Country Ln Ste 100
Hazard, KY 41701-9524
(606)439-1300
FAX: (606)435-7647

Henderson

Deaconess Henderson Hospital
1305 N Elm St
Henderson, KY 42420-2783
(270)827-7156
FAX: (270)831-7951

Owensboro Health Henderson Healthplex
1200 Barrett Blvd
Henderson, KY 42420-4950
(270)685-7100
FAX: (270)688-2275

Hopkinsville

Jennie Stuart Medical Center
320 W 18th St
Hopkinsville, KY 42240-6304
(270)887-0132
FAX: (270)887-0439

Jennie Stuart Medical Imaging Center
110 Nick Terhune Dr
Hopkinsville, KY 42240-8722
(270)887-8311
FAX: (270)887-8313

Horse Cave

The Medical Center At Caverna
1501 S Dixie St
Horse Cave, KY 42749-1480
(270)786-6644
FAX: (270)786-6646

Hyden

Mary Breckinridge Arh Hospital
PO Box 679
Hyden, KY 41749-0679
(606)672-2901
FAX: (606)672-1964

Irvine

Mercy Health-Marcum & Wallace Memorial Hospital, Llc
60 Mercy Ct
Irvine, KY 40336-1331
(606)726-2106
FAX: (606)726-2175

Jackson

Kentucky River Medical Center
540 Jett Dr
Jackson, KY 41339-9622
(606)666-6330
FAX: (606)666-6120

Lagrange

Baptist Health Lagrange
1025 New Moody Ln
Lagrange, KY 40031-9154
(502)222-3939
FAX: (502)222-3629

Lebanon

Spring View Hospital
320 N Loretto Rd
Lebanon, KY 40033-1323
(270)692-5267
FAX: (270)699-4601

Leitchfield

Owensboro Health Twin Lakes Medical Center
910 Wallace Ave, Radiology Department
Leitchfield, KY 42754-2414
(270)259-9490
FAX: (270)259-2950

Lexington

Baptist Health Lexington Breast Imaging Services
1760 Nicholasville Rd Ste 401
Lexington, KY 40503-1444
(859)260-6050
FAX: (859)260-4151

Baptist Health Lexington Breast Imaging Services Hamburg
1775 Alysheba Way Ste 110
Lexington, KY 40509-9024
(859)260-6050
FAX: (859)260-4151

Baptist Health Lexington Breast Imaging Services At Beaumont
3084 Lakecrest Cir Ste 150
Lexington, KY 40513-1973
(859)260-6050
FAX: (859)260-4151

Chi Health Saint Joseph Breast Care-Main
1401 Harrodsburg Rd Ste C45
Lexington, KY 40504-1779
(859)967-5563
FAX: (859)967-5617

Comprehensive Breast Care Center University Of Kentucky
234 Whitney-Hendrickson Bldg., 800 Rose St.
Lexington, KY 40536-0098
(859)323-2222
FAX: (859)323-6109

Lexington Clinic, East
100 N Eagle Creek Dr
Lexington, KY 40509-1833
(859)258-4937
FAX: (859)258-4246

New Lexington Clinic Psc
1221 S Broadway
Lexington, KY 40504-2771
(859)258-4932
FAX: (859)258-4246

Saint Joseph Breast Care At Saint Joseph East
160 N Eagle Creek Dr, Ste 101
Lexington, KY 40509-2121
(859)967-5874
FAX: (859)967-5874

Liberty

Casey County Hospital
187 Wolford Ave
Liberty, KY 42539-3278
(606)787-6275
FAX: (606)787-1425

London

London Women's Care
803 Meyers Baker Rd Ste 200
London, KY 40741-3040
(606)878-3240
FAX: (606)878-4308

Saint Joseph - London
1001 Saint Joseph Ln
London, KY 40741-8345
(606)330-6060
FAX: (606)330-6707

Louisa

Three Rivers Medical Center
Highway 644
Louisa, KY 41230
(606)638-1507
FAX: (606)638-4619

Louisville

All Women Ob/Gyn
4010 Dupont Cir Ste L07
Louisville, KY 40207-4812
(502)895-6559
FAX: (502)895-8994

Baptist Health Eastpoint Diagnostic Center
2400 Eastpoint Pkwy
Louisville, KY 40223-4154
(502)897-8888
FAX: (502)896-7729

Baptist Health Louisville
4000 Kresge Way, Women's Imaging Ctr
Louisville, KY 40207-4605
(502)897-8888
FAX: (502)259-4608

Baptist Health Medical Group - Medeast
4003 Kresge Way Ste 410
Louisville, KY 40207-4652
(502)893-7462
FAX: (502)212-7551

Baptist Health Medical Group Louisville Ob/Gyn
950 Breckenridge Ln, Ste 220
Louisville, KY 40207-5929
(502)893-6777
FAX: (502)895-1826

Baptist Health Medical Group/Partners In Womens Health
3940 Dupont Cir
Louisville, KY 40207-4806
(502)895-1111
FAX: (502)895-1085

Baptist Health Middletown Diagnostic Imaging Center
12010 Shelbyville Rd, Ste 600
Louisville, KY 40243-1499
(502)897-8888
FAX: (502)896-7266

Diagnostic Xray Physicians
5129 Dixie Hwy Ste 100
Louisville, KY 40216-1727
(502)447-8786
FAX: (502)447-8623

Heartland Imaging
7807 Shelbyville Rd
Louisville, KY 40222-5439
(502)429-6500
FAX: (502)429-0770

J.G. Brown Cancer Center - Breast Care Center
529 S Jackson St, Frnt
Louisville, KY 40202-3230
(502)562-4361
FAX: (502)562-4365

Jewish Hospital Medical Center East
3920 Dutchmans Ln
Louisville, KY 40207-4702
(502)587-4327
FAX: (502)259-6416

Mary & Elizabeth Hospital
4402 Churchman Ave Ste 101
Louisville, KY 40215-1192
(502)569-7951
FAX: (502)361-6080

Norton Audubon Hospital
1 Audubon Plaza Dr
Louisville, KY 40217-1397
(502)636-7180
FAX: (502)636-7190

Norton Breast Health Center - Brownsboro
4915 Norton Healthcare Blvd, Norton Medical Plaza Iii, Suite 102
Louisville, KY 40241-2860
(502)485-4700
FAX: (502)446-6615

Norton Diagnostic Center- Fern Creek
9344 Cedar Center Way
Louisville, KY 40291-4522
(502)753-3390
FAX: (502)753-3399

Norton Healthcare Pavilion Breast Center
315 E Broadway, Norton Medical Pavilion
Louisville, KY 40202-3700
(502)629-7050
FAX: (502)629-7004

Norton Prevention & Wellness
3999 Dutchmans Ln Ste 3C
Louisville, KY 40207-4747
(502)899-6890
FAX: (502)899-6852

Norton Women's And Children's Hospital
4001 Dutchmans Ln
Louisville, KY 40207-4714
(502)893-1292
FAX: (502)899-2696

Total Woman
4123 Dutchmans Ln Ste 500
Louisville, KY 40207-4730
(502)894-9494
FAX: (502)894-9404

Women First Of Louisville
3900 Kresge Way Ste 30
Louisville, KY 40207-4680
(502)891-8706
FAX: (502)891-8708

Women's Care Phys Of Louisville A Part Of Norton Womens Care
4130 Dutchmans Ln Ste 400
Louisville, KY 40207-4711
(502)897-0697
FAX: (502)897-0658

Women's Diagnostic Center - Baptist Health Lagrange
4004 Dupont Cir Ste 230
Louisville, KY 40207-4819
(502)893-1333
FAX: (502)899-9576

Madisonville

Baptist Health Women's Care
800 Hospital Dr, Department Of Mammography
Madisonville, KY 42431-1658
(270)326-3900
FAX: (270)326-4911

Owensboro Health Madisonville Healthplex
510 Ruby Dr
Madisonville, KY 42431-2168
(270)399-7900
FAX: (270)821-6446

Manchester

Adventhealth Manchester
210 Marie Langdon Dr
Manchester, KY 40962-6388
(606)598-1025
FAX: (606)598-1243

Marion

Crittenden Community Hospital
520 W Gum St
Marion, KY 42064-1516
(270)965-1073
FAX: (270)965-1072

Martin

Arh Our Lady Of The Way
11203 Main St
Martin, KY 41649-7999
(606)285-6480
FAX: (606)285-6489

Mayfield

Jackson Purchase Medical Center
1099 Medical Center Cir
Mayfield, KY 42066-1143
(270)251-4251
FAX: (270)251-4255

Maysville

Meadowview Regional Medical Center
989 Medical Park Dr
Maysville, KY 41056-8750
(833)248-1274
FAX: (606)759-5259

Mc Dowell

McDowell Appalachian Regional Hospital
PO Box 247, Ky Route 122
Mc Dowell, KY 41647-0247
(606)377-3442
FAX: (606)377-3441

Middlesboro

Middlesboro Arh Hospital
3600 Cumberland Ave
Middlesboro, KY 40965-2614
(606)242-1193
FAX: (606)242-1221

Monticello

Wayne County Hospital
166 Hospital St
Monticello, KY 42633-2416
(606)340-3236
FAX: (606)340-3294

Morehead

St. Claire Healthcare
222 Medical Cir
Morehead, KY 40351-1179
(606)783-6760
FAX: (606)783-6349

Morganfield

Deaconess Union County Hospital
4604 US Highway 60 W
Morganfield, KY 42437-6537
(270)389-5180
FAX: (270)389-5015

Mount Vernon

Rockcastle Regional Hospital
145 Newcomb Ave
Mount Vernon, KY 40456-2728
(606)256-7878
FAX: (606)256-7713

Mt Sterling

Saint Joseph Mount Sterling
225 Falcon Dr
Mt Sterling, KY 40353-9792
(859)497-5445
FAX: (859)497-5430

Murray

Murray-Calloway Co. Hospital
803 Poplar St
Murray, KY 42071-2467
(270)752-2171
FAX: (270)767-3606

Nicholasville

Baptist Hlth Lexington Breast Img Services Brannon Crossing
610 E Brannon Rd Ste 101
Nicholasville, KY 40356-6046
(859)260-6050
FAX: (859)260-4151

Center For Breast Care Jessamine Medical And Diag. Ctr
110 Village Pkwy
Nicholasville, KY 40356-2327
(859)258-4444
FAX: (859)258-4246

Saint Joseph Jessamine
1250 Keene Rd
Nicholasville, KY 40356-7600
(859)887-4100
FAX: (859)887-6858

Owensboro

Owensboro Health Muhlenberg Healthplex
PO Box 20007
Owensboro, KY 42304-0007
(270)685-7100
FAX: (270)688-2275

Owensboro Health OP Imaging Breckenridge
1000 Breckenridge St Ste 101
Owensboro, KY 42303-0840
(270)688-3679
FAX: (270)683-8309

Owensboro Health Outpatient Imaging - Springs
2200 E Parrish Ave Bldg D, Suite 200
Owensboro, KY 42303-1458
(270)926-8171
FAX: (270)852-7925

Owensboro Health Outpatient Imaging Ford
1006 Ford Ave
Owensboro, KY 42301-4677
(270)688-3679
FAX: (270)683-8309

Paducah

Baptist Health Paducah - Baptist Imaging Ctr
2705 Kentucky Ave
Paducah, KY 42003-3805
(270)575-2662
FAX: (270)415-7241

Lourdes Women's Center
1530 Lone Oak Rd, Ste 210
Paducah, KY 42003-7901
(270)444-2121
FAX: (270)538-5860

Lundberg Medical Imaging Psc
2421 Broadway St
Paducah, KY 42001-7115
(270)442-8272
FAX: (270)444-0539

Paintsville

Paul B. Hall Regional Medical Center
625 James Trimble Blvd
Paintsville, KY 41240-1055
(606)789-3511
FAX: (606)788-6462

Paris

Bourbon Community Hospital
9 Linville Dr
Paris, KY 40361-2196
(859)987-3600
FAX: (859)987-1073

Pikeville

Pikeville Medical Ctr Diagnostic Ctr
972 Bypass Rd
Pikeville, KY 41501
(606)218-1000
FAX: (606)218-1059

Pineville

Pineville Community Health Center
850 Riverview Ave
Pineville, KY 40977-1452
(606)337-3051
FAX: (606)654-2656

Powderly

Muhlenberg Medical Center
1010 Medical Center Dr
Powderly, KY 42367-5463
(270)377-2134
FAX: (270)377-1747

Prestonsburg

The Breast Center At Highlands Arh Regional Medical Center
5000 Ky Route 321
Prestonsburg, KY 41653-9113
(606)886-8511
FAX: (606)886-7610

Princeton

Caldwell Medical Center
100 Medical Center Dr
Princeton, KY 42445-2430
(270)365-0307
FAX: (270)365-4200

Richmond

Baptist Health Lexington Breast Imaging Services At Richmond
107 Meridian Way
Richmond, KY 40475-2878
(859)260-6050
FAX: (859)260-4151

Baptist Health Richmond
801 Eastern Byp
Richmond, KY 40475-2751
(859)625-3173
FAX: (859)625-3387

Russell Springs

Kentucky Breast Care
38 Joe T Petty Dr
Russell Springs, KY 42642-8533
(606)219-4184
FAX: (606)678-8368

Russell County Hospital
153 Dowell Rd
Russell Springs, KY 42642-4579
(270)866-4141
FAX: (270)866-8445

Russellville

Logan Memorial Hospital
1625 Nashville St
Russellville, KY 42276-8834
(270)725-4561
FAX: (270)725-4638

Salem

Livingston Hospital And Healthcare Services Inc
131 Hospital Dr
Salem, KY 42078-8043
(270)988-7212
FAX: (270)988-2771

Scottsville

Scottsville Medical Center
456 Burnley Rd
Scottsville, KY 42164-6355
(270)622-2872
FAX: (270)622-2983

Shelbyville

Uofl Health Shelbyville Hospital
727 Hospital Dr
Shelbyville, KY 40065-1660
(502)681-1405
FAX: (502)647-4038

Shepherdsville

Jewish Hospital Medical Center South
1903 W Hebron Ln
Shepherdsville, KY 40165-7425
(502)955-3315
FAX: (502)955-3397

Norton Medical Associates Shepherdsville
115 Huston Dr, Ste 1
Shepherdsville, KY 40165-7250
(502)955-7311
FAX: (502)957-0414

Somerset

Kentucky Breast Care
100 Sarahs Ln
Somerset, KY 42503-2774
(606)219-4184
FAX: (606)678-8368

Lake Cumberland Imaging Center
45 Tower Cir
Somerset, KY 42503-3476
(606)678-3545
FAX: (606)678-3432

Women's Care Of Lake Cumberland
333 Bogle St
Somerset, KY 42503-2873
(606)678-0705
FAX: (606)678-2807

South Williamson

Tug Valley Arh Regional Medical Center
260 Hospital Dr
South Williamson, KY 41503-4072
(606)237-1741
FAX: (606)237-1600

Stanford

Fort Logan Hospital
110 Metker Trl, Ste A
Stanford, KY 40484-1020
(606)365-4600
FAX: (606)365-4751

Tompkinsville

Monroe County Medical Center
529 Capp Harlan Rd
Tompkinsville, KY 42167-1840
(270)487-9231
FAX: (270)487-6033

Versailles

Bluegrass Community Hospital
360 Amsden Ave
Versailles, KY 40383-1286
(859)879-2359
FAX: (859)879-2410

West Liberty

Morgan County Appalachian Regional Hospital
476 Liberty Rd
West Liberty, KY 41472-2049
(606)743-3186
FAX: (606)743-4593

Whitesburg

Mountain Comprehensive Health Corporation
226 Medical Plaza Ln
Whitesburg, KY 41858-7425
(606)633-4871
FAX: (606)632-9107

Whitesburg Arh
240 Hospital Rd
Whitesburg, KY 41858-7627
(606)633-3500
FAX: (606)633-3583

Williamstown

St. Elizabeth Healthcare - Grant Co.
238 Barnes Rd
Williamstown, KY 41097-9482
(859)824-8238
FAX: (859)824-8109

Winchester

Clark Regional Medical Center
175 Hospital Dr
Winchester, KY 40391-9591
(859)737-8301
FAX: (859)737-6617

LOUISIANA

Abbeville

Abbeville General Hospital
118 N Hospital Dr, Radiology Department
Abbeville, LA 70510-4077
(337)898-6298
FAX: (337)898-6114

Alexandria

Alexandria Women's Center
3304 Masonic Dr Ste 4001
Alexandria, LA 71301-4255
(318)443-7222
FAX: (318)443-7641

Christus St Frances Cabrini Hosp Women's Life Ctr
3330 Masonic Dr
Alexandria, LA 71301-3841
(318)448-4005
FAX: (318)448-6772

Rapides Breast Imaging Center
501 Medical Center Dr Ste 1, Rapides Womens & Childrens Hospital
Alexandria, LA 71301-8124
(318)769-7040
FAX: (318)769-3858

Rapides Regional Medical Center
211 4th St Box 30101
Alexandria, LA 71301-8421
(318)769-3567
FAX: (318)769-3685

Bastrop

Morehouse General Hospital
PO Box 1060, 323 W Walnut St
Bastrop, LA 71221-1060
(318)283-3860
FAX: (318)239-8860

Baton Rouge

Associates In Women's Health
500 Rue De La Vie St Ste 310
Baton Rouge, LA 70817-5128
(225)201-0505
FAX: (225)201-9955

Baton Rouge General Imaging Center
2550 Oneal Ln
Baton Rouge, LA 70816-3310
(225)333-3564
FAX: (225)490-0292

Baton Rouge General Medical Center - Bluebonnet
8585 Picardy Ave
Baton Rouge, LA 70809-3748
(225)763-4631
FAX: (225)763-4470

Baton Rouge General Medical Center Mid - City
3600 Florida St
Baton Rouge, LA 70806-3889
(225)381-6505
FAX: (225)387-7017

Drs. Schwartzenburg, Lafranca, Guidry & Chapman
500 Rue De La Vie St Ste 210
Baton Rouge, LA 70817-5128
(225)214-4717
FAX: (225)928-5535

Elliott Breast Clinic
541 Shadows Ln, Ste C
Baton Rouge, LA 70806-6559
(225)755-3070
FAX: (225)755-3085

Lake Imaging Center
7135 Perkins Rd
Baton Rouge, LA 70808-4322
(225)765-6500
FAX: (225)765-2018

Louisiana Women's Health Care Associates, L.L.C.
500 Rue De La Vie St
Baton Rouge, LA 70817-5127
(225)201-2130
FAX: (225)201-2030

Lsu Health Baton Rouge North Clinic
5439 Airline Hwy
Baton Rouge, LA 70805-1712
(225)358-4853
FAX: (225)358-2428

Lsu Health Baton Rouge Perkins Surgery Center
9032 Perkins Rd
Baton Rouge, LA 70810-1507
(225)358-4853
FAX: (225)768-5854

Lsu Midcity Clinic
1401 N Foster Dr
Baton Rouge, LA 70806-1818
(225)358-4853
FAX: (225)987-9036

Ochsner Health Center - O'Neal
16777 Medical Center Dr Ste 100
Baton Rouge, LA 70816-3231
(225)761-5200
FAX: (225)761-5315

Ochsner Medical Complex-High Grove
10310 The Grove Blvd
Baton Rouge, LA 70836-6455
(225)761-5380
FAX: (225)761-5315

The Baton Rouge Clinic, Amc
7373 Perkins Rd
Baton Rouge, LA 70808-4373
(225)769-4044
FAX: (225)246-9120

Woman's Breast Center - Advanced Imaging
500 Rue De La Vie St Ste 110
Baton Rouge, LA 70817-5128
(225)924-8268
FAX: (225)924-8242

Woman's Hospital Breast Center
100 Womans Way
Baton Rouge, LA 70817-5100
(225)924-8267
FAX: (225)928-8829

Woman's Hospital On-Site Mammography - Mobile
100 Womans Way
Baton Rouge, LA 70817-5100
(225)924-8391
FAX: (225)924-8242

Benton

Wk Palmetto Breast Clinic
1001 Lackland Blvd Ste 100
Benton, LA 71006-2505
(318)935-1540
FAX: (318)935-1552

Bogalusa

Our Lady Of The Angels Hospital
433 Plaza St
Bogalusa, LA 70427-3729
(985)730-6803
FAX: (985)730-6806

Bossier City

Bossier Pavilion Imaging Ctr
2449 Hospital Dr Ste 120
Bossier City, LA 71111-1902
(318)212-8550
FAX: (318)212-7535

Christus Bossier Emergency Hospital
2531 Viking Dr
Bossier City, LA 71111-2103
(318)681-4100
FAX: (318)681-4433

Breaux Bridge

St. Martin Hospital
210 Champagne Blvd
Breaux Bridge, LA 70517-3700
(337)507-1209
FAX: (337)507-3986

Coushatta

Christus Coushatta Health Care Center
1635 Marvel St
Coushatta, LA 71019-9022
(318)932-2103
FAX: (318)932-2005

Covington

Diagnostic Imaging Services, Inc.Covington
71154 Highway 21
Covington, LA 70433-7161
(985)643-5476
FAX: (985)405-1330

Lakeview Regional Medical Center,A Campus Of Tulane Med Ctr
95 Judge Tanner Blvd
Covington, LA 70433-7507
(985)867-4049
FAX: (985)867-3895

Ochsner Health Systems Covington
1000 Ochsner Blvd
Covington, LA 70433-8107
(985)875-2828
FAX: (985)875-2731

Ochsner Women's Health Center
71380 Highway 21 Ste 100
Covington, LA 70433-7350
(985)809-5999
FAX: (985)898-7246

St Tammany Parish Hospital Women's Pavilion
301 N Highway 190 Ste C2
Covington, LA 70433-5057
(985)773-1500
FAX: (985)773-1513

Crowley

Ochsner Acadia General Hospital
1305 Crowley Rayne Hwy
Crowley, LA 70526-8202
(337)788-6584
FAX: (337)788-6437

Cut Off

Lady Of The Sea General Hospital
200 W 134th Pl
Cut Off, LA 70345-4143
(985)632-6401
FAX: (985)632-3846

Delhi

Richland Parish Hospital
407 Cincinnati St
Delhi, LA 71232-3007
(318)878-6306
FAX: (318)878-6406

Deridder

Beauregard Health System
600 S Pine St
Deridder, LA 70634-4942
(337)462-8782
FAX: (337)462-7437

Destrehan

St. Charles Parish Hospital - Outpatient Diagnostic Center
13100 River Rd Ste 150
Destrehan, LA 70047-5214
(985)235-5426
FAX: (985)785-3728

Donaldsonville

Prevost Memorial Hospital
301 Memorial Dr
Donaldsonville, LA 70346-4376
(225)474-2149
FAX: (225)474-2185

Eunice

Clhg-Acadian, Llc Dba Acadian Medical Center
3501 Highway 190
Eunice, LA 70535-5129
(337)580-7850
FAX: (337)580-7855

Farmerville

Union General Hospital
901 James Ave
Farmerville, LA 71241-2234
(318)368-7072
FAX: (318)368-6501

Ferriday

Trinity Medical
6569 Hwy 84
Ferriday, LA 71334
(318)757-6551
FAX: (318)757-0250

Fort Polk

Bayne-Jones Army Community Hospital
1585 3rd St
Fort Polk, LA 71459-5102
(337)531-3271
FAX: (337)531-3709

Franklin

Franklin Foundation Hospital
1097 Northwest Blvd
Franklin, LA 70538-3407
(337)355-1220
FAX: (337)828-0313

Franklinton

Riverside Medical Center
1900 Main St
Franklinton, LA 70438-3688
(985)795-4336
FAX: (985)795-4226

Gonzales

Our Lady Of The Lake Ascension
1125 W Highway 30
Gonzales, LA 70737-5004
(225)647-5008
FAX: (225)765-9808

Grand Coteau

Ogh Imaging Llc
1341 I-49 S Service Rd.
Grand Coteau, LA 70541
(337)407-4523
FAX: (337)662-2234

Gretna

Ochsner Medical Center - West Bank, Llc
2500 Belle Chasse Hwy
Gretna, LA 70056-7127
(504)391-5150
FAX: (504)391-5499

The Women's Medical Centers
515 Westbank Expy
Gretna, LA 70053-5644
(504)366-7233
FAX: (504)362-5529

Hammond

North Oaks Medical Center, Llc
15837 Paul Vega MD Dr
Hammond, LA 70403-1495
(985)230-7777
FAX: (985)230-6781

Ochsner Health Center Tangipahoa
41676 Veterans Ave
Hammond, LA 70403-1412
(985)543-3616
FAX: (985)543-3654

Homer

Claiborne Memorial Medical Center
620 E College St
Homer, LA 71040-3202
(318)371-3872
FAX: (318)927-4647

Houma

Breast Cancer Center At Physicians Medical Center
166 Corporate Dr
Houma, LA 70360-2766
(985)858-3333
FAX: (985)858-3342

Leonard J. Chabert Medical Center
1978 Industrial Blvd
Houma, LA 70363-7094
(985)850-2314
FAX: (985)873-2220

Terrebonne General Medical Center
8166 Main St
Houma, LA 70360-3498
(985)850-6052
FAX: (985)873-4280

Independence

Lsuhsc Lallie Kemp Medical Center
52579 Highway 51 S, Radiology
Independence, LA 70443-2231
(985)878-1450
FAX: (985)878-1527

Jefferson

Tansey Breast Imaging Center At Ochsner
1514 Jefferson Hwy
Jefferson, LA 70121-2429
(504)842-6409
FAX: (504)842-5679

Jena

Lasalle General Hospital
187 Ninth St
Jena, LA 71342-3900
(318)992-9200
FAX: (318)992-9245

Jennings

Jennings American Legion Hospital
1634 Elton Rd
Jennings, LA 70546-3614
(337)616-7190
FAX: (337)616-7197

Jonesboro

Jackson Parish Hospital
165 Beech Springs Rd
Jonesboro, LA 71251-2059
(318)395-4121
FAX: (318)259-5638

Kaplan

Abrom Kaplan Memorial Hospital
1310 W 7th St
Kaplan, LA 70548-2910
(337)643-5277
FAX: (337)643-5230

Kenner

Ochsner Diagnostic Center-Kenner
200 W Esplanade Ave
Kenner, LA 70065-2489
(504)712-2800
FAX: (504)464-2968

Lafayette

Breast Center Of Acadiana
935 Camellia Blvd Ste 100
Lafayette, LA 70508-7084
(337)504-5000
FAX: (337)504-5646

Lourdes Breast Center
2311 Kaliste Saloom Rd
Lafayette, LA 70508-6807
(337)470-7551
FAX: (337)289-2891

Ochsner Lafayette General Breast Center
1448 S College Rd
Lafayette, LA 70503-2920
(337)571-1300
FAX: (337)571-1301

Our Lady Of Lourdes Regional Medical Center
601 W Saint Mary Blvd Ste 104
Lafayette, LA 70506-3560
(337)470-7226
FAX: (337)289-2891

University Hospital And Clinics
2390 W Congress St
Lafayette, LA 70506-4205
(337)261-6279
FAX: (337)261-6769

Lake Charles

Breast Health Center Of Sw Louisiana At Lcmh
1701 Oak Park Blvd
Lake Charles, LA 70601-8911
(337)494-4755
FAX: (337)494-4757

Christus Ochsner Lake Area Hospital
4150 Nelson Rd Ste I
Lake Charles, LA 70605-4133
(337)475-4001
FAX: (337)475-4091

Christus Ochsner St. Patrick Women's Health Center
1601 Country Club Rd
Lake Charles, LA 70605-5325
(337)430-4444
FAX: (337)480-4841

Lake Charles Memorial Hospital For Women
1900 W Gauthier Rd
Lake Charles, LA 70605-7170
(337)480-7444
FAX: (337)480-7445

Laplace

Ochsner Medical Complex - River Parishes
1900 W Airline Hwy
Laplace, LA 70068-3338
(985)240-4454
FAX: (985)898-7155

Leesville

Leesville Diagnostic Center Dept Of Byrd Regional Hospital
506 S 6th St Ste C
Leesville, LA 71446-4482
(337)239-2992
FAX: (337)239-8543

Luling

St. Charles Parish Hospital
1057 Paul Maillard Rd
Luling, LA 70070-4349
(985)785-3662
FAX: (985)785-3728

Lutcher

St. James Parish Hospital
1645 Lutcher Ave
Lutcher, LA 70071-5150
(225)746-2953
FAX: (225)746-2986

Mamou

Savoy Medical Center
801 Poinciana Ave
Mamou, LA 70554-2298
(337)468-0166
FAX: (337)468-0435

Mandeville

St. Tammany Health System Mandeville Diagnostic Center
201 Saint Ann Dr Ste A
Mandeville, LA 70471-3472
(985)773-1500
FAX: (985)773-1513

Mansfield

Desoto Regional Health System
207 Jefferson St
Mansfield, LA 71052-2603
(318)871-3108
FAX: (318)872-0732

Marksville

Avoyelles Hospital
4231 Highway 1192
Marksville, LA 71351-4711
(318)240-6194
FAX: (318)240-6081

Marrero

Diagnostic Imaging Services Marrero
925 Avenue C
Marrero, LA 70072-3148
(504)888-5999
FAX: (504)883-5355

Ochsner Clinic Foundation Lapalco
4225 Lapalco Blvd
Marrero, LA 70072-4324
(504)391-5150
FAX: (504)595-8187

Women's Imaging & Breast Care Ctr
4521 Westbank Expy
Marrero, LA 70072-3120
(504)349-6300
FAX: (504)349-1959

Metairie

Diagnostic Imaging Services Women's Center
4241 Veterans Blvd., Ste. 100, Dis
Mammography Qa Coordinator
Metairie, LA 70006
(504)883-5999
FAX: (504)883-5355

East Jefferson General Hospital
4200 Houma Blvd, Domino Radiology
Dept/Breast Ctr
Metairie, LA 70006-2996
(504)503-6289
FAX: (504)503-5304

Ochsner Clinic Metairie
2005 Veterans Hwy.
Metairie, LA 70002
(504)842-6406
FAX: (504)842-5679

Ochsner Health Center Clearview
4500 Clearview Pkwy, Ste 102
Metairie, LA 70006-2350
(504)894-2800
FAX: (504)894-2214

Tulane-Lakeside Breast Center
4720 S I 10 Service Rd W Ste 100
Metairie, LA 70001-7403
(504)988-8106
FAX: (504)780-4545

Wjmc Imaging At Ridgelake
2121 Ridgelake Dr
Metairie, LA 70001-2080
(504)349-6300
FAX: (504)267-5698

Minden

Minden Medical Center - Breast Care Center
1 Medical Plaza Pl
Minden, LA 71055-3330
(318)371-2166
FAX: (318)371-7858

Monroe

Brfhh Monroe Llc Dba Ochsner Lsu Health
Monroe
4864 Jackson St
Monroe, LA 71202-6400
(318)330-7588
FAX: (318)330-7555

Kitty Degree Breast Health Center
2600 Tower Dr Ste 409
Monroe, LA 71201-5783
(318)812-7465
FAX: (318)966-7151

Monroe Surgical Hospital
2408 Broadmoor Blvd
Monroe, LA 71201-2994
(318)812-9517
FAX: (318)812-9571

Morgan City

Ochsner St. Mary
1125 Marguerite St
Morgan City, LA 70380-1855
(985)380-4443
FAX: (985)380-4310

Natchitoches

Natchitoches Regional Medical Center
501 Keyser Ave
Natchitoches, LA 71457-6018
(318)214-4265
FAX: (318)214-4275

New Iberia

Iberia Medical Center
600 N Lewis St
New Iberia, LA 70563-2043
(337)374-7616
FAX: (337)359-4510

New Orleans

East Jefferson General Hospital Imaging
Center- Lakeview
7030 Canal Blvd
New Orleans, LA 70124-3410
(504)454-4164
FAX: (504)456-8048

New Orleans East Hospital
5620 Read Blvd
New Orleans, LA 70127-3106
(504)592-6465
FAX: (504)592-6849

Ochsner - Outpatient Imaging Center
1601 Jefferson Hwy
New Orleans, LA 70121-2445
(504)842-3473
FAX: (504)842-5679

Ochsner Baptist A Campus Of Ochsner Medical
Center
2820 Napoleon Ave
New Orleans, LA 70115-6969
(504)894-2800
FAX: (504)894-2214

Ochsner Health Center-Lake Terrace
1532 Robert E Lee Blvd New Orleans
New Orleans, LA 70122-2146
(504)842-3473
FAX: (504)842-5679

Ochsner Main Campus- Primary Care And
Wellness
1401 Jefferson Hwy
New Orleans, LA 70121-2426
(504)842-3473
FAX: (504)842-5679

Touro Infirmary -Touro Imaging Center
2929 Napoleon Ave
New Orleans, LA 70115-6917
(504)897-8600
FAX: (504)897-8638

Touro Prytania Imaging Center
3437 Prytania St
New Orleans, LA 70115-3521
(504)210-4337
FAX: (504)210-4338

Tulane University Medical Center
1415 Tulane Ave
New Orleans, LA 70112-2600
(504)988-4030
FAX: (504)988-5223

University Medical Center Of New Orleans
2000 Canal St
New Orleans, LA 70112-3018
(504)702-5700
FAX: (504)702-5700

New Roads

Pointe Coupee General Hospital
2202 False River Dr
New Roads, LA 70760-2614
(225)638-5703
FAX: (225)638-5709

Oak Grove

West Carroll Memorial Hospital
706 Ross St
Oak Grove, LA 71263-9798
(318)428-6147
FAX: (318)428-8945

Oakdale

Oakdale Community Hospital
130 Hospital Dr, Radiology Department
Oakdale, LA 71463-3035
(318)215-3285
FAX: (318)215-3198

Olla

Hardtner Medical Center
1102 N Pine Rd
Olla, LA 71465-4804
(318)495-3131
FAX: (318)495-0746

Opelousas

Dr Gerald E Posner Ctr For Women's Hlth
Opelousas Gen Hlth
539 E Prudhomme St
Opelousas, LA 70570-6499
(337)407-4432
FAX: (337)943-7104

Plaquemine

Ochsner Medical Complex-Iberville
25455 Highway 1
Plaquemine, LA 70764-7513
(225)754-6845
FAX: (225)754-6806

Prairieville

Baton Rouge General Ascension
14105 Highway 73
Prairieville, LA 70769-3626
(225)763-4631
FAX: (225)763-4470

Ochsner Health Center - Prairieville
16220 Airline Hwy
Prairieville, LA 70769-4248
(225)761-5200
FAX: (225)761-5315

Raceland

Ochsner Bayou Llc Dba Ochsner St Anne Gen.
Hosp.
4608 Highway 1
Raceland, LA 70394-2623
(985)537-8298
FAX: (985)537-8259

Rayville

Richardson Medical Center
254 Highway 3048
Rayville, LA 71269-3624
(318)728-8358
FAX: (318)728-8126

Ruston

Clhg-Ruston, Llc Dba Northern La Medical Ctr
401 E Vaughn Ave
Ruston, LA 71270-5950
(318)254-2791
FAX: (318)254-2723

Green Clinic Breast Center
1200 S Farmerville St
Ruston, LA 71270-5941
(318)251-6380
FAX: (318)251-6145

Saint Francisville

West Feliciana Parish Hospital
5266 Commerce St
Saint Francisville, LA 70775-4409
(225)635-3811
FAX: (225)784-3499

Shreveport

Christus Breast Center Shreveport-Bossier
1505 E Bert Kouns Industrial Loop, Ste 201
Shreveport, LA 71105-5723
(318)681-4100
FAX: (318)681-4433

Lsuhsc - Shreveport - Partners In Wellness
2015 Fairfield Ave Ste 2B
Shreveport, LA 71104-2066
(318)813-4010
FAX: (318)675-0481

Ochsner Lsu Health Shreveport-Fwcc
1501 Kings Hwy
Shreveport, LA 71103-4228
(318)626-0802
FAX: (318)626-3083

Ochsnerlsu St Mary Medical Center
1 Saint Mary Pl
Shreveport, LA 71101-4307
(318)626-5000
FAX: (318)399-6193

W.K. Pierremont Health Center
8001 Youree Dr
Shreveport, LA 71115-2302
(318)212-3530
FAX: (318)212-3535

Willis-Knighton Breast Center South
2530 Bert Kouns Industrial Loop Ste 1
Shreveport, LA 71118-3132
(318)212-8550
FAX: (318)212-5249

Willis-Knighton Medical Center
2600 Greenwood Rd
Shreveport, LA 71103-3971
(318)212-8550
FAX: (318)212-8540

Wk Breast Health Center
7845 Youree Dr
Shreveport, LA 71105-5505
(318)212-8550
FAX: (318)212-3535

Slidell

Diagnostic Imaging Services, Inc.
1310 Gause Blvd
Slidell, LA 70458-3016
(985)643-5476
FAX: (985)643-2329

Ochsner Health Center Slidell
2750 Gause Blvd E
Slidell, LA 70461-4149
(985)639-3730
FAX: (985)639-3740

Ochsner Medical Center North Shore
100 Medical Center Dr
Slidell, LA 70461-5520
(985)646-5984
FAX: (985)646-5492

Smh Imaging
1495 Gause Blvd
Slidell, LA 70458-2205
(985)280-5229
FAX: (985)280-5216

Springhill

Smc/Doctors Clinic
401 11th St NE
Springhill, LA 71075-4503
(318)539-1068
FAX: (318)539-1072

Sulphur

West Calcasieu Cameron Hospital
701 Cypress St
Sulphur, LA 70663-5053
(337)527-4256
FAX: (337)527-4393

Thibodaux

Thibodaux Regional Health Sytem, Inc.
726 N Acadia Rd
Thibodaux, LA 70301-5051
(985)493-4304
FAX: (985)449-2539

Vidalia

Riverpark Imaging Center
107 Front St, Ste 1200
Vidalia, LA 71373-2834
(318)336-2220
FAX: (318)336-6060

Ville Platte

Ville Platte Medical Ctr Llc Dba Mercy Regional Medical Ctr
800 E Main St
Ville Platte, LA 70586-4618
(337)363-9485
FAX: (337)360-9680

Vivian

North Caddo Medical Center
815 S Pine St
Vivian, LA 71082-3314
(318)375-4038
FAX: (318)375-2886

Walker

Our Lady Of The Lake Livingston
5000 Odonavan Blvd
Walker, LA 70785-6351
(225)271-6062
FAX: (225)271-6104

West Monroe

Glenwood Regional Medical Center A Steward Family Hospital
102 Thomas Rd Ste 302
West Monroe, LA 71291-5547
(318)329-8585
FAX: (318)329-8544

Winnsboro

Franklin Medical Center
2106 Loop Rd, Frnt
Winnsboro, LA 71295-3342
(318)412-5237
FAX: (318)412-5487

Youngsville

Breast Center Of Acadiana-Youngsville
107 Centre Sarcelle Blvd, Ste 701
Youngsville, LA 70592-6368
(337)504-5000
FAX: (337)504-5646

Zachary

Lane Medical Plaza
6550 Main St, Mammo Dept
Zachary, LA 70791-4092
(225)658-6777
FAX: (225)658-4179

Lane Regional Medical Center
6300 Main St, Imaging Dept. - Mammo
Zachary, LA 70791-4037
(225)658-6777
FAX: (225)658-4179

MAINE

Augusta

Mainegeneral Medical Center - Alfond Center For Health
35 Medical Center Pkwy
Augusta, ME 04330-8160
(207)621-6422
FAX: (207)626-6875

Bangor

Breast And Osteoporosis Center Eastern Maine Med Ctr
489 State St
Bangor, ME 04401-6616
(207)973-8108
FAX: (207)973-8104

Breast And Osteoporosis Ctr At Emmc Healthcare Mall
925 Union St Ste 2, Imaging Center Of Maine
Bangor, ME 04401-3051
(207)973-8108
FAX: (207)973-8104

Regional Breast Care Center
900 Broadway Bldg 2
Bangor, ME 04401-1900
(207)907-1841
FAX: (207)907-1927

Bar Harbor

Mdi Hospital Breast Center
PO Box 8, 10 Wayman Ln
Bar Harbor, ME 04609-0008
(207)288-5082
FAX: (207)288-8436

Belfast

Mainehealth D/B/A Waldo County General Hospital
118 Northport Ave
Belfast, ME 04915-6072
(207)505-4500
FAX: (207)505-4901

Biddeford

Maine Health Doing Business As Southern Maine Health Care
PO Box 626, 1 Medical Center Dr
Biddeford, ME 04005-0626
(207)283-7171
FAX: (207)286-9773

Southern Maine Health Care - Healthcare Drive
9 Healthcare Dr
Biddeford, ME 04005-9449
(207)283-7171
FAX: (207)286-9773

Blue Hill

Blue Hill Memorial Hospital
57 Water St
Blue Hill, ME 04614-5231
(207)374-3999
FAX: (207)374-3974

Bridgton

Bridgton Hospital
10 Hospital Dr
Bridgton, ME 04009-1148
(207)647-6092
FAX: (207)647-6008

Brunswick

Martins Point Health Care Brunswick Bowdoin
74 Baribeau Dr
Brunswick, ME 04011-3218
(207)798-4968
FAX: (207)798-6552

Mid Coast Hospital-Women's Imaging Ctr
81 Medical Center Dr Ste 1200
Brunswick, ME 04011-2765
(207)373-6630
FAX: (207)373-6541

Caribou

Cary Medical Center
163 Van Buren Rd Ste 1
Caribou, ME 04736-3588
(207)498-1201
FAX: (207)498-1355

Damariscotta

Mainehealth D/B/A Lincolnhealth-Miles Campus
35 Miles St
Damariscotta, ME 04543-4047
(207)563-4343
FAX: (207)563-4463

Dover Foxcroft

Northern Light Mayo Hospital Imaging Center For Women
897 W Main St
Dover Foxcroft, ME 04426-1029
(207)564-4353
FAX: (207)564-4180

Ellsworth

Breast Clinic - Nlh Maine Coast Hospital
50 Union St
Ellsworth, ME 04605-1534
(207)664-5492
FAX: (207)664-5493

Falmouth

Mainehealth Dba Maine Medical Center, Falmouth Campus
5 Bucknam Rd Ste 1B
Falmouth, ME 04105-1208
(207)396-7750
FAX: (207)781-1717

Farmington

Franklin Memorial Hospital
111 Franklin Health Cmns, Mammography - Martha B. Webber Breast Ca
Farmington, ME 04938-6144
(207)779-2375
FAX: (207)779-2133

Fort Kent

Northern Maine Medical Center
194 E Main St
Fort Kent, ME 04743-1497
(207)834-1420
FAX: (207)834-3040

Gardiner

Mainegeneral Medical Center - Gardiner Campus
5 Central Maine Xing
Gardiner, ME 04345-6320
(207)621-6422
FAX: (207)626-6875

Gorham

Martin's Point Healthcare Gorham
575 Main St
Gorham, ME 04038-2623
(207)828-2494
FAX: (207)771-2647

Greenville

Northern Light Charles A. Dean Hospital
364 Pritham Ave
Greenville, ME 04441-7214
(207)695-5280
FAX: (207)695-5203

Houlton

Houlton Regional Hospital
20 Hartford St
Houlton, ME 04730-1859
(207)521-2193
FAX: (207)532-0902

Lewiston

Sam & Jennie Bennett Breast Care Center
12 High St Ste 103
Lewiston, ME 04240-7634
(207)795-2100
FAX: (207)795-2119

St. Mary's Regional Medical Center Womens Imaging Ctr
93 Campus Ave
Lewiston, ME 04240-6030
(207)777-4063
FAX: (207)777-4061

Lincoln

Penobscot Valley Hospital
7 Transalpine Rd
Lincoln, ME 04457-4222
(207)794-7234
FAX: (207)794-2834

Livermore Falls

Androscoggin Valley Medical Arts Ctr
21 Main St
Livermore Falls, ME 04254-1219
(207)779-2405
FAX: (207)779-2133

Machias

Down East Community Hospital
11 Hospital Dr
Machias, ME 04654-3325
(207)255-0474
FAX: (207)255-0238

Millinocket

Millinocket Regional Hospital
200 Somerset St
Millinocket, ME 04462-1298
(207)723-5161
FAX: (207)723-6498

Norway

Mainehealth D/B/A Stephens Memorial Hospital
181 Main St, Ste 1
Norway, ME 04268-5665
(207)744-6079
FAX: (207)743-5979

Pittsfield

Women's Health Center At Sebasticook Valley Health
447 N Main St
Pittsfield, ME 04967-3707
(207)487-4040
FAX: (207)487-4595

Portland

Intermed Mammography At Marginal Way
84 Marginal Way 10th Fl
Portland, ME 04101-2443
(207)523-3620
FAX: (207)774-1371

Maine Health Dba Maine Medial Center, Bramhall Campus
22 Bramhall St
Portland, ME 04102-3134
(207)396-7750
FAX: (207)396-7770

Martin's Point Health Care
331 Veranda St Bldg 6
Portland, ME 04103-5545
(207)828-2424
FAX: (207)828-2451

Northern Light Mercy Hospital Mammography Center
195 Fore River Pkwy, Medical Office Bldg., Ste. 260
Portland, ME 04102-2780
(207)879-3737
FAX: (207)553-6610

Presque Isle

The Aroostook Medical Center
140 Academy St
Presque Isle, ME 04769-3171
(207)768-4211
FAX: (207)768-4232

Rockport

Mainehealth D/B/A Pen Bay Medical Center
6 Glen Cove Dr, Radiology Department
Rockport, ME 04856-4272
(207)301-8520
FAX: (207)301-5295

Rumford

Rumford Hospital
420 Franklin St
Rumford, ME 04276-2145
(207)369-1131
FAX: (207)369-1017

Sanford

Maine Health Doing Business As Smhc Sanford
25 June St
Sanford, ME 04073-2621
(207)283-7171
FAX: (207)490-7920

Scarborough

Coastal Women's Healthcare
71 US Route 1 Ste A
Scarborough, ME 04074-7168
(207)885-8400
FAX: (207)885-8498

Mainehealth Dba Maine Medical Center, Scarborough Campus
100 Campus Dr Unit 121
Scarborough, ME 04074-7172
(207)396-7750
FAX: (207)396-6736

Skowhegan

Redington-Fairview General Hospital
46 Fairview Ave
Skowhegan, ME 04976-1481
(207)474-5121
FAX: (207)474-9256

South Portland

Intermed Imaging
50 Foden Rd
South Portland, ME 04106-1718
(207)523-3620
FAX: (207)761-3719

Topsham

Shields Imaging With Central Maine Health Llc
105 Topsham Fair Mall Rd
Topsham, ME 04086-1773
(800)258-4674
FAX: (800)253-7569

Waterville

Inland Hospital
180 Kennedy Memorial Dr, Ste 104
Waterville, ME 04901-4541
(207)861-3333
FAX: (207)861-3095

Mainegeneral Medical Center - Thayer
149 North St, Mammography
Waterville, ME 04901-4995
(207)872-1100
FAX: (207)872-1406

Wells

York Hospital In Wells
112 Sanford Rd
Wells, ME 04090-5533
(207)351-2023
FAX: (207)641-8940

Winthrop

Mainegeneral Medical Center Winthrop Outpatient Imaging
16 Commerce Plz, Ste 2C
Winthrop, ME 04364-1562
(207)621-6422
FAX: (207)626-6875

York

York Hospital
15 Hospital Dr
York, ME 03909-1099
(207)351-2023
FAX: (207)351-2036

MARYLAND

Abingdon

Kaiser Permanente Abingdon Medical Center
3400 Box Hill Corporate Center Dr
Abingdon, MD 21009-1290
(877)390-0033
FAX: (410)339-5692

Annapolis

Advanced Radiology - Annapolis
116 Defense Hwy Ste LI100
Annapolis, MD 21401-7626
(888)972-9700
FAX: (443)436-4875

Anne Arundel Diagnostics Breast Center
2000 Medical Pkwy Ste 202
Annapolis, MD 21401-3744
(443)481-5309
FAX: (443)481-5355

Chesapeake Medical Imaging
122 Defense Hwy, Ste 102
Annapolis, MD 21401-7044
(410)571-0350
FAX: (410)571-9348

Kaiser Permanente - Annapolis
888 Bestgate Rd Ste 102
Annapolis, MD 21401-2950
(301)548-5720
FAX: (301)548-5780

Baltimore

Advanced Radiology - Dundalk
1576 Merritt Blvd Ste 1
Baltimore, MD 21222-2114
(410)918-3150
FAX: (410)918-3161

Advanced Radiology - Medical Arts
9101 Franklin Square Dr Ste 102
Baltimore, MD 21237-4255
(410)918-3460
FAX: (410)918-3431

Advanced Radiology - Perry Hall
4211 Blakely Ave Ste 100
Baltimore, MD 21236-2456
(443)588-6221
FAX: (410)918-3359

Advanced Radiology- Maiden Choice
724 Maiden Choice Ln Ste 302
Baltimore, MD 21228-5966
(410)747-9303
FAX: (443)514-1290

Advanced Radiology- Pomona
1700 Reisterstown Rd Ste 112
Baltimore, MD 21208-2935
(410)580-2100
FAX: (410)580-2170

American Radiology Services At Fleet Street
3700 Fleet St Ste 110
Baltimore, MD 21224-4238
(410)298-0454
FAX: (443)663-2280

Johns Hopkins Breast Center Bayview Campus
301 Mason Lord Dr Ste 1300
Baltimore, MD 21224-3057
(410)550-8282
FAX: (410)550-0282

Johns Hopkins Breast Imaging
601 N Caroline St Rm 4008
Baltimore, MD 21287-0006
(410)955-2690
FAX: (410)614-7663

Johns Hopkins Imaging At White Marsh
4924 Campbell Blvd, Ste 105
Baltimore, MD 21236-5909
(443)442-2400
FAX: (443)442-2444

Kaiser Permanente - South Baltimore Medical Center
1701 Twin Springs Rd
Baltimore, MD 21227-3553
(877)390-0033
FAX: (301)548-5723

Kaiser Permanente - White Marsh
4920 Campbell Blvd
Baltimore, MD 21236-5916
(877)390-0033
FAX: (301)548-5780

Kaiser Permanente Baltimore Harbor Medical Center
815 E Pratt St
Baltimore, MD 21202-4889
(877)390-0033
FAX: (301)548-5723

Kaiser Permante - Woodlawn Facility
7141 Security Blvd
Baltimore, MD 21244-1811
(877)390-0033
FAX: (301)548-5780

Medstar Good Samaritan Hospital
5601 Loch Raven Blvd
Baltimore, MD 21239-2991
(443)444-4339
FAX: (443)444-4656

Medstar Harbor Hospital
3001 S Hanover St
Baltimore, MD 21225-1290
(410)350-3303
FAX: (410)350-3266

Medstar Union Memorial Hospital
201 E University Pkwy
Baltimore, MD 21218-2891
(410)554-2728
FAX: (410)554-6586

O'Brien Center For Women's Imaging At Mercy Medical Center
227 Saint Paul St
Baltimore, MD 21202-2001
(410)332-9102
FAX: (410)545-4047

Seton Imaging Center
3449 Wilkens Ave Ste 102
Baltimore, MD 21229-5216
(667)234-8675
FAX: (667)234-8688

Sinai Hospital Of Baltimore
2401 W Belvedere Ave
Baltimore, MD 21215-5270
(410)601-9729
FAX: (410)601-7403

University Of Maryland Medical Center
22 S Greene St, Department Of Radiology
Baltimore, MD 21201-1590
(410)328-3215
FAX: (410)328-8825

Bel Air

Advanced Radiology - Harford
201 Plumtree Rd, Ste 101
Bel Air, MD 21015-6055
(443)640-2501
FAX: (410)918-3302

Medstar Radiology Network At Bel Air
12 Medstar Blvd, Ste 150
Bel Air, MD 21015-1823
(443)625-5430
FAX: (443)356-4092

The Women's Center At Progressive Radiology-Bel Air
100 Fulford Ave
Bel Air, MD 21014-3812
(410)838-6767
FAX: (410)838-7895

University Of Maryland - Upper Chesapeake Medical Center
520 Upper Chesapeake Dr, Kcc-Breast Center
Bel Air, MD 21014-4339
(443)843-7000
FAX: (443)643-3022

Berlin

Atlantic General Hospital
9733 Healthway Dr
Berlin, MD 21811-1156
(410)641-9215
FAX: (410)641-9036

Bethesda

Community Radiology Associates
10215 Fernwood Rd Ste 620
Bethesda, MD 20817-1184
(240)800-2600
FAX: (301)530-0773

Johns Hopkins Medical Imaging Bethesda
6420 Rockledge Dr Ste 3100
Bethesda, MD 20817-7845
(301)897-5656
FAX: (301)896-6948

Walter Reed National Military Med Ctr - Breast Imaging Ctr
4954 North Palmer Road, Bldg 19 America Bldg, 3rd Fl
Bethesda, MD 20889-5600
(301)319-8502
FAX: (301)295-9076

Washington Radiology Associates
10215 Fernwood Rd Ste 103
Bethesda, MD 20817-1183
(301)564-1053
FAX: (301)493-8522

Bowie

Anne Arundel Diagnostics, Inc.
4175 N Hanson Ct Ste 102
Bowie, MD 20716-3179
(443)481-5000
FAX: (301)464-8410

Bowie Radiology Services
14999 Health Center Dr Ste 102
Bowie, MD 20716-1075
(301)860-1721
FAX: (301)860-1736

Community Radiology Associates Bowie South Imaging Ctr
4000 Mitchellville Rd Ste A100
Bowie, MD 20716-3123
(301)805-7002
FAX: (301)805-2968

Cambridge

Dorchester General Hospital
PO Box 439, 300 Byrn St
Cambridge, MD 21613-0439
(410)228-5511
FAX: (410)221-0864

Catonsville

Seton Imaging Route 40
6501 Baltimore National Pike
Catonsville, MD 21228-3923
(627)234-8675
FAX: (627)234-8688

Chester

Anne Arundel Diagnostics, Imaging
1630 Main St, Ste 104
Chester, MD 21619-2792
(410)604-2000
FAX: (410)604-2030

Chestertown

University Of Maryland Shore Medical Center At Chestertown
100 Brown St
Chestertown, MD 21620-1435
(410)778-3300
FAX: (410)810-7823

Chevy Chase

Washington Radiology Associates P.C.
4445 Willard Ave Ste 200
Chevy Chase, MD 20815-3696
(703)280-9800
FAX: (301)907-7414

Clinton

Clinton Imaging Center
9131 Piscataway Rd Ste 370
Clinton, MD 20735-2543
(240)846-6750
FAX: (301)868-4538

Ifrc, Llc Dba Fairfax Radiology Center At Heritage
8926 Woodyard Rd, Ste 401
Clinton, MD 20735-4233
(703)698-4444
FAX: (301)868-2481

Medstar Southern Maryland Imaging Center
7501 Surratts Rd Ste 105
Clinton, MD 20735-3362
(301)868-0972
FAX: (301)856-4559

Columbia

Advanced Radiology-Knoll Imaging
5500 Knoll North Dr, Ste 190
Columbia, MD 21045-2487
(443)917-2700
FAX: (410)917-4966

American Radiology Services At Howard County
8820 Columbia 100 Pkwy, Ste 100
Columbia, MD 21045-2169
(410)298-0454
FAX: (443)436-4188

Johns Hopkins Medical Imaging Columbia
11055 Little Patuxent Pkwy Ste L9
Columbia, MD 21044-2897
(443)574-5800
FAX: (443)730-4214

Kaiser Permanente - Columbia Gateway
7070 Samuel Morse Dr
Columbia, MD 21046-3424
(877)390-0033
FAX: (410)339-5692

Cumberland

Advanced Diagnostic Radiology, Llc
952 Seton Dr, Ste 210
Cumberland, MD 21502-1953
(301)777-3522
FAX: (301)777-1902

Upmc Diagnostic Center
12400 Willowbrook Rd
Cumberland, MD 21502-2559
(240)964-8888
FAX: (240)964-8110

Upmc Western Maryland
12500 Willowbrook Rd
Cumberland, MD 21502-6393
(240)964-8112
FAX: (240)964-8110

Denton

Denton Diagnostic Center
1140 Blades Farm Rd Ste 102
Denton, MD 21629-3488
(410)822-1000
FAX: (410)479-3527

Easton

Anne Arundel Diagnostic Imaging, Easton
28438 Marlboro Ave
Easton, MD 21601-2732
(443)481-5000
FAX: (410)690-3850

Chesapeake Medical Imaging
401 Purdy St Ste 104
Easton, MD 21601-4060
(410)822-1888
FAX: (410)822-6066

Diagnostic And Imaging Center
10 Martin Ct
Easton, MD 21601-4095
(410)822-1000
FAX: (410)770-8602

Eldersburg

Advanced Radiology - Eldersburg
1430 Progress Way, Ste 108 Ste 107-108
Eldersburg, MD 21784-6484
(443)436-1300
FAX: (443)436-7132

Elkton

Union Hospital
106 Bow St
Elkton, MD 21921-5596
(410)392-7075
FAX: (410)620-6173

Ellicott City

Advanced Radiology - Cross Roads
4801 Dorsey Hall Dr Ste 101
Ellicott City, MD 21042-7703
(443)436-1600
FAX: (443)436-1602

Fort George G Meade

Kimbrough Ambulatory Care Center
2480 Llewellyn Ave Ste 5800
Fort George G Meade, MD 20755-5129
(301)677-8488
FAX: (301)677-8191

Fort Washington

Adventist Healthcare Fort Washington Medical Center
11711 Livingston Rd
Fort Washington, MD 20744-5151
(301)203-2065
FAX: (301)292-2794

Frederick

Capital Women's Care, Frederick Ob/Gyn
61 Thomas Johnson Dr
Frederick, MD 21702-4301
(301)663-6171
FAX: (301)695-4469

Community Radiology Associates Frederick South Imaging Ctr
110 Baughmans Ln Ste 120
Frederick, MD 21702-4649
(301)662-0078
FAX: (301)662-1034

Community Radiology Frederick Imaging Center
67 Thomas Johnson Dr Ste 4
Frederick, MD 21702-4862
(301)624-1130
FAX: (301)831-4495

Frederick Health Imaging
1562 Opossumtown Pike
Frederick, MD 21702-4920
(240)566-3635
FAX: (240)566-3255

Frederick Health Imaging
7211 Bank Ct Ste 100-101
Frederick, MD 21703-2807
(240)566-3635
FAX: (240)566-3255

Kaiser Permanente - Frederick
7190 Crestwood Blvd, Ste 100
Frederick, MD 21703-7315
(877)390-0033
FAX: (301)548-5849

Fulton

Capital Women's Care
7625 Maple Lawn Blvd, Ste 1 Lower Lobby
Fulton, MD 20759-2565
(410)531-7557
FAX: (301)776-4348

Gaithersburg

Kaiser Permanente - Gaithersburg
655 Watkins Mill Rd
Gaithersburg, MD 20879-3301
(877)390-0033
FAX: (301)548-5849

Germantown

Community Radiology Associates - Holy Cross Imaging Center
19851 Observation Dr, Ste 155
Germantown, MD 20876-4142
(888)601-0943
FAX: (301)662-5870

Medical Faculty Associates Germantown
19731 Germantown Rd Ste 102
Germantown, MD 20874-1222
(301)590-8999
FAX: (301)444-8700

Glen Burnie

Advanced Radiology - Aiello
203 Hospital Dr Ste 100
Glen Burnie, MD 21061-6904
(410)918-3260
FAX: (410)918-3262

Advanced Radiology - Glen Burnie
200 Hospital Dr Ste Ll20
Glen Burnie, MD 21061-6436
(888)972-9700
FAX: (443)663-6980

Kaiser Permanente- North Arundel Medical Center
7670 Quarterfield Rd
Glen Burnie, MD 21061-3947
(800)777-7904
FAX: (410)508-7641

Greenbelt

Community Radiology Associates Greenbelt Imaging Ctr
7501 Greenway Center Dr Ste 200
Greenbelt, MD 20770-3514
(301)345-7690
FAX: (301)345-4878

Hagerstown

Capital Women's Care
1165 Imperial Dr, Ste 101
Hagerstown, MD 21740-6582
(240)513-6800
FAX: (240)513-6801

Robinwood Diagnostic Imaging Services Llc
11110 Medical Campus Rd Ste 245
Hagerstown, MD 21742-6797
(301)714-4200
FAX: (240)313-9780

Hanover

Advanced Radiology - Arundel Mills
7556 Teague Rd
Hanover, MD 21076-1213
(443)729-8100
FAX: (443)729-8102

Havre De Grace

University Of Maryland Harford Memorial Hospital
501 S Union Ave
Havre De Grace, MD 21078-3493
(443)843-5446
FAX: (443)843-6087

Hollywood

Medstar Medical Group-Southern Maryland, Llc
24035 Three Notch Rd
Hollywood, MD 20636-4871
(301)373-7300
FAX: (301)373-6300

Hyattsville

Kaiser Permanente Prince Georges
6525 Belcrest Rd
Hyattsville, MD 20782-2003
(877)390-0033
FAX: (301)548-5849

Jb Andrews

Malcolm Grow Medical Clinic And Surgery Center
1060 W Perimeter Rd
Jb Andrews, MD 20762-6602
(240)612-2040
FAX: (240)612-3380

Kensington

Kaiser Permanente - Kensington
10810 Connecticut Ave, Kensington Medical Center
Kensington, MD 20895-2145
(877)390-0033
FAX: (301)548-5849

Lanham

Greater Maryland Health System, Inc.
8116 Good Luck Rd, Ste 110
Lanham, MD 20706-3516
(301)552-8524
FAX: (240)542-3001

Laplata

University Of Maryland Diagnostic Radiology, Llc
5 N. Laplata Court Suite 104
Laplata, MD 20646
(703)356-4900
FAX: (703)356-4602

Largo

Dia -Mitchellville Radiology
1100 Mercantile Ln Ste 150
Largo, MD 20774-5366
(301)249-0022
FAX: (301)249-7640

Kaiser Permanente - Largo Medical Center
1221 Mercantile Ln
Largo, MD 20774-5374
(877)390-0033
FAX: (301)548-5780

Leonardtown

Medstar St. Mary's Hospital
25500 Point Lookout Rd
Leonardtown, MD 20650-2015
(240)434-7328
FAX: (240)434-7621

Lutherville

Advanced Radiology - Lutherville
1209 York Rd Ste 100
Lutherville, MD 21093-6208
(410)580-2240
FAX: (410)580-2270

Johns Hopkins Medical Imaging Green Spring
10803 Falls Rd, Ste 1100
Lutherville, MD 21093-4526
(443)997-7237
FAX: (410)583-2797

Kaiser Permanente - Towson
1447 York Rd Ste 100
Lutherville, MD 21093-6074
(877)390-0033
FAX: (301)548-5723

Saint Paul Place Specialists
1734 York Rd
Lutherville, MD 21093-5606
(443)275-5600
FAX: (443)275-5605

Millersville

Advanced Radiology-Shipley's Choice
8601 Veterans Hwy, Ste 100
Millersville, MD 21108-1571
(443)308-0300
FAX: (410)987-0251

Mount Airy

Community Radiology Associates - Mt Airy Imaging Center
504 E Ridgeville Blvd, Ste 130
Mount Airy, MD 21771-5942
(301)438-5011
FAX: (240)394-3181

Oakland

Oakland Mri & Diagnostics
259 N 4th St
Oakland, MD 21550-1375
(301)533-4674
FAX: (301)533-1077

Ocean City

Atlantic General Women's Imaging
12308 Ocean Gtwy, Ste 5
Ocean City, MD 21842-9341
(410)641-9173
FAX: (410)641-9036

Odenton

Anne Arundel Diagnostics
1106 Annapolis Rd Ste 110
Odenton, MD 21113-1738
(443)481-5000
FAX: (443)481-6444

Olney

Community Radiology Associates Of Olney
18111 Prince Philip Dr, Ste T20
Olney, MD 20832-1503
(240)559-3150
FAX: (301)570-4271

Medstar Health Breast & Imaging Center
18101 Prince Philip Dr, Ste 5200
Olney, MD 20832-1514
(301)260-3301
FAX: (301)260-3302

Owings Mills

Advanced Radiology - Owings Mills
21 Crossroads Dr Ste 120
Owings Mills, MD 21117-5497
(888)972-9700
FAX: (410)654-1166

Oxon Hill

Tower Radiology
251 National Harbor Blvd
Oxon Hill, MD 20745-1052
(301)638-4606
FAX: (301)638-4608

Potomac

Washington Radiology
12505 Park Potomac Ave Ste 120
Potomac, MD 20854-6812
(703)280-9800
FAX: (240)223-4701

Prince Frederick

Ars An Affiliate Of Maryland Imaging Network
130 Hospital Rd Ste Ll100
Prince Frederick, MD 20678-4029
(443)295-9225
FAX: (410)414-5361

Ifrc, Llc Dba Fairfax Radiology Center At Patuxent
230 W Dares Beach Rd
Prince Frederick, MD 20678-3150
(301)855-9754
FAX: (301)855-1367

Queenstown

Shore Medical Pavillion Ste 130 Imaging
125 Shoreway Dr
Queenstown, MD 21658-1680
(410)822-1000
FAX: (410)827-3156

Randallstown

Northwest Hospital
5401 Old Court Rd
Randallstown, MD 21133-5185
(410)521-5913
FAX: (410)521-5915

Rockville

Community Radiology Assoc - Rockville Imaging
15225 Shady Grove Rd Ste 105
Rockville, MD 20850-3201
(301)438-5135
FAX: (301)947-0701

Kaiser Permanente-Shady Grove
1396 Piccard Dr
Rockville, MD 20850-4302
(877)390-0033
FAX: (301)548-5849

Medical Faculty Associates Shady Grove Breast Center
9711 Medical Center Dr Ste 201
Rockville, MD 20850-3383
(301)762-1116
FAX: (301)762-5524

Medical Faculty Associates Shady Grove Medical Pavilion
9601 Blackwell Rd, Ste 150
Rockville, MD 20850-6474
(301)590-8999
FAX: (240)864-1125

Medical Faculty Associates, Inc. North Bethesda
6000 Executive Blvd, Ste 309
Rockville, MD 20852-3803
(301)590-8999
FAX: (301)230-1542

Salisbury

Peninsula Breast Center Of Tidalhealth Peninsula Regional
804 Snow Hill Rd
Salisbury, MD 21804-1938
(410)543-7596
FAX: (410)543-7598

Peninsula Imaging, L.L.C
1655 Woodbrooke Dr Ste 101
Salisbury, MD 21804-2317
(410)749-1123
FAX: (410)543-1063

Severna Park

Bay Radiology Llc
537 Baltimore Annapolis Blvd Ste B
Severna Park, MD 21146-3826
(410)544-3331
FAX: (410)544-3329

Silver Spring

Community Radiology Associates, Inc.
3801 International Dr Ste 103
Silver Spring, MD 20906-1550
(240)516-7850
FAX: (301)598-6439

Community Radiology Associates, Inc.
2121 Medical Park Dr, Suite 1 And 2
Silver Spring, MD 20902-4054
(301)681-8242
FAX: (301)681-6315

Community Radiology Associates-White Oak
11120 New Hampshire Ave, Rms 100 & 105
Silver Spring, MD 20904-2633
(240)247-2960
FAX: (301)681-8087

Holy Cross Hospital Of Silver Spring, Inc
1500 Forest Glen Rd
Silver Spring, MD 20910-1484
(301)754-7360
FAX: (301)754-7477

Kaiser Permanente- Silver Spring
12201 Plum Orchard Dr
Silver Spring, MD 20904-7803
(877)390-0033
FAX: (301)548-5849

Medical Faculty Associates White Oak Breast Center
12008 Cherry Hill Rd
Silver Spring, MD 20904-1985
(301)590-8999
FAX: (301)572-8134

Suitland

Kaiser Permanente-Marlow Heights
5100 Auth Way
Suitland, MD 20746-4276
(877)390-0033
FAX: (301)548-5780

Temple Hills

Kaiser Permanente Camp Springs
6104 Old Branch Ave
Temple Hills, MD 20748-2557
(877)390-0033
FAX: (240)632-4451

Timonium

Advanced Radiology - Timonium
2080 York Rd Ste 160
Timonium, MD 21093-4249
(443)436-4700
FAX: (443)436-4780

Towson

Advanced Radiology - Gbmc Pavilion
6701 N Charles St, Ste 3103
Towson, MD 21204-6808
(410)580-2301
FAX: (410)580-2321

Advanced Radiology - St. Joe's
7501 Osler Dr, Bldg A Ste 204
Towson, MD 21204-7733
(410)580-6000
FAX: (410)427-2552

Waldorf

American Radiology Services At Waldorf
3510 Old Washington Rd Ste 101
Waldorf, MD 20602-3234
(301)638-2862
FAX: (443)663-6582

Ifrc,Llc Dba Fairfax Radiology Center At Pembrooke
11345 Pembrooke Sq Ste 104
Waldorf, MD 20603-4804
(301)870-8434
FAX: (301)932-4137

Medstar Medical Grp-So MD Llc Dba Medstar Shah Medical Grp
10 Saint Patricks Dr
Waldorf, MD 20603-4527
(240)448-2949
FAX: (240)448-2950

Westminster

Advanced Radiology-Fisher
193 Stoner Ave Ste 200
Westminster, MD 21157-5794
(443)487-5701
FAX: (443)436-1328

Capital Women's Care, Westminster
844 Washington Rd, Ste 302
Westminster, MD 21157-6664
(410)876-2003
FAX: (410)848-3009

White Plains

Tower Radiology
4255 Altamont Pl Ste 104
White Plains, MD 20695-3066
(301)638-4606
FAX: (301)638-4608

MASSACHUSETTS

Amesbury

Amesbury Health Center
24 Morrill Pl
Amesbury, MA 01913-3585
(978)834-8301
FAX: (978)834-8139

Amherst

Amherst Community Health Ctr. Cooley Dickinson Hosp.
170 University Dr Ste 103
Amherst, MA 01002-2272
(413)582-2200
FAX: (413)253-0447

Amherst Medical Center-Valley Medical Group
31 Hall Dr, Ste 1
Amherst, MA 01002-2778
(413)256-8561
FAX: (413)256-4443

Andover

Lawrence General Hospital Women's Health Imaging
323 Lowell St Ste 301
Andover, MA 01810-4659
(978)475-5213
FAX: (978)946-8352

Arlington

Mount Auburn Radiology At Arlington
22 Mill St Ste 106
Arlington, MA 02476-4738
(617)499-5407
FAX: (617)499-5434

Athol

Athol Memorial Hospital
2033 Main St
Athol, MA 01331-3598
(978)514-1623
FAX: (978)249-5630

Attleboro

Sturdy Memorial Hospital
211 Park St, Radiology Department
Attleboro, MA 02703-3137
(508)236-7770
FAX: (508)236-7760

Auburn

St. Vincent Hospital At Auburn Grove Medical
250 Hampton St
Auburn, MA 01501-2584
(508)363-9729
FAX: (508)363-7071

Ayer

Nashoba Valley Medical Center A Steward Family Hospital, Inc
200 Groton Rd, Mammography Department
Ayer, MA 01432-1168
(978)784-9272
FAX: (978)784-9550

Barnstable

Cuda Center Wilkens Medical Complex
35 Wilkens Lane
Barnstable, MA 02620
(508)957-1623
FAX: (508)957-1707

Barre

Umass Memorial Barre Family Health Ctr
151 Worcester Rd
Barre, MA 01005-9099
(978)355-6321
FAX: (978)355-6295

Beverly

Women's Health Medical & Arts Center
83 Herrick St
Beverly, MA 01915-2757
(978)922-3000
FAX: (978)304-8015

Boston

Avon Comprehensive Breast Center Mgh
15 Parkman St
Boston, MA 02114-3117
(617)724-9729
FAX: (617)726-1074

Beth Israel Deaconess Medical Center
330 Brookline Ave
Boston, MA 02215-5491
(617)254-9500
FAX: (617)754-9510

Boston Medical Center - Belkin Breast Imaging
830 Harrison Ave, Moakley Bldg, Ste 1300
Boston, MA 02118-2905
(617)414-8163
FAX: (617)638-8136

Brigham & Women's Hospital - Lee Bell Ctr
75 Francis St 206 Cwn
Boston, MA 02115-6106
(617)732-6248
FAX: (617)264-5150

Dana Farber Cancer Institute
450 Brookline Ave
Boston, MA 02215-5450
(857)215-0349
FAX: (617)632-3991

Dana-Farber's Mammography Van - Mobile
450 Brookline Ave, Dana-Farber Cancer Institute
Boston, MA 02215-5450
(857)215-0349
FAX: (617)632-2655

Fenway Health
1340 Boylston St, 4th Fl
Boston, MA 02215-4302
(857)313-6563
FAX: (617)867-8646

Harvard Vanguard Medical Assoc - Kenmore Practice
133 Brookline Ave
Boston, MA 02215-3904
(617)421-1372
FAX: (617)421-2134

Sagoff Breast Imaging And Diagnostic Centre
1153 Centre St, Brigham And Women's Faulkner Hospital
Boston, MA 02130-3446
(617)983-7272
FAX: (617)983-7091

South Cove Community Health Center
145 South St, Fl 4
Boston, MA 02111-2826
(617)521-6720
FAX: (617)521-6729

Steward St Elizabeth Med Ctr
736 Cambridge St Rm 5073, St. Margaret's Center/Mammography
Boston, MA 02135-2907
(617)789-3160
FAX: (617)562-7518

Tufts Medical Center
800 Washington St, Radiology Department
Boston, MA 02111-1552
(617)636-9774
FAX: (617)636-9214

Bourne

Inmed Diagnostic Services Of Ma, Llc
2 Technology Park Dr, Ste B
Bourne, MA 02532-8341
(508)759-8191
FAX: (508)759-8178

Brockton

Signature Healthcare Brockton Hospital 110 Liberty Street
110 Liberty St
Brockton, MA 02301-5674
(508)894-0440
FAX: (508)894-0381

Signature Healthcare - Brockton Hospital
680 Centre St, Women's Imaging Dept
Brockton, MA 02302-3395
(508)894-0440
FAX: (508)941-6107

Brookline

Hmfp Radiology
1101 Beacon St Ste 3
Brookline, MA 02446-5587
(617)754-0450
FAX: (617)754-0460

Burlington

Lahey Clinic
41 Mall Rd
Burlington, MA 01805-0002
(781)744-8595
FAX: (781)744-3738

Cambridge

M.I.T. Health Services Center
25 Carleton St, E23 Rm 144
Cambridge, MA 02142-1323
(617)253-4905
FAX: (617)253-5512

Mount Auburn Hospital
330 Mount Auburn St
Cambridge, MA 02138-5597
(617)499-5407
FAX: (617)499-5434

Mount Auburn Radiology At Concord Ave
725 Concord Ave Ste 3400
Cambridge, MA 02138-1055
(617)499-6789
FAX: (617)499-6779

The Cambridge Health Alliance
1493 Cambridge St
Cambridge, MA 02139-1099
(617)665-2019
FAX: (617)665-2035

Charlton

Harrington Healthcare At Charlton
10 N Main St
Charlton, MA 01507-1590
(508)765-3020
FAX: (508)909-7723

Chelmsford

Atrius Health
228 Billerica Rd
Chelmsford, MA 01824-3604
(978)250-6280
FAX: (978)250-6309

Women's Imaging Center
4 Meeting House Rd, Ste 13
Chelmsford, MA 01824-2775
(978)937-6023
FAX: (978)323-2829

Chelsea

Beth Israel Deaconess Healthcare Chelsea
1000 Broadway
Chelsea, MA 02150-2247
(617)754-9540
FAX: (617)975-6039

Chestnut Hill

Brigham And Women's Ambulatory Care Center
850 Boylston St Ste 560
Chestnut Hill, MA 02467-2405
(617)732-9801
FAX: (617)731-8064

Chicopee

Trinity Health Of New England Medical Group
444 Montgomery St
Chicopee, MA 01020-1969
(413)598-7161
FAX: (413)598-7164

Clinton

Health Alliance - Clinton Hospital, Clinton Campus
201 Highland St
Clinton, MA 01510-1037
(978)466-2620
FAX: (978)368-3844

Concord

Hermel Breast Health Center Emerson Hospital
747 Main St Ste 101
Concord, MA 01742-3329
(978)287-8107
FAX: (978)287-8104

Danvers

Lahey Outpatient Center, Danvers
480 Maple St
Danvers, MA 01923-4065
(978)922-3000
FAX: (978)304-8125

Mgh/Northshore Center For Outpatient Care
102 Endicott St
Danvers, MA 01923-3623
(978)882-6161
FAX: (978)882-6141

Nsmc Breast Health Center / Outpatient Services
1 Hutchinson Dr
Danvers, MA 01923-3748
(978)354-4900
FAX: (978)777-5957

Dedham

Dedham Medical Associates
1 Lyons St
Dedham, MA 02026-5599
(781)493-3521
FAX: (781)407-7752

Dorchester

Boston Medical Center Radiology At Uphams Corner Health Ctr.
415 Columbia Rd
Dorchester, MA 02125-2424
(617)287-8000
FAX: (617)287-1500

Codman Square Health Center
637 Washington St
Dorchester, MA 02124-3510
(617)822-8147
FAX: (617)822-8226

Dothouse Health
1353 Dorchester Ave, Department Of Radiology
Dorchester, MA 02122-2932
(617)288-3230
FAX: (617)825-6279

Steward Carney Hospital
2100 Dorchester Ave, Radiology Department
Dorchester, MA 02124-5666
(617)296-4000
FAX: (617)506-2033

East Boston

East Boston Neighborhood Health Center
10 Gove St
East Boston, MA 02128-1931
(617)568-4667
FAX: (617)568-4058

East Bridgewater

Smg Compass Medical
1 Compass Way, Ste 200
East Bridgewater, MA 02333-1464
(508)350-2200
FAX: (508)350-2312

Easthampton

Valley Medical Group Easthampton Health Ctr
238 Northampton St
Easthampton, MA 01027-1046
(413)282-3872
FAX: (413)282-3871

Everett

Cambridge Health Alliance Women's Health Center
96 Garland St, Mammography Ste
Everett, MA 02149-5067
(617)665-2039
FAX: (617)665-2035

Fall River

Primacare Diagnostic Center
289 Pleasant St Ste 101
Fall River, MA 02721-3005
(508)646-0006
FAX: (508)646-0004

Robert Stoico Fed Ctr For Breast Care St Anne's Hosp
795 Middle St
Fall River, MA 02721-1798
(508)235-5353
FAX: (508)235-5360

Southcoast Health Breast Center
235 Hanover St
Fall River, MA 02720-5246
(508)973-3900
FAX: (508)973-9805

Southcoast Hospitals Group Radiology Services - Healthfirst
387 Quarry St Ste 104
Fall River, MA 02723-1026
(508)973-3900
FAX: (508)973-9305

Falmouth

Falmouth Hospital - Seifer Imaging Center
90 Ter Heun Dr
Falmouth, MA 02540-2533
(508)457-3551
FAX: (508)457-3861

Fitchburg

Health Alliance-Clinton Hospital, Burbank Campus
275 Nichols Rd
Fitchburg, MA 01420-2360
(978)343-5090
FAX: (978)466-2684

Foxboro

Norwood Hospital Mammography At Foxboro
70 Walnut St
Foxboro, MA 02035-5312
(781)278-6118
FAX: (508)698-3249

Foxborough

Brigham And Women's / Mass General Health Care Ctr
20 Patriot Pl Bldg C
Foxborough, MA 02035-1375
(508)718-4025
FAX: (508)718-4026

Framingham

Charles River Medical Associates
571 Union Ave First Floor
Framingham, MA 01702-5855
(508)848-2164
FAX: (508)202-9515

Metrowest Medical Center - Framingham Campus
115 Lincoln St
Framingham, MA 01702-6358
(508)383-8400
FAX: (508)383-8521

Metrowest Wellness Center
761 Worcester Rd
Framingham, MA 01701-5232
(508)383-8400
FAX: (508)383-8470

Franklin

Milford Regional Franklin Diagnostic Imaging
1280 W Central St, Ste 103
Franklin, MA 02038-3110
(508)422-2665
FAX: (508)482-7303

Gardner

Heywood Hospital
242 Green St
Gardner, MA 01440-1373
(978)630-5070
FAX: (978)630-6123

Gloucester

Addison Gilbert Hospital
298 Washington St
Gloucester, MA 01930-4889
(978)283-4000
FAX: (978)491-6576

Great Barrington

Fairview Hospital
29 Lewis Ave
Great Barrington, MA 01230-1796
(413)528-8600
FAX: (413)854-9794

Greenfield

Baystate Franklin Medical Center
164 High St
Greenfield, MA 01301-2613
(413)773-2348
FAX: (413)773-2139

Valley Medical Group Greenfield Health Center
329 Conway St, Ste 1
Greenfield, MA 01301-1522
(413)774-3308
FAX: (413)772-3393

Harwich

Fontaine Medical Center
525 Long Pond Dr
Harwich, MA 02645-1236
(508)957-1623
FAX: (508)430-3216

Haverhill

Anna Jaques Hospital At Parkway Imaging
1 Park Way
Haverhill, MA 01830-6278
(978)834-8210
FAX: (978)372-1303

Holyoke

Holyoke Medical Center Women's Center
2 Hospital Dr Ste 202
Holyoke, MA 01040-6619
(413)534-2771
FAX: (413)534-2773

Jamaica Plain

Lemuel Shattuck Hospital
170 Morton St
Jamaica Plain, MA 02130-3735
(617)971-3366
FAX: (617)971-3856

Lawrence

Lawrence General Hospital
1 General St
Lawrence, MA 01841-2997
(978)683-4000
FAX: (978)946-8146

Leominster

Health Alliance-Clinton Hospital, Leominster Campus
60 Hospital Rd
Leominster, MA 01453-2205
(978)466-2660
FAX: (978)466-2684

Reliant Medical Group
225 New Lancaster Rd
Leominster, MA 01453-4958
(978)466-3242
FAX: (978)514-8831

Lexington

Beth Israel Deaconess Healthcare Lexington
482 Bedford St
Lexington, MA 02420-1402
(781)528-2560
FAX: (781)528-2565

Lahey Lexington
16 Hayden Ave
Lexington, MA 02421-7929
(781)744-8000
FAX: (781)372-7086

Longmeadow

Baystate Radiology & Imaging
21 Dwight Rd
Longmeadow, MA 01106-1765
(413)827-7400
FAX: (413)827-7407

Lowell

Lowell General Hospital
295 Varnum Ave, Radiology Department
Lowell, MA 01854-2193
(978)937-6023
FAX: (978)937-6825

Lowell General Hospital Saints Campus
1 Hospital Dr
Lowell, MA 01852-1311
(978)937-6023
FAX: (978)937-6825

Lynn

Nsmc Breast Health Lynn Community Health Center
269 Union St
Lynn, MA 01901-1314
(978)354-4900
FAX: (978)777-5957

Salem Hospital Outpatient Services - Lynn
480 Lynnfield St
Lynn, MA 01904-1419
(978)354-4900
FAX: (781)477-3601

Marlborough

Charles River Medical Associates
246 Maple St, Ste 3
Marlborough, MA 01752-3235
(508)251-0303
FAX: (508)820-8360

Umass Memorial Marlborough Hospital Women's Imaging Center
207 Union St
Marlborough, MA 01752-1246
(508)486-5599
FAX: (508)597-2257

Mattapan

Boston Medical Center Radiology At Mattapan Health Center
1575 Blue Hill Ave Ste 1-15
Mattapan, MA 02126-2122
(617)898-9076
FAX: (617)898-1290

Medford

Lawrence Memorial Hospital
170 Governors Ave
Medford, MA 02155-1643
(781)338-7111
FAX: (781)338-6472

Melrose

Melrosewakefield Healthcare, Inc Melrose Campus
830 Main St
Melrose, MA 02176-2741
(781)665-8300
FAX: (781)662-7887

Methuen

Holy Family Hospital
70 East St
Methuen, MA 01844-4597
(978)686-6492
FAX: (978)681-0654

Middleboro

Morton Health Services
511 W Grove St Ste 208
Middleboro, MA 02346-1479
(508)828-7690
FAX: (508)946-9833

Smg Compass Medical
8 Commerce Blvd
Middleboro, MA 02346-1030
(774)260-9200
FAX: (774)260-9205

Milford

Milford Regional Medical Center
14 Prospect St
Milford, MA 01757-3003
(508)422-2665
FAX: (508)482-7303

Milton

Beth Israel Deaconess Hospital Milton
199 Reedsdale Rd
Milton, MA 02186-3926
(617)313-1700
FAX: (617)313-1526

N Dartmouth

Steward Medical Group Inc.
531 Faunce Corner Rd
N Dartmouth, MA 02747-1242
(508)961-0855
FAX: (508)961-0825

Nantucket

Nantucket Cottage Hospital
57 Prospect St
Nantucket, MA 02554-4396
(508)825-8382
FAX: (508)825-8390

Natick

Newton-Wellesley Ambulatory - Care Ctr - Natick
307 W Central St
Natick, MA 01760-3719
(617)243-5345
FAX: (617)243-5838

Needham

Beth Israel Deaconess Hospital Needham
148 Chestnut St
Needham, MA 02492-2523
(781)453-3044
FAX: (781)453-5789

New Bedford

Southcoast Hospitals Group Radiology Services - Gnbchc
874 Purchase St
New Bedford, MA 02740-6232
(508)992-6553
FAX: (508)973-9305

Newburyport

Anna Jaques Hospital
25 Highland Ave, Radiology Department
Newburyport, MA 01950-3894
(978)834-8301
FAX: (978)463-1171

Newton

Beth Israel Deaconess - Chestnut Hill
200 Boylston St
Newton, MA 02467-2012
(617)278-8550
FAX: (617)278-8555

Dana Farber Cancer Institute - Chestnut Hill
300 Boylston St
Newton, MA 02467-1959
(857)215-0349
FAX: (617)632-2655

Newton Wellesley Hospital
2014 Washington St
Newton, MA 02462-1699
(617)243-5345
FAX: (617)243-5838

North Adams

Northern Berkshire Health Center Of Berkshire Medical Center
71 Hospital Ave
North Adams, MA 01247-2504
(413)447-2451
FAX: (413)496-6856

North Dartmouth

Southcoast Hospitals Group Radiology Services - Cwh
300B Faunce Corner Rd, Center For Womens Health
North Dartmouth, MA 02747-1257
(508)973-9300
FAX: (508)973-9305

North Easton

Good Samaritan Medical Center - Womens Imaging
15 Roche Brothers Way, Ste 120
North Easton, MA 02356-1000
(508)427-2665
FAX: (508)427-2855

Northampton

Baystate Radiology And Imaging - Northampton
325 King St Ste B
Northampton, MA 01060-2370
(413)827-7400
FAX: (413)827-7447

Cooley Dickinson Hospital
30 Locust St
Northampton, MA 01060-2093
(413)582-5000
FAX: (413)582-4993

Norwell

Inmed Diagnostic Services Of Ma, Llc
600 Longwater Dr Ste 105
Norwell, MA 02061-1639
(781)878-4004
FAX: (781)878-4075

South Shore Medical Center
143 Longwater Dr
Norwell, MA 02061-1683
(781)261-4702
FAX: (781)681-1715

Norwood

Guild Imaging Center Of Norwood Hospital
825 Washington St Ste 210
Norwood, MA 02062-3489
(781)762-5595
FAX: (781)762-9966

Steward Norwood Hospital, Inc.
800 Washington St, Ste 1
Norwood, MA 02062-3487
(781)278-6397
FAX: (781)278-6944

Oak Bluffs

Martha's Vineyard Hospital
1 Hospital Rd
Oak Bluffs, MA 02557-1406
(508)957-9421
FAX: (508)696-7376

Peabody

Lahey Medical Center Peabody
1 Essex Center Dr
Peabody, MA 01960-2901
(978)538-4662
FAX: (781)744-8595

Pembroke

Brigham And Women's Healthcare Center, Pembroke
15 Corporate Park Dr
Pembroke, MA 02359-1966
(844)783-3736
FAX: (617)732-9649

Pittsfield

Berkshire Medical Center, Medical Art Complex
777 North St, Ste 337
Pittsfield, MA 01201-4172
(413)447-2451
FAX: (413)447-2148

Plymouth

Beth Israel Deaconess Hospital- Plymouth
275 Sandwich St
Plymouth, MA 02360-2183
(508)830-3000
FAX: (508)830-2359

Beth Israel Deaconess Hospital-Plymouth Imaging At The Park
45 Resnik Rd, Ste 106
Plymouth, MA 02360-4843
(508)830-3000
FAX: (508)747-1383

Provincetown

Outer Cape Health Service
49 Harry Kemp Way
Provincetown, MA 02657-1618
(774)538-3314
FAX: (774)539-3392

Quincy

Biocare Diagnostics Crown Colony Medical Center
300 Congress St, Ste 103
Quincy, MA 02169-0907
(617)770-9300
FAX: (617)770-3463

Smg Compass Medical
54 Miller St
Quincy, MA 02169-4725
(617)481-3200
FAX: (508)350-2200

Reading

Hallmark Health Medical Center Reading
30 New Crossing Rd
Reading, MA 01867-3270
(781)213-5100
FAX: (781)213-5105

Revere

Mgh Hlthcare Ctr-Revere Massachusetts General Hosp
300 Ocean Ave
Revere, MA 02151-3675
(781)485-6180
FAX: (781)485-6188

Rowley

North Shore Physicians Group Imaging Services
414 Haverhill St
Rowley, MA 01969-1919
(978)354-4900
FAX: (978)348-5200

Roxbury

Dana-Farber Cancer Institute Atwhittier Street Health Center
1290 Tremont St - Mammography Suite
Roxbury, MA 02120-3432
(857)215-0349
FAX: (617)632-2655

Salem

Nsmc Brudnick Breast Health Center
81 Highland Ave, Nsmc - Salem Hospital
Salem, MA 01970-2714
(978)354-4900
FAX: (978)354-4840

Shrewsbury

Umass Memorial - Shrewsbury Mammography
26 Julio Dr Ste 104
Shrewsbury, MA 01545-3020
(508)334-9900
FAX: (508)845-9011

Somerville

Atrius Health
40 Holland St 3rd Fl
Somerville, MA 02144-2705
(617)629-6150
FAX: (617)629-6158

South Boston

South Boston Community Health Center
409 W Broadway 1st Fl
South Boston, MA 02127-2249
(617)464-7624
FAX: (617)464-7598

South Dennis

Inmed Diagnostic Services Of Ma, Llc
434 Route 134 Ste C2
South Dennis, MA 02660-3433
(508)398-3617
FAX: (508)398-3763

South Easton

Smg Compass Medical
21 Bristol Dr, Ste 102
South Easton, MA 02375-1199
(508)565-7200
FAX: (508)565-7240

South Hadley

Baystate Radiology & Imaging
470 Granby Rd Ste 5
South Hadley, MA 01075-3215
(413)827-7400
FAX: (413)827-7447

South Weymouth

South Shore Hosp Diag Imaging & Women's Specialty Ctr
101 Columbian St Level 1
South Weymouth, MA 02190-1601
(781)624-4714
FAX: (781)624-5012

Southborough

Reliant Medical Group
24 Newton St 28
Southborough, MA 01772-1215
(508)853-2716
FAX: (508)852-1365

Southbridge

Harrington Memorial Hospital
100 South St
Southbridge, MA 01550-4047
(508)765-3020
FAX: (508)909-7723

Springfield

Baystate Breast & Wellness Center
100 Wason Ave Ste 300
Springfield, MA 01107-1179
(413)794-9564
FAX: (413)794-9460

Center For Mammography At Mercy Hospital
299 Carew St
Springfield, MA 01104-2301
(413)748-9101
FAX: (413)748-9081

Stoneham

Melrosewakefield Healthcare, Inc. - Breast Health Center
41 Montvale Ave, 4th Fl
Stoneham, MA 02180-2445
(781)224-5806
FAX: (781)224-5807

Taunton

Morton Hospital A Steward Family Hospital
88 Washington St, Radiology Department
Taunton, MA 02780-2465
(508)828-7690
FAX: (508)828-7988

Uxbridge

Tri River Family Health Center
281 E Hartford Ave
Uxbridge, MA 01569-1253
(508)278-8529
FAX: (508)278-8433

Walpole

Newton Wellesley Ambulatory Care Ctr-Walpole
111 Norfolk St
Walpole, MA 02081-1703
(617)243-5345
FAX: (617)243-6776

Waltham

Mass General Imaging - Waltham
52 2nd Ave, Ste 300
Waltham, MA 02451-1127
(781)487-6030
FAX: (781)487-6144

Mount Auburn Healthcare Waverley Oaks
355 Waverley Oaks Rd
Waltham, MA 02452-8474
(781)314-7650
FAX: (781)314-7676

Ware

Baystate Mary Lane Outpatient Center
85 South St, Radiology Department
Ware, MA 01082-1625
(866)531-8378
FAX: (413)967-2330

Wareham

Southcoast Hospitals Group Radiology Services
100 Rosebrook Way, Ste 101
Wareham, MA 02571-1140
(508)973-3900
FAX: (508)973-9305

Webster

Harrington Healthcare At Webster
340 Thompson Rd
Webster, MA 01570-1509
(508)765-3020
FAX: (508)949-3988

Wellesley Hills

Boston Breast Diagnostic Center
165 Worcester St
Wellesley Hills, MA 02481-3615
(617)553-5300
FAX: (617)553-5353

West Yarmouth

Cape Diagnostic Imaging
21 Aarons Way
West Yarmouth, MA 02673-2596
(508)771-5200
FAX: (508)771-5202

Westfield

Burk Women's Imaging Center At Baystate Noble Hospital
115 W Silver St
Westfield, MA 01085-3678
(413)571-0140
FAX: (413)572-5133

Westford

Emerson Hospital Health Center-Westford
133 Littleton Rd Ste 105
Westford, MA 01886-3198
(978)287-8107
FAX: (978)287-8104

Westwood

Brigham And Womens Healthcare Cntr Westwood
100 Brigham Way
Westwood, MA 02090-2445
(877)937-8182
FAX: (508)718-4026

Weymouth

Atrius Health, Inc - Imaging Dept
51 Performance Dr, Ste 100
Weymouth, MA 02189-3141
(781)682-0550
FAX: (781)682-0565

Wilmington

Winchester Hospital Family Medical Center
500 Salem St
Wilmington, MA 01887-1200
(978)988-6040
FAX: (978)657-5826

Woburn

Winchester Hospital Breast Care Center
200 Unicorn Park Dr, Ste 302
Woburn, MA 01801-3342
(781)756-2308
FAX: (781)756-4798

Worcester

Family Health Center Of Worcester, Inc.
26 Queen St
Worcester, MA 01610-2478
(508)860-7995
FAX: (508)860-7863

Neary-Hunter Ob/Gyn, Llc
67 Belmont St Ste 101
Worcester, MA 01605-2608
(508)752-1491
FAX: (508)459-3032

Physicians For Women's Health, Llc
328 Shrewsbury St Ste 100
Worcester, MA 01604-5465
(508)755-4861
FAX: (508)752-1392

Reliant Medical Group
5 Neponset St
Worcester, MA 01606-2714
(508)853-2716
FAX: (508)365-6588

Saint Vincent Women's Wellness Center
1 Eaton Pl
Worcester, MA 01608-1232
(508)363-5000
FAX: (508)363-9236

Umass Memorial - Memorial Campus
119 Belmont St 1st Floor Jaquith Bld, Diagnostic Center
Worcester, MA 01605-2982
(508)334-9900
FAX: (774)441-6429

Umass Memorial Medical Center - Hahnemann Campus
281 Lincoln St, Mammography
Worcester, MA 01605-2138
(774)441-6408
FAX: (774)441-6429

Umass Memorial Medical Center Ambulatory Care Center
55 Lake Ave N, Mammography 5th Floor
Worcester, MA 01655-0002
(508)334-9900
FAX: (774)441-6429

MICHIGAN

Adrian

Promedica Bixby Hospital
5640 N Adrian Hwy
Adrian, MI 49221-8318
(517)265-0271
FAX: (517)265-0378

Promedica Hickman Hosp - Women's Health Center
5640 N Adrian Hwy
Adrian, MI 49221-8318
(517)577-0271
FAX: (517)424-3613

Allegan

Ascension Allegan Hospital
555 Linn St
Allegan, MI 49010-1524
(269)686-4210
FAX: (269)686-4215

Alma

Midmichigan Medical Center Gratiot
300 E Warwick Dr
Alma, MI 48801-1096
(989)466-3343
FAX: (989)466-7250

Alpena

Midmichigan Medical Center Alpena
1501 W Chisholm St
Alpena, MI 49707-1498
(989)356-8001
FAX: (989)356-7551

Ann Arbor

East Ann Arbor Health Center Breast Imaging
PO Box 2712, 4260 Plymouth Rd
Ann Arbor, MI 48106-2712
(734)936-6274
FAX: (734)615-8327

University Of Michigan - Briarwood Radiology
1901 Briarwood Cir, Bldg 9
Ann Arbor, MI 48108-1679
(734)936-6274
FAX: (734)615-8327

University Of Michigan Health System
1500 E Medical Center Dr, Cancer Center B2-353
Ann Arbor, MI 48109-5000
(734)936-6274
FAX: (734)615-8327

West Ann Arbor Health Center
380 Parkland Plz, Radiology
Ann Arbor, MI 48103-6201
(734)936-4500
FAX: (734)615-8327

Atlanta

Mid Michigan Medical Health-Thunder Bay Clinic Atlanta Mi
11899 M 32
Atlanta, MI 49709-9374
(989)785-5940
FAX: (989)356-7551

Auburn Hills

Ascension Providence Rochester Center For Breast Health
2251 N Squirrel Rd Ste 201
Auburn Hills, MI 48326-4602
(248)652-5437
FAX: (248)475-1725

Bad Axe

Huron Memorial Hospital Dba McLaren Thumb Region
1100 S Van Dyke Rd
Bad Axe, MI 48413-9615
(989)269-9521
FAX: (989)269-5209

Battle Creek

Borgess Health Park Battle Creek
3035 Capital Ave SW
Battle Creek, MI 49015-4334
(269)565-9233
FAX: (269)565-9236

Bronson Battle Creek
300 North Ave
Battle Creek, MI 49017-3396
(269)245-8167
FAX: (269)245-8087

Bay City

Ascension St. Mary's Of Michigan Bay City
4040 N Euclid Ave
Bay City, MI 48706-2484
(989)684-4300
FAX: (989)684-3931

McLaren Bay Region
3175 Professional Ct
Bay City, MI 48706-2823
(989)667-6350
FAX: (989)667-6359

Bellaire

Bellaire Family Health Center
4955 S M 88 Hwy
Bellaire, MI 49615-9082
(231)533-8649
FAX: (231)533-6778

Berrien Springs

University Medical Specialties
9045 US Highway 31
Berrien Springs, MI 49103-1666
(269)473-2222
FAX: (269)473-6880

Big Rapids

Spectrum Health Big Rapids Hospital
605 Oak St
Big Rapids, MI 49307-2048
(231)592-4440
FAX: (231)592-4481

Birmingham

Beaumont Health - Mammography- Birmingham
35046 Woodward Ave, LL Mammography Ste.
Birmingham, MI 48009-0964
(800)328-8542
FAX: (248)855-7470

Bloomfield Hills

Henry Ford Medical Center Bloomfield Township
1961 S Telegraph Rd
Bloomfield Hills, MI 48302-0246
(248)325-3400
FAX: (248)325-3863

Boyne City

Munson Healthcare Boyne Area Health Center
223 N Park St
Boyne City, MI 49712-1220
(231)547-7123
FAX: (231)582-5338

Brighton

Brighton Center For Speciality Care
7500 Challis Rd, Radiology- Breast Imaging
Brighton, MI 48116-9416
(734)936-4500
FAX: (734)615-8327

Saint Joseph Mercy Breast Imaging
7575 Grand River Rd, Ste 110
Brighton, MI 48114-7389
(734)712-1313
FAX: (734)712-5944

Brownstown

Henry Ford Health Center Brownstown
23050 West Rd, Ste 110
Brownstown, MI 48183-1470
(734)671-1440
FAX: (734)671-1614

Burton

Ascension Genesys Ambulatory Imaging
1096 S Belsay Rd Ste J, Suite J
Burton, MI 48509-1948
(810)715-0803
FAX: (810)715-1301

Byron Center

Saint Mary's Southwest
2373 64th St SW
Byron Center, MI 49315-7974
(616)685-4000
FAX: (616)685-3939

Cadillac

Munson Health Care Cadillac Hospital
400 Hobart St
Cadillac, MI 49601-2389
(231)935-7200
FAX: (231)876-7855

Canton

Beaumont Medical Center Canton
7300 N Canton Center Rd, Radiology Department
Canton, MI 48187-1579
(734)454-8029
FAX: (734)454-0416

St. Joseph Mercy Breast Imaging - Canton
1600 S Canton Center Rd
Canton, MI 48188-1992
(734)712-1313
FAX: (734)712-5944

University Of Michigan - Canton Health Center
1051 N Canton Center Rd
Canton, MI 48187-5097
(734)936-6274
FAX: (734)615-8327

Caro

Caro Community Hospital D/B/A McLaren Caro Region
401 N Hooper St
Caro, MI 48723-1476
(989)672-5111
FAX: (989)672-5789

Carson City

Sparrow Carson Hospital
406 E Elm St
Carson City, MI 48811-9693
(989)584-3131
FAX: (989)584-2161

Cass City

Hills & Dales General Hospital
4675 Hill St
Cass City, MI 48726-1099
(989)912-6374
FAX: (989)912-6127

Charlevoix

Munson Healthcare Charlevoix Hospital
14700 Lake Shore Dr
Charlevoix, MI 49720-1931
(231)547-8774
FAX: (231)547-8082

Charlotte

Sparrow Eaton Hospital
321 E Harris St
Charlotte, MI 48813-1629
(517)543-1050
FAX: (517)541-5820

Cheboygan

McLaren Northern Michigan - Cheboygan Campus
748 S Main St
Cheboygan, MI 49721-2220
(231)487-4189
FAX: (231)627-1530

Chelsea

Saint Joseph Mercy Chelsea, Inc
775 S Main St
Chelsea, MI 48118-1383
(734)593-5540
FAX: (734)593-5505

Chesterfield Township

Henry Ford Hospital - Macomb Chesterfield Hlth Ctr
30795 Twenty Three Mile Road
Chesterfield Township, MI 48047
(586)203-1600
FAX: (586)421-3117

Clare

Midmichigan Medical Center- Clare
703 N McEwan St
Clare, MI 48617-1440
(989)802-5194
FAX: (989)802-8425

Clarkston

Clarkston Imaging Center
7210 N Main St, Ste 211
Clarkston, MI 48346-1575
(248)858-6092
FAX: (248)858-6720

McLaren Oakland-Clarkston
5701 Bow Pointe Dr Ste 255
Clarkston, MI 48346-5402
(248)922-6810
FAX: (248)922-6811

Clinton Township

Henry Ford Macomb Health Center Fraser
15717 15 Mile Rd
Clinton Township, MI 48035-2101
(586)203-1600
FAX: (586)285-3873

Henry Ford Macomb Hospital
16151 19 Mile Rd Ste 110
Clinton Township, MI 48038-1157
(586)203-1600
FAX: (586)263-2509

Henry Ford Mobile Mammography
15855 19 Mile Rd
Clinton Township, MI 48038-3504
(248)325-3404
FAX: (586)336-2401

Clinton Twp

McLaren Macomb - Clinton
36561 Harper Ave, Ste F
Clinton Twp, MI 48035-2012
(586)493-3790
FAX: (586)493-3796

Clio

Ascension Genesys Ambulatory Imaging
4154 W Vienna Rd
Clio, MI 48420-2809
(810)564-1100
FAX: (810)564-2645

Coldwater

Community Health Center Of Branch County
274 E Chicago St
Coldwater, MI 49036-2088
(517)279-5017
FAX: (517)279-5449

Commerce

Huron Valley - Sinai Hospital
1 William Carls Dr
Commerce, MI 48382-2283
(248)937-3800
FAX: (248)937-3810

Davison

Regional Medical Imaging
1141 S State Rd, Ste 4 Ste 26
Davison, MI 48423-1964
(810)732-1919
FAX: (810)732-1945

Dearborn

Basha Diagnostics, P.C.
4407 Roemer St
Dearborn, MI 48126-3405
(313)584-0768
FAX: (248)435-8099

Beaumont Breast Care Center, Dearborn
18100 Oakwood Blvd Ste 200, Dearborn Medical Park
Dearborn, MI 48124-4085
(313)438-7715
FAX: (313)438-7720

Dearborn Obstetrical & Gyn Assoc. Pc
25080 Michigan Ave
Dearborn, MI 48124-1740
(313)730-8880
FAX: (877)550-8437

Henry Ford Medical Center-Fairlane
19401 Hubbard Dr
Dearborn, MI 48126-2699
(313)982-8650
FAX: (313)982-8575

Deckerville

Deckerville Community Hospital
3559 Pine St
Deckerville, MI 48427-7703
(810)376-7020
FAX: (810)376-7033

Detroit

Henry Ford Cancer Center
2800 W Grand Blvd, Radiology
Detroit, MI 48202-2610
(313)916-9624
FAX: (313)916-9625

Henry Ford Hospital
2799 W Grand Blvd
Detroit, MI 48202-2689
(313)916-2932
FAX: (313)916-9625

Henry Ford Medical Center-Detroit Northwest
7800 W Outer Dr
Detroit, MI 48235-3461
(313)653-2550
FAX: (313)753-2680

Karmanos Cancer Center -Walt Comprehensive Breast Ctr
4100 John R St
Detroit, MI 48201-2013
(800)527-6266
FAX: (313)576-9319

Vhs, Sinai-Grace Hospital Inc
6001 W Outer Dr Ste 206, Professional Building
Detroit, MI 48235-2626
(313)966-6060
FAX: (313)966-3641

Dowagiac

Ascension Borgess-Lee Hospital
420 W High St
Dowagiac, MI 49047-1943
(269)783-3030
FAX: (269)783-3056

East China

Ascension River District Hospital
4100 River Rd
East China, MI 48054-2914
(810)329-5390
FAX: (810)326-4757

East Jordan

East Jordan Family Health Center
601 Bridge St
East Jordan, MI 49727-9383
(231)536-2206
FAX: (231)536-7150

East Lansing

Msu Health Care
4660 S Hagadorn Rd Ste 600
East Lansing, MI 48823-5383
(517)884-9000
FAX: (517)884-0000

Eaton Rapids

Eaton Rapids Medical Center
1500 S Main St
Eaton Rapids, MI 48827-1952
(517)633-9426
FAX: (517)663-9428

Escanaba

Marquette Medical Clinic Escanaba
710 S Lincoln Rd Ste 600
Escanaba, MI 49829-1487
(906)786-1839
FAX: (906)789-8797

OSF St. Francis Hospital
3401 Ludington St
Escanaba, MI 49829-1377
(906)786-3311
FAX: (906)789-4489

Farmington Hills

Ascension Providence Farmington Hills
30055 Northwestern Hwy
Farmington Hills, MI 48334-3230
(248)864-4111
FAX: (248)865-4083

Botsford Breast Center
27900 Grand River Ave Ste 110
Farmington Hills, MI 48336-5965
(947)521-4435
FAX: (248)473-4995

Botsford Hospital North Professional Building
28050 Grand River Ave, Ste 101
Farmington Hills, MI 48336-5919
(947)521-4435
FAX: (248)473-4995

Karmanos Cancer Center - Farmington Hills
31995 Northwestern Hwy
Farmington Hills, MI 48334-1625
(800)527-6266
FAX: (313)576-9960

Millennium Diagnostic Center
32255 Northwestern Hwy, Ste 100
Farmington Hills, MI 48334-1573
(248)945-0000
FAX: (248)945-1819

Fenton

McLaren-Flint
2420 Owen Rd
Fenton, MI 48430-3417
(810)496-2430
FAX: (810)342-4839

Regional Medical Imaging
221 W Roberts St
Fenton, MI 48430-2634
(810)720-7550
FAX: (810)732-1945

Flint

McLaren Flint
501 S Ballenger Hwy Ste B
Flint, MI 48532-3606
(810)342-4800
FAX: (810)342-4839

Park Plaza Radiology
G1071 N Ballenger Hwy, Ste 102
Flint, MI 48504-4453
(810)244-5450
FAX: (810)235-8928

Regional Medical Imaging
3346 Lennon Rd, Ste 2
Flint, MI 48507-1082
(810)732-1919
FAX: (810)732-1945

Regional Medical Imaging
5059 Villa Linde Pkwy Ste 25
Flint, MI 48532-3438
(810)732-1919
FAX: (810)732-1945

Fort Gratiot

Lake Huron Medical Center- North Campus
4190 24th Ave
Fort Gratiot, MI 48059-3882
(810)216-1572
FAX: (810)216-1676

Frankenmuth

Covenant Breast Health Center Frankenmuth
600 N Main St
Frankenmuth, MI 48734-1152
(989)583-6279
FAX: (989)583-5269

Frankfort

Munson Paul Oliver Memorial Hospital
224 Park Ave
Frankfort, MI 49635-9036
(800)968-9292
FAX: (231)352-2222

Fremont

Spectrum Health Gerber Memorial
212 S Sullivan Ave
Fremont, MI 49412-1548
(231)924-1100
FAX: (231)924-1136

Garden City

Prime Healthcare Services Garden City Llc
6245 Inkster Rd
Garden City, MI 48135-4001
(734)458-7210
FAX: (734)458-3249

Gaylord

Munson Healthcare Otsego Memorial Hospital
825 N Center Ave
Gaylord, MI 49735-1592
(989)731-2100
FAX: (989)731-2479

Gladwin

Mid-Michigan Medical Center - Gladwin
515 Quarter St, Radiology Department
Gladwin, MI 48624-1967
(989)246-6488
FAX: (989)246-6484

Grand Blanc

Ascension Genesys Ambulatory Imaging
600 Health Park Blvd Ste B
Grand Blanc, MI 48439-2558
(810)606-1601
FAX: (810)606-1610

Regional Medical Imaging
8483 Holly Rd Ste 101
Grand Blanc, MI 48439-1840
(810)732-1919
FAX: (810)694-1921

Grand Haven

Health Pointe
15100 Whittaker Way
Grand Haven, MI 49417-8696
(616)935-6240
FAX: (616)935-6245

North Ottawa Community Health Systems
1309 Sheldon Rd
Grand Haven, MI 49417-2488
(616)847-5430
FAX: (616)847-5611

Grand Ledge

McLaren Greater Lansing
1035 Charlevoix Dr Ste 200
Grand Ledge, MI 48837-2223
(517)626-3106
FAX: (517)626-3105

Grand Rapids

Metro Health Park East
4055 Cascade Rd SE
Grand Rapids, MI 49546-2149
(616)252-7515
FAX: (616)252-6286

Spectrum Health Integrated Care Campus Beltline
2750 E Beltline Ave NE
Grand Rapids, MI 49525-8614
(616)774-7998
FAX: (616)486-6034

Spectrum Health Lemmen Holton Cancer Pavilion
145 Michigan St NE Ste 4200MC 202
Grand Rapids, MI 49503-2562
(616)267-2626
FAX: (616)486-6034

Spectrum Health Medical Group
4069 Lake Dr SE Ste 116
Grand Rapids, MI 49546-8816
(616)267-2626
FAX: (616)486-6034

Spectrum Hlth Hosp Betty Ford Breast Care
1840 Wealthy St SE
Grand Rapids, MI 49506-2921
(616)774-7998
FAX: (616)486-6034

Spectrum Hlth Hospitals Women's Hlth Center
555 Midtowne St NE Ste 101
Grand Rapids, MI 49503-5730
(616)774-7998
FAX: (616)486-6035

Spectrum Hlth Mobile-Betty Ford Breast Care Svcs-Mobile
1345 Monroe Ave NW
Grand Rapids, MI 49505-4671
(616)774-7998
FAX: (616)486-6035

Spectrum Hlth-South Campus - Betty Ford Breast Care Servs.
80 68th St SE
Grand Rapids, MI 49548-6980
(616)774-7998
FAX: (616)486-6034

Trinity Health-Michigan D/B/A Mercy Health Saint Mary's
1471 E Beltline Ave NE Ste 103
Grand Rapids, MI 49525-4548
(616)685-4000
FAX: (616)685-3086

Trinity Health-Michigan D/B/A Mercy Health Saint Mary's
250 Cherry St SE Ste 2500
Grand Rapids, MI 49503-4608
(616)685-4000
FAX: (616)685-3086

Grayling

Munson Healthcare Grayling Hospital
1100 E Michigan Ave
Grayling, MI 49738-1312
(800)968-9292
FAX: (989)348-0426

Greenville

Spectrum Health United Hospital
615 S Bower St
Greenville, MI 48838-2614
(616)225-9090
FAX: (616)754-2946

Grosse Pointe

Ascension St. John Hospital Health Center At Kercheval
17141 Kercheval Ave
Grosse Pointe, MI 48230-1660
(313)642-5020
FAX: (313)642-4975

Beaumont Hospital Grosse Pointe
468 Cadieux Rd
Grosse Pointe, MI 48230-1507
(313)473-1876
FAX: (313)473-1806

Grosse Pointe Farms

Henry Ford Medical Center Cottage
159 Kercheval Ave
Grosse Pointe Farms, MI 48236-3610
(313)640-2182
FAX: (313)640-2316

Grosse Pointe Woods

Ascension St. John Hospital, Liggett Breast Center
19229 Mack Ave Ste 31
Grosse Pointe Woods, MI 48236-2857
(866)501-3627
FAX: (313)647-3310

Grosse Pointe Physicians X-Ray Center, P.C.
21003 Mack Ave
Grosse Pointe Woods, MI 48236-1397
(313)881-0411
FAX: (313)881-3099

Hancock

Up Health System Portage
500 Campus Dr, Ste 100
Hancock, MI 49930-1453
(906)483-1499
FAX: (906)483-1417

Harbor Beach

Harbor Beach Community Hospital
210 S 1st St
Harbor Beach, MI 48441-1236
(989)479-3201
FAX: (989)479-5022

Haslett

Cima Breast Ctr An Affiliate Of Cima, P.C.
1650 Haslett Rd
Haslett, MI 48840-7615
(517)853-5588
FAX: (517)999-0358

Hastings

Spectrum Health Pennock
1009 W Green St
Hastings, MI 49058-1790
(269)945-1212
FAX: (269)945-4295

Spectrum Health Pennock State Street Center
1108 W State St
Hastings, MI 49058-9711
(269)945-1212
FAX: (269)945-4295

Hillsdale

Hillsdale Hospital
168 S Howell St
Hillsdale, MI 49242-2081
(517)437-4895
FAX: (517)437-5156

Holland

Holland Hospital Breast Health Services
844 Washington Ave Ste 2100
Holland, MI 49423-7136
(616)355-3865
FAX: (616)396-2453

Holland Hospital Breast Health Services-Hmic
3299 N Wellness Dr Bldg C
Holland, MI 49424-7269
(616)355-3865
FAX: (616)392-1428

Houghton

Aspirus Houghton Clinic
1000 Cedar St
Houghton, MI 49931-1978
(906)337-6151
FAX: (906)337-6532

Houghton Lake

Midmichigan Community Health Services
9249 W Lake City Rd
Houghton Lake, MI 48629-9602
(989)422-2171
FAX: (989)422-2623

Howell

Ascension Livingston Ambulatory Medical Center
1225 S Latson Rd
Howell, MI 48843-7643
(517)338-2335
FAX: (517)338-2337

Saint Joseph Mercy Breast Imaging
620 Byron Rd
Howell, MI 48843-1002
(734)712-1313
FAX: (734)712-5944

Indian River

Munson Healthcare Omh Medical Group-Indian River
3860 S Straits Hwy
Indian River, MI 49749-5146
(989)731-2174
FAX: (989)731-2479

Ionia

Sparrow Ionia Hospital
3565 S State Rd
Ionia, MI 48846-9416
(616)523-1354
FAX: (616)526-1555

Iron Mountain

Bellin Health Iron Mountain
440 Woodward Ave
Iron Mountain, MI 49801-4631
(920)445-7272
FAX: (906)774-0871

Dickinson County Healthcare System
1721 S Stephenson Ave
Iron Mountain, MI 49801-3637
(906)776-5383
FAX: (906)776-5523

Iron River

Aspirus Iron River Hospital And Clinics
1400 W Ice Lake Rd
Iron River, MI 49935-9526
(906)265-0463
FAX: (906)265-3593

Ironwood

Aspirus Ironwood Hospital
N10561 Grandview Ln
Ironwood, MI 49938-9622
(906)932-6211
FAX: (906)932-7380

Ishpeming

Up Health System Bell
901 Lakeshore Dr
Ishpeming, MI 49849-2197
(906)485-2632
FAX: (906)485-2370

Jackson

Henry Ford Allegiance Diagnostic Center-Professional Bldg
1100 E Michigan Ave, Ste 104
Jackson, MI 49201-1800
(517)205-4905
FAX: (517)205-7845

Henry Ford Allegiance Health
205 N East Ave
Jackson, MI 49201-1753
(517)205-4905
FAX: (517)205-7769

Henry Ford Allegiance Mobile Health-Mobile
1201 E Michigan Ave
Jackson, MI 49201-1852
(517)205-4905
FAX: (517)205-7769

Henry Ford Allegiance Women's Health Center
3305 Spring Arbor Rd Ste 500
Jackson, MI 49203-3795
(517)205-4905
FAX: (517)205-7325

Kalamazoo

Ascension Borgess Hospital Breast Imaging Center
1535 Gull Rd Ste 30
Kalamazoo, MI 49048-1628
(269)226-6999
FAX: (269)226-7271

Ascension Borgess Westside Radiology
6565 W Main St
Kalamazoo, MI 49009-6114
(269)567-1771
FAX: (269)353-6155

Bronson Advanced Radiology Services
524 S Park St
Kalamazoo, MI 49007-5118
(269)341-8700
FAX: (269)341-7308

Bronson Breast Health Center
601 John St Ste M-515
Kalamazoo, MI 49007-5352
(269)341-8700
FAX: (269)341-7914

Bronson Mammography Oshtemo
2854 S 11th St
Kalamazoo, MI 49009-2129
(269)341-8700
FAX: (269)341-7308

Kalkaska

Kalkaska Memorial Health Center
419 S Coral St, Ste A
Kalkaska, MI 49646-2503
(231)258-7510
FAX: (231)258-7769

Kentwood

Kent Radiology, P.C.
2080 44th St SE
Kentwood, MI 49508-5299
(616)455-4049
FAX: (616)455-3246

Spectrum Hlth Hosp Betty Ford Breast Care Services- Kentwood
4600 Breton Rd SE Ste 203
Kentwood, MI 49508-5221
(616)774-7998
FAX: (616)486-6034

Lake Orion

Beaumont Medical Center, Lake Orion
1455 S Lapeer Rd Ste 10
Lake Orion, MI 48360-1468
(248)577-9700
FAX: (248)964-5199

Lake Orion Diagnostic Imaging
1375 S Lapeer Rd Ste 104
Lake Orion, MI 48360-1421
(248)858-6092
FAX: (248)858-6720

Women's Excellence
1410 S Lapeer Rd
Lake Orion, MI 48360-1437
(248)731-5442
FAX: (248)693-3683

Lanse

Baraga County Memorial Hospital
18341 US Highway 41
Lanse, MI 49946-8024
(906)524-3343
FAX: (906)524-3404

Lansing

McLaren Greater Lansing
1540 Lake Lansing Rd Ste 107
Lansing, MI 48912-3757
(517)913-3800
FAX: (517)913-3801

McLaren Greater Lansing-Breast Care Center
401 W Greenlawn Ave
Lansing, MI 48910-2819
(517)975-6425
FAX: (517)975-6430

Sparrow Health Center Lansing
2909 E Grand River Ave Ste 103
Lansing, MI 48912-4335
(517)364-3659
FAX: (517)485-0646

Sparrow Health System - Sparrow Professional Building
1200 E Michigan Ave
Lansing, MI 48912-1800
(517)253-6300
FAX: (517)364-5562

Lapeer

Lapeer Imaging Center
3273 Davison Rd Ste 3
Lapeer, MI 48446-4307
(810)245-5675
FAX: (810)245-6650

Lapeer Medical Diagnostics
944 Baldwin Rd Ste F
Lapeer, MI 48446-3089
(810)245-7812
FAX: (810)245-7821

McLaren Lapeer Region
1375 N Main St
Lapeer, MI 48446-1350
(810)667-5760
FAX: (810)667-5741

Regional Medical Imaging
1794 N Lapeer Rd, Ste B
Lapeer, MI 48446-7664
(810)732-1919
FAX: (810)732-1945

Laurium

Aspirus Keweenaw Hospital
205 Osceola St
Laurium, MI 49913-2134
(906)337-6531
FAX: (906)337-6532

Lenox Township

McLaren Macomb - Lenox/Richmond
66440 Gratiot Ave
Lenox Township, MI 48050-2032
(586)493-3790
FAX: (586)493-3796

McLaren Macomb-Bay River
36267 26 Mile Rd
Lenox Township, MI 48048-3253
(586)591-1401
FAX: (586)493-3796

Lewiston

Munson Healthcare Omh Medical Group Lewiston Clinic
3040 Bourn St
Lewiston, MI 49756-8134
(989)731-2176
FAX: (989)731-2479

Livonia

Ascension Medical Center Livonia
37595 7 Mile Rd
Livonia, MI 48152-1003
(734)432-6134
FAX: (734)432-6055

Henry Ford Medical Center - Livonia
29200 Schoolcraft Rd
Livonia, MI 48150-2228
(734)523-1720
FAX: (734)523-1783

Livonia Medical Center
19000 St Joe's Parkway
Livonia, MI 48152
(734)655-2765
FAX: (734)655-2077

St. Mary Mercy Hospital
36475 5 Mile Rd
Livonia, MI 48154-1988
(734)655-2765
FAX: (734)655-2011

U Of M Health System Livonia Center For Specialty Care
19900 Haggerty Rd Ste 101
Livonia, MI 48152-1054
(734)936-6274
FAX: (734)615-8327

Ludington

Mem Med Ctr West Mi D/B/A Spectrum Hlth Ludington Hospital
1 Atkinson Dr
Ludington, MI 49431-1906
(231)845-5210
FAX: (231)845-5233

Macomb

Beaumont Medical Center Macomb Township
15979 Hall Rd, Ste 200
Macomb, MI 48044-5360
(248)577-9700
FAX: (248)964-5199

Macomb Township

Ascension St. John Hospital Health Center At 23 Mile
17700 23 Mile Rd Ste 175
Macomb Township, MI 48044-1159
(866)501-3627
FAX: (586)416-7531

Madison Heights

Oakland Imaging Diagnostic Center
27483 Dequindre Rd Ste 101
Madison Heights, MI 48071-5700
(248)544-9050
FAX: (248)544-2331

Manistee

Munson Healthcare Manistee Hospital
1465 E Parkdale Ave
Manistee, MI 49660-9709
(231)398-1114
FAX: (231)398-1427

Manistique

Schoolcraft Memorial Hospital
7870 W Us. Highway 2
Manistique, MI 49854
(906)341-3262
FAX: (906)341-3255

Marlette

Marlette Regional Hospital
2770 Main St, Radiology Department
Marlette, MI 48453-1141
(989)635-4332
FAX: (989)635-4354

Marquette

Dlp Marquette General Hospital
850 W Baraga Ave
Marquette, MI 49855-4550
(906)449-1440
FAX: (906)449-1813

Marshall

Womens Diagnostic Center
103 E Mansion St
Marshall, MI 49068-1117
(269)789-8982
FAX: (269)789-8983

Midland

Midmichigan Medical Ctr-Midland Ctr For Womens Health
4320 Campus Ridge Dr
Midland, MI 48640-6104
(989)837-9066
FAX: (989)837-9065

Monroe

Promedica Monroe Regional Hospital Womens Health Center
730 N Macomb St, Ste 110
Monroe, MI 48162-2904
(734)240-4188
FAX: (734)240-4210

Mount Clemens

McLaren Macomb - Mount Clemens
1000 Harrington St
Mount Clemens, MI 48043-2920
(586)493-3790
FAX: (586)493-3796

Mount Pleasant

McLaren Central Michigan
1221 South Dr, Lbby
Mount Pleasant, MI 48858-3258
(989)309-0103
FAX: (989)779-5272

Mt Pleasant

Midmichigan Medical Center - Mt. Pleasant
4851 E Pickard St, Suite 1780 Imaging Services
Mt Pleasant, MI 48858-2029
(989)956-5174
FAX: (989)775-1652

Munising

Munising Memorial Hospital
1500 Sandpoint Rd
Munising, MI 49862-1497
(906)387-4110
FAX: (906)387-4553

Muskegon

Mercy Health Mercy Campus
1500 E Sherman Blvd
Muskegon, MI 49444-1849
(231)672-6246
FAX: (231)672-3006

Radiology Muskegon, P.C. Breast Imaging Center
3535 Park St Ste 105, Breast Imaging Center
Muskegon, MI 49444-3792
(231)739-7191
FAX: (231)737-0237

Newberry

Helen Newberry Joy Hospital
502 W Harrie St
Newberry, MI 49868-1209
(906)293-9134
FAX: (906)293-9135

Niles

Lakeland Hospital Niles
31 N Saint Joseph Ave
Niles, MI 49120-2287
(269)556-2844
FAX: (269)556-2861

Norton Shores

Mercy Health Comprehensive Breast Center
6401 Prairie St
Norton Shores, MI 49444-7840
(231)727-7947
FAX: (231)724-7844

Novi

Ascension Providence Hospital - Novi Campus
47601 Grand River Ave
Novi, MI 48374-1233
(866)501-3627
FAX: (248)465-4881

Envision Diagnostic Center Pllc
39475 Lewis Dr Ste 200
Novi, MI 48377-2980
(248)471-0675
FAX: (248)254-3874

Regional Medical Imaging, Pc
24285 Karim Blvd
Novi, MI 48375-2952
(810)732-1919
FAX: (248)536-0420

Okemos

Sparrow Imaging Sparrow Meridian One Building
1600 W Grand River Ave Ste 3, Sparrow-Meridian One Building
Okemos, MI 48864-2394
(517)364-5621
FAX: (517)364-5562

Ontonagon

Aspirus Ontonagon Hospital
601 S 7th St
Ontonagon, MI 49953-1496
(906)884-8000
FAX: (906)884-2639

Owosso

Memorial Diagnostic Center
100 Health Park Dr
Owosso, MI 48867-1296
(989)725-8847
FAX: (989)725-9958

Memorial Healthcare
826 W King St
Owosso, MI 48867-2120
(989)729-4876
FAX: (989)729-6150

Oxford

Ascension Providence Hospital Imaging At S. Washington
72 S Washington St Ste 101
Oxford, MI 48371-6421
(248)969-3200
FAX: (248)969-3206

McLaren Oakland - Oxford
385 N Lapeer Rd
Oxford, MI 48371-3610
(248)620-5012
FAX: (248)628-8927

Paw Paw

Bronson Lakeview Hospital
408 Hazen St, Radiology Department
Paw Paw, MI 49079-1019
(269)341-8700
FAX: (269)657-1023

Petoskey

McLaren Northern Michigan
416 Connable Ave
Petoskey, MI 49770-2212
(231)487-3100
FAX: (231)487-7885

Visconti Imaging And Vein Institute
1114 Charlevoix Ave
Petoskey, MI 49770-9701
(231)439-9700
FAX: (231)439-9709

Pigeon

Scheurer Hospital
170 N Caseville Rd
Pigeon, MI 48755-9781
(989)453-5250
FAX: (989)453-4476

Plainwell

Ascesnion Borgess-Pipp Hospital
411 Naomi St
Plainwell, MI 49080-1222
(269)685-0762
FAX: (269)685-0842

Plymouth

St. Joseph Mercy Breast Imaging
990 W Ann Arbor Trl Ste 301
Plymouth, MI 48170-6202
(734)712-1313
FAX: (734)712-5944

Pontiac

McLaren Oakland
50 N Perry St
Pontiac, MI 48342-2217
(248)338-5604
FAX: (248)338-5605

St. Joseph Mercy Hospital - Oakland
44405 Woodward Ave Ste 201, Ambulatory Care Center
Pontiac, MI 48341-5023
(248)858-6092
FAX: (248)858-6720

Port Huron

Lake Huron Medical Center
2601 Electric Ave
Port Huron, MI 48060-6587
(810)216-1856
FAX: (810)216-1859

McLaren Port Huron
1221 Pine Grove Ave
Port Huron, MI 48060-3511
(810)985-2663
FAX: (810)989-3174

Portage

Ascension Borgess At Woodbridge Hills
7901 Angling Rd
Portage, MI 49024-0714
(269)324-8597
FAX: (269)324-8462

Bronson Diagnostics At Woodbridge
2640 W Centre Ave
Portage, MI 49024-4828
(269)341-8700
FAX: (269)327-0068

Prudenville

Munson Healthcare Prudenville Community Health Center
2585 W Houghton Lake Dr
Prudenville, MI 48651-9624
(800)968-9292
FAX: (989)348-0426

Reed City

Spectrum Health - Reed City Hospital
300 N Patterson Rd
Reed City, MI 49677-8041
(231)832-7135
FAX: (231)832-0214

Rochester

Ascension Providence Rochester Hospital
1101 W University Dr
Rochester, MI 48307-1863
(248)652-5325
FAX: (248)652-9731

Rochester Hills

Ascension Providence Rochester Barclay Imaging Center
355 Barclay Cir, Ste B
Rochester Hills, MI 48307-5816
(248)601-6161
FAX: (248)853-1613

Oakland Imaging Diagnostic Center North
633 South Blvd E, Ste 1250
Rochester Hills, MI 48307-5470
(248)243-3565
FAX: (248)243-3575

Oakland Macomb Obstetrics And Gynecology, P.C.
1701 South Blvd E Ste LI50
Rochester Hills, MI 48307-6122
(248)997-5805
FAX: (248)844-2957

William Beaumont Hospital Rochester Hills
6700 N Rochester Rd, Rochester Hills Medical Office Bldg
Rochester Hills, MI 48306-4362
(248)577-9700
FAX: (248)964-5199

Rockford

Spectrum Health Betty Ford Breast Care Services-Rockford
8501 Meadowcreek Drive
Rockford, MI 49341
(616)774-7998
FAX: (616)486-6034

Rogers City

Northern Michigan Medical Management
573 N Bradley Hwy
Rogers City, MI 49779-1508
(989)734-2171
FAX: (989)734-2312

Roseville

Eastside Gynecology-Obstetrics, P.C.
29751 Little Mack Ave Ste B
Roseville, MI 48066-6504
(586)415-6200
FAX: (586)415-6217

Royal Oak

Basha Diagnostics, P.C.
30701 Woodward Ave
Royal Oak, MI 48073-0987
(248)288-1600
FAX: (248)435-8099

Beaumont Hospital Imaging Center
3601 W 13 Mile Rd, Imaging Center 2nd Floor
Royal Oak, MI 48073-6712
(800)328-8542
FAX: (248)551-1850

Regional Medical Imaging
26454 Woodward Ave, Ste 100
Royal Oak, MI 48067-0969
(734)281-6600
FAX: (734)281-7481

Saginaw

Ascension St. Mary's Of Michigan Towne Centre
4599 Towne Centre Rd
Saginaw, MI 48604-2804
(989)907-8222
FAX: (989)497-3120

Covenant Breast Health Center
5400 Mackinaw Rd
Saginaw, MI 48604-9515
(989)583-6278
FAX: (989)583-5269

Covenant Breast Health Center-State St
5570 State St Ste 3
Saginaw, MI 48603-3582
(989)583-6279
FAX: (989)583-0118

Saint Ignace

Mackinac Straits Health System
1140 N State St, Ste 1788
Saint Ignace, MI 49781-1048
(906)643-0440
FAX: (906)328-2123

Saint Johns

Clinton County Medical Center
1005 S US Highway 27 Ste 100
Saint Johns, MI 48879-2423
(989)224-3000
FAX: (989)224-1424

Sparrow Clinton Hospital
805 S Oakland St
Saint Johns, MI 48879-2253
(517)227-3391
FAX: (989)227-3421

Sandusky

McKenzie Health System
120 N Delaware St, Radiology Department
Sandusky, MI 48471-1087
(810)648-6175
FAX: (810)648-4204

Sault S Marie

Chippewa County War Memorial Hospital
500 Osborn Blvd
Sault S Marie, MI 49783-1884
(906)635-4439
FAX: (906)253-1383

Sault Sainte Marie

Sault Ste Marie Tribe Of Chippewa Indians Health Center
2864 Ashmun St, Department Of Health & Social Services
Sault Sainte Marie, MI 49783-3740
(906)632-5237
FAX: (906)632-5262

Shelby

Mercy Health Partners Aka Mhp Lakeshore Campus
72 S State St
Shelby, MI 49455-1228
(231)861-3008
FAX: (231)861-3006

Shelby Township

McLaren Macomb - Shelby Creek
8180 26 Mile Rd Ste 120
Shelby Township, MI 48316-5139
(586)493-3790
FAX: (586)493-3796

Sheridan

Sheridan Community Hospital
301 N Main St
Sheridan, MI 48884-9235
(989)291-6336
FAX: (989)291-3046

South Haven

Bronson South Haven
955 S Bailey Ave
South Haven, MI 49090-6743
(269)639-2828
FAX: (269)639-2829

Southfield

Ascension Providence Hospital Southfield Campus
22250 Providence Dr, Mammography Center Lower Level
Southfield, MI 48075-4825
(866)501-3627
FAX: (248)849-2784

Epic Primary Care
18591 W 10 Mile Rd
Southfield, MI 48075-2619
(248)621-9443
FAX: (248)416-1355

Farmbrook Radiology
29829 Telegraph Rd Ste L105
Southfield, MI 48034-1376
(248)352-9525
FAX: (248)357-2959

Northland Radiology, Inc.
20905 Greenfield Rd, Ste 105
Southfield, MI 48075-5344
(248)569-0296
FAX: (248)569-3390

Southgate

Beaumont Imaging Services - Southgate
15777 Northline Rd Ste 104, Diagnostic Services
Southgate, MI 48195-2300
(734)246-8140
FAX: (734)246-8143

Regional Medical Imaging Pc
15300 Trenton Rd
Southgate, MI 48195-2027
(734)281-6600
FAX: (810)732-1945

St Clair Shores

Ascension St. John Hospital Health Center At 12 Mile
21000 E 12 Mile Rd Ste 116
St Clair Shores, MI 48081-1156
(866)501-3627
FAX: (586)447-5104

Beaumont St. Clair Shores Medical Office Building
25631 Little Mack Ave
St Clair Shores, MI 48081-2100
(586)443-2950
FAX: (586)443-2951

St Joseph

Center For Outpatient Services
3900 Hollywood Rd
St Joseph, MI 49085-9149
(269)556-2810
FAX: (269)556-2861

South Shore Women's Health Care
2690 S Cleveland Ave
St Joseph, MI 49085-3002
(269)428-2800
FAX: (269)428-7177

Standish

Ascension-Standish Hospital
805 W Cedar St
Standish, MI 48658-9257
(800)605-9141
FAX: (989)846-3537

Sterling Heights

Basha Diagnostics, P.C.
13753 19 Mile Rd
Sterling Heights, MI 48313-2703
(586)566-8680
FAX: (586)566-8730

Henry Ford Medical Center-Lakeside
14500 Hall Rd M-59
Sterling Heights, MI 48313-1229
(586)247-2920
FAX: (586)247-2939

Henry Ford Medical Center-Sterling Heights
3500 15 Mile Rd
Sterling Heights, MI 48310-5353
(586)977-9972
FAX: (586)977-6408

Sturgis

Sturgis Hospital
916 Myrtle St, Radiology Department
Sturgis, MI 49091-2391
(269)659-4461
FAX: (269)659-4498

Tawas City

Ascension St. Joseph Hospital
PO Box 659, 200 Hemlock St
Tawas City, MI 48764-0659
(989)362-9897
FAX: (989)362-5270

Taylor

Henry Ford Medical Center-Taylor
24555 Haig St
Taylor, MI 48180-3322
(313)375-2350
FAX: (313)375-2356

Three Rivers

Ascension Borgess, Promed Physicians Three Rivers
1241 W Broadway St
Three Rivers, MI 49093-8319
(269)273-9539
FAX: (269)279-1491

Three Rivers Health
701 S Health Parkway
Three Rivers, MI 49093-9306
(269)273-9638
FAX: (269)273-9622

Traverse City

Munson Healthcare Smith Family Breast Health Center
4100 Park Forest Dr
Traverse City, MI 49684-7331
(231)935-2185
FAX: (231)935-0432

Women's Imaging Center - Munson Medical Center
1105 Sixth St
Traverse City, MI 49684-2345
(231)392-7100
FAX: (231)935-3473

Trenton

Beaumont Trenton-Karen Colina Smithbauer Breast Care Ctr
5400 Fort St, Ste 170
Trenton, MI 48183-4632
(734)362-6787
FAX: (734)642-2130

Troy

Troy Internal Medicine A Div Of Arcturus Hlthcare Plc
4600 Investment Dr, Ste 300
Troy, MI 48098-6368
(248)267-5000
FAX: (248)267-5001

William Beaumont Hospital
44201 Dequindre Rd
Troy, MI 48085-1198
(248)577-9700
FAX: (248)964-5199

Walker

Kent Radiology P.C. - Northwest
933 3 Mile Rd NW Ste 106
Walker, MI 49544-1673
(616)785-3603
FAX: (616)784-3932

Warren

Ascension - Macomb Breast Center
27472 Schoenherr Rd Ste 120
Warren, MI 48088-6675
(586)582-7900
FAX: (586)582-7901

Beaumont Health Warren
8545 Common Rd Ste 104
Warren, MI 48093-6776
(800)328-8542
FAX: (248)855-7470

Washington Twp

Henry Ford Macomb - Washington Township
12150 30 Mile Rd Ste 103
Washington Twp, MI 48095-2035
(586)203-1600
FAX: (586)203-1601

Watervliet

Lakeland Hospital Watervliet
400 Medical Park Dr
Watervliet, MI 49098-9225
(269)556-2810
FAX: (269)463-4805

Wayne

Beaumont Breast Care Center - Wayne
33101 Annapolis St
Wayne, MI 48184-2405
(734)467-6770
FAX: (734)467-6775

West Bloomfield

Beaumont Health- West Bloomfield
6900 Orchard Lake Rd Ste 110
West Bloomfield, MI 48322-3424
(800)328-8542
FAX: (248)855-7470

Henry Ford West Bloomfield Hospital
6777 W Maple Rd
West Bloomfield, MI 48322-3013
(248)325-3828
FAX: (248)325-3863

St Joseph Mercy - Oakland Diag. Ctr. - West Bloomfield
2300 Haggerty Rd Ste 1050
West Bloomfield, MI 48323-2186
(248)858-6092
FAX: (248)858-3027

Womens Health And Menopause Center
5777 W Maple Rd, Ste 200
West Bloomfield, MI 48322-2271
(248)932-9223
FAX: (877)550-8437

West Branch

McLaren Bay West Branch
2110 S M 76, Ste 8
West Branch, MI 48661-8821
(989)516-5081
FAX: (989)894-6143

Midmichigan Medical Center West Branch
2463 S M 30
West Branch, MI 48661-9312
(989)343-3200
FAX: (989)343-3237

Westland

Millennium West Diagnostic Center
6149 N Wayne Rd
Westland, MI 48185-7128
(734)728-2130
FAX: (734)728-2626

Wyoming

Dms Imaging Inc - Mobile 6
5900 Byron Center Ave SW
Wyoming, MI 49519-9606
(616)252-4461
FAX: (616)252-6990

Metro Health University Of Michigan Health
5900 Byron Center Ave SW
Wyoming, MI 49519-9606
(616)252-4461
FAX: (616)252-6990

Spectrum Health W. Pavilion Betty Ford Breast Care Svcs
6105 Wilson Ave SW
Wyoming, MI 49418-9714
(616)267-2626
FAX: (616)486-6034

Ypsilanti

Saint Joseph Mercy Breast Imaging
5320 Elliott Dr Ste 100
Ypsilanti, MI 48197-1032
(734)712-1313
FAX: (734)712-5944

Womens Huron Valley Correctional Facility
3201 Bemis Rd, East Building
Ypsilanti, MI 48197-9307
(734)434-2984
FAX: (734)434-8009

Zeeland

Holland Hospital Breast Health Services-Zeeland
8300 Westpark Way
Zeeland, MI 49464-7901
(616)355-3865
FAX: (616)396-2453

Spectrum Health Zeeland Community Hospital
8333 Felch St
Zeeland, MI 49464-2608
(616)772-5761
FAX: (616)772-5770

MINNESOTA

Aitkin

Riverwood Healthcare Center
200 Bunker Hill Dr
Aitkin, MN 56431-1865
(218)927-2121
FAX: (218)927-5528

Albert Lea

Mayo Clinic Heath System-Albert Lea
404 W Fountain St
Albert Lea, MN 56007-2437
(507)373-6347
FAX: (507)377-6351

Alexandria

Alexandria Cdi
111 17th Ave E
Alexandria, MN 56308-5273
(320)762-6040
FAX: (320)762-6038

Alexandria Clinic A Service Of Alomere Health
610 30th Ave W
Alexandria, MN 56308-3426
(320)759-4011
FAX: (320)759-4044

Sanford Health Broadway Clinic
1527 Broadway St
Alexandria, MN 56308-2537
(320)762-6816
FAX: (320)762-5789

Anoka

Healthpartners Riverway Anoka Clinic
601 Jacob Ln
Anoka, MN 55303-1776
(952)967-7075
FAX: (763)587-4228

Apple Valley

Allina Health - Apple Valley
14655 Galaxie Ave
Apple Valley, MN 55124-8602
(651)241-3850
FAX: (651)241-3871

Fairview Oxboro Clinic - Mobile
15650 Cedar Ave
Apple Valley, MN 55124-7283
(612)336-2670
FAX: (952)885-6022

Arden Hills

Health Partners - Arden Hills
3930 Northwoods Dr
Arden Hills, MN 55112-6963
(952)967-7860
FAX: (651)523-8509

Healthpartners Mobile
3930 Northwoods Dr
Arden Hills, MN 55112-6974
(651)402-6308
FAX: (608)839-9057

Arlington

Ridgeview Sibley Medical Center
601 W Chandler St
Arlington, MN 55307-2127
(952)777-4471
FAX: (507)964-8467

Austin

Mayo Clinic Health System-Austin
1000 1st Dr NW
Austin, MN 55912-2941
(507)434-1402
FAX: (507)434-1468

Baudette

Lakewood Health Center
600 Main Ave S
Baudette, MN 56623-2855
(218)634-3402
FAX: (218)634-3480

Baxter

Essentia Health St Joseph's Baxter Clinic
13060 Isle Dr
Baxter, MN 56425-8331
(218)454-5803
FAX: (218)828-7629

Bemidji

Sanford Clinic - Bemidji
1233 34th St NW
Bemidji, MN 56601-5112
(218)333-4624
FAX: (218)333-4941

Benson

Swift County-Benson Hospital
1815 Wisconsin Ave
Benson, MN 56215-1653
(320)843-4232
FAX: (320)843-4708

Bigfork

Bigfork Valley Hospital
258 Pine Tree Dr.
Bigfork, MN 56628
(218)743-4132
FAX: (218)743-4258

Blaine

Midwest Radiology Outpatient Imaging, Llc
11855 Ulysses St NE Ste 130
Blaine, MN 55434-4178
(763)786-9460
FAX: (763)786-6408

Bloomington

Fairview Clinics-Bloomington Oxboro
600 W 98th St
Bloomington, MN 55420-4773
(952)881-2651
FAX: (952)885-6022

Health Partners Bloomington Clinic
8600 Nicollet Ave S
Bloomington, MN 55420-2824
(952)541-2867
FAX: (952)541-2855

Park Nicollet Bloomington
5320 Hyland Greens Dr
Bloomington, MN 55437-3934
(952)993-3700
FAX: (952)993-0319

Blue Earth

United Hospital District, Inc
PO Box 160, 515 S Moore St
Blue Earth, MN 56013-0160
(507)526-7953
FAX: (507)526-7987

Brainerd

Essentia Health St. Joseph's Medical Center
523 N 3rd St
Brainerd, MN 56401-3054
(218)454-5803
FAX: (218)828-7629

Breckenridge

St. Francis Healthcare Campus
2400 St Francis Dr
Breckenridge, MN 56520-1025
(218)643-0238
FAX: (218)643-0868

Brooklyn Center

Healthpartners Brooklyn Center Clinic
6845 Lee Ave N
Brooklyn Center, MN 55429-1717
(651)254-8200
FAX: (763)503-4425

Brooklyn Park

Fairview Fridley Clinic - Mobile
10000 Zane Ave N
Brooklyn Park, MN 55443-1400
(763)586-5816
FAX: (763)586-5888

Hennepin Healthcare Brooklyn Park
7650 Zane Ave N
Brooklyn Park, MN 55443-3151
(612)873-2500
FAX: (612)904-4545

Buffalo

Buffalo Hospital
303 Catlin St
Buffalo, MN 55313-4507
(763)684-7560
FAX: (763)684-7555

Stellis Health, P.A.
1700 Highway 25 N
Buffalo, MN 55313-1930
(763)684-3600
FAX: (763)684-3623

Burnsville

M Health Fairview Breast Center Burnsville
303 E Nicollet Blvd Ste 220
Burnsville, MN 55337-4592
(952)892-2273
FAX: (952)892-2919

Midwest Radiology Outpatient Imaging
Burnsville
14000 Nicollet Ave Ste 204
Burnsville, MN 55337-5796
(952)898-2333
FAX: (952)898-6270

Park Nicollet Clinic Burnsville
14050 Fairview Dr
Burnsville, MN 55337-5713
(952)993-9800
FAX: (652)993-8604

Cambridge

Cambridge Medical Center
701 Dellwood St S
Cambridge, MN 55008-1923
(763)688-9966
FAX: (763)688-7771

Canby

Sanford Canby Medical Center
112 Saint Olaf Ave S
Canby, MN 56220-1433
(507)223-7277
FAX: (507)223-7305

Cannon Falls

Mayo Clinic Health System-Cannon Falls
32021 County 24 Blvd
Cannon Falls, MN 55009-5003
(507)263-9782
FAX: (507)263-9650

Cass Lake

Cass Lake Indian Health Service Hospital
425 7th St NW
Cass Lake, MN 56633-3360
(218)335-3274
FAX: (218)335-3363

Chanhassen

Park Nicollet Clinic Chanhassen
300 Lake Dr E
Chanhassen, MN 55317-9302
(952)993-4445
FAX: (952)993-4447

Chaska

Two Twelve Medical Ctr - Ridgeview Imaging Ctr
111 Hundertmark Rd Ste 130
Chaska, MN 55318-1195
(952)777-4471
FAX: (952)361-2453

Cloquet

Cloquet Community Memorial Hospital
512 Skyline Blvd
Cloquet, MN 55720-1199
(218)878-7015
FAX: (218)878-7085

Cook

Cook Hospital
10 5th St SE
Cook, MN 55723-9745
(218)666-6217
FAX: (218)666-6226

Coon Rapids

Allina Health Coon Rapids Clinic
9055 Springbrook Dr NW
Coon Rapids, MN 55433-5841
(763)236-1156
FAX: (763)236-1128

Healthpartners Coon Rapids Clinic
11475 Robinson Dr NW
Coon Rapids, MN 55433-3746
(651)254-8200
FAX: (763)587-9136

Midwest Radiology Outpatient Imaging, Llc
8990 Springbrook Dr NW Ste 125
Coon Rapids, MN 55433-5879
(763)786-9460
FAX: (763)795-0710

Piper Breast Center - Mercy Hospital
11850 Blackfoot St NW Ste 300
Coon Rapids, MN 55433-2772
(763)236-0818
FAX: (763)236-6065

Crookston

Altru Clinic - Crookston
400 S Minnesota St
Crookston, MN 56716-1808
(218)281-9100
FAX: (218)281-9861

Riverview Health
323 S Minnesota St
Crookston, MN 56716-1601
(218)281-9428
FAX: (218)281-9264

Crosby

Cuyuna Regional Medical Center
320 E Main St
Crosby, MN 56441-1690
(218)546-2317
FAX: (218)546-2343

Dawson

Johnson Memorial Health Services
1282 Walnut St
Dawson, MN 56232-2333
(320)769-4323
FAX: (320)769-4576

Deer River

Essentia Health-Deer River
115 10th Ave NE, Radiology Department
Deer River, MN 56636-8795
(218)246-3023
FAX: (218)246-3094

Detroit Lakes

Essentia Health St. Mary's Detroit Lakes
1027 Washington Ave
Detroit Lakes, MN 56501-3409
(218)847-0833
FAX: (218)847-0838

Sanford Clinic Detroit Lakes
1245 Washington Ave
Detroit Lakes, MN 56501-3905
(218)846-2108
FAX: (218)846-2149

Duluth

Essentia Health Duluth Clinic
420 E 1st St
Duluth, MN 55805-1901
(218)786-1019
FAX: (218)786-8375

Essentia Health West Duluth Clinic
4212 Grand Ave
Duluth, MN 55807-2737
(218)786-1019
FAX: (218)786-8375

St. Luke's Regional Breast Center
915 E 1st St, Radiology Department
Duluth, MN 55805-2107
(218)249-5593
FAX: (218)249-5365

Eagan

Fairview Clinics-Eagan
3305 Central Park Village Dr, Ste 110
Eagan, MN 55121-7707
(651)406-8789
FAX: (651)406-8946

East Grand Forks

Sanford Health East Grand Forks
621 Demers Ave
East Grand Forks, MN 56721-1812
(218)773-5857
FAX: (218)773-5991

Edina

Crl Imaging Southdale
6525 France Ave S Ste 110
Edina, MN 55435-2158
(952)915-4320
FAX: (952)915-4338

Edina Family Physicians
5301 Vernon Ave S
Edina, MN 55436-2303
(952)925-2200
FAX: (952)925-0335

Fairview Center For Women-Edina
6525 France Ave S
Edina, MN 55435-2148
(952)927-4021
FAX: (952)927-4026

M Health Fairview Breast Center Edina
6545 France Ave S Ste 250, Southdale Medical Center
Edina, MN 55435-2118
(952)836-3620
FAX: (952)836-3601

Elk River

Allina Health Elk River Clinic
14181 Business Center Dr NW
Elk River, MN 55330-4654
(763)236-0500
FAX: (763)236-0535

Riverway Clinics Elk River
530 3rd St NW
Elk River, MN 55330-8863
(952)967-7075
FAX: (763)587-4880

Ely

Ely Bloomenson Community Hospital
328 W Conan St
Ely, MN 55731-1198
(218)365-8737
FAX: (218)365-8744

Fairmont

Mayo Clinic Health System - Fairmont
800 Medical Center Dr
Fairmont, MN 56031-4575
(507)238-8184
FAX: (507)238-8677

Faribault

District One Hospital
200 State Ave
Faribault, MN 55021-6398
(507)497-3518
FAX: (507)497-3517

Mayo Clinic Health System - Faribault
300 State Ave
Faribault, MN 55021-6319
(507)333-3300
FAX: (507)333-3221

Fergus Falls

Lake Region Healthcare Corp.
PO Box 728, 712 S Cascade St
Fergus Falls, MN 56538-0728
(218)736-8341
FAX: (218)736-8723

Forest Lake

Allina Health Forest Lake Clinic
1540 Lake St S
Forest Lake, MN 55025-2628
(651)464-7100
FAX: (651)241-1515

Fosston

First Care Medical Services Dba Essentia Health-Fosston
900 Hilligoss Blvd SE
Fosston, MN 56542-1542
(218)435-7648
FAX: (218)435-6573

Fridley

Fairview Fridley Clinic
6401 University Ave NE Ste 150
Fridley, MN 55432-4341
(763)586-5884
FAX: (763)502-4884

North Memorial Health Clinic Fridley
480 Osborne Rd NE Ste 100
Fridley, MN 55432-2781
(763)581-0604
FAX: (763)581-0619

Garrison

Riverwood Garrison Clinic
PO Box 426, 27278 State Hwy 18
Garrison, MN 56450-0426
(218)429-3902
FAX: (218)927-5528

Glencoe

Glencoe Regional Health Services
1805 Hennepin Ave N
Glencoe, MN 55336-1416
(320)864-7080
FAX: (320)864-7968

Glenwood

Glacial Ridge Health System
10 4th Ave SE
Glenwood, MN 56334-1898
(320)634-2273
FAX: (320)634-2005

Graceville

Essentia Health Holy Trinity Hospital
115 W 2nd St
Graceville, MN 56240-4845
(320)748-8219
FAX: (320)748-8233

Grand Marais

North Shore Health
515 5th Ave W
Grand Marais, MN 55604-3017
(218)387-3268
FAX: (218)387-3270

Grand Rapids

Essentia Health-Grand Rapids Clinic
1542 Golf Course Rd, Ste 204
Grand Rapids, MN 55744-3537
(218)999-7000
FAX: (218)999-7099

Grand Itasca Clinic And Hospital
1601 Golf Course Rd
Grand Rapids, MN 55744-8648
(218)999-1655
FAX: (218)999-1654

Granite Falls

Avera Granite Falls
345 10th Ave
Granite Falls, MN 56241-1442
(320)564-6241
FAX: (320)564-2358

Hastings

Regina Hospital, Part Of Allina Health
1175 Nininger Rd
Hastings, MN 55033-1056
(651)404-1004
FAX: (651)404-1655

Hendricks

Hendricks Community Hospital
PO Box 106, 503 E Lincoln St
Hendricks, MN 56136-0106
(507)275-3141
FAX: (507)275-2268

Hermantown

Essentia Health Hermantown Breast Ctr
4855 W Arrowhead Rd
Hermantown, MN 55811-3936
(218)786-1743
FAX: (218)786-8375

Hibbing

Essentia Health Hibbing Clinic
730 E 34th St
Hibbing, MN 55746-5109
(218)262-3425
FAX: (218)262-5670

Hibbing Family Medical Clinic
1120 E 34th St
Hibbing, MN 55746-2909
(218)362-7118
FAX: (218)362-7144

Range Regional Health Services Mesaba Clinic Hibbing
750 E 34th St
Hibbing, MN 55746-4511
(218)362-6207
FAX: (218)362-6699

Hutchinson

Hutchinson Health
1095 Highway 15 S
Hutchinson, MN 55350-3182
(320)234-5000
FAX: (320)234-5125

International Falls

Essentia Health International Falls Clinic
2501 Keenan Dr
International Falls, MN 56649-2181
(877)201-3461
FAX: (218)285-6245

Rainy Lake Medical Center
1400 Hwy. 11-71
International Falls, MN 56649
(218)283-5418
FAX: (218)283-5526

Lake City

Mayo Clinic Health System - Lake City
500 W Grant St
Lake City, MN 55041-1143
(651)345-1163
FAX: (651)345-6724

Lakeville

Center For Diagnostic Imaging
10438 185th St W, Ste 100
Lakeville, MN 55044-5307
(952)345-3878
FAX: (952)469-4542

Le Sueur

Ridgeview Le Sueur Medical Center
621 S 4th St
Le Sueur, MN 56058-2203
(507)665-8780
FAX: (507)665-8696

Litchfield

Meeker Memorial Hospital And Clinics
612 S Sibley Ave
Litchfield, MN 55355-3340
(320)693-4519
FAX: (320)693-4540

Little Falls

St. Gabriel's Hospital
815 2nd St SE
Little Falls, MN 56345-3596
(320)631-5140
FAX: (320)631-5006

Long Prairie

Centracare Health - Long Prairie
50 Centracare Dr
Long Prairie, MN 56347-2100
(320)732-7237
FAX: (320)732-7293

Luverne

Sanford Luverne Medical Center
1600 N Kniss Ave
Luverne, MN 56156-1067
(507)449-1290
FAX: (507)283-4671

Madelia

Madelia Community Hospital
121 Drew Ave SE
Madelia, MN 56062-1841
(507)642-5221
FAX: (507)642-3848

Mahnomen

Mahnomen Health Center
414 W Jefferson Ave
Mahnomen, MN 56557-4912
(218)935-2511
FAX: (218)935-5463

Mankato

Mankato Clinic
1230 E Main St
Mankato, MN 56001-8001
(507)389-8570
FAX: (507)625-1697

Mayo Clinic Health System In Mankato Eastridge
101 Martin Luther King Dr
Mankato, MN 56001-6460
(507)594-7770
FAX: (507)594-7775

Maple Grove

Park Nicollet Clinic Maple Grove
9555 Upland Ln N
Maple Grove, MN 55369-4485
(952)993-3700
FAX: (952)993-0319

The Breast Center Of Maple Grove
9855 Hospital Dr Ste 150
Maple Grove, MN 55369-4776
(763)398-6363
FAX: (763)398-6364

University Of Minnesota Health, Maple Grove Clinics
14500 99th Ave N
Maple Grove, MN 55369-4730
(763)898-1000
FAX: (763)898-1294

Maplewood

Healthpartners Maplewood Clinic
2165 White Bear Ave N
Maplewood, MN 55109-2707
(651)523-9800
FAX: (651)523-9831

M Health Fairview Breast Center Maplewood
2945 Hazelwood St, Ste 305
Maplewood, MN 55109-1244
(651)471-9300
FAX: (651)471-9399

Maplewood Imaging Center- St Paul Radiology
2945 Hazelwood St Ste 110
Maplewood, MN 55109-1242
(651)632-5700
FAX: (651)747-4501

Minnesota Women's Care, P.A.
2603 White Bear Ave N
Maplewood, MN 55109-5110
(651)600-3035
FAX: (877)550-8437

Marshall

Avera Marshall Regional Medical Center
300 S Bruce St
Marshall, MN 56258-1934
(507)537-9189
FAX: (507)537-9259

McGregor

Riverwood Clinic McGregor
PO Box 340, 2 E Center Ave
McGregor, MN 55760-0340
(218)429-3902
FAX: (218)927-5528

Melrose

Centracare Health - Melrose
525 Main St W, Imaging Department
Melrose, MN 56352-1043
(320)256-4231
FAX: (320)256-1784

Minneapolis

Abbott Northwestern Hospital Piper Breast Center
800 E 28th St, Piper Bldg., Suite 402
Minneapolis, MN 55407-3799
(612)863-1248
FAX: (612)863-3286

Hcmc Whittier Clinic
2810 Nicollet Ave
Minneapolis, MN 55408-3160
(612)873-2500
FAX: (612)904-4545

Hennepin County Medical Center
715 S 8th St, Hennepin Healthcare Breast Center
Minneapolis, MN 55404-1210
(612)873-2500
FAX: (612)904-4545

Northpoint Health & Wellness Center
1313 Penn Ave N
Minneapolis, MN 55411-3047
(612)543-2677
FAX: (612)677-6405

University Of Minnesota - Mammography Services, West Bank
606 24th Ave S Ste 300, Rm 3-345
Minneapolis, MN 55454-1437
(612)676-4256
FAX: (612)676-4756

University Of Minnesota Health Breast Center
909 Fulton St SE, Mail Code 2121A
Minneapolis, MN 55455-4800
(612)676-4200
FAX: (612)676-4756

Minnetonka

North Memorial Health Clinic - Minnetonka Medical Center
15450 Highway 7
Minnetonka, MN 55345-3522
(763)581-8905
FAX: (763)581-8902

Premier Obgyn Of Minnesota Pa
14001 Ridgedale Dr, Ste 200
Minnetonka, MN 55305-1747
(952)249-2000
FAX: (952)905-3045

Montevideo

Chippewa County - Montevideo Hospital
824 N 11th St
Montevideo, MN 56265-1629
(320)321-8185
FAX: (320)321-8190

Monticello

Centracare Health - Monticello
1013 Hart Blvd
Monticello, MN 55362-8575
(763)271-2288
FAX: (763)271-2463

Stellis Health, Pa
1001 Hart Blvd Ste 100
Monticello, MN 55362-8929
(763)271-3800
FAX: (763)271-3806

Moorhead

Sanford Clinic Moorhead
4000 28th St S
Moorhead, MN 56560-7460
(701)234-7100
FAX: (701)234-7481

Moose Lake

Essentia Health-Moose Lake
4572 County Road 61
Moose Lake, MN 55767-9401
(218)485-5578
FAX: (218)485-5678

Mora

Welia Health
301 Highway 65 S
Mora, MN 55051-1899
(320)225-3447
FAX: (320)225-3458

Morris

Stevens Community Medical Center
400 E 1st St
Morris, MN 56267-1408
(320)589-1313
FAX: (320)589-7694

New Prague

Mayo Clinic Health System In New Prague
301 2nd St NE
New Prague, MN 56071-1709
(952)758-4431
FAX: (952)758-8125

New Ulm

New Ulm Medical Center
1324 5th St N
New Ulm, MN 56073-1514
(507)217-5154
FAX: (507)217-5379

North St Paul

Center For Diagnostic Imaging
2601 Centennial Dr, Ste 108
North St Paul, MN 55109-3087
(651)287-4132
FAX: (651)202-2997

Northfield

Allina Medical Clinic - Northfield, Part Of Allina Health
1400 Jefferson Rd
Northfield, MN 55057-3081
(507)663-9000
FAX: (651)241-0575

Northfield Hospital
2000 North Ave
Northfield, MN 55057-1697
(507)646-1143
FAX: (507)646-1144

Ogema

White Earth Phs Ihs
40520 County Highway 34
Ogema, MN 56569-9612
(218)983-6310
FAX: (218)983-6393

Olivia

Olivia Hospital & Clinic
100 Healthy Way
Olivia, MN 56277-1117
(320)523-3445
FAX: (320)523-8352

Onamia

Mille Lacs Health System-Cmdi
200 Elm St N
Onamia, MN 56359-7901
(320)532-2550
FAX: (320)532-2579

Ortonville

Ortonville Area Health Services
450 Eastvold Ave
Ortonville, MN 56278-1133
(320)839-4274
FAX: (320)839-4010

Owatonna

Mayo Clinic Health System - Owatonna
2200 NW 26th St
Owatonna, MN 55060-5503
(507)451-1120
FAX: (507)446-5120

Park Rapids

Chi St. Joseph's Health
600 Pleasant Ave S
Park Rapids, MN 56470-1431
(218)616-3030
FAX: (218)616-3013

Paynesville

Centracare-Paynesville
200 W 1st St
Paynesville, MN 56362-1445
(320)243-7711
FAX: (320)243-2446

Perham

Perham Health
1000 Coney St W, Radiology Department
Perham, MN 56573-2102
(218)347-1375
FAX: (218)347-1377

Pine City

Welia Health
1425 Main St N
Pine City, MN 55063-6026
(320)225-3447
FAX: (320)225-3458

Pipestone

Pipestone County Medical Center
916 4th Ave SW
Pipestone, MN 56164-1065
(507)825-6065
FAX: (507)825-5914

Plymouth

Imaging Center Of Plymouth
2800 Campus Dr, Ste 30
Plymouth, MN 55441-2669
(763)398-6390
FAX: (763)398-6369

Piper Breast Center Westhealth
2855 Campus Dr
Plymouth, MN 55441-2649
(763)577-7133
FAX: (763)577-7224

Voyage Healthcare Formerly North Clinic
15655 37th Ave N, Ste 180
Plymouth, MN 55446-4008
(763)587-7932
FAX: (763)587-7988

Princeton

M Health Fairview Northland Medical Center
911 Northland Dr
Princeton, MN 55371-2173
(763)389-6432
FAX: (763)389-6431

Red Wing

Mayo Clinic Health System - Red Wing
PO Box 95, 701 Hewitt Blvd
Red Wing, MN 55066-0095
(651)267-5258
FAX: (651)267-5907

Redlake

Red Lake Indian Hospital
Hwy 1, 24760 Hospital Dr
Redlake, MN 56671
(218)679-3912
FAX: (218)679-0195

Redwood Falls

Carris Health - Redwood, Llc
101 Caring Way
Redwood Falls, MN 56283-2624
(320)231-6776
FAX: (320)214-6257

Richfield

Allina Health Richfield Clinic
407 W 66th St
Richfield, MN 55423-2304
(612)798-8800
FAX: (612)798-8816

Hennepin Healthcare Richfield
790 W 66th St
Richfield, MN 55423-2203
(612)873-2500
FAX: (612)904-4545

Robbinsdale

North Memorial Health Breast Center
3366 Oakdale Ave N Ste LL
Robbinsdale, MN 55422-2961
(763)581-3554
FAX: (763)581-3581

Rochester

Mayo Clinic
200 1st St SW
Rochester, MN 55905-0002
(507)284-5968
FAX: (507)538-6035

Olmsted Medical Center
1650 4th St SE
Rochester, MN 55904-4717
(507)292-7096
FAX: (507)292-7097

Roseau

Lifecare Medical Center
715 Delmore Dr
Roseau, MN 56751-1599
(218)463-4753
FAX: (218)463-4766

Roseville

Center For Diagnostic Imaging
1835 County Road C W Ste 180
Roseville, MN 55113-1368
(651)287-4132
FAX: (952)738-7709

Saint Cloud

Alliance Imaging
3351 Roosevelt Rd
Saint Cloud, MN 56301-6270
(320)255-6530
FAX: (320)255-6535

Center For Diagnostic Imaging
251 County Road 120
Saint Cloud, MN 56303-4872
(320)251-0609
FAX: (320)229-4651

Centracare Clinic River Campus
1200 6th Ave N
Saint Cloud, MN 56303-2736
(320)240-2115
FAX: (320)240-7895

St. Cloud Hospital Breast Center
1900 Centracare Cir Ste 1500, Centracare Health Plaza
Saint Cloud, MN 56303-5000
(320)229-4919
FAX: (320)229-5102

Saint Paul

Allina Health Bandana Square Clinic
1021 Bandana Blvd E, Ste 100
Saint Paul, MN 55108-5109
(651)241-9758
FAX: (651)241-9769

Healtheast Rice Street Clinic
980 Rice St
Saint Paul, MN 55117-4949
(651)326-9020
FAX: (651)326-8030

Healthpartners - St. Paul Clinic
205 Wabasha St S
Saint Paul, MN 55107-1805
(651)293-8105
FAX: (651)293-8108

Healthpartners Como Clinic
2500 Como Ave
Saint Paul, MN 55108-1494
(651)641-3163
FAX: (651)632-8974

Healthpartners Health Center For Women
2635 University Ave W Ste 160
Saint Paul, MN 55114-8665
(651)254-2760
FAX: (651)254-2761

M Health Fairview Midway Clinic
1390 University Ave W
Saint Paul, MN 55104-4001
(651)232-4800
FAX: (651)326-9609

M Health Fairview Roselawn Clinic
1983 Sloan Pl Ste 1
Saint Paul, MN 55117-2095
(651)326-5729
FAX: (651)326-9788

Piper Breast Center-United
310 Smith Ave N, Ste 300
Saint Paul, MN 55102-2383
(651)241-8300
FAX: (651)241-8391

Regions Breast Health Center
640 Jackson St
Saint Paul, MN 55101-2502
(651)254-4600
FAX: (651)254-4639

Sandstone

Essentia Health Sandstone
705 Lundorff Dr
Sandstone, MN 55072-5099
(320)245-6760
FAX: (320)245-5650

Sartell

Center For Diagnostic Imaging
166 19th St S Ste 100
Sartell, MN 56377-2154
(320)251-0609
FAX: (320)251-0657

Sauk Centre

Centracare Health - Sauk Centre
425 Elm St N, Radiology Dept
Sauk Centre, MN 56378-1010
(320)352-2221
FAX: (320)351-1744

Savage

St. Francis Health Center - Savage
6350 W 143rd St Ste 102
Savage, MN 55378-2890
(952)428-2268
FAX: (952)428-2666

Shakopee

St. Francis Regional Medical Center
1455 Saint Francis Ave
Shakopee, MN 55379-3380
(952)428-2268
FAX: (952)428-2666

Slayton

Murray County Medical Center
2042 Juniper Ave
Slayton, MN 56172-1008
(507)836-6153
FAX: (507)836-1243

Sleepy Eye

Sleepy Eye Medical Center
400 4th Ave NW
Sleepy Eye, MN 56085-1109
(507)794-3571
FAX: (507)794-2840

Springfield

Springfield Clinic-New Ulm Medical Center
625 N Jackson Ave
Springfield, MN 56087-1714
(507)217-6201
FAX: (507)217-8178

St James

Mayo Clinic Health System In St. James
1101 Moulton And Parsons Dr
St James, MN 56081-5550
(507)375-3391
FAX: (507)375-8674

St Louis Park

Center For Diagnostic Imaging
5775 Wayzata Blvd, Ste 190
St Louis Park, MN 55416-1236
(651)287-4132
FAX: (651)202-2997

Park Nicollet Clinic Jane Brattain Breast Center
3850 Park Nicollet Blvd
St Louis Park, MN 55416-2527
(952)993-3700
FAX: (952)993-3998

Park Nicollet Hvc Women's Center
6500 Excelsior Blvd
St Louis Park, MN 55426-4702
(952)993-3701
FAX: (952)993-1750

Park Nicollet Mobile Mammography
6600 Excelsior Blvd
St Louis Park, MN 55426-4744
(952)993-9800
FAX: (952)993-8604

St Peter

River's Edge Hospital And Clinic
1900 Sunrise Dr
St Peter, MN 56082-5376
(507)934-7632
FAX: (507)934-6130

Staples

Lakewood Health System
49725 County 83
Staples, MN 56479-5280
(218)894-8465
FAX: (218)894-8721

Stillwater

Curve Crest Mammography
1500 Curve Crest Blvd W
Stillwater, MN 55082-6040
(651)430-8589
FAX: (651)430-4611

Lakeview Hospital
927 Churchill St W
Stillwater, MN 55082-5999
(651)430-4612
FAX: (651)430-4691

Thief River Falls

Sanford Thief River Falls Medical Center
3001 Sanford Pkwy
Thief River Falls, MN 56701-2700
(218)683-2785
FAX: (218)683-2611

Two Harbors

Lake View Memorial Hospital, Inc
1010 4th St
Two Harbors, MN 55616-1200
(218)834-7700
FAX: (218)834-7727

Virginia

Essentia Health Virginia, Llc
901 9th St N, Ste 215
Virginia, MN 55792-2375
(218)749-9463
FAX: (218)749-9587

Laurentian Medical Clinic
8373 Unity Dr
Virginia, MN 55792-4005
(218)748-7470
FAX: (218)748-7485

Wabasha

Gundersen St Elizabeth's Hospital And Clinics
1200 Grant Blvd W
Wabasha, MN 55981-1042
(651)565-5556
FAX: (651)565-5674

Waconia

Lakeview Clinic, Ltd.
424 W State Highway 5
Waconia, MN 55387-1795
(952)442-4461
FAX: (952)442-5751

Ridgeview Medical Center
500 S Maple St
Waconia, MN 55387-1791
(952)777-4471
FAX: (952)442-6556

Wadena

Tri County Hospital
415 Jefferson St N
Wadena, MN 56482-1297
(218)631-7466
FAX: (218)631-7519

Walker

Sanford Health Walker
614 Michigan Ave W
Walker, MN 56484-2276
(218)547-7700
FAX: (218)547-7729

Waseca

Mayo Clinic Health System - Waseca
501 State St N, Radiology Department
Waseca, MN 56093-2811
(507)781-8276
FAX: (507)781-8158

Wayzata

Park Nicollet Wayzata
250 Central Ave N Ste 226
Wayzata, MN 55391-1208
(952)993-8216
FAX: (952)993-8217

West St Paul

Center For Diagnostic Imaging
232 Wentworth Ave E
West St Paul, MN 55118-3525
(651)287-4132
FAX: (651)202-2997

White Bear Lake

Healthpartners White Bear Clinic
1430 Highway 96 E
White Bear Lake, MN 55110-3653
(651)653-2134
FAX: (651)653-2137

Willmar

Carris Health Llc - Willmar
101 Willmar Ave SW
Willmar, MN 56201-3591
(320)231-6776
FAX: (320)214-6257

Carris Health Llc - Willmar Lakeland Clinic
502 2nd St SW
Willmar, MN 56201-3337
(320)231-6776
FAX: (320)214-6257

Windom

Avera Medical Group Windom
PO Box 338, 2020 Hospital Dr Suite 2
Windom, MN 56101-0338
(507)831-1703
FAX: (507)831-5668

Windom Area Hospital
2150 Hospital Dr
Windom, MN 56101-1287
(507)831-2400
FAX: (507)407-3269

Winona

Gundersen Winona Campus
1122 W Highway 61
Winona, MN 55987-1957
(800)362-9567
FAX: (608)775-6175

Winona Health Services
855 Mankato Ave
Winona, MN 55987-4868
(507)457-4320
FAX: (507)474-3046

Woodbury

Allina Health Woodbury Clinic
8675 Valley Creek Rd
Woodbury, MN 55125-2337
(651)241-3155
FAX: (651)241-3168

Health Partners - Woodbury Clinic
8450 Seasons Pkwy
Woodbury, MN 55125-4402
(651)702-5321
FAX: (651)702-5355

M Health Fairview Ww
1925 Woodwinds Dr
Woodbury, MN 55125-4445
(651)232-0967
FAX: (651)232-0221

Worthington

Avera Medical Group Worthington
1216 Ryans Rd
Worthington, MN 56187-1780
(507)372-6515
FAX: (507)372-6506

Sanford Worthington Medical Center
1018 6th Ave
Worthington, MN 56187-2202
(507)372-3366
FAX: (507)372-3322

Wyoming

M Health Fairview Lakes
5200 Fairview Blvd
Wyoming, MN 55092-8013
(651)982-7630
FAX: (651)982-7633

MISSISSIPPI

Amory

North Mississippi Medical Gilmore-Amory
1105 Earl Frye Blvd, Radiology Department
Amory, MS 38821-5500
(662)256-6023
FAX: (662)305-4276

Batesville

Panola Medical Center
303 Medical Center Dr
Batesville, MS 38606-8608
(662)712-2299
FAX: (662)712-2242

Bay St Louis

Ochsner Medical Center Hnacock
149 Drinkwater Rd, Radiology Department
Bay St Louis, MS 39520-1658
(228)467-8793
FAX: (228)467-8720

Biloxi

Coastal Family Health Center
715A Division St
Biloxi, MS 39530-2209
(228)374-2494
FAX: (228)374-2713

Memorial Diagnostic Center Cedar Lake
1756 Popps Ferry Rd
Biloxi, MS 39532-2118
(228)867-4395
FAX: (228)867-4029

North Bay Diagnostics
1720A Medical Park Dr Ste 110
Biloxi, MS 39532-2122
(228)809-5184
FAX: (228)392-9932

Booneville

Baptist Memorial Hospital - Booneville
100 Hospital St
Booneville, MS 38829-3354
(662)720-5017
FAX: (662)720-3015

Brandon

Crossgates River Oaks Hospital Dba Merit Health Rankin
350 Crossgates Blvd
Brandon, MS 39042-2601
(601)824-8377
FAX: (601)824-8378

Brookhaven

Brookhaven Ob - Gyn Associates P.A.
1012 D A Biglane Dr
Brookhaven, MS 39601-2331
(601)833-8157
FAX: (601)833-1633

Kings Daughters Medical Center: Mammography Dept
427 Highway 51 N
Brookhaven, MS 39601-2350
(601)835-9292
FAX: (601)835-9291

Canton

Merit Health Madison
161 River Oaks Dr
Canton, MS 39046-5375
(601)855-4511
FAX: (601)855-4330

Carthage

Baptist Memorial Leake
1100 Highway 16 E
Carthage, MS 39051-4222
(601)267-1100
FAX: (601)267-1261

Centreville

Field Health System
178 Highway 24
Centreville, MS 39631-4217
(601)890-0613
FAX: (601)645-5433

Clarksdale

Delta Health-Northwest Regional
1970 Hospital Dr
Clarksdale, MS 38614-7202
(662)624-3464
FAX: (662)624-3124

The Woman's Clinic
2000 N State St
Clarksdale, MS 38614-6100
(662)627-7361
FAX: (662)627-4793

Cleveland

Phc-Cleveland Dba Bolivar Medical Center
901 E Sunflower Rd, Highway 8 East
Cleveland, MS 38732-2833
(662)846-2523
FAX: (662)846-2467

Columbus

Baptist Memorial Hospital-Golden Triangle
2520 5th St N, Out Patient Pavilion Mammography
Columbus, MS 39705-2008
(662)244-1540
FAX: (662)244-1541

Imaging Center Of Columbus
2526 5th St N
Columbus, MS 39705-2019
(662)328-8402
FAX: (662)328-1554

Corinth

Magnolia Regional Health Center
611 Alcorn Dr
Corinth, MS 38834-9388
(662)293-1460
FAX: (662)293-4210

Diamondhead

Memorial Diagnostic Center Diamondhead
4300 Leisure Time Dr
Diamondhead, MS 39525-3241
(228)867-4395
FAX: (228)867-4029

Diberville

Compass Imaging
3200 Mallett Rd, Ste E2
Diberville, MS 39540-9305
(228)314-7226
FAX: (228)314-5038

Eupora

North Mississippi Medical Center - Eupora
70 Medical Plz
Eupora, MS 39744-4018
(662)258-9397
FAX: (662)258-9290

Flowood

East Lakeland Ob Gyn Associates
1020 River Oaks Dr, Ste 320
Flowood, MS 39232-9512
(601)936-1400
FAX: (601)936-3435

Jackson Healthcare For Women
291 E Layfair Dr
Flowood, MS 39232-9527
(601)936-9190
FAX: (601)326-6018

Lakeland Premier Women's Clinic
2506 Lakeland Dr, Ste 600
Flowood, MS 39232-7640
(601)939-1600
FAX: (601)939-1606

University Physicians At Grant's Ferry
1010 Lakeland Pl
Flowood, MS 39232-6678
(601)815-4723
FAX: (601)815-8950

Women's Health Associates, Pllc
1050 River Oaks Dr Ste 110
Flowood, MS 39232-9564
(601)420-0134
FAX: (601)936-9245

Forest

Lackey Memorial Hospital
330 N Broad St
Forest, MS 39074-3508
(601)469-4151
FAX: (601)469-3348

Greenville

Delta Regional Medical Center
1400 E Union St
Greenville, MS 38703-3246
(662)725-2620
FAX: (662)725-2113

Greenwood

Greenwood Leflore Hospital
1401 River Rd
Greenwood, MS 38930-4030
(662)459-2769
FAX: (662)459-2706

Grenada

Ummc Grenada Imaging Center
1300 Sunset Dr Ste U
Grenada, MS 38901-4082
(662)226-9326
FAX: (662)226-9328

Gulfport

Acadian Plaza Diagnostic Ctr - Memorial Hosp Gulfport
12261 Highway 49 Ste 12
Gulfport, MS 39503-2976
(228)867-4395
FAX: (228)867-4288

Compass Imaging
14245 Dedeaux Rd
Gulfport, MS 39503-3369
(228)314-7226
FAX: (228)314-7227

Memorial Hospital - Gulfport
4500 13th St
Gulfport, MS 39501-2569
(228)867-4395
FAX: (228)867-4029

Ochsner Health Center Downtown
4502 Old Pass Rd
Gulfport, MS 39501-2585
(228)863-9977
FAX: (228)863-2125

Singing River - Gulfport
15200 Community Rd
Gulfport, MS 39503-3085
(228)575-7175
FAX: (228)575-7499

Hattiesburg

Lake Serene Mammography Hbc
6813 U S Highway 98
Hattiesburg, MS 39402-8446
(601)268-5744
FAX: (601)268-5868

Merit Health Wesley Breast Care Center
5001 Hardy St
Hattiesburg, MS 39402-1308
(601)296-3400
FAX: (601)261-6755

The Breast Center
421 S 28th Ave Ste 100, 28th Pl Breast Ctr
Hattiesburg, MS 39401-7208
(601)268-5744
FAX: (601)268-5868

Women's Pavilion Of South Mississippi
6524 US Hwy 98
Hattiesburg, MS 39402
(601)268-9393
FAX: (601)450-4863

Hazlehurst

Copiah County Medical Center
27190 Highway 28
Hazlehurst, MS 39083-2224
(601)574-7129
FAX: (601)574-7134

Holly Springs

Alliance Healthcare System
1430 Hwy 4E
Holly Springs, MS 38635
(662)252-1222
FAX: (662)252-2921

Houston

Trace Regional Health System
1002 E Madison St
Houston, MS 38851-2428
(662)456-1070
FAX: (662)456-0130

Indianola

South Sunflower County Hospital
121 E Baker St, Radiology Department
Indianola, MS 38751-2498
(662)887-5235
FAX: (662)887-4485

Iuka

Iuka Hospital
PO Box 860, 1777 Curtis Dr
Iuka, MS 38852-0860
(662)423-4502
FAX: (662)423-4051

Jackson

Center For Breast Health
1225 N State St West Tower
Jackson, MS 39202-2064
(601)973-3180
FAX: (601)973-1697

Center For Womens Health St Dominic
Dominican Plaza
970 Lakeland Dr Ste 33
Jackson, MS 39216-4640
(601)200-6732
FAX: (601)200-4945

Merit Health Central
1860 Chadwick Dr Ste 150
Jackson, MS 39204-3486
(601)376-1748
FAX: (601)376-1742

Merit Health Woman's Hospital
1026 N Flowood Dr
Jackson, MS 39232-9599
(601)933-6426
FAX: (601)936-9500

Southern Womens Health Pllc
1020 River Oaks Dr Ste 310
Jackson, MS 39232-9512
(601)932-5006
FAX: (601)932-4548

The Woman's Clinic
501 Marshall St Ste 400
Jackson, MS 39202-1687
(601)354-0869
FAX: (601)352-6521

Uhc - Jackson Medical Mall Breast Imaging Center
350 W Woodrow Wilson Ave
Jackson, MS 39213-7681
(601)815-4723
FAX: (601)815-8972

Uhc- Medical Pavilion
1410 E Woodrow Wilson Ave
Jackson, MS 39216-5114
(601)984-6280
FAX: (601)815-3378

Keesler Afb

Keesler Air Force Base
301 Fisher St, 81st Mdg/ Mdts/Sgqx Mammography
Keesler Afb, MS 39534-2508
(228)376-0475
FAX: (228)376-0178

Kosciusko

Baptist Medical Center Attala
220 Highway 12 W
Kosciusko, MS 39090-3208
(662)290-3295
FAX: (662)290-3347

Laurel

South Central Regional Medical Center
1300 Jefferson St
Laurel, MS 39440
(601)426-4048
FAX: (601)426-4517

Leland

The Indianola Clinic, Llc Dba Leland Medical Clinic
201 Baker Blvd
Leland, MS 38756-3401
(662)626-4121
FAX: (662)686-4770

Lexington

Holmes County Hospital And Clinics
239 Bowling Green Rd
Lexington, MS 39095-5167
(662)834-5123
FAX: (662)834-5145

Louisville

Winston Medical Center
17550 E Main St
Louisville, MS 39339-2772
(662)446-1100
FAX: (662)446-1172

Lucedale

George Regional Hospital
859 Winter St
Lucedale, MS 39452-6603
(601)947-9123
FAX: (601)947-9198

Madison

St Dominic's Madison Medical Imaging
106 Highland Way Ste 100
Madison, MS 39110-6930
(601)853-9149
FAX: (601)605-4814

The Womans Clinic
401 Baptist Dr Ste 402
Madison, MS 39110-2009
(601)354-0869
FAX: (601)352-6487

Magee

Magee General Hospital Diagnostic Imaging
300 3rd Ave SE
Magee, MS 39111-3665
(601)849-7312
FAX: (601)849-7329

McComb

Diagnostic Imaging Services
1510 Harrison Ave
McComb, MS 39648-2716
(601)249-1157
FAX: (601)249-1830

Southwest Mississippi Regional Medical Center
215 Marion Ave
McComb, MS 39648-2705
(601)249-5197
FAX: (601)249-1830

Meridian

Anderson Regional Breast Center
2124 14th St
Meridian, MS 39301-4040
(601)553-6595
FAX: (601)581-1878

Rush Imaging Center
1800 12th St
Meridian, MS 39301-4158
(601)703-9544
FAX: (601)703-4321

Women's Healthcare Center
1730A 14th St
Meridian, MS 39301-4140
(601)703-4395
FAX: (601)703-4394

Natchez

Merit Health Natchez
54 Sgt Prentiss Dr
Natchez, MS 39120-4726
(601)443-2230
FAX: (601)442-9304

New Albany

Baptist Memorial Hospital - Union County
200 State Highway 30 W
New Albany, MS 38652-3197
(662)538-2133
FAX: (662)538-2123

Ocean Springs

Ocean Springs Hospital Ocean Springs Imaging Center
3535 Bienville Blvd
Ocean Springs, MS 39564-5705
(228)818-4201
FAX: (228)818-4202

Oxford

Baptist Memorial Hospital - North Mississippi
1100 Belk Blvd
Oxford, MS 38655-5242
(662)636-4252
FAX: (662)636-1663

Oxford Clinic For Women, Pllc
2610 S Lamar Blvd
Oxford, MS 38655-5243
(662)234-1731
FAX: (662)236-2392

Oxford Diagnostic Center
504 Azalea Dr, Ste B
Oxford, MS 38655-5397
(662)636-1201
FAX: (662)636-1699

Pascagoula

Singing River Medical Park
3101 Denny Ave Ste 300
Pascagoula, MS 39581-5307
(228)471-1410
FAX: (228)471-1425

Philadelphia

Choctaw Health Center
210 Hospital Cir
Philadelphia, MS 39350-6781
(601)389-4350
FAX: (601)389-4351

Neshoba County General Hospital
1001 Holland Ave
Philadelphia, MS 39350-2161
(601)781-2281
FAX: (601)781-2288

Picayune

Highland Community Hospital
130 Highland Pkwy
Picayune, MS 39466-5574
(601)358-9535
FAX: (601)358-9757

Pontotoc

Nmmc Pontotoc
176 S Main St
Pontotoc, MS 38863-3311
(662)488-7619
FAX: (662)488-7690

Ruleville

Sunflower Diagnostic Center
101 E Floyce St
Ruleville, MS 38771-3915
(662)756-4000
FAX: (662)756-1750

Southaven

Baptist Memorial Hospital - Desoto Womens Center
7601 Southcrest Pkwy
Southaven, MS 38671-4739
(901)227-4433
FAX: (662)772-2141

Desoto Imaging Specialists
7420 Guthrie Dr N Ste 106
Southaven, MS 38671-5857
(662)349-4321
FAX: (662)349-3263

Diagnostic Ultrasound Consultants, P.C.
7640 Clarington Cv Ste A
Southaven, MS 38671-5652
(662)349-3420
FAX: (662)349-3422

Memphis Obgyn Association, P.C.
7900 Airways Blvd, Bldg C2 Suite 2
Southaven, MS 38671-4114
(662)349-5554
FAX: (662)349-5570

Methodist Diagnostic Center-Southaven
7400 Airways Blvd
Southaven, MS 38671-5863
(662)996-2122
FAX: (662)996-2101

Starkville

Center For Breast Health And Imaging
102 Doctors Park
Starkville, MS 39759-2570
(662)615-3800
FAX: (662)615-3807

Tupelo

North Ms Medical Center Breast Care Center
4376 S Eason Blvd
Tupelo, MS 38801-6516
(662)377-4910
FAX: (662)377-2071

North Ms Medical Center Breast Care Suite
830 S Gloster St
Tupelo, MS 38801-4934
(662)377-4910
FAX: (662)377-2071

Obstetrics - Gynecology Associates, P.A.
1793 Cliff Gookin Blvd
Tupelo, MS 38801-6723
(662)842-1161
FAX: (662)842-6375

Sanders Clinic For Women, P.A.
1041 S Madison St
Tupelo, MS 38801-6391
(662)844-8754
FAX: (662)844-1973

The Imaging Center
320 S Gloster St
Tupelo, MS 38801-4748
(662)377-7880
FAX: (662)821-1888

Union

Laird Hospital
25117 Highway 15
Union, MS 39365-9099
(601)774-1565
FAX: (601)774-5090

Vicksburg

The Women's Imaging Center
2100 Highway 61 N
Vicksburg, MS 39183-8211
(601)883-5000
FAX: (601)883-5475

Water Valley

Yalobusha General Hospital
604 S Main St
Water Valley, MS 38965-3468
(662)473-4050
FAX: (662)473-5258

Waynesboro

Wayne General Hospital
950 Matthew Dr
Waynesboro, MS 39367-2590
(601)735-7109
FAX: (601)735-7183

West Point

Nmmc-West Point
150 Medical Center Dr
West Point, MS 39773-0428
(662)495-2331
FAX: (662)495-2397

Winona

Tyler Holmes Memorial Hospital
409 Tyler Holmes Dr
Winona, MS 38967-1599
(662)283-6133
FAX: (662)283-6135

Yazoo City

Baptist Medical Center - Yazoo, Inc.
823 Grand Ave
Yazoo City, MS 39194-3233
(662)751-8164
FAX: (662)751-8287

MISSOURI

Albany

Mosaic Medical Center- Albany
705 N College St
Albany, MO 64402-1433
(660)726-3941
FAX: (660)726-3944

Aurora

Mercy Hospital Aurora
500 Porter Ave
Aurora, MO 65605-2365
(417)678-7880
FAX: (417)678-7828

Ballwin

Mercy Breast Center Clayton Clarkson
15945 Clayton Rd Ste 110
Ballwin, MO 63011-2490
(314)251-6300
FAX: (636)256-5343

St. Louis Breast Center Llc
884 Woods Mill Rd Ste 203
Ballwin, MO 63011-3657
(636)779-8008
FAX: (636)779-8010

Belton

Belton Regional Medical Center Midamerica Division
17065 South 71 Hwy
Belton, MO 64012
(816)348-1224
FAX: (816)348-1296

Bethany

Harrison County Community Hospital
2600 Miller St
Bethany, MO 64424-2701
(660)425-0274
FAX: (660)425-7892

Bloomsdale

Bloomsdale Medical Centre
255 Boderman Ste 1C
Bloomsdale, MO 63627-9099
(573)883-7720
FAX: (573)883-7721

Blue Springs

Saint Lukes's Mammography-Blue Springs
600 NE Adams Dairy Pkwy, Ste 195
Blue Springs, MO 64014-5497
(816)347-4904
FAX: (816)347-5645

St. Mary's Medical Center
201 NW R D Mize Rd
Blue Springs, MO 64014-2513
(816)655-5515
FAX: (816)943-5770

Bolivar

Citizens Memorial Hospital Breast Care Center
1155 W Parkview St, Ste 1D
Bolivar, MO 65613-8279
(417)328-7860
FAX: (417)328-1138

Mercy Bolivar Multi-Specialty
3817 S Springfield Ave Ste 160
Bolivar, MO 65613-9129
(417)885-3492
FAX: (417)885-3491

Branson

Coxhealth Women's Imaging Branson
525 Branson Landing Blvd Ste 408
Branson, MO 65616-2192
(417)335-7733
FAX: (417)335-7732

Bridgeton

Ssm/Cdi Imaging Center Llc
3440 De Paul Ln Ste 100
Bridgeton, MO 63044-3546
(314)739-0924
FAX: (314)739-0832

Brookfield

Pershing Memorial Hospital
130 E Lockling St
Brookfield, MO 64628-2337
(660)258-1119
FAX: (660)258-1011

Butler

Bates County Memorial Hospital
PO Box 370, 615 W Nursery
Butler, MO 64730-0370
(660)200-7085
FAX: (660)200-7084

Cameron

Cameron Regional Medical Center
1600 E Evergreen St
Cameron, MO 64429-2400
(816)649-3228
FAX: (816)649-3224

Cape Girardeau

Breast Care And Diagnostic Ctr Llc
60 Doctors Park
Cape Girardeau, MO 63703-4928
(573)519-4900
FAX: (573)986-6693

Cape Radiology Group Llc
70 Doctors Park
Cape Girardeau, MO 63703-4928
(573)334-6071
FAX: (573)334-2990

Saint Francis Medical Center - Womancare
211 Saint Francis Dr
Cape Girardeau, MO 63703-5049
(573)331-5175
FAX: (573)331-5175

Carrollton

Carroll County Memorial Hospital
1502 N Jefferson St
Carrollton, MO 64633-1999
(660)542-1695
FAX: (660)542-6079

Carthage

Mercy Hospital Carthage
3125 Dr Russell Smith Way, Radiology Department
Carthage, MO 64836-7402
(417)359-1320
FAX: (417)237-7283

Cassville

Mercy Hospital Inc.-Cassville
94 Main St
Cassville, MO 65625-1610
(417)847-6015
FAX: (417)847-6016

Chesterfield

St. Luke's Hospital
232 S Woods Mill Rd, Ste 200 East
Chesterfield, MO 63017-3485
(314)205-6480
FAX: (314)205-6998

St. Lukes Women's Center
6 McBride And Son Center Dr, Ste 102
Chesterfield, MO 63005-1418
(636)530-5505
FAX: (636)530-5510

Chillicothe

Hedrick Medical Center
2799 N Washington St
Chillicothe, MO 64601-1599
(660)214-8325
FAX: (660)214-8324

Clinton

Golden Valley Memorial Hospital
1600 N 2nd St
Clinton, MO 64735-1297
(660)890-7145
FAX: (660)885-8217

Columbia

Boone Hospital Center- Nifong Medical Plaza
900 W Nifong Blvd
Columbia, MO 65203-4467
(573)815-8150
FAX: (573)815-3750

Boone Hospital Center-Harris Breast Center
1600 E Broadway
Columbia, MO 65201-5844
(573)815-3523
FAX: (573)815-8590

Ellis Fischel Cancer Center
1 Hospital Dr
Columbia, MO 65212-1001
(573)882-8089
FAX: (573)884-5249

Creve Coeur

Berland Diagnostic Imaging Center Of Creve Coeur
774 N New Ballas Rd
Creve Coeur, MO 63141-6716
(314)567-1656
FAX: (314)567-0622

Dexter

Southeast Health Center Of Stoddard County
1200 N One Mile Rd
Dexter, MO 63841-1000
(573)614-9440
FAX: (573)614-9453

Eldorado Springs

Cedar County Memorial Hospital
1401 S Park St
Eldorado Springs, MO 64744-2037
(417)876-3542
FAX: (417)876-3957

Ellisville

Bjc Outpatient Center - Ellisville
15838 Fountain Plaza Dr., Suite B
Ellisville, MO 63011
(636)484-5200
FAX: (636)484-5201

Excelsior Springs

Excelsior Springs Hospital
1700 Rainbow Blvd
Excelsior Springs, MO 64024-1190
(816)629-2700
FAX: (816)629-3630

Fairfax

Community Hospital Association, Inc.
PO Box 107, 26136 US Hwy 59
Fairfax, MO 64446-0107
(660)686-2360
FAX: (660)686-2753

Farmington

Parkland Health Center - Bjc
1101 W Liberty St, Dept. Of Mammography
Farmington, MO 63640-1921
(573)760-8460
FAX: (573)760-8358

Fenton

Ssm St Clare Hospital
1015 Bowles Ave
Fenton, MO 63026-2394
(636)496-2803
FAX: (636)496-4928

Festus

Mercy Imaging Services
1500 Calvary Church Rd
Festus, MO 63028-4125
(636)933-1234
FAX: (636)933-5740

Florissant

Metro Imaging
125 Dunn Rd
Florissant, MO 63031-8007
(314)333-6742
FAX: (314)432-0178

Northwest Healthcare
1225 Graham Rd
Florissant, MO 63031-8012
(314)653-4530
FAX: (314)953-6916

Fort Leonard Wood

General Leonard Wood Army Community Hospital
4430 Missouri Ave
Fort Leonard Wood, MO 65473-9098
(573)596-0029
FAX: (573)596-1683

Fredericktown

Madison Medical Center
611 W Main St, Ste A
Fredericktown, MO 63645-1120
(573)783-3341
FAX: (573)783-1011

Gladstone

Encompass Medical Group-Premier Imaging Englewood
101 NW Englewood Rd
Gladstone, MO 64118-4054
(816)414-4486
FAX: (913)495-3714

Grandview

Encompass Medical Group - Hickman Mills
7201 E 147th St
Grandview, MO 64030-4204
(816)348-2260
FAX: (913)495-3734

Hannibal

Hannibal Clinic Operations
100 Medical Dr
Hannibal, MO 63401-6877
(573)231-3290
FAX: (573)231-3731

Hannibal Regional Hospital
6000 Hospital Dr
Hannibal, MO 63401-6887
(573)248-5300
FAX: (573)248-5302

Harrisonville

Cass Regional Medical Center
2800 E Rock Haven Rd
Harrisonville, MO 64701-4411
(816)380-5888
FAX: (816)887-0730

Hazelwood

Mercy Imaging Hazelwood
801 Hazelwest Dr Ste 400
Hazelwood, MO 63042-1754
(314)251-6300
FAX: (314)919-2779

Hermann

Hermann Area District Hospital
509 W 18th St
Hermann, MO 65041-1547
(573)486-2191
FAX: (573)486-5018

Houston

Texas County Memorial Hospital
1333 S Sam Houston Blvd
Houston, MO 65483-2046
(417)967-1276
FAX: (417)967-1313

Independence

Centerpoint Medical Center Of Independence, Llc
19600 E 39th St S
Independence, MO 64057-2301
(816)836-6686
FAX: (816)698-8815

Diagnostic Imaging Centers - Independence
4911 S Arrowhead Dr Ste 100
Independence, MO 64055-7008
(816)795-7040
FAX: (816)795-0821

Encompass Medical Group - Premier Imaging - Independence
4811 S Arrowhead Dr
Independence, MO 64055-6981
(816)356-5000
FAX: (816)356-5875

Medical Imaging Eastland Truman Medical Center Lakewood
19000 E Eastland Center Ct, Ste 100
Independence, MO 64055-7023
(816)876-2900
FAX: (816)876-2903

Jackson

Cape Radiology Group, Llc
1404 Old Cape Rd, Ste 204
Jackson, MO 63755-2390
(573)334-6071
FAX: (573)339-0329

Jefferson City

Capital Region Medical Center
1125 Madison St
Jefferson City, MO 65101-5200
(573)632-5152
FAX: (573)632-5820

Jefferson City Medical Group
1241 W Stadium Blvd
Jefferson City, MO 65109-6023
(573)556-7755
FAX: (573)761-3599

Ssm Health St. Mary's Hospital Women's Imaging
2505 Mission Dr Ste 100
Jefferson City, MO 65109-9508
(573)681-3181
FAX: (573)681-3662

Joplin

Freeman Health System, Freeman Women's Pavilion
1532 W 32nd St Ste 101
Joplin, MO 64804-1642
(417)347-4934
FAX: (417)347-9164

Mercy Hospital Joplin
100 Mercy Way, Ste 260
Joplin, MO 64804-4524
(417)556-2273
FAX: (417)659-6399

Kansas City

Diagnostic Imaging Centers North
303 NE Englewood Rd, Ste A
Kansas City, MO 64118-4501
(816)455-5959
FAX: (816)455-3728

Diagnostic Imaging Centers Pa - Plaza
4801 Main St Ste 200
Kansas City, MO 64112-2582
(816)561-5151
FAX: (913)696-0040

Diagnostic Imaging Centers, P.A. Liberty
9151 NE 81st Ter, Ste 250
Kansas City, MO 64158-1307
(816)883-2590
FAX: (816)883-2597

Element Medical Imaging
9778 North Ash
Kansas City, MO 64157
(913)469-8998
FAX: (913)469-5695

Encompass Medical Group - Premier Imaging
373 W 101st Ter
Kansas City, MO 64114-4498
(816)941-1400
FAX: (816)941-1129

Imaging For Women, Llc
630 NW Englewood Rd
Kansas City, MO 64118-3973
(816)453-2700
FAX: (816)453-9943

North Kansas City Hospital Dba Medical Imaging
9501 N Oak Trfy
Kansas City, MO 64155-2241
(816)455-0661
FAX: (816)876-2960

Research Medical Center
2316 E Meyer Blvd
Kansas City, MO 64132-1199
(816)276-4141
FAX: (816)276-3692

Research Medical Center Brookside Campus
6675 Holmes Rd, Outpatient Imaging
Kansas City, MO 64131-1150
(816)276-4088
FAX: (816)276-4572

Samuel U. Rodgers Community Health Center
825 Euclid Ave
Kansas City, MO 64124-2398
(816)889-4674
FAX: (816)889-1804

St Lukes Hospital Breast Center
4401 Wornall Rd
Kansas City, MO 64111-3241
(816)502-8500
FAX: (816)502-8575

St. Joseph Medical Center
1000 Carondelet Dr
Kansas City, MO 64114-4865
(816)943-3173
FAX: (816)943-4571

St. Luke's North Breast And Imaging Center
5820 NW Barry Rd, Ste 100
Kansas City, MO 64154-2578
(816)891-2273
FAX: (816)891-6762

Swope Health Services
3801 Blue Pkwy
Kansas City, MO 64130-2807
(816)599-5870
FAX: (816)599-5976

Truman Medical Center Hospital Hill
2301 Holmes St
Kansas City, MO 64108-2677
(816)404-0698
FAX: (816)404-0699

University Health
2101 Charlotte St, Ste 1
Kansas City, MO 64108-2728
(816)404-0751
FAX: (816)404-0701

Kirksville

Northeast Regional Medical Center
315 S Osteopathy Ave
Kirksville, MO 63501-6401
(660)785-1267
FAX: (660)785-1270

Lake St Louis

St. Joseph Hospital West
400 Medical Plz Ste 50
Lake St Louis, MO 63367-1491
(636)949-9600
FAX: (636)625-5398

Lamar

Cox Barton County Hospital
29 NW 1st Ln
Lamar, MO 64759-8105
(417)681-5162
FAX: (417)681-5521

Lebanon

Mercy Hospital Lebanon
100 Hospital Dr
Lebanon, MO 65536-9210
(417)533-6094
FAX: (417)533-6001

Lees Summit

Diagnostic Imaging Centers - Lee's Summit
301 NE Mulberry St Ste 100
Lees Summit, MO 64086-6016
(816)444-9989
FAX: (816)444-9957

Element Medical Imaging
3210 NE Carnegie Dr
Lees Summit, MO 64064-3201
(913)469-8998
FAX: (913)469-5695

Encompass Medical Group Lee's Summit Clinic
615 SW 3rd St
Lees Summit, MO 64063-2212
(816)524-3799
FAX: (913)495-3727

Lee's Summit Medical Center
2100 SE Blue Pkwy
Lees Summit, MO 64063-1007
(816)282-5608
FAX: (816)282-5602

Saint Luke's East Hospital
110 NE Saint Lukes Blvd Ste 300
Lees Summit, MO 64086-6075
(816)347-4904
FAX: (816)347-5645

Lexington

Lafayette Regional Health Center
1500 State St
Lexington, MO 64067-1107
(660)259-6863
FAX: (660)259-6806

Liberty

Breast Care Center At Liberty Hospital
2529 Glenn Hendren Dr Ste 206
Liberty, MO 64068-9607
(816)792-7016
FAX: (816)415-5108

Louisiana

Pike County Memorial Hospital
2305 Georgia St
Louisiana, MO 63353-2559
(573)754-5531
FAX: (573)754-3492

Marshall

Fitzgibbon Hospital
2305 S 65 Hwy.
Marshall, MO 65340
(660)831-3208
FAX: (660)886-3420

Maryville

Mosaic Medical Center - Maryville
2016 S Main St
Maryville, MO 64468-2655
(660)562-7907
FAX: (660)562-7956

Memphis

Scotland County Hospital
450 E Sigler Ave
Memphis, MO 63555-1726
(660)465-8511
FAX: (660)465-7419

Mexico

Audrain Community Hospital
620 E Monroe St
Mexico, MO 65265-2919
(573)582-8539
FAX: (573)582-3727

Moberly

Moberly Diagnostics
1509 Union Ave
Moberly, MO 65270-9407
(660)263-8986
FAX: (660)263-8993

Monett

Cox Monett Hospital, Inc.
1000 E US Highway 60
Monett, MO 65708-1698
(417)354-1137
FAX: (417)354-1140

Mountain View

Mercy St. Francis Hospital
100 W. Hwy. 60
Mountain View, MO 65548
(417)934-7156
FAX: (417)934-7089

Neosho

Freeman Women's Pavilion - Neosho
336 S Jefferson St
Neosho, MO 64850-1769
(417)347-4512
FAX: (417)347-6266

Nevada

Nevada City Hospital Dba Nevada Regional Med Center
800 S Ash St
Nevada, MO 64772-3224
(417)448-2468
FAX: (417)448-3670

North Kansas City

North Kansas City Hospital
2790 Clay Edwards Dr
North Kansas City, MO 64116-3276
(816)346-7620
FAX: (816)346-7577

Ofallon

Mercy Imaging O'Fallon
300 Winding Woods Dr, Ste 106
Ofallon, MO 63366-4772
(314)251-6300
FAX: (636)379-4302

Progress West Hospital
2 Progress Point Pkwy
Ofallon, MO 63368-2205
(636)344-1702
FAX: (636)344-1716

St. Lukes Center For Diagnostic Imaging
5551 Winghaven Blvd Ste 60
Ofallon, MO 63368-3618
(636)625-4434
FAX: (636)625-4432

Osage Beach

Lake Regional Imaging Partners, Llc
1075 Nichols Rd
Osage Beach, MO 65065-3093
(573)348-6161
FAX: (573)348-6162

Osceola

Golden Valley Memorial Healthcare - Osceola
675 3rd St
Osceola, MO 64776-2934
(417)646-2231
FAX: (417)646-2338

Perryville

Perry County Memorial Hospital
434 N West St
Perryville, MO 63775-1398
(573)768-3295
FAX: (573)547-3026

Poplar Bluff

Bluff Imaging And Women's Center
2588 N Westwood Blvd
Poplar Bluff, MO 63901-2339
(573)785-6610
FAX: (573)785-3699

Saint Francis Medical Partners Kneibert Clinic
686 Lester St
Poplar Bluff, MO 63901-5025
(573)778-7234
FAX: (573)686-7878

Saint Francis Outpatient Center - Pb
223 Physicians Park
Poplar Bluff, MO 63901-3956
(573)778-2637
FAX: (573)712-2778

Potosi

Washington County Memorial Hospital
300 Health Way Dr
Potosi, MO 63664-1499
(573)438-5451
FAX: (573)438-1866

Richmond

Ray County Memorial Hospital
904 Wollard Blvd
Richmond, MO 64085-2243
(816)470-5432
FAX: (816)470-7303

Richmond Heights

Metro Imaging Richmond Heights
6520 Clayton Rd
Richmond Heights, MO 63117-1706
(314)333-5777
FAX: (314)333-5888

Ssm Health St. Mary's Hospital
1031 Bellevue Ave Ste 100
Richmond Heights, MO 63117-1855
(314)768-2500
FAX: (314)768-7123

Rolla

Mercy Hospital Lebanon Imaging Services - Rolla
1605 Martin Springs Dr Ste 110A
Rolla, MO 65401-2982
(573)458-6625
FAX: (573)458-6628

Phelps Health
1050 W 10th St, Medical Office Bldg
Rolla, MO 65401-2905
(573)364-8899
FAX: (573)458-8481

Saint Charles

Ssm Health Outpatient Center- St Charles
711 Veterans Memorial Pkwy, Dept. Of Radiology
Saint Charles, MO 63303-2106
(636)669-2410
FAX: (636)669-2448

Ssm St Joseph Hospital Outpatient Center
1475 Kisker Rd, Ste 170
Saint Charles, MO 63304-8786
(636)498-7900
FAX: (636)498-7925

Saint Joseph

Diagnostic Imaging Centers, P.A. St. Joe
3937 Sherman Ave
Saint Joseph, MO 64506-3649
(816)676-0625
FAX: (816)676-0627

Mosaic Life Care At St Joseph Mammography
802 N Riverside Rd, Plaza I Suite G10
Saint Joseph, MO 64507-2502
(816)271-1278
FAX: (816)271-6632

Saint Louis

American Multispecialty Group Dba Esse Health Excel Imaging
9930 Watson Rd
Saint Louis, MO 63126-1845
(314)984-8827
FAX: (314)984-0736

Barnes - Jewish Hospital
4921 Parkview Pl, Breast Health Center
Saint Louis, MO 63110-1032
(314)454-7500
FAX: (314)454-5676

Barnes Jewish Hospital, Center For Advanced Medicine-South
5201 Mid America Plz Ste 1600
Saint Louis, MO 63129-0002
(314)454-7500
FAX: (314)454-5676

Barnes-Jewish Hospital At Highlands Plaza 3
1110 Highlands Plaza Dr E, Ste 325
Saint Louis, MO 63110-1352
(314)454-7500
FAX: (314)454-5676

Barnes-Jewish West County Hospital
969 N Mason Rd Ste 110
Saint Louis, MO 63141-6338
(314)996-8080
FAX: (314)996-8620

Breast Healthcare Center Rock Hill Mammography
9450 Manchester Rd Ste 206
Saint Louis, MO 63119-1452
(314)996-5170
FAX: (314)737-5182

Breast Healthcare Center At Missouri Baptist Medical Ctr.
3023 N Ballas Rd, Ste 210D Bldg D
Saint Louis, MO 63131-2330
(314)996-7534
FAX: (314)996-7560

Carestl Health
5471 Dr Martin Luther King Dr
Saint Louis, MO 63112-4265
(314)367-5820
FAX: (314)361-8355

Christian Hospital - Northeast Division
11133 Dunn Rd
Saint Louis, MO 63136-6163
(314)653-4530
FAX: (314)653-4151

Mercy Breast Center Mercy Hospital St Louis
621 S New Ballas Rd Ste 23
Saint Louis, MO 63141-8232
(314)251-6300
FAX: (314)251-5892

Mercy Imaging Old Tesson
12348 Old Tesson Rd Ste 120
Saint Louis, MO 63128-2251
(314)467-3864
FAX: (314)467-3861

Mercy Imaging Services- Kennerly
10010 Kennerly Rd, Radiology Department
Saint Louis, MO 63128-2106
(314)525-1300
FAX: (314)525-4969

Mercy Imaging Services-7345 Watson Road
7345 Watson Rd, Ll2
Saint Louis, MO 63119-9804
(314)525-1300
FAX: (314)752-7225

Mercy Rooney Breast Center
10050 Kennerly Rd, Ste 1400
Saint Louis, MO 63128-2106
(314)525-1300
FAX: (314)525-4969

Metro Imaging
11615 Olive Blvd, Ste D
Saint Louis, MO 63141-7095
(314)993-9555
FAX: (314)993-9550

Metro Imaging South County
13303 Tesson Ferry Rd Ste 30
Saint Louis, MO 63128-4062
(314)843-5888
FAX: (314)843-1905

Midwest Breast Care Center
450 N New Ballas Rd, Ste 250
Saint Louis, MO 63141-6817
(314)567-4449
FAX: (314)567-0762

People's Health Centers, Inc.
5701 Delmar Blvd
Saint Louis, MO 63112-2617
(314)367-7848
FAX: (314)367-5271

Ssm Health Breast Care At Saint Louis University Hospital
3655 Vista Ave, West Pavillion/First Floor
Saint Louis, MO 63110-2539
(314)257-8300
FAX: (314)577-6026

St. Luke's Des Peres Hospital
2345 Dougherty Ferry Rd
Saint Louis, MO 63122-3313
(314)966-9384
FAX: (314)966-9622

Watson Imaging Center
3915 Watson Rd Ste Ll2
Saint Louis, MO 63109-1251
(314)781-9711
FAX: (314)781-9768

Salem

Salem Memorial District Hospital
35629 Highway 72
Salem, MO 65560-7217
(573)729-5917
FAX: (573)739-1902

Sedalia

Bothwell Diagnostic Center-Winchester
990 Winchester Dr
Sedalia, MO 65301-2416
(660)827-7910
FAX: (660)829-0361

Sikeston

Missouri Delta Medical Center
1008 N Main St
Sikeston, MO 63801-5099
(573)472-7330
FAX: (573)472-7735

Springfield

Coxhealth Breast Care Clinic
3850 S National Ave Ste 300, Hulston Cancer Center
Springfield, MO 65807-5287
(417)269-5239
FAX: (417)269-6992

Coxhealth Breast Care Clinic - North
1423 N Jefferson Ave
Springfield, MO 65802-1917
(417)269-5239
FAX: (417)269-5139

Mercy Breast Center - Mobile
2055 S Fremont Ave
Springfield, MO 65804-2206
(417)820-2395
FAX: (417)820-8155

Mercy Breast Center O'Reilly Cancer Center
2055 S Fremont Ave, Breast Center Suite 120
Springfield, MO 65804-2206
(417)820-2395
FAX: (417)820-8155

St Peters

Barnes-Jewish St. Peter's Hospital
10 Hospital Dr
St Peters, MO 63376-1691
(636)916-9320
FAX: (636)916-9618

Metro Imaging St. Peters
4750 Mexico Rd
St Peters, MO 63376-1663
(636)498-4555
FAX: (636)498-2555

Sullivan

Mercy Hospitals East Communities Dba Mercy Hosp Washington
1326 S Service Rd W
Sullivan, MO 63080-2306
(636)239-8265
FAX: (573)468-1621

Missouri Baptist Hospital - Sullivan
751 Sappington Bridge Rd
Sullivan, MO 63080-2354
(573)468-4151
FAX: (573)468-1364

Sunset Hills

Missouri Baptist Outpatient Center - Sunset Hills
3844 S Lindbergh Blvd, Ste 140
Sunset Hills, MO 63127-1369
(314)525-0505
FAX: (314)525-0507

Trenton

Saint Lukes Hospital Dba Wright Memorial Hospital
191 Iowa Blvd
Trenton, MO 64683-8343
(660)358-5793
FAX: (660)358-5876

Troy

Mercy Hospital Lincoln
1000 E Cherry St
Troy, MO 63379-1513
(636)528-3488
FAX: (636)528-3487

Unionville

Putnam County Memorial Hospital
1926 Oak St
Unionville, MO 63565-1180
(660)947-2411
FAX: (660)947-2187

Warrensburg

Western Missouri Medical Center
403 Burkarth Rd
Warrensburg, MO 64093-3101
(660)262-7370
FAX: (660)747-2432

Warsaw

Bothwell Health Center - Truman Lake
1765 Commercial St
Warsaw, MO 65355-3096
(660)438-6800
FAX: (660)438-6525

Golden Valley Medical Warsaw
1771 Commercial St
Warsaw, MO 65355-3096
(660)438-5193
FAX: (660)438-2833

Washington

Mercy Hospital Washington
851 E 5th St Ste 100
Washington, MO 63090-3128
(636)239-8250
FAX: (636)390-7484

Mercy Hospitals East Communities Dba Mercy Hosp Washington
901 Patients First Dr
Washington, MO 63090-4700
(636)390-1771
FAX: (636)390-1772

Waynesville

Phelps Health
1000 Gw Ln
Waynesville, MO 65583-2339
(573)458-8899
FAX: (573)458-8497

Wentzville

Ssm Health Wentzville Outpatient Center
1598 W Meyer Rd
Wentzville, MO 63385-3653
(636)332-8042
FAX: (636)332-8034

West Plains

Ozarks Healthcare
1111 N Kentucky Ave
West Plains, MO 65775-2028
(417)257-5901
FAX: (417)257-5896

MONTANA

Anaconda

Community Hospital Of Anaconda
401 W Pennsylvania Ave, Medical Imaging Department
Anaconda, MT 59711-1999
(406)563-8660
FAX: (406)563-8663

Baker

Fallon Medical Complex
202 S 4th St W
Baker, MT 59313-9156
(406)778-5347
FAX: (406)778-5354

Billings

Billings Clinic Center For Breast Health
801 N 29th St
Billings, MT 59101-0905
(406)238-2501
FAX: (406)435-7269

Billings Clinic West
2675 Central Ave, Ste 14
Billings, MT 59102-6661
(406)238-2501
FAX: (406)238-2948

Scl Health Montana St Vincent Breast Center
2900 12th Ave N Ste 276W
Billings, MT 59101-7598
(406)237-4373
FAX: (406)237-4275

Bozeman

Advanced Medical Imaging
905 Highland Blvd Ste 4100
Bozeman, MT 59715-6901
(406)414-5200
FAX: (406)414-5205

Butte

3d Mammography Of Southwest Montana, Inc.
800 W Platinum St, Unit D
Butte, MT 59701-2200
(406)299-3302
FAX: (406)299-3304

St. James Healthcare - Intermountain Imaging Ctr
400 S Clark St
Butte, MT 59701-2328
(406)723-2950
FAX: (406)723-2854

Columbus

Stillwater Billings Clinic
710 11th St N
Columbus, MT 59019-7215
(406)322-1000
FAX: (406)322-8450

Deer Lodge

Deer Lodge Medical Center
1100 Hollenbeck Ln
Deer Lodge, MT 59722-2317
(406)846-7701
FAX: (406)415-1044

Dillon

Barrett Hospital & Healthcare
600 Mt Highway 91 S
Dillon, MT 59725-7379
(406)683-3266
FAX: (406)683-3112

Ennis

Madison Valley Medical Center
305 N Main St
Ennis, MT 59729-8001
(406)682-6612
FAX: (406)682-6650

Glasgow

Frances Mahon Deaconess Hospital
621 3rd St S
Glasgow, MT 59230-2699
(406)228-3630
FAX: (406)228-3531

Glendive

Glendive Medical Center
202 Prospect Dr
Glendive, MT 59330-1999
(406)345-3306
FAX: (406)345-3334

Great Falls

Benefis Hospitals South Tower
1101 26th St S
Great Falls, MT 59405-5161
(406)731-8400
FAX: (406)731-8433

Great Falls Clinic Hospital
3000 15th Ave S, Great Falls Clinic Spec Bldg
Great Falls, MT 59405-5240
(406)771-3159
FAX: (406)268-3803

Hamilton

Marcus Daly Memorial Hospital
1200 Westwood Dr
Hamilton, MT 59840-2395
(406)375-4426
FAX: (406)375-4704

Hardin

Big Horn Hospital Association
17 N Miles Ave
Hardin, MT 59034-2323
(406)665-2310
FAX: (406)665-2138

Harlem

Ft. Belknap Center Ihs
669 Agency Main St
Harlem, MT 59526-9455
(406)353-3142
FAX: (406)353-3260

Havre

Northern Montana Hospital
30 13th St
Havre, MT 59501-5222
(406)262-1218
FAX: (406)262-1617

Helena

Helena Imaging Center
25 Medical Park Dr
Helena, MT 59601-4949
(406)442-7227
FAX: (406)442-4863

St. Peter's Health - Mammography Department
2475 E Broadway St
Helena, MT 59601-4928
(406)495-6721
FAX: (406)495-6729

Kalispell

Kalispell Regional Medical Center
310 Sunnyview Ln
Kalispell, MT 59901-3199
(406)751-7523
FAX: (406)752-8390

Logan Health Kalispell
320 Sunnyview Ln
Kalispell, MT 59901-3129
(406)751-9729
FAX: (406)752-8390

Lewistown

Central Montana Medical Center
408 Wendell Ave
Lewistown, MT 59457-2261
(406)535-6205
FAX: (406)535-6335

Libby

Cabinet Peaks Medical Center
209 Health Park Dr
Libby, MT 59923-2001
(406)283-7080
FAX: (406)293-8027

Livingston

Livingston Healthcare
320 Alpenglow Ln
Livingston, MT 59047-8506
(406)823-6441
FAX: (406)823-6449

Miles City

Billings Clinic Miles City
620 S Haynes Ave
Miles City, MT 59301-4769
(406)233-7039
FAX: (406)233-7077

Holy Rosary Healthcare
2600 Wilson St
Miles City, MT 59301-5016
(406)233-2677
FAX: (406)233-2694

Missoula

Advanced Imaging Center
3275 N Reserve St Ste A
Missoula, MT 59808-1562
(406)327-5120
FAX: (406)327-3855

Advanced Imaging Center
2803 South Ave W
Missoula, MT 59804-5103
(406)327-3950
FAX: (406)327-3955

Broadway Imaging Center
500 W Broadway St, Broadway Building
Missoula, MT 59802-4008
(406)329-5757
FAX: (406)327-1715

Broadway Imaging Center - Now Care
2901 Brooks St, Now Care Southgate Mall
Missoula, MT 59801-7703
(406)543-7271
FAX: (406)327-1715

Broadway Imaging Center- Grant Creek
3075 N Reserve St
Missoula, MT 59808-1389
(406)329-5757
FAX: (406)327-1715

Plains

Clark Fork Valley Hospital
10 Kruger Rd
Plains, MT 59859
(406)826-4980
FAX: (406)826-4924

Plentywood

Sheridan Memorial Hospital
440 W Laurel Ave
Plentywood, MT 59254-1596
(406)765-3739
FAX: (406)765-1495

Polson

Providence St. Joseph Medical Center
6 13th Ave E
Polson, MT 59860-5315
(406)883-8402
FAX: (406)883-8244

Red Lodge

Beartooth Billings Clinic
2525 N Broadway Ave
Red Lodge, MT 59068-9222
(406)446-2345
FAX: (406)446-1660

Ronan

St. Luke Community Healthcare
107 6th Ave SW
Ronan, MT 59864-2634
(406)523-5272
FAX: (406)676-0105

Sidney

Sidney Health Center
216 14th Ave SW
Sidney, MT 59270-3586
(406)488-2168
FAX: (406)488-2172

Stevensville

Advanced Imaging
3920 US Highway 93 N, Ste F
Stevensville, MT 59870-6478
(406)327-3950
FAX: (406)327-3955

Superior

Mineral Community Hospital
1208 6th Ave
Superior, MT 59872-9667
(406)822-3705
FAX: (406)822-4961

Whitefish

North Valley Hospital
1600 Hospital Way
Whitefish, MT 59937-2990
(406)863-3576
FAX: (406)863-3676

Wolf Point

Northeast Montana Health Services, Inc.
315 Knapp St
Wolf Point, MT 59201-1826
(406)653-6538
FAX: (406)653-6597

NEBRASKA

Ainsworth

Brown County Hospital
945 E Zero St
Ainsworth, NE 69210-1547
(402)387-2800
FAX: (402)387-2745

Albion

Boone County Health Center
PO Box 151, 723 W Fairview
Albion, NE 68620-0151
(402)395-3137
FAX: (402)395-3119

Alliance

Box Butte General Hospital
2101 Box Butte Ave
Alliance, NE 69301-4444
(308)761-4357
FAX: (308)762-5488

Alma

Harlan County Health System
717 Brown St
Alma, NE 68920-2180
(308)928-3008
FAX: (308)928-2816

Atkinson

West Holt Memorial Hospital
406 W Neely St
Atkinson, NE 68713-5112
(402)925-2811
FAX: (402)925-5230

Auburn

Nemaha County Hospital 2022 13th Auburn Ne 68305
2022 13th St
Auburn, NE 68305-1701
(402)274-6127
FAX: (402)274-4399

Aurora

Memorial Hospital
1423 7th St
Aurora, NE 68818-1197
(402)694-8258
FAX: (402)694-3177

Bassett

Rock County Hospital
102 E South St
Bassett, NE 68714-5512
(402)684-3908
FAX: (402)684-2607

Beatrice

Beatrice Community Hospital & Health Center
4800 Hospital Pkwy
Beatrice, NE 68310-6906
(402)228-3344
FAX: (402)223-6531

Bellevue

Nebraska Medicine Bellevue
2500 Bellevue Medical Center Dr
Bellevue, NE 68123-1591
(402)763-3200
FAX: (402)763-3198

Benkelman

Dundy County Hospital
1313 N Cheyenne St
Benkelman, NE 69021-3074
(308)423-7009
FAX: (308)423-5749

Blair

Memorial Community Hospital
810 N 22nd St
Blair, NE 68008-1199
(402)426-1166
FAX: (402)426-1483

Broken Bow

Jennie M. Melham Memorial Medical Center
145 Memorial Dr
Broken Bow, NE 68822-1378
(308)872-4138
FAX: (308)872-4183

Callaway

Callaway District Hospital
211 E Kimball St
Callaway, NE 68825-2597
(308)836-2228
FAX: (308)836-2380

Cambridge

Tri Valley Health System
1305 Highway 6 34
Cambridge, NE 69022-6616
(308)697-3329
FAX: (308)697-3204

Central City

Merrick Medical Center
PO Box 417
Central City, NE 68826-0417
(308)946-3015
FAX: (308)946-5536

Chadron

Chadron Community Hosp And Health Services
825 Centennial Dr
Chadron, NE 69337-9400
(308)432-5586
FAX: (308)432-0269

Columbus

Columbus Community Hospital
PO Box 1800, 4600 38th St
Columbus, NE 68602-1800
(402)562-3180
FAX: (402)562-3187

Cozad

Cozad Community Hospital
300 E 12th St
Cozad, NE 69130-1532
(308)784-2261
FAX: (308)784-2218

Creighton

Avera Creighton Hospital
1503 Main St
Creighton, NE 68729-3019
(402)358-5700
FAX: (402)358-5707

Crete

Crete Area Medical Center
2910 Betten Dr
Crete, NE 68333-3084
(402)826-6579
FAX: (402)826-7955

David City

Butler County Health Care Center
372 S 9th St
David City, NE 68632-2116
(402)367-1235
FAX: (855)681-8976

Elkhorn

Methodist Health System Imaging Services
717 N 190th Plz Ste 2300, 717 Medical Office Building
Elkhorn, NE 68022-3985
(402)354-4001
FAX: (402)815-1070

Fairbury

Jefferson Community Health & Life
2200 H St
Fairbury, NE 68352-1119
(402)729-3351
FAX: (402)729-3917

Falls City

Community Medical Center, Inc.
3307 Barada St
Falls City, NE 68355-2470
(402)245-6556
FAX: (402)245-6639

Fremont

Methodist Fremont Health
450 E 23rd St
Fremont, NE 68025-2387
(402)727-3731
FAX: (402)727-3513

Geneva

Fillmore County Hospital
1900 F St
Geneva, NE 68361-2229
(402)759-3252
FAX: (402)759-4656

Gordon

Gordon Memorial Health Services
300 E 8th St
Gordon, NE 69343-1123
(308)282-0401
FAX: (308)282-6237

Gothenburg

Gothenburg Health
910 20th St
Gothenburg, NE 69138-1253
(308)537-3661
FAX: (308)537-4040

Grand Island

Chi Health St. Francis
2620 W Faidley Ave, Department Of Radiology
Grand Island, NE 68803-4205
(308)398-5674
FAX: (308)398-5353

Grand Island Regional Medical Center
3533 Prairieview St
Grand Island, NE 68803-4409
(308)675-5000
FAX: (308)675-5212

Mary Lanning Healthcare
1010 N Diers Ave Ste 3B
Grand Island, NE 68803-4906
(308)398-1712
FAX: (308)398-1715

Grant

Perkins County Health Services
900 Lincoln Ave
Grant, NE 69140-3128
(308)352-7233
FAX: (308)352-7299

Hastings

Family Medical Center Of Hastings
1021 W 14th St
Hastings, NE 68901-3046
(402)463-2423
FAX: (402)463-9697

Hastings Medical Imaging
2207 Osborne Dr W Ste 200
Hastings, NE 68901-9111
(402)462-4070
FAX: (402)461-8460

Hebron

Thayer County Health Services
120 Park Ave
Hebron, NE 68370-2019
(402)768-7203
FAX: (402)768-4647

Henderson

Henderson Health Care Services Inc.
1621 Front St
Henderson, NE 68371-8902
(402)723-4512
FAX: (402)723-4493

Holdrege

Phelps Memorial Health Center
1215 Tibbals St
Holdrege, NE 68949-1261
(308)995-2891
FAX: (308)995-2892

Imperial

Chase County Community Hospital
PO Box 819, 600 W 12th St
Imperial, NE 69033-0819
(308)882-7240
FAX: (308)882-7280

Kearney

Chi Health Good Samaritan
10 E 31st St
Kearney, NE 68847-2908
(308)865-7559
FAX: (308)865-2721

Contemporary Obstetrics And Gynecology, P.C.
101 W 24th St, Ste 1
Kearney, NE 68847-5358
(308)865-2740
FAX: (308)865-2747

Kearney Regional Medical Center
804 22nd Ave
Kearney, NE 68845-2206
(308)455-8346
FAX: (308)455-3968

La Vista

Medical Imaging Consultants, P.C.
7950 Harrison St
La Vista, NE 68128-2912
(402)592-0711
FAX: (402)934-9242

Lexington

Lexington Regional Health Center
1201 N Erie St
Lexington, NE 68850-1560
(308)324-8346
FAX: (308)324-8328

Lincoln

Advanced Medical Imaging
7601 Pioneers Blvd
Lincoln, NE 68506-4675
(402)484-6677
FAX: (402)484-4802

Bryan Medical Center, Bryan West Campus
2300 S 16th St
Lincoln, NE 68502-3704
(402)481-5121
FAX: (402)481-5177

Bryan Medical Center, Pine Lake Campus
3901 Pine Lake Rd Ste 110
Lincoln, NE 68516-5497
(402)481-5121
FAX: (402)481-5177

Bryan Medical Plaza Radiology Department
1500 S 48th St
Lincoln, NE 68506-1276
(402)481-5121
FAX: (402)481-5177

Chi Health St. Elizabeth
555 S 70th St
Lincoln, NE 68510-2462
(402)219-7895
FAX: (402)219-8964

Women's Clinic Of Lincoln, P.C.
200 Lyncrest Dr
Lincoln, NE 68510-2229
(402)434-3385
FAX: (402)489-0249

McCook

Community Hospital
1301 E H St
McCook, NE 69001-3498
(308)344-8285
FAX: (308)344-8283

Minden

Kearney County Health Services
727 E 1st St
Minden, NE 68959-1705
(308)832-3400
FAX: (308)832-3419

Nebraska City

Chi Health St. Mary's
PO Box 70, 1301 Grundman Blvd
Nebraska City, NE 68410-0070
(402)873-8912
FAX: (402)873-8949

Neligh

Antelope Memorial Hospital
PO Box 229, 102 W 9th St
Neligh, NE 68756-0229
(402)887-6269
FAX: (402)887-6360

Norfolk

Faith Regional Health Services
2700 W Norfolk Ave
Norfolk, NE 68701-4438
(402)644-7121
FAX: (402)644-7612

Faith Regional Health Services South
2701 W Norfolk Ave
Norfolk, NE 68701-4407
(402)844-8074
FAX: (402)644-7612

Midwest Health Partners
1410 N 13th St
Norfolk, NE 68701-2669
(402)379-2322
FAX: (402)379-0888

North Platte

Great Plains Health Imaging Center
1101 S Oak St
North Platte, NE 69101-6522
(308)568-7951
FAX: (308)568-7959

Oakland

Mercyone Oakland Medical Center
601 E 2nd St
Oakland, NE 68045-1400
(402)685-7513
FAX: (402)685-7578

Offutt Afb

Ehrling Bergquist Clinic
55th Medical Group Acc, Radiology Dept.
Offutt Afb, NE 68113
(402)294-7405
FAX: (402)294-8644

Ogallala

Ogallala Community Hospital
2601 N Spruce St
Ogallala, NE 69153-2471
(308)284-7221
FAX: (308)284-7224

Omaha

Chi Health Creighton University Medical Center-Bergan Mercy
7500 Mercy Rd, Radiology Department
Omaha, NE 68124-2319
(402)717-2222
FAX: (402)398-6636

Chi Health Immanuel
6901 N 72nd St
Omaha, NE 68122-1709
(402)572-2339
FAX: (402)572-2504

Chi Health Lakeside Hospital
16901 Lakeside Hills Ct
Omaha, NE 68130-2318
(402)717-2222
FAX: (402)717-8150

Methodist Breast Care Center
8303 Dodge St Ste 302
Omaha, NE 68114-4108
(402)354-4001
FAX: (402)354-3211

Methodist Physicians Clinic Indian Hills Imaging Center
8901 W Dodge Rd, Ste 200
Omaha, NE 68114-3321
(402)354-4001
FAX: (402)354-0950

Methodist Physicians Clinic Regency
10060 Regency Cir
Omaha, NE 68114-3732
(402)354-1430
FAX: (402)354-1585

Mhs Mobile
8303 Dodge St, Methodist Hospital, Mecc Suite 302
Omaha, NE 68114-4108
(402)354-4001
FAX: (402)354-3211

Nebraska Medicine
44th And Emile, Rm 4699 University Tower
Omaha, NE 68198-3265
(402)559-1046
FAX: (402)559-1146

Nebraska Medicine At Village Pointe
111 N 175th St
Omaha, NE 68118-3579
(402)552-3019
FAX: (402)552-3019

Think Aksarben, Llc
7100 W Center Rd
Omaha, NE 68106-2714
(402)506-9000
FAX: (402)506-9001

Oneill

Avera St Anthony's Hospital
300 N 2nd St
Oneill, NE 68763-1514
(402)336-2611
FAX: (402)336-5117

Ord

Valley County Health System
2707 L St
Ord, NE 68862-1665
(308)728-4249
FAX: (308)728-3228

Osceola

Annie Jeffrey Memorial County Health Center
531 Beebe St
Osceola, NE 68651-5537
(402)747-2031
FAX: (402)747-1441

Papillion

Chi Health Midlands
11111 S 84th St
Papillion, NE 68046-4122
(402)717-2222
FAX: (402)593-3812

Pawnee City

Pawnee County Memorial Hospital
600 I St
Pawnee City, NE 68420-3001
(402)852-0303
FAX: (402)852-0313

Pender

Pender Community Hospital
PO Box 100, 100 Hospital Dr
Pender, NE 68047-0100
(402)385-4069
FAX: (402)385-4094

Schuyler

Chi Health Schuyler
104 W 17th St
Schuyler, NE 68661-1304
(402)352-4052
FAX: (402)352-4082

Scottsbluff

Regional West Medical Center
3911 Avenue B Ste 3200
Scottsbluff, NE 69361-4617
(308)630-2700
FAX: (308)630-1923

Seward

Memorial Health Care Systems
300 N Columbia Ave
Seward, NE 68434-2228
(402)643-2971
FAX: (402)646-4671

Sidney

Sidney Regional Medical Center
1000 Pole Creek Xing
Sidney, NE 69162-2901
(308)254-5825
FAX: (308)254-4886

St Paul

Howard County Medical Center
PO Box 406, 1113 Sherman
St Paul, NE 68873-0406
(308)754-4421
FAX: (308)754-2309

Superior

Brodstone Memorial Hospital
520 E 10th St, Radiology Department
Superior, NE 68978-1225
(402)879-4432
FAX: (402)879-3503

Syracuse

Syracuse Area Health
2731 Healthcare Dr
Syracuse, NE 68446-7880
(402)269-7590
FAX: (402)269-3132

Tecumseh

Johnson County Hospital
202 High St
Tecumseh, NE 68450-2443
(402)335-6345
FAX: (402)335-6358

Valentine

Cherry County Hospital
510 N Green St
Valentine, NE 69201-1932
(402)376-2525
FAX: (402)376-3288

Wahoo

Saunders Medical Center
1760 County Road J
Wahoo, NE 68066-4152
(402)443-1424
FAX: (402)443-1434

Wayne

Providence Medical Center
1200 Providence Rd
Wayne, NE 68787-1299
(402)375-3800
FAX: (402)375-7650

West Point

St. Francis Memorial Hospital
430 N Monitor St
West Point, NE 68788-1595
(402)372-6735
FAX: (402)372-6758

Winnebago

Twelve Clans Unity Hospital-Wchs
225 South Bluff St
Winnebago, NE 68071
(402)878-3487
FAX: (402)878-2695

York

York General Healthcare Services
2222 N Lincoln Ave
York, NE 68467-1095
(402)362-6671
FAX: (402)362-0405

NEVADA

Boulder City

Center For Diagnostics
895 Adams Blvd
Boulder City, NV 89005-2235
(702)293-0406
FAX: (702)293-0192

Carson City

Carson Tahoe Breast Center
1400 Medical Pkwy
Carson City, NV 89703-4624
(775)445-5500
FAX: (775)885-8568

Elko

High Desert Imaging
976 Mountain City Hwy, Ste 100
Elko, NV 89801-2728
(775)621-5800
FAX: (775)621-5801

Northeastern Nevada Regional Hospital
2001 Errecart Blvd
Elko, NV 89801-8333
(775)748-2243
FAX: (775)748-2031

Ely

William Bee Ririe Hospital
1500 Avenue H
Ely, NV 89301-2699
(775)289-3467
FAX: (775)289-6392

Fallon

Banner Churchill Community Hospital
801 E Williams Ave
Fallon, NV 89406-3052
(775)867-7150
FAX: (775)423-7390

Gardnerville

Carson Valley Medical Center
1107 US Highway 395 N
Gardnerville, NV 89410-5304
(775)782-1533
FAX: (775)782-1543

Henderson

Desert Radiology - Horizon Ridge
2811 W Horizon Ridge Pkwy
Henderson, NV 89052-4394
(702)759-8600
FAX: (702)616-3563

Pueblo Medical Imaging
100 N Green Valley Pkwy Ste 130
Henderson, NV 89074-6392
(702)228-0031
FAX: (702)228-7253

Smi Imaging , Llc - Henderson
6301 Mountain Vista St, Ste 103
Henderson, NV 89014-2365
(702)433-7216
FAX: (702)433-7298

Southwest Medical
2845 Siena Heights Dr, Ste 1100
Henderson, NV 89052-4161
(702)877-5390
FAX: (702)878-3614

Southwest Medical
3175 Saint Rose Pkwy Ste 200
Henderson, NV 89052-3507
(702)877-5390
FAX: (702)878-3614

St. Rose Dominican Hospital Siena Campus
3001 Saint Rose Pkwy
Henderson, NV 89052-3839
(702)616-5585
FAX: (702)616-5488

Steinberg Diagnostic Medical Imaging
4 Sunset Way Ste D
Henderson, NV 89014-2016
(702)240-1232
FAX: (702)243-7531

Steinberg Diagnostic Medical Imaging
2850 Siena Heights Dr
Henderson, NV 89052-4154
(702)732-6000
FAX: (702)732-6035

Steinberg Diagnostic Medical Imaging Centers
800 N Gibson Rd Ste 110
Henderson, NV 89011-1706
(702)732-6000
FAX: (702)243-7531

Las Vegas

Desert Radiologist-Nellis
31 N Nellis Blvd
Las Vegas, NV 89110-5330
(702)835-4950
FAX: (702)794-2143

Desert Radiologists - Cathedral Rock
7200 Cathedral Rock Dr Ste 230
Las Vegas, NV 89128-0441
(702)387-6900
FAX: (702)256-2253

Desert Radiologists - Eastern
3920 S Eastern Ave Ste 100
Las Vegas, NV 89119-5171
(702)387-6900
FAX: (702)794-2143

Desert Radiologists - Palomino
2020 Palomino Ln Ste 100
Las Vegas, NV 89106-4894
(702)759-8720
FAX: (702)598-3439

Desert Radiology Centra Point
6675 South Cimarron Road, Suite 105
Las Vegas, NV 89113
(702)759-4433
FAX: (702)912-4220

Desert Radiology South Rainbow
3025 S Rainbow Blvd
Las Vegas, NV 89146-6582
(702)759-8600
FAX: (702)333-4893

Las Vegas Radiology
7500 Smoke Ranch Rd Ste 100
Las Vegas, NV 89128-0373
(702)254-5004
FAX: (702)405-8435

Mike O'Callaghan Military Medical Center, Nellis Afb Nv
4700 Las Vegas Blvd N, 99th Medical Group Msgs/Sgcr
Las Vegas, NV 89191-6600
(702)653-2150
FAX: (702)653-2515

Nevada Health Centers Mammovan-Mobile
1799 Mount Mariah Dr
Las Vegas, NV 89106-1501
(887)581-6266
FAX: (702)220-3679

Pueblo Medical Imaging
2628 W Charleston Blvd Ste B
Las Vegas, NV 89102-2176
(702)228-0031
FAX: (702)228-7253

Pueblo Medical Imaging
5495 S Rainbow Blvd Ste 101
Las Vegas, NV 89118-1872
(702)228-0031
FAX: (702)228-7253

Pueblo Medical Imaging
8551 W Lake Mead Blvd Ste 150
Las Vegas, NV 89128-7649
(702)228-0031
FAX: (702)228-7253

Red Rock Radiology A Department Of Mountainview Hosp.
7130 Smoke Ranch Rd
Las Vegas, NV 89128-3157
(702)962-7775
FAX: (877)330-0432

Smi Imaging , Llc - Centennial
7540 Oso Blanca Rd Ste 140
Las Vegas, NV 89149-1417
(702)658-4300
FAX: (702)436-5459

Smi Imaging , Llc - Flamingo
3560 E Flamingo Rd Ste 100
Las Vegas, NV 89121-5088
(702)433-6100
FAX: (702)433-9489

Smi Imaging , Llc Dba Simonmed Imaging - Southwest
8530 W Sunset Rd, Ste 120
Las Vegas, NV 89113-2244
(702)522-8780
FAX: (702)436-5453

Smi Imaging, Llc - Summerlin
7455 W Washington Ave, Ste 120
Las Vegas, NV 89128-4338
(702)433-6455
FAX: (702)433-6508

Southern Hills Medical Center
9300 W Sunset Rd
Las Vegas, NV 89148-4844
(702)916-7282
FAX: (702)880-2951

Southwest Medical
540 N Nellis Blvd
Las Vegas, NV 89110-5368
(702)877-5390
FAX: (702)878-3614

Southwest Medical
4835 S Durango Dr
Las Vegas, NV 89147-8171
(702)877-5390
FAX: (702)878-3614

Southwest Medical
2300 W Charleston Blvd
Las Vegas, NV 89102-2149
(702)877-5286
FAX: (702)878-3614

Southwest Medical
4750 W Oakey Blvd
Las Vegas, NV 89102-1535
(702)877-5390
FAX: (702)878-3614

Southwest Medical
2704 N Tenaya Way
Las Vegas, NV 89128-0424
(702)877-5390
FAX: (702)878-3614

Southwest Medical
10105 Banburry Cross Dr Ste 150
Las Vegas, NV 89144-6647
(702)877-5390
FAX: (702)878-3614

Southwest Medical
4475 S Eastern Ave
Las Vegas, NV 89119-7826
(702)877-5286
FAX: (702)877-5259

Southwest Medical - Mobile
2704 N Tenaya Way
Las Vegas, NV 89128-0424
(702)877-5390
FAX: (702)878-3614

Steinberg Diagnostic Medical Imaging
2767 N Tenaya Way
Las Vegas, NV 89128-0425
(702)732-6000
FAX: (702)243-7531

Steinberg Diagnostic Medical Imaging
9070 W Post Rd
Las Vegas, NV 89148-2419
(702)240-1232
FAX: (702)243-7531

Steinberg Diagnostic Medical Imaging
2950 S Maryland Pkwy
Las Vegas, NV 89109-2257
(702)240-1232
FAX: (702)243-7531

Steinberg Diagnostic Medical Imaging
6925 N Durango Dr
Las Vegas, NV 89149-4410
(702)732-6000
FAX: (702)243-7531

Steinberg Diagnostic Medical Imaging Centers
800 Shadow Ln
Las Vegas, NV 89106-4123
(702)732-6000
FAX: (702)243-7531

Summerlin Hospital Medical Center
657 N Town Center Dr
Las Vegas, NV 89144-6367
(702)233-7337
FAX: (702)233-7340

Sunrise Hospital And Medical Center
3006 S Maryland Pkwy Ste 250
Las Vegas, NV 89109-6213
(702)961-7250
FAX: (702)961-7248

Mesquite

Mesa View Regional Hospital
1299 Bertha Howe Ave
Mesquite, NV 89027-7500
(702)345-4265
FAX: (702)345-4221

Minden

Carson-Tahoe Imaging
925 Ironwood Dr Ste 1106
Minden, NV 89423-5179
(775)445-5500
FAX: (775)888-4444

N Las Vegas

Steinberg Diagnostic Medical Imaging
1650 W Craig Rd
N Las Vegas, NV 89032-0219
(702)732-6000
FAX: (702)243-7531

Pahrump

Dvh Hospital Alliance, Llc
360 S Lola Ln
Pahrump, NV 89048-0884
(775)751-7567
FAX: (775)751-7555

Reno

Reno Diagnostic Center
590 Eureka Ave
Reno, NV 89512-3425
(775)323-5083
FAX: (775)785-8731

Reno Diagnostic Centers
625 Sierra Rose Dr
Reno, NV 89511-2060
(775)323-5083
FAX: (775)785-8731

Renown Breast Health Center
901 E 2nd St Ste 103
Reno, NV 89502-1176
(775)982-4186
FAX: (775)982-4803

Renown Health X-Ray And Imaging Services At South McCarran
6630 S McCarran Blvd, Ste 27
Reno, NV 89509-6186
(775)982-8100
FAX: (775)982-6690

Saint Mary's Medical Group Inc
411 W 6th St
Reno, NV 89503-4415
(775)770-3187
FAX: (775)770-7310

Saint Mary's Medical Group, Inc.
411 W 6th St
Reno, NV 89503-4415
(775)770-3187
FAX: (775)770-7310

Saint Mary's Outpatient Imaging Center
645 N Arlington Ave Ste 250
Reno, NV 89503-4442
(775)770-3546
FAX: (775)770-3371

Sparks

Northern Nevada Med. Ctr - Diagnostic Breast Care Ctr
2385 E Prater Way Ste 107
Sparks, NV 89434-9663
(775)356-5800
FAX: (775)356-6161

Renown Imaging And X-Ray At Vista
910 Vista Blvd
Sparks, NV 89434-6501
(775)982-5585
FAX: (775)982-5104

Winnemucca

Humboldt General Hospital
118 E Haskell St
Winnemucca, NV 89445-3299
(775)623-5222
FAX: (775)625-8532

NEW HAMPSHIRE

Bedford

Catholic Medical Center Breast Care Center
9 Washington Pl Ste 203
Bedford, NH 03110-6750
(603)663-5270
FAX: (603)663-5342

Derry Medical Center,Pa Dba Derry Imaging Center At Bedford
160 S River Rd Ste 2100
Bedford, NH 03110-6927
(603)537-1363
FAX: (603)537-1324

Southern New Hampshire Radiology Consultants, Pc
703 Riverway Pl
Bedford, NH 03110-6768
(603)627-1663
FAX: (603)669-6944

Berlin

Androscoggin Valley Hospital
59 Page Hill Rd
Berlin, NH 03570-3542
(603)326-5720
FAX: (603)326-5732

Claremont

Valley Regional Hospital
243 Elm St
Claremont, NH 03743-4999
(603)542-3478
FAX: (603)542-1820

Colebrook

Upper Connecticut Valley Hospital
181 Corliss Ln
Colebrook, NH 03576-3207
(603)388-4231
FAX: (603)388-4141

Concord

Concord Imaging At Horseshoe Pond
60 Commercial St Ste 101
Concord, NH 03301-5096
(603)415-9444
FAX: (603)415-9440

Concord Imaging Center
248 Pleasant St Ste 102
Concord, NH 03301-7562
(603)225-0425
FAX: (603)224-9933

Dartmouth-Hitchcock Clinic - Concord
253 Pleasant St
Concord, NH 03301-2593
(603)229-5060
FAX: (603)229-5058

Derry

Derry Medical Center, Pa Dba Derry Imaging Center
6 Tsienneto Rd Ste 100LL
Derry, NH 03038-1584
(603)537-1375
FAX: (603)537-1324

Dover

New England Mammography
770 Central Ave
Dover, NH 03820-3469
(603)742-0101
FAX: (603)743-3171

Exeter

Exeter Hospital
5 Alumni Dr
Exeter, NH 03833-2160
(603)580-6867
FAX: (603)580-7024

Franklin

Concord Hospital-Franklin
15 Aiken Ave, Mammography Department
Franklin, NH 03235-1259
(603)934-2060
FAX: (603)934-1468

Keene

The Cheshire Medical Center
580 Court St
Keene, NH 03431-1729
(603)354-5454
FAX: (603)354-6831

Laconia

Concord Hospital Obgyn - Laconia
734 N Main St
Laconia, NH 03246-2777
(603)527-1855
FAX: (603)527-1872

Concord Hospital- Laconia
80 Highland St
Laconia, NH 03246-3235
(603)527-2992
FAX: (603)527-2943

Lancaster

Weeks Medical Center
173 Middle St
Lancaster, NH 03584-3508
(603)788-5011
FAX: (603)788-5062

Lebanon

Alice Peck Day Memorial Hospital
10 Alice Peck Day Dr
Lebanon, NH 03766-2650
(603)448-7486
FAX: (603)443-9561

Dartmouth Hitchcock Medical Center
1 Medical Center Dr
Lebanon, NH 03756-0001
(603)650-8260
FAX: (603)727-7821

Littleton

Littleton Regional Healthcare
600 Saint Johnsbury Rd
Littleton, NH 03561-3443
(603)444-9536
FAX: (603)444-2343

Londonderry

Elliot Imaging Center At Londonderry
40 Buttrick Rd
Londonderry, NH 03053-3381
(603)663-2180
FAX: (603)552-1489

Manchester

Dartmouth Hitchcock Manchester
100 Hitchcock Way
Manchester, NH 03104-4125
(603)695-2850
FAX: (603)695-2856

Elliot Breast Imaging Center At River's Edge
185 Queen City Ave
Manchester, NH 03101-7121
(603)663-8487
FAX: (603)663-8494

Senior Health Radiology
138 Webster St
Manchester, NH 03104-2512
(603)663-2180
FAX: (603)663-7028

Milford

St. Joseph Hospital - Milford Campus Milford Nh
442 Nashua St
Milford, NH 03055-4915
(603)595-5700
FAX: (603)578-5004

Nashua

Dartmouth Hitchcock - Nashua
2300 Southwood Dr
Nashua, NH 03063-1899
(603)577-4070
FAX: (603)577-4090

Denicola Breast Health Center
PO Box 2014, 8 Prospect St
Nashua, NH 03061-2014
(603)577-2830
FAX: (603)577-2649

St Joseph Hospital
172 Kinsley St
Nashua, NH 03060-3688
(603)595-5700
FAX: (603)578-5004

New London

New London Hospital
273 County Rd
New London, NH 03257-7700
(603)526-5249
FAX: (603)526-5394

Newport

Newport Health Center
11 John Stark Hwy
Newport, NH 03773-1807
(603)863-4100
FAX: (603)863-3585

North Conway

Memorial Hospital
3073 White Mountain Hwy
North Conway, NH 03860-7101
(603)356-5461
FAX: (603)356-8880

Peterborough

Monadnock Community Hospital
452 Old Street Rd
Peterborough, NH 03458-1295
(603)924-4699
FAX: (603)924-1715

Plaistow

Exeter Hospital
127 Plaistow Rd
Plaistow, NH 03865-2811
(603)580-6035
FAX: (603)580-7024

Plymouth

Speare Memorial Hospital
16 Hospital Rd
Plymouth, NH 03264-1199
(603)238-2141
FAX: (603)536-5063

Portsmouth

The Breast Center At Portsmouth Regional Hospital
155 Borthwick Ave, Ste 101 West
Portsmouth, NH 03801-7156
(603)559-4190
FAX: (603)957-5479

Wentworth-Douglass Hospital Breast Health Center
67 Corporate Dr, Bldg A
Portsmouth, NH 03801-2847
(603)742-6673
FAX: (603)742-6757

Salem

Salem Radiology A Department Of Parkland Medical Center
31 Stiles Rd Ste 1200
Salem, NH 03079-2958
(603)890-2813
FAX: (603)890-2831

Somersworth

Women's Life Imaging Center
200 Route 108 Ste 3
Somersworth, NH 03878-1117
(603)742-6673
FAX: (603)742-6757

Windham

Derry Medical Center Dba Derry Imaging Center At Windham
49 Range Rd Ste 103
Windham, NH 03087-2029
(603)537-1363
FAX: (603)537-1324

Wolfeboro

Huggins Hospital
240 S Main St, Radiology Department
Wolfeboro, NH 03894-4455
(603)569-7529
FAX: (603)569-7531

Woodsville

Cottage Hospital
90 Swiftwater Rd
Woodsville, NH 03785-1446
(603)747-9213
FAX: (603)747-2953

NEW JERSEY

Annandale

Hunterdon Radiological Associates Pa
1 Dogwood Dr.
Annandale, NJ 08801
(908)237-5395
FAX: (908)735-6532

Atlantic City

Atlanticare Regional Medical Center - City Division
1925 Pacific Ave
Atlantic City, NJ 08401-6713
(609)383-2800
FAX: (609)572-8356

Avenel

Njin Of Woodbridge
1500 Saint Georges Ave
Avenel, NJ 07001-1000
(732)574-1414
FAX: (732)574-0845

Basking Ridge

Memorial Sloan Kettering Cancer Center Basking Ridge
136 Mountainview Blvd
Basking Ridge, NJ 07920-3444
(908)542-3000
FAX: (908)542-3211

Bayonne

Bayonne Medical Center
29 E 29th St
Bayonne, NJ 07002-4695
(201)858-6572
FAX: (201)858-5303

New Jersey Imaging Network Of Bayonne
519 Broadway
Bayonne, NJ 07002-3713
(201)608-6250
FAX: (201)608-6260

Bedminster

University Radiology Group, P.C.
1 Robertson Dr, Ste 16
Bedminster, NJ 07921-1716
(732)955-8820
FAX: (908)470-3680

Belleville

New Jersey Imaging Network Of Belleville
36 Newark Ave Ste 100
Belleville, NJ 07109-4120
(973)844-4170
FAX: (973)844-4192

Berkeley Hts

Summit Medical Group, P.A.
1 Diamond Hill Rd
Berkeley Hts, NJ 07922-2104
(908)988-2287
FAX: (908)277-8774

Brick

Atlantic Medical Imaging Women's Imaging Center
495 Jack Martin Blvd
Brick, NJ 08724-7778
(732)840-6500
FAX: (732)840-6459

Womens Imaging Pavilion At Ocean Medical Center
425 Jack Martin Blvd
Brick, NJ 08724-7732
(732)836-4083
FAX: (732)206-8387

Bridgeton

Atlantic Medical Imaging
1119 Highway 77 Bldg 2
Bridgeton, NJ 08302-3620
(856)453-1555
FAX: (856)453-0255

Bridgewater

Hunterdon Advanced Imaging At Bridgewater
1121 US Highway 22, Ste 103
Bridgewater, NJ 08807-2982
(908)782-4700
FAX: (908)284-5222

Regional Women's Health Group, Llc - Bridgewater
215 Union Ave
Bridgewater, NJ 08807-3063
(908)722-2900
FAX: (908)722-1856

University Radiology Group, P.C.
33 Monroe St
Bridgewater, NJ 08807-3043
(908)725-1291
FAX: (908)725-8335

Camden

Cooper Breast Imaging Center At MD Anderson
2 Cooper Plz, 400 Haddon Ave Suite C1104
Camden, NJ 08103-1461
(856)342-2380
FAX: (856)735-6412

Cooper University Radiology At 3 Cooper Plaza
3 Cooper Plz Rm 100
Camden, NJ 08103-1407
(856)342-2380
FAX: (856)968-8265

Virtua Our Lady Of Lourdes Hospital
1600 Haddon Ave
Camden, NJ 08103-3117
(877)277-8547
FAX: (856)365-7971

Cape May Court House

Aims Diagnostic Imaging Of South Jersey, Llc
13 Mechanic St 15
Cape May Court House, NJ 08210-4221
(609)465-7800
FAX: (609)465-4419

Atlantic Medical Imaging
421 Route 9 N
Cape May Court House, NJ 08210-1960
(609)677-9729
FAX: (609)465-0918

Cape Radiology Cmch
223 N Main St Ste 103
Cape May Court House, NJ 08210-2182
(609)463-2273
FAX: (609)778-2358

Cherry Hill

Cooper University Radiology At Kings Highway
1103 Kings Hwy N Ste 103
Cherry Hill, NJ 08034-1983
(856)348-6110
FAX: (856)482-0398

Jefferson Health Cherry Hill
2201 Chapel Ave W
Cherry Hill, NJ 08002-2048
(856)406-4100
FAX: (856)488-6419

Penn Medicine Cherry Hill
1865 Marlton Pike E
Cherry Hill, NJ 08003-2005
(856)433-2768
FAX: (856)528-5221

South Jersey Radiology Associates
315 Marlton Pike E, Ste B
Cherry Hill, NJ 08034-2408
(856)428-4344
FAX: (856)428-0356

Virtua Health And Wellness - Cherry Hill
1 Brace Rd
Cherry Hill, NJ 08034-2600
(877)277-8547
FAX: (856)824-3051

Clark

Atlantic Imaging Services At Clark
140 Central Ave, Ste 600
Clark, NJ 07066-1121
(732)943-5030
FAX: (732)943-5031

Clifton

Allwood Imaging Pa
914 Clifton Ave
Clifton, NJ 07013-2708
(973)777-5022
FAX: (973)594-4769

Njin Of Clifton
1339 Broad St
Clifton, NJ 07013-4219
(973)778-9600
FAX: (973)778-4846

St. Joseph's Regional Med. Ctr. Ambulatory Imaging Ctr.
1135 Broad St
Clifton, NJ 07013-3346
(973)569-6300
FAX: (973)569-6301

Colts Neck

Jacqueline M Wilentz Comp. Breast Ctr At Colts Neck
310 Rte 34 2nd Fl
Colts Neck, NJ 07722
(732)923-7700
FAX: (732)923-7710

Cranford

Njin Of Cranford
25 S Union Ave
Cranford, NJ 07016-2843
(908)709-1323
FAX: (908)709-1329

Denville

Denville Diagnostics
161 E Main St
Denville, NJ 07834-2647
(973)586-1212
FAX: (973)586-6555

Dover

Breast Health Center At Rockaway
333 Mount Hope Avenue, Suite 130
Dover, NJ 07801
(973)895-6609
FAX: (973)895-5381

Saint Clare's Hospital/Dover General
400 W Blackwell St
Dover, NJ 07801-2599
(973)537-5665
FAX: (973)537-5660

East Brunswick

Regional Women's Health Group, Llc - East Brunswick
620 Cranbury Rd, Ste 206
East Brunswick, NJ 08816-4000
(732)967-0033
FAX: (877)932-1244

University Radiology Group, P.C.
483 Cranbury Rd
East Brunswick, NJ 08816-3610
(732)390-0033
FAX: (732)390-5383

East Orange

East Orange General Hospital
300 Central Ave
East Orange, NJ 07018-2897
(973)266-4415
FAX: (973)266-8482

East Windsor

Penn Med. Princeton Med.Ctr. Breast Health Center
300B Princeton Hightstown Rd Ste 102, East Windsor Medical Commons 2
East Windsor, NJ 08520-1400
(609)688-2700
FAX: (609)688-2701

Windsor Radiology, Llc
300 Princeton Hightstown Rd Ste 101, Building A
East Windsor, NJ 08520-1411
(609)426-9200
FAX: (609)426-9211

Edison

Jfk University Medical Center Breast Center
60 James St
Edison, NJ 08820-3988
(732)321-7540
FAX: (732)321-7544

Njin Of Edison
3830 Park Ave
Edison, NJ 08820-2562
(732)494-9061
FAX: (732)494-5960

University Radiology Group
3900 Park Ave
Edison, NJ 08820-3032
(732)548-6800
FAX: (732)548-6920

Egg Harbor Township

Atlantic Medical Imaging
6529 Black Horse Pike
Egg Harbor Township, NJ 08234-4509
(609)646-6102
FAX: (609)646-5469

Elizabeth

Trinitas Regional Medical Center
225 Williamson St
Elizabeth, NJ 07202-3625
(908)994-5196
FAX: (908)994-5118

Union County Healthcare Associates, MD Urgent Care
637 Westfield Ave
Elizabeth, NJ 07208-1325
(732)381-3740
FAX: (732)215-4344

University Radiology At Trinitas, Llc
415 Morris Ave
Elizabeth, NJ 07208-3612
(908)351-7600
FAX: (908)351-4406

Elmer

Inspira Health Network
501 Front St
Elmer, NJ 08318-2101
(856)363-1550
FAX: (856)358-0762

Emerson

Advanced Medical Img. Of Englewood Hosp & Med. Ctr
452 Old Hook Rd, Ste 301
Emerson, NJ 07630-1391
(201)894-3146
FAX: (201)608-2413

Englewood

Bergen Imaging Center, P.A.
180 N Dean St, Ste 3S
Englewood, NJ 07631-2541
(201)568-4242
FAX: (201)568-1298

Leslie Simon Breast Care And Cytodiagnosis Center
350 Engle St, 4th Fl Berrie Bldg
Englewood, NJ 07631-1808
(201)894-3000
FAX: (201)608-2413

Englewood Cliffs

New Jersey Imaging Network Of Englewood
401 Sylvan Ave
Englewood Cliffs, NJ 07632-2703
(201)541-5401
FAX: (201)541-5400

Englishtown

Princeton Radiology Associates
176 US Highway 9 1st Fl, Northpoint Bldg.
Englishtown, NJ 07726-9218
(732)577-2750
FAX: (732)536-0805

Fair Lawn

Denville Diagnostic Imaging & Open Mri, Llc
20-100 28th Street
Fair Lawn, NJ 07410
(201)475-1300
FAX: (201)475-1709

Englewood Hospital Imaging At Fair Lawn
22-02 Broadway, Ste 201
Fair Lawn, NJ 07410-3016
(551)299-2900
FAX: (201)608-2413

Fair Lawn Imaging
19-04 Fair Lawn Ave
Fair Lawn, NJ 07410-2341
(201)794-3132
FAX: (201)794-6291

Flemington

Hunterdon Womens Imaging Center
121 State Route 31 Ste 1100
Flemington, NJ 08822-5755
(908)782-4700
FAX: (908)782-0076

Pink Breast Center
3 Walter E. Foran Blvd., Suite 312
Flemington, NJ 08822
(908)284-2300
FAX: (908)442-7432

Florham Park

Summit Medical Group
140 Park Ave
Florham Park, NJ 07932-1049
(973)404-9738
FAX: (973)377-0874

Summit Medical Group Pa
150 Park Ave
Florham Park, NJ 07932-1049
(973)437-2685
FAX: (973)660-1838

Forked River

University Radiology Group
833 Lacey Rd
Forked River, NJ 08731-1200
(609)242-2334
FAX: (609)242-2402

Freehold

Centrastate Medical Center The Women's Health Center
901 W Main St
Freehold, NJ 07728-2549
(732)294-2778
FAX: (732)294-2627

Princeton Radiology
901 W Main St, Medical Arts Building
Freehold, NJ 07728-2537
(732)462-4844
FAX: (732)462-9482

University Radiology Group Pc
900 W Main St
Freehold, NJ 07728-2156
(732)462-1900
FAX: (732)462-1848

Galloway

Atlantic Medical Imaging
44 E Jimmie Leeds Rd Ste 101
Galloway, NJ 08205-4470
(609)677-9729
FAX: (609)652-6512

Glen Rock

Valley Medical Group Breast Health Center
385 S Maple Ave, Ste 201
Glen Rock, NJ 07452-1545
(201)670-4550
FAX: (201)670-6318

Hackensack

Hmh Hospitals Corporation
20 Prospect Ave Ste 513
Hackensack, NJ 07601-1962
(551)996-2220
FAX: (201)525-0843

Njin Of Hackensack
385 Prospect Ave, First Floor
Hackensack, NJ 07601-2570
(201)488-4808
FAX: (201)488-9558

Hackettstown

Hackettstown Medical Center
651 Willow Grove St, Ste A
Hackettstown, NJ 07840-1797
(908)850-6843
FAX: (908)979-8787

Radiology Associates Of Hackettstown Llc
57 US Highway 46, Ste 212
Hackettstown, NJ 07840-2695
(908)979-1621
FAX: (908)852-2393

Haddon Heights

Njin Of Haddon Heights
17 White Horse Pike
Haddon Heights, NJ 08035-1299
(856)546-1177
FAX: (856)546-0666

Haddon Township

Inspira Imaging Center Haddon Township
400 W Cuthbert Blvd
Haddon Township, NJ 08108-3327
(856)696-7979
FAX: (856)696-7961

Haddonfield

South Jersey Radiology Associates
807 N Haddon Ave Ste 5
Haddonfield, NJ 08033-1749
(856)616-1130
FAX: (856)616-9481

Hamilton

Mercer Diagnostic Imaging, Llc
1245 Whitehorse Mercerville Rd, Ste 403
Hamilton, NJ 08619-3831
(609)581-2727
FAX: (609)581-3772

Robert Wood Johnson University Hospital At Hamilton
1 Hamilton Health Pl
Hamilton, NJ 08690-3599
(609)584-6400
FAX: (609)584-5908

Hamilton Township

Radiology Affiliates Imaging/Capital Health Imaging, Llc
2501 Kuser Rd
Hamilton Township, NJ 08691-3386
(609)585-8800
FAX: (609)585-1825

Hammonton

Ami - Atlanticare Partners In Imaging
219 N White Horse Pike
Hammonton, NJ 08037-1896
(609)878-9729
FAX: (609)561-1758

Hillsborough

Hillsborough Radiology Centers, Llc
105 Raider Blvd, Ste 100
Hillsborough, NJ 08844-1528
(908)874-7600
FAX: (908)874-7052

Hoboken

Hoboken University Medical Center
308 Willow Ave
Hoboken, NJ 07030-3808
(201)418-3220
FAX: (201)418-1877

Holmdel

Bayshore Medical Center Women's Center
727 N Beers St
Holmdel, NJ 07733-1514
(732)739-5982
FAX: (732)962-7234

Holmdel Imaging Llc
100 Commons Way, Ste 110
Holmdel, NJ 07733-2937
(732)671-6618
FAX: (732)671-7353

Howell

Jacqueline Wilentz Breast Center At Howell Site
4013 US Highway 9 Ste 2S
Howell, NJ 07731-4022
(732)923-7700
FAX: (732)923-7710

Iselin

Open Mri Radiology Llc, Dba Imagecare At Woodbridge
530 Green St
Iselin, NJ 08830-2654
(732)326-1515
FAX: (732)326-1522

Jackson

Health Village Imaging
27 S Cooks Bridge Rd, Ste 1-6
Jackson, NJ 08527-2460
(732)497-1200
FAX: (732)928-0388

Jersey City

Cristie Kerr Women's Health Center
377 Jersey Ave, Ste 110
Jersey City, NJ 07302-4396
(201)915-2400
FAX: (201)309-2410

D/B/A Carepoint Health -Christ Hospital
176 Palisade Ave, Radiology Dept 3rd Fl.
Jersey City, NJ 07306-1121
(201)795-0700
FAX: (201)795-8167

Hudson River Radiology Center
550 Newark Ave Ste 102
Jersey City, NJ 07306-1353
(201)656-5050
FAX: (800)706-0381

Montclair Radiology
550 Summit Ave
Jersey City, NJ 07306-2707
(973)661-4674
FAX: (973)439-6885

Womens Health Center
116 Newark Ave, Ste 3
Jersey City, NJ 07302-2960
(201)915-2400
FAX: (201)915-2232

Lakewood

Center For Health Education Medicine & Dentistry
1771 Madison Ave
Lakewood, NJ 08701-1242
(732)364-2144
FAX: (732)364-3559

Jacqueline M Wilentz Breast Center Mmc Southern Campus
600 River Ave
Lakewood, NJ 08701-5237
(732)923-7700
FAX: (732)923-7715

Shore Imaging Pc
PO Box 49
Lakewood, NJ 08701-0049
(732)364-9565
FAX: (732)364-9730

Lawrenceville

Radiology Affiliates Lawrenceville
3120 Princeton Pike, Fl 1A
Lawrenceville, NJ 08648-2325
(609)219-1000
FAX: (609)219-1448

Linden

Jersey Diagnostics Imaging
929 N Wood Ave
Linden, NJ 07036-4068
(908)241-5222
FAX: (908)241-0332

Little Silver

Red Bank Radiologists, P.A.
200 White Rd Ste 115
Little Silver, NJ 07739-1160
(732)741-9595
FAX: (732)741-0985

Livingston

Barnabas Health Ambulatory Care Center
200 S Orange Ave
Livingston, NJ 07039-5817
(973)322-7888
FAX: (973)322-7829

Summit Medical Group
75 E Northfield Rd
Livingston, NJ 07039-4532
(973)436-1380
FAX: (973)533-1298

Long Branch

Jacqueline M. Wilentz Comprehensive Breast Ctr At Mmc
300 2nd Ave
Long Branch, NJ 07740-6303
(732)923-7700
FAX: (732)923-7710

Lyndhurst

The Radiology Center
736 Page Ave
Lyndhurst, NJ 07071-2541
(201)729-1234
FAX: (201)729-1150

Mahwah

Valley Center For Health And Wellness
1400 Macarthur Blvd
Mahwah, NJ 07430-3618
(201)447-8200
FAX: (201)316-8453

Manahawkin

Ami-Atlanticare
517 Route 72 W
Manahawkin, NJ 08050-2821
(609)384-7729
FAX: (609)384-7040

Health Village Imaging
1301 Route 72 W Ste 100
Manahawkin, NJ 08050-2483
(609)660-9729
FAX: (609)978-2076

Manalapan

Atrium Diagnostic Imaging
224 Taylors Mills Rd Ste 108
Manalapan, NJ 07726-3281
(732)431-7600
FAX: (732)431-1606

Manasquan

Atlantic Medical Imaging
2399 Highway 34 Bldg B
Manasquan, NJ 08736-1500
(732)223-9729
FAX: (732)292-9950

Maplewood

University Radiology Group
2130 Millburn Ave, Ste A8
Maplewood, NJ 07040-3723
(973)912-0404
FAX: (973)912-0444

Marlton

South Jersey Radiology Associates
1000 Lincoln Dr E Ste 1
Marlton, NJ 08053-1566
(856)983-1818
FAX: (856)983-3226

Maywood

Hmh Hospitals Corporation
87 State Rt 17 N
Maywood, NJ 07607-1017
(551)996-2222
FAX: (201)525-0843

Medford

Larchmont Imaging Associates
103 Old Marlton Pike Ste 115
Medford, NJ 08055-8772
(609)261-4500
FAX: (609)261-2519

Mercerville

Capital Health-Hamilton Outpatient Services
1445 Whitehorse Mercerville Rd, Ste 102
Mercerville, NJ 08619-3834
(609)588-5073
FAX: (609)588-5077

Princeton Radiology
8 Quakerbridge Plz, Ste A
Mercerville, NJ 08619-1255
(609)921-8211
FAX: (609)890-0823

Metuchen

University Radiology Group
260 Amboy Ave
Metuchen, NJ 08840-2441
(732)548-2322
FAX: (732)548-3392

Middletown

Memorial Sloan Kettering Cancer Center - Monmouth
480 Red Hill Rd
Middletown, NJ 07748-3052
(848)225-6035
FAX: (201)691-6697

Middletown Venture Assocs Llc, Dba Imagecare At Middletown
1275 State Route 35
Middletown, NJ 07748-2040
(732)275-0999
FAX: (732)275-0979

Millburn

Imagecare Center At Millburn
120 Millburn Ave, Ste 101
Millburn, NJ 07041-1935
(908)377-0391
FAX: (973)376-0010

Monroe

Princeton Radiology Associates, P.A.
9 Centre Dr Ste 110
Monroe, NJ 08831-5153
(609)921-3345
FAX: (609)655-4016

Monroe Township

University Radiology Group
111 Union Valley Rd, Ste 101
Monroe Township, NJ 08831-6000
(609)395-3470
FAX: (609)395-1718

Montclair

Hackensack Meridian Mountainside Medical Center
1 Bay Ave, Radiology Department
Montclair, NJ 07042-4837
(973)873-7787
FAX: (973)680-7946

Montclair Breast Center, P.C.
37 N Fullerton Ave, Ste 3
Montclair, NJ 07042-3446
(973)509-1818
FAX: (973)509-0532

Montclair Radiological Associates, P.A.
116 Park St
Montclair, NJ 07042-2930
(973)746-2525
FAX: (973)746-5802

Montvale

Memorial Sloan Kettering Cancer Center Bergen
225 Summit Ave
Montvale, NJ 07645-1523
(201)775-7000
FAX: (201)691-6645

Moorestown

Larchmont Imaging Assoc.
401 Young Ave Ste 185
Moorestown, NJ 08057-3140
(609)261-4500
FAX: (609)261-2519

Morristown

Carol W. And Julius A. Rippel Screening Center
435 South St Ste 305
Morristown, NJ 07960-6422
(973)971-5321
FAX: (973)290-7432

Hirsch And Ratakonda, M.D. P.A.
290 Madison Ave, Ste 4
Morristown, NJ 07960-7401
(973)538-8181
FAX: (973)538-6565

Hirsch, Ratakonda, M.D. P.A.
261 James St, Ste 1E
Morristown, NJ 07960-6348
(973)631-1158
FAX: (973)631-1156

Image Care Morristown
95 Madison Ave, Ste B03
Morristown, NJ 07960-6023
(973)984-1111
FAX: (973)261-5787

Morristown Medical Center
100 Madison Ave, Radiology Department
Morristown, NJ 07960-6136
(973)971-5321
FAX: (973)290-7325

The Radiology Center At Harding
1201 Mount Kemble Ave, Ste 1
Morristown, NJ 07960-6667
(908)221-0603
FAX: (908)221-0631

Mount Holly

Virtua Memorial Hospital
175 Madison Ave
Mount Holly, NJ 08060-2099
(609)914-6006
FAX: (609)914-7355

Mount Laurel

Larchmont Imaging Associates
210 Ark Rd, Ste 106
Mount Laurel, NJ 08054-3188
(609)261-4500
FAX: (609)261-2519

Mountain Lakes

Medical Park Imaging Mountain Lakes
333 US Highway 46
Mountain Lakes, NJ 07046-1743
(973)625-3690
FAX: (973)625-5896

Mullica Hill

Inspira Imaging Center Tomlin Station
201 Tomlin Station Rd Ste A
Mullica Hill, NJ 08062-1612
(856)241-2555
FAX: (856)241-2575

Inspira Leading Edge Cancer Center
698 Mullica Hill Rd
Mullica Hill, NJ 08062-4452
(856)508-1000
FAX: (856)221-4174

Neptune

Jersey Shore Imaging
2100 Corlies Avenue
Neptune, NJ 07753
(732)988-1234
FAX: (732)502-0368

New Brunswick

The Women's Imaging Ctr. At St. Peter's Univ. Hosp.
254 Easton Ave, Mammography Department
New Brunswick, NJ 08901-1766
(732)745-8600
FAX: (732)745-8610

University Radiology At Robert Wood Johnson
10 Plum St, Ste 910
New Brunswick, NJ 08901-2066
(800)758-5545
FAX: (732)955-8870

New Providence

Summit Medical Group
890 Mountain Ave, Imaging, 1st Floor
New Providence, NJ 07974-1218
(973)404-9738
FAX: (973)377-0874

Newark

Frank Aguirre, MD
195 Lafayette St
Newark, NJ 07105-1864
(973)465-3044
FAX: (973)465-3032

Newark Beth Israel Medical Center
201 Lyons Ave, L3
Newark, NJ 07112-2094
(973)926-7466
FAX: (973)391-8930

St Michael's Medical Center
111 Central Ave
Newark, NJ 07102-1909
(973)465-2792
FAX: (973)877-5205

University Hospital - Center For Breast Imaging
205 S Orange Ave C-1123
Newark, NJ 07103-2785
(973)972-2880
FAX: (973)972-8439

Newfoundland

Medical Park Imaging Of Newfoundland
2713 State Rt 23, Ste 1
Newfoundland, NJ 07435-1415
(973)697-1755
FAX: (973)440-1890

Newton

Newton Medical Center
175 High St
Newton, NJ 07860-1004
(973)579-8720
FAX: (973)383-0064

The Imagecare Ctr At Newton Radiologic Assoc Of Nnj
222 High St Ste 101
Newton, NJ 07860-9604
(973)729-0002
FAX: (973)383-2774

North Bergen

Hackensack Meridian Health Palisades Medical Center
7650 River Rd Ste 240
North Bergen, NJ 07047-6526
(201)854-5014
FAX: (201)520-4798

Northfield

Advanced Shore Imaging Associates
2605 Shore Rd Ste 101& 102
Northfield, NJ 08225-2136
(609)380-4175
FAX: (609)377-8249

Nutley

Montclair Radiological Associates, P.A.
20 High St
Nutley, NJ 07110-1198
(973)661-4674
FAX: (973)284-0269

Old Bridge

Atlantic Medical Imaging
3548 US Highway 9 Ste 2
Old Bridge, NJ 08857-2963
(732)349-2867
FAX: (732)349-3810

Jfk Advanced Medical Imaging Of Old Bridge
3548 US Highway 9, Ste 2
Old Bridge, NJ 08857-2963
(732)970-0420
FAX: (732)970-0517

Raritan Bay Medical Center Old Bridge Division
2 Hospital Plz Ste 150, Old Bridge Medical Offices Bldg. Suite 1
Old Bridge, NJ 08857-3153
(732)360-4252
FAX: (732)360-4231

Oradell

New Century Imaging- Oradell
555 Kinderkamack Rd, Ste 1
Oradell, NJ 07649-1517
(201)599-1311
FAX: (201)599-8333

Paramus

Bergen New Bridge Medical Center
230 E Ridgewood Ave
Paramus, NJ 07652-4142
(201)967-4064
FAX: (201)967-4288

Robert And Audrey Luckow Pavillion
1 Valley Health Plz
Paramus, NJ 07652-3628
(201)447-8600
FAX: (201)447-8404

Parsippany

Saint Clare's Imaging Center At Parsippany Commons
3219 US Highway 46 Ste 110
Parsippany, NJ 07054-1283
(973)625-6649
FAX: (973)334-1008

Passaic

Prime Healthcare Services - St. Mary's Passaic, Llc
350 Boulevard
Passaic, NJ 07055-2840
(973)365-5251
FAX: (973)916-2033

Paterson

Pink Breast Center
680 Broadway Ste 111
Paterson, NJ 07514-1526
(973)977-6662
FAX: (973)341-1128

St. Joseph's Regional Medical Center
703 Main St
Paterson, NJ 07503-2621
(973)754-4343
FAX: (973)754-3181

Pennington

Capital Health Medical Center - Hopewell
1 Capital Way
Pennington, NJ 08534-2520
(609)303-4178
FAX: (609)303-4135

Pennsville

Pennsville Radiology
248 S Broadway, Ste 3
Pennsville, NJ 08070-2740
(856)678-8118
FAX: (856)678-8130

Perth Amboy

Perth Amboy Diagnostic Imaging
607 Amboy Ave
Perth Amboy, NJ 08861-2595
(732)442-5444
FAX: (732)442-2626

Raritan Bay Medical Center Pad
530 New Brunswick Ave
Perth Amboy, NJ 08861-3685
(732)324-6055
FAX: (732)324-4661

Phillipsburg

St. Luke's Warren Hospital
185 Roseberry St
Phillipsburg, NJ 08865-1684
(908)859-6740
FAX: (908)859-6818

Plainsboro

Penn Medicine Princeton Medical Center
1 Plainsboro Rd
Plainsboro, NJ 08536-1913
(609)853-7070
FAX: (609)683-6853

Point Pleasant

University Radiology Group Pc
3822 River Rd, Point Pleasant Facility
Point Pleasant, NJ 08742-2067
(732)892-1200
FAX: (732)892-1202

Pomona

Atlanticare Regional Medical Center - Mainland Div
65 W Jimmie Leeds Rd
Pomona, NJ 08240-9102
(609)383-2800
FAX: (609)748-7275

Pompton Plains

The Breast Center Of Chilton Medical Center
97 W Parkway
Pompton Plains, NJ 07444-1647
(973)831-5201
FAX: (973)831-5467

Princeton

Princeton Radiology Associates, P.A.
419 N Harrison St
Princeton, NJ 08540-3594
(609)921-3345
FAX: (609)683-8847

Rahway

Robert Wood Johnson University Hospital Rahway
865 Stone St
Rahway, NJ 07065-2742
(844)795-4968
FAX: (732)815-7615

Randolph

Njin Of Randolph
121 Center Grove Rd, Ste 7
Randolph, NJ 07869-4453
(973)989-8400
FAX: (973)989-5208

Red Bank

Riverview Medical Center
1 Riverview Plz
Red Bank, NJ 07701-1872
(732)530-2305
FAX: (732)224-8410

Ridgewood

The Valley Hospital
223 N Van Dien Ave
Ridgewood, NJ 07450-2736
(201)447-8600
FAX: (201)447-8404

Womens Diagnostic Imaging
79 Chestnut St, Ste 100
Ridgewood, NJ 07450-2533
(201)444-4484
FAX: (201)444-4148

Rio Grande

Cape Radiology
4011 Route 9 S, Ste 100
Rio Grande, NJ 08242-1917
(609)778-1009
FAX: (609)463-3191

Rutherford

Njin Of Rutherford
69 Orient Way
Rutherford, NJ 07070-2011
(201)559-4140
FAX: (201)933-5662

Salem

Womens Diag Imaging Ctr At Salem Medical Center
310 Woodstown Road
Salem, NJ 08079
(856)878-6893
FAX: (856)935-1297

Secaucus

Hudson Regional Hospital
55 Meadowlands Pkwy
Secaucus, NJ 07094-2977
(201)392-3518
FAX: (201)392-3239

Sewell

Jefferson Health Opic
900 Medical Center Dr Ste 101, Outpatient Medical Imaging
Sewell, NJ 08080-2358
(856)582-3130
FAX: (856)582-3132

Jefferson Univ. Rad Assoc.,Dba/Jefferson Outpatient Imaging
243 Hurffville Crosskeys Rd, Ste 102
Sewell, NJ 08080-4011
(215)503-4900
FAX: (215)503-4921

South Jersey Radiology Associates
105 Kings Way W, Washington Township
Sewell, NJ 08080-2233
(856)589-6646
FAX: (856)589-8461

Sicklerville

Inspira Imaging Center Sicklerville
485 Williamstown Rd
Sicklerville, NJ 08081-1777
(856)241-2555
FAX: (856)241-2575

Somers Point

Atlantic Medical Imaging Llc
30 E Maryland Ave
Somers Point, NJ 08244-2451
(609)653-0209
FAX: (609)926-1307

Shore Medical Center
100 Medical Center Way
Somers Point, NJ 08244-2300
(609)653-4600
FAX: (609)653-3740

Somerset

University Radiology Group, P.C.
75 Veronica Ave Ste 102
Somerset, NJ 08873-5002
(800)758-5545
FAX: (732)545-0758

Somerville

Sanofi Us Breast Care Center
30 Rehill Ave Ste 3100
Somerville, NJ 08876-2549
(908)243-8648
FAX: (908)203-5971

Sparta

Women's Diagnostic Center
89 Sparta Ave Ste 120
Sparta, NJ 07871-1790
(973)729-0002
FAX: (973)726-4456

Stratford

Jefferson Health Stratford
18 E Laurel Rd
Stratford, NJ 08084-1327
(856)406-4100
FAX: (856)346-6689

Summit

The Breast Center At Overlook Medical Center
11 Overlook Rd Ste Ll103
Summit, NJ 07901-3577
(908)522-6135
FAX: (908)522-5883

Teaneck

Holy Name Medical Center
718 Teaneck Rd
Teaneck, NJ 07666-4281
(201)833-7100
FAX: (201)833-7248

University Radiology Group
699 Teaneck Rd, Ste 105
Teaneck, NJ 07666-4244
(201)836-2500
FAX: (201)836-7921

Tinton Falls

University Radiology Atlantic
48 N Gilbert St
Tinton Falls, NJ 07701-4905
(732)530-5750
FAX: (732)530-5848

Toms River

Atlantic Medical Imaging
864 Route 37 W, West Hills Plaza
Toms River, NJ 08755-5033
(732)223-9729
FAX: (732)240-3795

Atlantic Medical Imaging Toms River Women's Center
222 Oak Ave Ste 1
Toms River, NJ 08753-3348
(848)221-8209
FAX: (732)608-8969

Community Medical Center-Nexus Properties
368 Lakehurst Rd, Ste 102
Toms River, NJ 08755-7339
(732)557-8150
FAX: (732)557-3916

Njin Of Toms River West & Women's Imaging
9 Mule Rd, Ste 17
Toms River, NJ 08755-5053
(732)240-1400
FAX: (732)914-1760

Toms River X-Ray Ct & Mri Center
154 Route 37 W
Toms River, NJ 08755-8059
(732)244-0777
FAX: (732)244-1428

Trenton

Capital Health System At Regional Medical Center
750 Brunswick Ave
Trenton, NJ 08638-4143
(609)394-6695
FAX: (609)303-4135

St. Francis Medical Center
601 Hamilton Ave
Trenton, NJ 08629-1915
(609)599-5550
FAX: (609)599-6487

Turnersville

Njin Of Washington Township
157 Fries Mill Rd
Turnersville, NJ 08012-2017
(856)677-1010
FAX: (856)677-1020

South Jersey Radiology Associates
901 Route 168, Suites 301-305, Washington Professional Campus II
Turnersville, NJ 08012
(856)770-0504
FAX: (856)227-8537

Union

Njin Of Union Women's Imaging
2770 Morris Ave
Union, NJ 07083-4827
(908)933-9116
FAX: (908)686-7099

Overlook Medical Center Imaging Union Campus
PO Box 13, 1000 Galloping Hill Rd
Union, NJ 07083-0013
(908)522-6280
FAX: (908)964-2163

Women's Healthcare Imaging Corp
1896 Morris Ave
Union, NJ 07083-3535
(908)964-0004
FAX: (908)964-0034

Union City

Bergenline X - Ray Diagnostic Center
400 43rd St 402
Union City, NJ 07087-5010
(201)348-6060
FAX: (201)348-2064

Hudson River Radiology Center
120 48th St, Ste 2 152
Union City, NJ 07087-6439
(201)665-8707
FAX: (800)706-0381

Njin Of Union City
3196 Kennedy Blvd, Ste 3
Union City, NJ 07087-2468
(201)865-6100
FAX: (201)865-6102

Vernon

Radiologic Associates Of Northern New Jersey, P.A. Vernon
212 State Rt 94 Ste 1-B
Vernon, NJ 07462-3324
(973)729-0002
FAX: (973)827-0117

Vineland

Atlantic Medical Imaging
1450 E Chestnut Ave, Ste 1E Bldg 4 Suite A
Vineland, NJ 08361-8467
(856)794-1700
FAX: (856)794-1788

Inspira Medical Center Vineland
1505 W Sherman Ave
Vineland, NJ 08360-7059
(856)641-7950
FAX: (856)641-7679

Inspira Medical Center, Inc South Delsea Imaging
2848 S Delsea Dr, Ste C1-A
Vineland, NJ 08360-7042
(856)285-7777
FAX: (856)285-5576

Voorhees

Cooper Breast Imaging At Ripa
6100 Main St
Voorhees, NJ 08043-4643
(856)342-2380
FAX: (856)673-4207

Cooper University Radiology At Voorhees
900 Centennial Blvd Ste B
Voorhees, NJ 08043-4637
(856)342-2380
FAX: (856)325-6588

South Jersey Radiology Associates Women's Center At Virtua
200 Bowman Dr, Ste E152
Voorhees, NJ 08043-9647
(856)768-3123
FAX: (856)768-2037

South Jersey Radiology Women's Center
100 Carnie Blvd Ste A4
Voorhees, NJ 08043-4513
(856)751-5522
FAX: (856)751-5650

Women's Imaging Of South Jersey
2401 E Evesham Rd, Ste A2
Voorhees, NJ 08043-9590
(856)489-5700
FAX: (856)489-5722

Waldwick

Radiology Associates Of Ridgewood, P.A.
20 Franklin Tpke
Waldwick, NJ 07463-1744
(201)445-8822
FAX: (201)857-1101

Warren

University Radiology Group
16 Mountain Blvd
Warren, NJ 07059-5614
(908)769-7200
FAX: (908)769-9141

Wayne

Hudson River Radiology Center
516 Hamburg Tpke Ste 6
Wayne, NJ 07470-2063
(201)656-5050
FAX: (800)706-0381

Medical Park Imaging
330 Ratzer Rd, Ste A6A
Wayne, NJ 07470-7703
(973)696-5770
FAX: (973)633-1204

University Imaging - St. Joseph's Wayne Hospital
246 Hamburg Tpke, Ste 105
Wayne, NJ 07470-2159
(973)595-1300
FAX: (973)790-7397

West Caldwell

Montclair Radiological Associates, P.A.
1140 Bloomfield Ave
West Caldwell, NJ 07006-7130
(973)439-9729
FAX: (973)439-6885

West New York

Ricardo T. Baldonado, M.D., North Jersey Imaging Center
307 60th St
West New York, NJ 07093-5412
(201)854-1200
FAX: (201)854-3333

West Orange

Image Care Of West Orange Llc
61 Main St
West Orange, NJ 07052-5352
(973)736-1680
FAX: (862)930-7397

New Jersey Imaging Network Of West Orange
772 Northfield Ave
West Orange, NJ 07052-1100
(973)325-0002
FAX: (973)325-8140

Regional Women's Health Group, Llc - West Orange
101 Old Short Hills Rd, Ste 101
West Orange, NJ 07052-1023
(973)736-1100
FAX: (877)302-1202

Summit Medical Group
375 Mount Pleasant Ave, Ste 206
West Orange, NJ 07052-2751
(973)436-4749
FAX: (973)533-1298

Westfield

Summit Medical Group
574 Springfield Ave
Westfield, NJ 07090-1001
(908)277-8673
FAX: (908)232-3156

Westwood

Hackensack Meridian Health Pascack Valley Medical Center
250 Old Hook Rd
Westwood, NJ 07675-3123
(201)781-1400
FAX: (201)383-1976

Whiting

Cmc Radiology At Whiting
65 Lacey Rd, Ste G
Whiting, NJ 08759-2985
(732)557-2550
FAX: (732)557-3916

Willingboro

Larchmont Imaging Associates
219 Sunset Rd
Willingboro, NJ 08046-1109
(609)261-4500
FAX: (609)261-2519

Virtua Willingboro Hospital
218A Sunset Rd
Willingboro, NJ 08046-1110
(609)835-3191
FAX: (609)835-3190

Woodbury

South Jersey Radiology Associates
748 Kings Hwy
Woodbury, NJ 08096-3190
(856)848-4998
FAX: (856)853-7362

Woodbury Heights

Penn Medicine Woodbury
1006 Mantua Pike, Ste 2
Woodbury Heights, NJ 08097-1225
(856)686-8282
FAX: (856)686-8280

Woodland Park

McBride Imaging Center
1167 McBride Ave, Ste 3
Woodland Park, NJ 07424-2543
(973)837-8100
FAX: (973)638-1300

Wrightstown

Virtua Health And Wellness- New Hanover
25 Wrightstown Cookstown Rd
Wrightstown, NJ 08562-2341
(609)835-2900
FAX: (609)835-5431

NEW MEXICO

Alamogordo

Alamogordo Imaging Center
2539 Medical Dr Ste 101
Alamogordo, NM 88310-8720
(575)434-1353
FAX: (575)434-1398

Albuquerque

Breast Imaging Center
4630 Jefferson Ln NE, Ste C
Albuquerque, NM 87109-2151
(505)998-1912
FAX: (505)998-1906

Davita Medical Group - Journal Center Clinic
5150 Journal Center Blvd NE
Albuquerque, NM 87109-5900
(505)232-1535
FAX: (505)262-3272

High Resolution
4411 The 25 Way NE Ste 150
Albuquerque, NM 87109-5888
(505)332-5800
FAX: (505)332-5801

Lovelace Westside Hospital
10501 Golf Course Rd NW
Albuquerque, NM 87114-5000
(505)727-8966
FAX: (505)727-9186

Lovelace Women's Hospital
4705 Montgomery Blvd NE, Ste 105
Albuquerque, NM 87109-1246
(505)727-6929
FAX: (505)727-9179

Northwest Imaging Center
10200 Corrales Rd NW Ste B4
Albuquerque, NM 87114-9261
(505)559-5812
FAX: (505)559-5817

Unm Hospitals
1213 University Blvd NE
Albuquerque, NM 87102-1703
(505)272-4545
FAX: (505)925-4947

Artesia

Artesia General Hospital
702 N 13th St
Artesia, NM 88210-1199
(575)736-8164
FAX: (575)748-8381

Carlsbad

Carlsbad Medical Center
2430 W Pierce St
Carlsbad, NM 88220-3597
(575)887-4481
FAX: (575)887-4582

Clovis

Assured Imaging Women's Wellness Of Southern Arizona, Llc
2105 W 21st St
Clovis, NM 88101-4017
(520)744-6121
FAX: (520)572-7138

Plains Regional Medical Center - Clovis
PO Box 1688, 2100 N Dr Martin Luther King Jr Blvd
Clovis, NM 88102-1688
(575)769-7341
FAX: (575)769-7296

Plains Regional Mob
2200 W 21st St
Clovis, NM 88101-2011
(575)769-6313
FAX: (575)769-6312

Crownpoint

Crownpoint Healthcare Facility Indian Health Service
Highway 371 And Navajo Route 9
Crownpoint, NM 87313
(505)786-6206
FAX: (505)786-6419

Deming

Mimbres Memorial Hospital
900 W Ash St
Deming, NM 88030-4098
(575)546-5872
FAX: (575)543-6920

Espanola

Espanola Hospital - Radiology Department
1010 Spruce St
Espanola, NM 87532-2724
(505)753-1524
FAX: (505)753-1527

Farmington

San Juan Regional Medical Center
801 W Maple St
Farmington, NM 87401-5630
(505)609-6228
FAX: (505)609-6066

San Juan Regional Medical Ctr Outpatient Diagnostic Ctr
2300 E 30th St Bldg C
Farmington, NM 87401-8991
(505)609-6228
FAX: (505)609-6066

X-Ray Associates Of Farmington
1750 E 30th St
Farmington, NM 87401-9020
(505)327-0123
FAX: (505)327-0127

Gallup

Gallup Indian Medical Center
516 E Nizhoni Blvd
Gallup, NM 87301-5748
(505)722-1162
FAX: (505)722-1192

Rehoboth McKinley Christian Hospital
1901 Red Rock Dr
Gallup, NM 87301-5683
(505)863-7015
FAX: (505)863-7324

Grants

Cibola General Hospital
1016 E Roosevelt Ave
Grants, NM 87020-2118
(505)287-5255
FAX: (505)287-5287

Hobbs

Covenant Health Hobbs Hospital
5419 N Lovington Hwy
Hobbs, NM 88240-9100
(577)492-5155
FAX: (575)492-5151

Las Cruces

Assured Imaging Women's Wellness Of Southern Arizona, Llc
3530 Foothills Rd, Ste I
Las Cruces, NM 88011-3621
(888)233-6121
FAX: (520)572-7138

Memorial Healthplex
2735 Northrise Dr
Las Cruces, NM 88011-1698
(575)521-5270
FAX: (866)278-6782

Mountain View Regional Medical Center
4351 E Lohman Ave, Ste 101
Las Cruces, NM 88011-8258
(575)556-7257
FAX: (575)556-7258

Sun View Imaging Llc
2525 S Telshor Blvd
Las Cruces, NM 88011-5071
(575)522-6236
FAX: (575)522-1246

Las Vegas

Alta Vista Regional Hospital
104 Legion Dr
Las Vegas, NM 87701-4804
(505)426-3610
FAX: (505)426-3548

Los Alamos

Los Alamos Medical Center
3917 West Rd, Ste G21
Los Alamos, NM 87544-2278
(505)661-9181
FAX: (505)661-9151

Los Lunas

Assured Imaging Women's Wellness Of Southern Arizona, Llc
1400 Main St NW, Ste K
Los Lunas, NM 87031-4866
(888)233-6121
FAX: (520)572-7138

Lovington

Nor-Lea General Hospital
1600 N Main Ave
Lovington, NM 88260-2871
(575)396-6611
FAX: (575)396-2908

Portales

Roosevelt General Hospital
PO Box 868, 42121 US Hwy 70
Portales, NM 88130-0868
(575)359-1800
FAX: (575)356-7109

Rio Rancho

High Resolution Rust
2400 Unser Blvd SE, Ste 28200
Rio Rancho, NM 87124-4741
(505)332-5800
FAX: (505)332-5801

Unm Sandoval Regional Medical Center
3001 Broadmoor Blvd NE
Rio Rancho, NM 87144-2100
(505)994-7230
FAX: (505)994-7260

Roswell

Medical Arts Complex
601 W Country Club Rd
Roswell, NM 88201-5224
(505)624-8761
FAX: (575)624-5657

Rio Pecos Medical Associates, Ltd.
PO Box 2608, 305 W Country Club Rd
Roswell, NM 88202-2608
(575)622-6322
FAX: (575)623-3565

Ruidoso

Lincoln County Medical Center
211 Sudderth Dr
Ruidoso, NM 88345-6043
(575)257-8292
FAX: (575)630-4294

Santa Fe

High Resolution Santa Fe
4801 Beckner Rd Ste 2700
Santa Fe, NM 87507-3641
(505)332-5800
FAX: (505)332-5801

Santa Fe Imaging, L.L.C.
1640 Hospital Dr
Santa Fe, NM 87505-4754
(505)983-9350
FAX: (505)955-8738

Xray Associates At Santa Fe
490A W Zia Rd Ste 110
Santa Fe, NM 87505-7007
(505)983-9139
FAX: (505)983-9645

Shiprock

Northern Navajo Medical Center
PO Box 160, US Highway 491 North
Shiprock, NM 87420-0160
(505)368-7150
FAX: (505)368-6403

Silver City

Gila Regional Medical Center
1313 E 32nd St
Silver City, NM 88061-7244
(575)538-4129
FAX: (575)538-4876

Taos

Holy Cross Medical Center
1397 Weimer Rd
Taos, NM 87571-6253
(575)737-3231
FAX: (575)737-3232

Truth Or Consequences

Sierra Vista Hospital
800 E 9th Ave
Truth Or Consequences, NM 87901-1961
(575)743-1280
FAX: (575)894-1038

Tucumcari

Dr. Dan C. Trigg Memorial Hospital
301 E Miel De Luna Ave
Tucumcari, NM 88401-3810
(575)461-7050
FAX: (575)461-7277

Zuni

Zuni Comprehensive Community Health Center
Route 301 North, Box 467
Zuni, NM 87327
(505)782-4431
FAX: (505)782-7310

NEW YORK

Albany

Albany Medical Center South Clinical Campus
25 Hackett Blvd
Albany, NY 12208-3462
(518)262-1259
FAX: (518)262-1112

St Peter's Breast Center - Washington Ave Mammography
1365 Washington Ave, Ste 202
Albany, NY 12206-1098
(518)525-1401
FAX: (518)525-5288

St. Peter's Breast Imaging Center
317 S Manning Blvd Ste 305
Albany, NY 12208-1738
(518)525-7700
FAX: (518)525-1200

Alexandria Bay

River Hospital Inc
4 Fuller St
Alexandria Bay, NY 13607-1391
(315)482-1156
FAX: (315)482-2015

Amherst

Buffalo Mri
4925 Main St, Ste 101
Amherst, NY 14226-4000
(716)839-3333
FAX: (716)839-3338

Seton Imaging
3730 Sheridan Dr
Amherst, NY 14226-1732
(716)633-8675
FAX: (716)633-9231

Amsterdam

St. Mary's Healthcare Rao Outpatient Pavilion
4950 State Highway 30
Amsterdam, NY 12010-7520
(518)841-7224
FAX: (518)839-0558

Armonk

White Plains Hospital Imaging At Armonk
99 Business Park Dr
Armonk, NY 10504-1720
(914)849-7979
FAX: (914)848-7978

Astoria

Lenox Hill Radiology, Pc - Astoria
2916 Astoria Blvd
Astoria, NY 11102-1742
(718)204-5800
FAX: (718)721-4572

The Mount Sinai Hospital Of Queens
2510 30th Ave
Astoria, NY 11102-2418
(718)808-7500
FAX: (718)808-7988

Wruble N D, M.D.
2184 Steinway St
Astoria, NY 11105-1805
(718)726-9600
FAX: (718)726-0808

Auburn

Auburn Community Hospital
17 Lansing St
Auburn, NY 13021-1943
(315)255-7440
FAX: (315)255-7063

Diagnostic Imaging Center
37 W Garden St Ste 107
Auburn, NY 13021-2663
(315)255-2828
FAX: (315)255-3503

St. Joseph's Imaging Associates
615 N Seward Ave
Auburn, NY 13021-2107
(315)760-3913
FAX: (315)452-2559

Baldwinsville

St. Joseph's Imaging Assoc. Baldwinsville
8280 Willett Pkwy Ste 100
Baldwinsville, NY 13027-1331
(315)635-6814
FAX: (315)635-6816

Batavia

Elizabeth Wende Breast Care, L.L.C.
203 Summit St, Ste 1
Batavia, NY 14020-1680
(585)442-2190
FAX: (585)758-7085

United Memorial Jerome Center
16 Bank St
Batavia, NY 14020-2260
(585)344-5225
FAX: (585)344-7475

Bath

Ira Davenport Memorial Hospital
7571 State Route 54
Bath, NY 14810-9590
(607)737-8152
FAX: (607)737-8196

Bay Shore

Zwanger-Pesiri Radiology
160 Brentwood Rd
Bay Shore, NY 11706-6948
(631)666-7040
FAX: (631)666-9168

Bayshore

Lenox Hill Radiology & Medical Associates, P.C.
375 E Main St Ste 12
Bayshore, NY 11706-8418
(631)665-2275
FAX: (631)665-5535

Bayside

Main Street Radiology At Bayside
4401 Francis Lewis Blvd
Bayside, NY 11361-3028
(718)428-1500
FAX: (718)352-0292

Zwanger Pesiri Radiology
21302 Northern Blvd
Bayside, NY 11361-3344
(631)444-5544
FAX: (631)870-8732

Bethpage

Lenox Hill Radiology-Bethpage
1055 Stewart Ave, Ste 100C
Bethpage, NY 11714-3596
(631)277-1600
FAX: (718)629-4493

Prohealth Radiology Behtpage
4277 Hempstead Tpke, Ste 200
Bethpage, NY 11714-5706
(516)796-4340
FAX: (516)579-4163

Binghamton

Lourdes Hospital
169 Riverside Dr, Depaul Pavilion
Binghamton, NY 13905-4198
(607)798-5723
FAX: (607)798-6111

Brewster

Caremount Medical, P.C.
185 Route 312, SE Executive Park
Brewster, NY 10509-2337
(888)656-4723
FAX: (845)278-3514

Northeast Radiology
3839 Danbury Rd
Brewster, NY 10509-5412
(845)278-6200
FAX: (845)278-3340

Brockport

Ide Imaging Partners Inc Dba Borg & Ide Imaging Pc
6668 4th Section Rd, Unity At Brockport
Brockport, NY 14420-2448
(585)241-6400
FAX: (585)241-6689

University Of Rochester Med Ctr, Strong Memorial Hospital
156 West Ave
Brockport, NY 14420-1229
(585)487-3300
FAX: (585)276-1067

Bronx

Bronxcare Health & Wellness Center
199 Mount Eden Pkwy 2nd Fl
Bronx, NY 10457-7703
(718)960-4518
FAX: (718)960-2050

Bronxcare Health System
1650 Grand Concourse, Dept Of Radiology
Bronx, NY 10457-7606
(718)960-1396
FAX: (718)960-2050

Distinguished Diagnostic Imaging
625 E Fordham Rd
Bronx, NY 10458-5049
(718)828-6800
FAX: (718)828-6586

Jacobi Medical Center
1400 Pelham Pkwy S Rm 4N15, Department Of Radiology
Bronx, NY 10461-1197
(718)918-4717
FAX: (718)918-7535

Lenox Hill Radiology P.C.-Fordham
410 E 189th St
Bronx, NY 10458-5507
(917)804-3039
FAX: (973)767-0258

Lenox Hill Radiology P.C.-Pelham
3250 Westchester Ave
Bronx, NY 10461-4500
(718)444-3777
FAX: (718)629-4493

Lincoln Medical And Mental Health Center
234 E 149th St
Bronx, NY 10451-5504
(718)579-5684
FAX: (718)579-4649

Madison Avenue Radiology Center 3055 3rd Avenue
3055 3rd Ave, Ste A
Bronx, NY 10451-4861
(212)860-3500
FAX: (212)860-3531

Montefiore Advanced Imaging, Medical Arts Pavillion
3400 Bainbridge Ave Lowr Level, Ste 300
Bronx, NY 10467-2404
(866)662-9729
FAX: (718)658-5402

Montefiore Breast Center
1500 Blondell Ave Ste 2
Bronx, NY 10461-2643
(718)920-5481
FAX: (718)655-4732

Montefiore Medical Center North Division
600 E 233rd St, Radiology Dept
Bronx, NY 10466-2604
(718)920-9449
FAX: (718)920-9940

Montefiore Medical Group
2300 Westchester Ave
Bronx, NY 10462-5071
(718)409-8950
FAX: (718)409-8961

Montefiore Medical Group Grand Concourse
2532 Grand Concourse, Radiology / Cellar Level
Bronx, NY 10458-4902
(718)960-1590
FAX: (718)960-2110

Montefiore Medical Group-Chcc
305 E 161st St
Bronx, NY 10451-3535
(718)579-2500
FAX: (718)410-0834

Morris Heights Health Center Harrison Circle Radiology
57 W Burnside Ave
Bronx, NY 10453-4038
(718)716-4400
FAX: (718)299-2958

Morrisania Diagnostic And Treatment Center
1225 Gerard Ave
Bronx, NY 10452-8015
(718)960-2701
FAX: (718)960-2707

Mosholu Park Radiology, P.C.
3130 Grand Concourse Ste 1P
Bronx, NY 10458-1263
(718)933-6969
FAX: (718)933-6970

North Central Bronx Hospital
3424 Kossuth Ave, Rm 2F01
Bronx, NY 10467-2489
(718)519-3086
FAX: (718)519-3777

Saint Joseph's Imaging At Riverdale
3050 Corlear Ave
Bronx, NY 10463-5180
(347)842-2250
FAX: (347)842-2240

Segundo Ruiz Belvis Diagnostic Treatment Ctr Nychhc
545 E 142nd St
Bronx, NY 10454-2110
(718)579-4010
FAX: (718)579-1842

St. Barnabas Hospital
4507 3rd Ave
Bronx, NY 10457-1515
(718)960-6162
FAX: (718)960-3612

St. Barnabas Hospital - Mobile
4422 3rd Ave
Bronx, NY 10457-2594
(718)960-6162
FAX: (718)960-3601

Starling Diagnositcs
1480 East Ave
Bronx, NY 10462-7502
(718)319-1610
FAX: (716)810-1991

Third Avenue Imaging Llc
2781 3rd Ave
Bronx, NY 10455-4002
(718)402-0300
FAX: (718)742-1643

University Diagnostic Medical Imaging, P.C.
1200 Waters Pl Rm M108
Bronx, NY 10461-0377
(718)931-5620
FAX: (718)824-0706

Urban Health Plan, Inc
1065 Southern Blvd
Bronx, NY 10459-2417
(718)589-4755
FAX: (718)589-4793

Zwanger Pesiri Radiology
1888 Westchester Ave
Bronx, NY 10472-3000
(631)225-7200
FAX: (631)870-8732

Bronxville

Newyork-Presbyterian Lawrence Hospital
55 Palmer Ave
Bronxville, NY 10708-3491
(914)787-5008
FAX: (914)787-5058

Brooklyn

Advantage Radiology
3049 Ocean Pkwy, Ste 303
Brooklyn, NY 11235-8367
(718)265-1000
FAX: (718)265-1002

Bay Ridge Medical Imaging At Dyker Heights
7117 - 7121 - 13th Avenue
Brooklyn, NY 11228
(718)238-7000
FAX: (718)759-1450

Bay Ridge Medical Imaging, Pc
9920 4th Ave Ste 105
Brooklyn, NY 11209-8379
(718)921-0333
FAX: (718)759-1450

Bay Ridge Medical Imaging, P.C.
7601 4th Ave, Ste 1
Brooklyn, NY 11209-3269
(718)238-7000
FAX: (718)759-1450

Boro Park Medical
1379 54th St Ste 2
Brooklyn, NY 11219-4259
(718)436-1600
FAX: (718)436-2085

Brmi At Boro Park/Division Of Prohealthcare
3802 14th Ave
Brooklyn, NY 11218-3610
(718)854-5400
FAX: (718)759-1450

Brmi At Midwood
2005 Coney Island Ave
Brooklyn, NY 11223-2328
(718)238-7000
FAX: (718)759-1450

Brmi At Stillwell - Division Of Prohealth
1783 Stillwell Ave, Bay Ridge Medical Imaging
Brooklyn, NY 11223-1006
(718)238-7000
FAX: (718)759-1450

Brookdale Family Care Center
1095 Flatbush Ave
Brooklyn, NY 11226-6141
(718)240-8800
FAX: (718)240-6398

Brookdale University Hospital & Medical Center
1 Brookdale Plz, Radiology Department
Brooklyn, NY 11212-3198
(718)240-8270
FAX: (718)240-6398

Brooklyn Heights Imaging
161 Atlantic Ave
Brooklyn, NY 11201-6792
(718)802-0400
FAX: (718)802-0409

City Wide Health Facility, Inc.
6817 Bay Pkwy
Brooklyn, NY 11204-5507
(718)236-6800
FAX: (718)236-4696

Community Radiology Ny
849 57th St, Lower Level
Brooklyn, NY 11220-3797
(929)234-3150
FAX: (212)349-2760

Comprehensive Breast Care
9711 3rd Ave
Brooklyn, NY 11209-7717
(718)921-3800
FAX: (718)921-1168

Coney Island Hospital
2601 Ocean Pkwy
Brooklyn, NY 11235-7791
(718)616-3738
FAX: (718)616-3747

Cumberland Diagnostic & Treatment Center
100 N Portland Ave
Brooklyn, NY 11205-2005
(718)260-7656
FAX: (718)260-4850

East New York Diagnostic And Treatment Center
2094 Pitkin Ave, Kings County Hospital Center - Dept. Of
Brooklyn, NY 11207-3509
(718)240-0529
FAX: (718)245-3155

Excelsior Integrated Medical Group, Pllc
758 61st St
Brooklyn, NY 11220-4212
(718)522-1118
FAX: (212)335-0320

Interfaith Medical Center
1545 Atlantic Ave
Brooklyn, NY 11213-1166
(718)613-4408
FAX: (718)613-4721

Kings County Hospital Center
451 Clarkson Ave S2nd Flr
Brooklyn, NY 11203-2097
(718)245-5503
FAX: (718)245-4416

Kingsbrook Jewish Medical Center
585 Schenectady Ave
Brooklyn, NY 11203-1891
(718)604-5461
FAX: (718)363-6884

Lenox Hill Radiology - Crown Heights
546 Eastern Pkwy
Brooklyn, NY 11225-1604
(855)547-4227
FAX: (917)246-4973

Lenox Hill Radiology - Downtown
447 Atlantic Ave
Brooklyn, NY 11217-1702
(646)680-1848
FAX: (718)491-4081

Lenox Hill Radiology And Medical Imaging
2095 Flatbush Ave
Brooklyn, NY 11234-4338
(718)338-6868
FAX: (718)252-3650

Lenox Hill Radiology P.C. -Bond St
9 Bond St Fl 4
Brooklyn, NY 11201-5801
(718)222-3000
FAX: (718)765-4081

Lenox Hill Radiology P.C. -Midwood
1230 Avenue R
Brooklyn, NY 11229-1016
(718)444-3777
FAX: (718)629-4493

Lenox Hill Radiology P.C.-Millbasin
2475 Ralph Ave
Brooklyn, NY 11234-5521
(718)444-3303
FAX: (718)629-4493

Lenox Hill Radiology- Bayridge
405 91st St
Brooklyn, NY 11209-5913
(718)491-7822
FAX: (718)491-7800

Lenox Hill Radiology- Cobble Hill
205 Smith St
Brooklyn, NY 11201-6410
(718)732-7232
FAX: (718)282-7068

Lenox Hill Radiology-Bensonhurst
2215 79th St
Brooklyn, NY 11214-2004
(718)444-1069
FAX: (718)629-4493

Lenox Hill Radiology-Brooklyn Avenue
1014 Brooklyn Ave
Brooklyn, NY 11203-4003
(718)444-3777
FAX: (718)282-7068

Lenox Hill Radiology-East New York
101 Pennsylvania Ave
Brooklyn, NY 11207-2428
(917)453-0426
FAX: (718)629-1438

Lerman Diagnostic Imaging
6511 Fort Hamilton Pkwy
Brooklyn, NY 11219-5524
(718)491-4545
FAX: (718)491-4123

Maimonides Comprehensive Cancer Center
745 64th St
Brooklyn, NY 11220-4745
(718)765-2560
FAX: (718)765-2564

Marine Park Radiology, P.C.
2270 Kimball St Ste 102
Brooklyn, NY 11234-5158
(718)253-6616
FAX: (718)253-7059

Mount Sinai Brooklyn Heights Medical Group
300 Cadman Plz W Fl 18
Brooklyn, NY 11201-3226
(929)210-6330
FAX: (646)537-1486

Mount Sinai- Beth Israel Brooklyn
3201 Kings Hwy
Brooklyn, NY 11234-2625
(718)951-2717
FAX: (718)951-2718

New York-Presbyterian Brooklyn Methodist Hospital
506 6th St
Brooklyn, NY 11215-3609
(718)780-5029
FAX: (718)780-3778

Nyu Langone Radiology- Avenue P
1300 Avenue P, Ground Floor
Brooklyn, NY 11229
(718)954-3840
FAX: (718)954-3850

Nyu Lutheran Medical Center
150 55th St, Department Of Radiology
Brooklyn, NY 11220-2559
(718)630-7400
FAX: (718)630-6453

Pinnacle Diagnostic Radiology At Bay Parkway
6010 Bay Pkwy
Brooklyn, NY 11204-6079
(718)307-5020
FAX: (718)232-4761

Radiology Associates Of Brooklyn
762 Bedford Ave
Brooklyn, NY 11205-1573
(718)947-2570
FAX: (718)947-2571

Radiology Associates Of Brooklyn Llp
1421 57th St 23
Brooklyn, NY 11219-4664
(718)436-7337
FAX: (718)436-7713

Radiology Associates Of Brooklyn, Llp
2021 Avenue X
Brooklyn, NY 11235-2905
(718)332-6800
FAX: (718)332-4209

Rs Nuclear Medicine Pc
835 61st St, Unit 101-102
Brooklyn, NY 11220-4312
(718)686-0895
FAX: (347)715-3532

Select Diagnostic Imaging
2350 Ocean Ave Ste 4
Brooklyn, NY 11229-3044
(516)676-4550
FAX: (718)676-4557

Suny/Downstate Medical Center University Hospital
450 Clarkson Ave, Department Of Radiology - 1208
Brooklyn, NY 11203-2012
(718)270-7333
FAX: (718)221-6168

The Brooklyn Hospital Center
121 Dekalb Ave
Brooklyn, NY 11201-5493
(718)250-6304
FAX: (718)250-6656

Urban Radiology Pc
2809 Ocean Pkwy
Brooklyn, NY 11235-7802
(718)332-6401
FAX: (718)332-6411

Woodhull Medical & Mental Health Center
760 Broadway
Brooklyn, NY 11206-5317
(718)630-3205
FAX: (718)963-5800

Wyckoff Heights Medical Center
374 Stockholm St
Brooklyn, NY 11237-4006
(718)963-7373
FAX: (718)963-6511

Wyckoff Heights Medical Center, Women's Health Center.
110 Wyckoff Ave
Brooklyn, NY 11237-3904
(718)963-7373
FAX: (718)963-6511

Xxi Century Radiology And Imaging
3140 Coney Island Ave
Brooklyn, NY 11235-6228
(718)333-0022
FAX: (718)333-0054

Xxi Century Radiology And Imaging P.C.
8686 Bay Pkwy Ste M3
Brooklyn, NY 11214-5193
(718)333-0022
FAX: (718)333-0054

Zwanger Pesiri Radiology
1128 Eastern Pkwy
Brooklyn, NY 11213-4108
(631)225-7200
FAX: (631)870-8732

Buffalo

Amherst Radiology/Breast Screening Center Of Western Ny
2828 Main St
Buffalo, NY 14214-1722
(716)838-1300
FAX: (716)837-7725

Buffalo General Medical Center
100 High St
Buffalo, NY 14203-1154
(716)859-5258
FAX: (716)859-2962

Roswell Park Cancer Institute Mammography Center
666 Elm St, Elm & Carlton Streets
Buffalo, NY 14263-0001
(716)845-3014
FAX: (716)845-3011

Sisters Of Charity Hospital - Main Street Campus
2157 Main St
Buffalo, NY 14214-2692
(716)862-1182
FAX: (716)862-1564

Western New York Breast Health - Mobile Mammography
462 Grider St, C/O Erie County Medical Center Ecmc Foun
Buffalo, NY 14215-3021
(716)632-7465
FAX: (716)632-7464

Western New York Mri
1021 Broadway St
Buffalo, NY 14212-1460
(716)580-2860
FAX: (716)855-2860

Western New York Mri
222 Genesee St
Buffalo, NY 14203-1512
(716)855-2866
FAX: (716)855-2860

Callicoon

Garnet Health Medical Center - Catskills Grover Hermann Div
8881 State Route 97
Callicoon, NY 12723-5052
(845)794-3300
FAX: (845)794-0141

Cambria Heights

Lenox Hill Radiology-Cambria Heights
20620 Linden Blvd
Cambria Heights, NY 11411-1524
(646)680-5629
FAX: (516)791-2472

Camillus

St. Joseph's Imaging Associates
5700 W Genesee St Ste 12
Camillus, NY 13031-3262
(315)631-6555
FAX: (315)631-6559

Canandaigua

Thompson Health Breast Imaging Center
195 Parrish St, Ste 103
Canandaigua, NY 14424-1693
(585)396-6631
FAX: (585)396-6004

Canton

Noble Mammography Unit
80 E Main St
Canton, NY 13617-1450
(315)261-5240
FAX: (315)261-6416

Carmel

Putnam Hospital Center
670 Stoneleigh Ave
Carmel, NY 10512-3997
(845)790-8855
FAX: (845)278-5544

Carthage

Elizabeth Wende Breast Care, L.L.C.
3 Bridge St Ste 1
Carthage, NY 13619-1353
(585)442-2190
FAX: (585)758-7085

Catskill

Greene Medical Imaging
159 Jefferson Hts Ste D106
Catskill, NY 12414-1205
(518)943-0212
FAX: (518)943-0422

Central Square

Central Square Medical Center
3045 East Ave
Central Square, NY 13036-2726
(315)668-5290
FAX: (315)668-5299

Clifton Park

Capital Imaging Assoc, P.C.
3 Emma Ln
Clifton Park, NY 12065-3763
(518)785-7373
FAX: (518)785-5859

Carenet Medical Group
2 Chelsea Pl
Clifton Park, NY 12065-3227
(518)381-1121
FAX: (518)381-3930

Imagecare Clifton Park
1783 Route 9, Ste 104
Clifton Park, NY 12065-2465
(518)836-2428
FAX: (518)836-2413

St. Peter's Medical Imaging
1 Tallow Wood Dr
Clifton Park, NY 12065-2807
(518)373-4448
FAX: (518)373-4556

Clifton Springs

Finger Lakes Breast Care
4 Coulter Rd
Clifton Springs, NY 14432-1122
(315)462-1750
FAX: (315)462-2167

Cobleskill

Bassett Hospital Of Schoharie County
178 Grandview Dr
Cobleskill, NY 12043-1533
(518)254-3351
FAX: (518)254-3360

Cold Spring

The Medical Center At Cold Spring
1756 Route 9D
Cold Spring, NY 10516-2619
(845)265-3642
FAX: (845)265-4324

Commack

Memorial Sloan Kettering Cancer Center At Suffolk
650 Commack Rd
Commack, NY 11725-5404
(631)623-4300
FAX: (631)864-3092

St Catherine Diagnostic
500 Commack Rd Unit 150C
Commack, NY 11725-5009
(934)223-7171
FAX: (934)223-6399

Stony Brook Medicine Advanced Imaging At Commack
500 Commack Rd, Unit 206 Ste 101
Commack, NY 11725-5022
(631)638-2600
FAX: (631)638-0018

Zwanger-Pesiri Radiology
763 Larkfield Rd, Ste 103
Commack, NY 11725-3131
(631)225-7200
FAX: (631)870-8732

Cooperstown

Bassett Healthcare Network
1 Atwell Rd, Mammography Department
Cooperstown, NY 13326-1394
(607)547-3600
FAX: (607)547-6554

Coram

Zwanger Pesiri Radiology
347 Middle Country Rd
Coram, NY 11727-4403
(631)225-7200
FAX: (631)870-8732

Corning

Arnot Health - Corning Medical Office Building
123 Conhocton St
Corning, NY 14830-2959
(607)737-8140
FAX: (607)737-8153

Guthrie Corning Hospital Breast Care Center
1 Guthrie Dr
Corning, NY 14830-3696
(607)937-7060
FAX: (607)937-7358

Cortland

Cayuga Medical Center - Commons Imaging
1129 Commons Ave
Cortland, NY 13045-1639
(607)758-7770
FAX: (607)758-7869

Guthrie Cortland Medical Center
134 Homer Ave
Cortland, NY 13045-1206
(607)756-3793
FAX: (607)756-3802

St Josephs Imaging Associates
1259 Fisher Ave, Department Of Radiology
Cortland, NY 13045-1012
(607)756-4600
FAX: (607)753-6266

Cortlandt Manor

Newyork-Presbyterian/Hudson Valley Hospital
1978 Crompond Rd
Cortlandt Manor, NY 10567-4111
(914)734-3674
FAX: (914)734-3614

Croton On Hudson

Croton Diagnostic
35 S Riverside Ave
Croton On Hudson, NY 10520-2653
(914)271-9481
FAX: (914)271-9404

Phelps Hospital Croton On Hudson
440 S Riverside Ave
Croton On Hudson, NY 10520-3059
(914)366-3464
FAX: (914)366-1214

Dansville

Nicholas H. Noyes Memorial Hospital
111 Clara Barton St
Dansville, NY 14437-9527
(585)335-4235
FAX: (585)335-7952

Delhi

O'Connor Hospital
460 Andes Rd
Delhi, NY 13753-7443
(607)746-0375
FAX: (607)746-0380

Depew

Windsong Radiology Group At Lancaster
4893 Transit Rd Ste 500
Depew, NY 14043-4690
(716)631-2500
FAX: (716)631-4051

Dobbs Ferry

Phelps Hospital At Dobbs Ferry
11 Ashford Ave 17
Dobbs Ferry, NY 10522-1822
(914)366-3464
FAX: (914)366-1214

St. John's Riverside Hospital-Dobbs Ferry Pavilion
128 Ashford Ave
Dobbs Ferry, NY 10522-1924
(914)964-4329
FAX: (914)693-0639

Dunkirk

Brooks Memorial Hospital
529 Central Ave
Dunkirk, NY 14048-2599
(716)363-3933
FAX: (716)363-3947

E Patchogue

Long Island Community Hospital Women's Imaging Services
100 Hospital Rd, Ste 100
E Patchogue, NY 11772-8811
(631)654-7448
FAX: (631)687-2928

East Aurora

Mercy Diagnostic Center - East Aurora
94 Olean St
East Aurora, NY 14052-2531
(716)828-2373
FAX: (716)655-2215

East Hampton

University Hospital Stony Brook Southampton Hospital Campus
200 Pantigo Pl
East Hampton, NY 11937-5920
(631)726-8285
FAX: (631)726-8483

East Islip

Lenox Hill Radiology - East Islip
369 E Main St Ste 16, Building III
East Islip, NY 11730-2800
(631)277-1600
FAX: (631)277-1638

East Meadow

Nassau Univ. Med. Center Breast Imaging Center
2201 Hempstead Tpke
East Meadow, NY 11554-1859
(516)572-6635
FAX: (516)296-4997

East Patchogue

Zwanger Pesiri Radiology
285 Sills Rd Ste A B C Bld 15
East Patchogue, NY 11772-4869
(631)225-7200
FAX: (631)870-8732

East Syracuse

Cny Diagnostic Imaging Assoc.
4939 Brittonfield Pkwy Ste 102
East Syracuse, NY 13057-9211
(315)634-6690
FAX: (315)634-6691

Crouse Medical Imaging Services
5000 Brittonfield Pkwy Ste A114
East Syracuse, NY 13057-9228
(315)234-4680
FAX: (315)463-4614

Elizabethtown

Uvmhn-Elizabethtown Community Hospital
75 Park St
Elizabethtown, NY 12932
(518)873-3036
FAX: (518)873-9192

Ellenville

Ellenville Regional Hospital
10 Healthy Way, Radiology Dept
Ellenville, NY 12428-5612
(845)647-6400
FAX: (845)647-1394

Elmhurst

Apollo Imaging Management Llc
4036 74th St, Ste A
Elmhurst, NY 11373-5619
(718)426-6600
FAX: (718)374-5348

Elmhurst Hospital Center
7901 Broadway, Radiology E1-18
Elmhurst, NY 11373-1368
(718)334-3318
FAX: (718)334-5089

Lenox Hill Radiology, P.C. Elmhurst
8940 56th Ave
Elmhurst, NY 11373-4933
(718)335-5532
FAX: (718)426-9268

Lenox Hill Radiology- Elmhurst Queens Blvd
8812 Queens Blvd
Elmhurst, NY 11373-4489
(718)335-5532
FAX: (718)426-9268

Elmira

Arnot Ogden Medical Center - Health Center For Women
600 Fitch St
Elmira, NY 14905-1634
(607)737-8153
FAX: (607)737-8196

Guthrie Medical Group Southport
1336 Cedar St
Elmira, NY 14904-2951
(607)734-3929
FAX: (607)734-0781

Elmont

Zwanger-Pesiri Radiology
1390 Hempstead Tpke
Elmont, NY 11003-2539
(516)992-6437
FAX: (516)798-8354

Fairport

Rghs Imaging At Cross Keys
100 Cross Keys Office Park Ste 170
Fairport, NY 14450-3509
(585)922-2160
FAX: (585)223-0701

Far Rockaway

St. John's Episcopal Hospital
327 Beach 19th St
Far Rockaway, NY 11691-4423
(718)869-7780
FAX: (718)869-7134

Fayetteville

St. Joseph's Imaging Associates
4117 Medical Center Dr, Ste 117
Fayetteville, NY 13066-6600
(315)329-7555
FAX: (315)329-7559

St. Joseph's Imaging, Associates
4109 Medical Center Dr
Fayetteville, NY 13066-6608
(315)329-7555
FAX: (315)329-7559

Fishkill

Caremount Medical, P.C.
600 Westage Business Ctr Dr
Fishkill, NY 12524-2281
(888)656-4723
FAX: (914)242-1394

Dra, A Division Of Vassar Brothers Medical Center
200 Westage Business Ctr Dr
Fishkill, NY 12524-2264
(845)790-8855
FAX: (845)454-5128

Flushing

Central Radiology, Pc Flushing Imaging Center
13710 Northern Blvd
Flushing, NY 11354-4122
(718)888-9180
FAX: (718)888-9260

Flushing Hospital Medical Center
4500 Parsons Blvd
Flushing, NY 11355-2205
(718)670-5453
FAX: (718)670-3039

Flushing Pet/Ct & Biopsy Services, Pc
14238 37th Ave, Ste 2D
Flushing, NY 11354-4580
(718)353-5555
FAX: (718)353-1777

Jib Medical Pc
15811 Jewel Ave
Flushing, NY 11365-3085
(718)591-2014
FAX: (718)591-9528

Lenox Hill Radiology Pc-Flushing
4355 147th St
Flushing, NY 11355-1736
(718)762-0900
FAX: (718)886-5659

Lenox Hill Radiology-Flushing North
14015 Sanford Ave
Flushing, NY 11355-2686
(917)885-4688
FAX: (718)888-8881

Main Street Radiology At Bayside III Dba Radiology Assoc.
13625 37th Ave 2nd Fl
Flushing, NY 11354-4110
(718)428-1500
FAX: (718)907-2321

Newyork-Presbyterian/Queens
5645 Main St
Flushing, NY 11355-5045
(718)670-1050
FAX: (718)670-1901

Richmond Hill Radiology Pc
4125 Kissena Blvd Ste 122
Flushing, NY 11355-3150
(718)321-2849
FAX: (347)438-1600

Forest Hills

Forest Hills Hospital - Long Island Jewish
10201 66th Rd
Forest Hills, NY 11375-7624
(718)830-4747
FAX: (718)830-4349

Lenox Hill Radiology-Forest Hills
9610 Metropolitan Ave
Forest Hills, NY 11375-6625
(917)903-2617
FAX: (718)629-4493

Neighborhood Radiology Service, Pc
11302 Queens Blvd
Forest Hills, NY 11375-6468
(718)544-3066
FAX: (718)544-3123

Nyu Langone-Qmi-Forest Hills
6915 Austin St
Forest Hills, NY 11375-4255
(718)544-5100
FAX: (718)575-1926

Freeport

Zwanger Pesiri Radiology
375 W Sunrise Hwy
Freeport, NY 11520-3120
(516)544-5003
FAX: (631)870-8732

Fulton

Fulton Medical Imaging An Affilate Of Oswego Health
510 S 4th St
Fulton, NY 13069-2951
(315)349-5540
FAX: (315)592-3548

Garden City

Complete Womens Imaging Pc
990 Stewart Ave Ste 100
Garden City, NY 11530-4838
(516)222-4294
FAX: (516)222-4885

Northwell Health Imaging At Garden City
711 Stewart Ave
Garden City, NY 11530-4731
(516)321-3456
FAX: (516)321-3450

Nyu Langone-Metropolitan-Garden City
224 7th St
Garden City, NY 11530-5781
(516)747-0161
FAX: (516)747-0166

Nyu Langone-Nrad Garden City
765 Stewart Ave
Garden City, NY 11530-4713
(516)222-2022
FAX: (516)222-2004

Nyu Winthrop Breast Center At Zeckendorf
777 Zeckendorf Blvd
Garden City, NY 11530-2126
(516)663-2400
FAX: (516)663-3960

Garden City Park

Square Care Mammography At New Hyde Park
191 Herricks Rd
Garden City Park, NY 11040-5236
(561)486-8853
FAX: (561)423-0675

Geneseo

Elizabeth Wende Breast Care
126 Court St
Geneseo, NY 14454-1036
(585)442-2190
FAX: (585)758-7085

Noyes Health Services
50 E South St
Geneseo, NY 14454-1300
(585)991-6016
FAX: (585)991-6022

Geneva

Geneva General Hospital Women's Health Services
196 North St
Geneva, NY 14456-1694
(315)787-4555
FAX: (315)787-4403

Glen Cove

Northwell Health Imaging At Glen Cove
10 Medical Plz Ste 106
Glen Cove, NY 11542-2101
(516)674-1616
FAX: (516)674-7912

Glendale

Emusc, Llc
8340 Woodhaven Blvd
Glendale, NY 11385-7824
(718)850-4368
FAX: (718)849-6523

Main Street Radiology
8314 Cooper Ave
Glendale, NY 11385-7722
(718)428-1500
FAX: (718)907-2391

Glens Falls

Glens Falls Hospital Breast Center
100 Park St
Glens Falls, NY 12801-4447
(518)926-5333
FAX: (518)926-6628

Irongate Family Practice Associates Pllc
3 Irongate Ctr
Glens Falls, NY 12801-3473
(518)793-4409
FAX: (518)793-5886

North Country Imaging Ctr. Adirondack Radiology Assoc, P.C.
11 Murray St
Glens Falls, NY 12801-4311
(518)793-1000
FAX: (518)793-1976

Womens Care Ob/Gyn
45 Hudson Ave
Glens Falls, NY 12801-4313
(518)793-4477
FAX: (518)793-5643

Gloversville

Nathan Littauer Hospital And Nursing Home
99 E State St
Gloversville, NY 12078-1293
(518)775-4250
FAX: (518)773-5632

Gouverneur

Gouverneur Hospital
77 W Barney St
Gouverneur, NY 13642-1040
(315)261-5712
FAX: (315)535-9268

Great Neck

Northwell Health Imaging At Great Neck
935 Northern Blvd Ste 200
Great Neck, NY 11021-5327
(516)829-4414
FAX: (516)829-7754

Nyu Langone-Ngr-Great Neck
560 Northern Blvd Ste 102
Great Neck, NY 11021-5100
(516)504-1600
FAX: (516)504-6398

Zwanger Pesiri Radiology
907 Northern Blvd
Great Neck, NY 11021-5304
(631)225-7200
FAX: (631)870-8732

Greenlawn

Mount Sinai Doctors, Long Island
5 Cuba Hill Rd
Greenlawn, NY 11740-1624
(631)628-5000
FAX: (631)628-5708

Northwell Health Reichert Family Imaging At Huntington
284 Pulaski Rd
Greenlawn, NY 11740-1602
(631)670-3400
FAX: (631)670-3498

Greenport

Stony Brook Eastern Long Island Hospital
201 Manor Pl
Greenport, NY 11944-1298
(631)477-5152
FAX: (631)477-5845

Greenvale

St. Francis Hospital Dematteis Center Womens Hlth Ctr
101 Northern Blvd
Greenvale, NY 11548-1340
(516)629-2011
FAX: (516)629-2116

Greenwich

Greenwich Regional Medical Center
1134 State Route 29
Greenwich, NY 12834-6107
(518)926-5333
FAX: (518)926-6628

Hamburg

Southtowns Radiology Associates, L.L.C.
3040 Amsdell Rd
Hamburg, NY 14075-5835
(716)649-9000
FAX: (716)649-9005

Windsong Radiology Group At Hamburg
4855 Camp Rd
Hamburg, NY 14075-2600
(716)631-2500
FAX: (716)202-4341

Hamilton

Community Memorial Hospital
150 Broad St
Hamilton, NY 13346-9518
(315)824-6181
FAX: (315)824-6534

Hampton Bays

University Hospital Stony Brook Southampton Hospital Campus
182 W Montauk Hwy Ste B
Hampton Bays, NY 11946-4210
(631)723-1232
FAX: (631)723-1268

Harris

Garnet Health Medical Center-Catskills Women's Imaging
68 Harris-Bushville Road
Harris, NY 12742
(845)794-3300
FAX: (845)794-0141

Hartsdale

Hartsdale Imaging
141 S Central Park Avenue
Hartsdale, NY 10530
(914)761-4030
FAX: (914)949-2931

Hawthorne

Westchester Medical Center Advance Imaging
19 Bradhurst Ave Ste 3700
Hawthorne, NY 10532-2140
(914)597-3744
FAX: (914)493-2550

Henrietta

Henrietta Medical Campus
50 Middle Rd Imaging Department
Henrietta, NY 14467-9312
(585)922-9729
FAX: (585)336-5006

Herkimer

Bassett Healthcare Network - Herkimer
321 E Albany St
Herkimer, NY 13350-2016
(315)867-2792
FAX: (315)867-2820

Hewlett

Lenox Hill Radiology Pc - Hewlett
1137 Broadway
Hewlett, NY 11557-2321
(516)569-8885
FAX: (516)791-4318

Neighborhood Radiology Services, Pc
227 Franklin Ave
Hewlett, NY 11557-1902
(516)295-5500
FAX: (516)295-9251

Hicksville

Zwanger-Pesiri Radiology
272 N Broadway
Hicksville, NY 11801-2911
(631)225-7200
FAX: (631)225-9550

Hornell

Ur Women's Imaging And Breast Center
7309 Seneca Rd N, Suite 113 Enterance E
Hornell, NY 14843-9691
(607)324-8245
FAX: (607)324-8270

Horseheads

Arnot Ogden Med. Ctr. - Horseheads Medical Office Bldg.
100 John Roemmelt Dr
Horseheads, NY 14845-8301
(607)737-8140
FAX: (607)737-8196

Guthrie Medical Group Big Flats
31 Arnot Rd
Horseheads, NY 14845-8533
(607)739-3874
FAX: (607)795-5166

Howard Beach

South Shore Radiology A Division Of Prohealthcare Howard Bch
15636A Crossbay Blvd
Howard Beach, NY 11414-2745
(718)738-0700
FAX: (718)738-4177

Hudson

Columbia Memorial Hospital
71 Prospect Ave
Hudson, NY 12534-2907
(518)828-8109
FAX: (518)828-8191

Huntington

Lenox Hill Radiology & Medical Associates, P.C.
214 Wall St, Fl 2
Huntington, NY 11743-7804
(631)427-8869
FAX: (631)427-5414

Pro Healthcare Associates, Llp
339 Main St
Huntington, NY 11743-6958
(631)470-9090
FAX: (631)470-9091

Huntington Station

Nyu Langone Huntington Medical Group
180 E Pulaski Rd, Department Of Radiology
Huntington Station, NY 11746-1915
(631)425-2175
FAX: (631)425-2274

Zwanger Pesiri Radiology
326 Walt Whitman Rd
Huntington Station, NY 11746-8703
(631)225-7200
FAX: (631)870-8732

Islip

Northwell Health Imaging At Great South Bay
620 Main St
Islip, NY 11751-3516
(631)439-7237
FAX: (631)439-7292

Ithaca

Cayuga Medical Center At Ithaca
101 Dates Dr
Ithaca, NY 14850-1383
(607)274-4255
FAX: (607)274-4564

Cayuga Medical Center At Ithaca-Women's Imaging Ctr
10 Arrowood Dr
Ithaca, NY 14850-1857
(607)274-4255
FAX: (607)252-3724

Guthrie Medical Group Ithaca
1780 Hanshaw Rd
Ithaca, NY 14850-9105
(607)257-5858
FAX: (607)257-1718

Jackson Heights

Lenox Hill Radiology Pc -Jackson Heights
3717 76th St
Jackson Heights, NY 11372-6533
(917)903-2617
FAX: (718)765-4081

Main Street Radiology 4
7206 Northern Blvd, 1st Fl
Jackson Heights, NY 11372-1049
(718)907-2383
FAX: (718)907-2384

Jamaica

Apollo Medical Diagnostic Services Pllc
17010 Cedarcroft Rd
Jamaica, NY 11432-2732
(718)262-8300
FAX: (914)462-4759

Jamaica Hospital Medical Center
8900 Van Wyck Expy
Jamaica, NY 11418-2897
(718)206-6000
FAX: (718)206-8992

Lenox Hill Radiology-Jamaica Estates
18005 Hillside Ave
Jamaica, NY 11432-4727
(917)903-2617
FAX: (718)629-4493

Multi-Diagnostic Services, Inc. - Mobile
13916 91st Ave
Jamaica, NY 11435-4219
(718)454-8556
FAX: (718)454-7950

Nyu Langone-Nrad-Hillcrest
8015 164th St
Jamaica, NY 11432-1119
(718)380-6010
FAX: (718)969-8108

Queens Hospital Center
8268 164th St, Radiology Dept.Room G-52
Jamaica, NY 11432-1104
(718)883-4400
FAX: (718)883-6198

Jamestown

Upmc Chautauqua At Wca
PO Box 840, 207 Foote Ave
Jamestown, NY 14702-0840
(716)664-8448
FAX: (716)485-7894

Katonah

Caremount Medical, P.C.
111 Bedford Rd
Katonah, NY 10536-2115
(888)656-4723
FAX: (914)232-4495

Kenmore

Kenmore Mercy Hospital
2950 Elmwood Ave, Mammography
Kenmore, NY 14217-1390
(716)447-6111
FAX: (716)447-6282

Kew Gardens

Lenox Hill Radiologyp.C.-Kew Gardens
8002 Kew Gardens Rd
Kew Gardens, NY 11415-3600
(718)444-3777
FAX: (718)629-4493

Kingston

Fern Feldman Anolick Center For Breast Health
111 Marys Ave Ste 1
Kingston, NY 12401-5853
(845)334-3088
FAX: (845)334-8928

Nuvance Health Medical Practice, Pc
1240 Ulster Ave
Kingston, NY 12401-1517
(845)443-8720
FAX: (845)336-5016

River Radiology
45 Pine Grove Ave
Kingston, NY 12401-5472
(845)340-4500
FAX: (845)340-4501

Lake Grove

Medical Arts Radiology
570 Smith Haven Mall
Lake Grove, NY 11755-1206
(631)652-3424
FAX: (631)390-0041

Suffolk Breast Imaging, P.C.
2780 Middle Country Rd Ste 210
Lake Grove, NY 11755-2129
(631)588-4500
FAX: (631)588-4595

Lake Katrine

Caremount Medical
1561 Ulster Ave
Lake Katrine, NY 12449-5173
(888)656-4723
FAX: (845)592-7713

Lake Success

Breast Imaging Center Of Northwell Health
450 Lakeville Rd
Lake Success, NY 11042-1118
(516)734-8281
FAX: (516)734-8270

Lenox Hill Radiology-Lake Success
1991 Marcus Ave 2nd Fl
Lake Success, NY 11042-2057
(646)680-5632
FAX: (718)629-4493

Nyu Langone-Nrad Lake Success
6 Ohio Dr Ste 205
Lake Success, NY 11042-1129
(516)222-2022
FAX: (516)730-2081

Prohealth Women's Imaging & Bone Densitometry
1 Dakota Dr, Ste 215
Lake Success, NY 11042-1136
(516)622-2998
FAX: (516)608-6812

Latham

Capital Imaging Associates
PO Box 1130, 1001 Loudon Rd
Latham, NY 12110-0079
(518)785-7373
FAX: (518)785-1132

Imagecare Latham
713 Troy Schenectady Rd, Ste 120
Latham, NY 12110-2490
(518)786-1600
FAX: (518)213-0674

Laurelton

Zwanger Pesiri Radiology
23135 Merrick Blvd
Laurelton, NY 11413-2111
(631)225-7200
FAX: (631)870-8732

Lawrence

Zwanger Pesiri Radiology
625 Rockaway Tpke
Lawrence, NY 11559-1029
(631)219-2585
FAX: (631)870-8732

Levittown

Zwanger-Pesiri Radiology
3235 Hempstead Tpke
Levittown, NY 11756-1319
(516)544-5001
FAX: (516)544-5002

Lewiston

Mount St. Mary's Hospital
5300 Military Rd
Lewiston, NY 14092-1997
(716)298-2370
FAX: (716)298-3785

Lindenhurst

Nassau Suffolk Radiological Assoc Lindenhurst Xray
20 W John St
Lindenhurst, NY 11757-3759
(631)226-2230
FAX: (631)226-3024

Zwanger-Pesiri Radiology Group, Llp
150 Sunrise Hwy
Lindenhurst, NY 11757-2539
(631)225-7200
FAX: (631)225-9550

Little Falls

Bassett Healthcare Network Little Falls Hospital
140 Burwell St
Little Falls, NY 13365-1725
(315)823-5232
FAX: (315)823-5319

Liverpool

Cny Diagnostic Imaging Associates
8100 Oswego Rd, Clay Medical Center
Liverpool, NY 13090-1666
(315)652-1020
FAX: (315)652-4578

St. Joseph's Imaging Associates
5100 W Taft Rd Ste 2A
Liverpool, NY 13088-4886
(315)452-2555
FAX: (315)452-2559

Lockport

Eastern Niagara Hospital- Imaging Center
5875 S Transit Rd
Lockport, NY 14094-6340
(716)514-5823
FAX: (716)514-5817

Long Island City

Nyhtc - Queens Health Center
3711 Queens Blvd
Long Island City, NY 11101-1725
(718)361-5100
FAX: (718)361-5173

Lowville

Lewis County General Hospital
7785 N State St
Lowville, NY 13367-1297
(315)376-5213
FAX: (315)376-3636

Lynbrook

Zwanger Pesiri Radiology
443 Sunrise Hwy
Lynbrook, NY 11563-3017
(631)225-7200
FAX: (631)870-8732

Malone

Alice Hyde Medical Center
133 Park St
Malone, NY 12953-1241
(518)483-3000
FAX: (518)481-2482

Malta

Malta Medical Imaging A Service Of Saratoga Hospital
6 Medical Park Dr, Ste 204
Malta, NY 12020-5053
(518)886-5266
FAX: (518)886-5260

Manhasset

Square Care Mammography At Manhasset
1615 Northern Blvd, Ste 102
Manhasset, NY 11030-3033
(516)738-5602
FAX: (561)423-0675

Manorville

Northwell Health Imaging Grossman Imaging At Manorville
496 County Road 111 Bldg F1
Manorville, NY 11949-3388
(631)405-3240
FAX: (631)281-0303

Margaretville

Margaretville Hospital
42084 State Highway 28
Margaretville, NY 12455-2820
(845)586-2631
FAX: (845)586-1786

Massapequa

Lenox Hill Radiology & Medical Associates, P.C.
4160 Merrick Rd
Massapequa, NY 11758-6000
(631)626-2731
FAX: (516)797-8463

Zwanger Pesiri Radiology
126 Hicksville Rd
Massapequa, NY 11758-5822
(516)798-4242
FAX: (631)870-8732

Massena

Massena Hospital, Inc.
1 Hospital Dr
Massena, NY 13662-1097
(315)769-4228
FAX: (315)769-4370

Medford

Zwanger-Pesiri Radiology
1729 N Ocean Ave
Medford, NY 11763-2649
(631)444-5544
FAX: (631)870-8732

Medina

Medina Memorial Hospital
200 Ohio St
Medina, NY 14103-1095
(585)798-8054
FAX: (585)798-8150

Merrick

Zwanger Pesiri Radiology Group
2012 Sunrise Hwy
Merrick, NY 11566-3825
(516)225-7200
FAX: (516)870-8732

Middletown

Crystal Run Healthcare Llp
95 Crystal Run Rd
Middletown, NY 10941-7001
(845)703-6366
FAX: (845)703-3849

Garnet Health Medical Center Ray W. Moody,MD Breast Center
707 E Main St
Middletown, NY 10940-2650
(845)333-7040
FAX: (845)333-7042

Middletown Medical, P.C.
60 Dunning Rd
Middletown, NY 10940-2215
(845)342-4774
FAX: (845)342-2520

Mineola

Nyu Winthrop Hosp Breast Imaging & Diagnostic Ste
120 Mineola Blvd Ste 550
Mineola, NY 11501-4061
(516)663-2400
FAX: (516)663-3960

Monroe

Crystal Run Healthcare Llp
855 State Route 17M
Monroe, NY 10950-1600
(845)796-5474
FAX: (845)358-1948

Hudson Valley Imaging
745 State Route 17M Ste 106
Monroe, NY 10950-2663
(845)220-2222
FAX: (845)784-3755

Orange Radiology Mri Of Orange
505 State Route 208 Ste 18
Monroe, NY 10950-1607
(845)783-3444
FAX: (845)783-2498

Montour Falls

Schuyler Hospital
220 Steuben St
Montour Falls, NY 14865-9709
(607)535-8613
FAX: (607)535-4186

Mount Kisco

Caremount Medical, P.C.
90 S Bedford Rd
Mount Kisco, NY 10549-3412
(888)666-4723
FAX: (914)242-2989

Caremount Medical, P.C.
105 S Bedford Rd Ste 103R
Mount Kisco, NY 10549-3441
(888)656-4723
FAX: (914)242-1389

Northeast Radiology
666 Lexington Ave
Mount Kisco, NY 10549-3632
(914)666-6692
FAX: (914)666-6553

Northern Westchester Hospital
400 E Main St
Mount Kisco, NY 10549-3477
(914)666-1445
FAX: (914)242-8136

Mount Vernon

Montefiore Mount Vernon Hospital
12 N 7th Ave
Mount Vernon, NY 10550-2098
(914)664-8000
FAX: (914)664-0456

New City

Mid Rockland Imaging
18 Squadron Blvd
New City, NY 10956-5210
(845)634-9729
FAX: (845)634-6442

New Hartford

Oxford Medical Imaging, P.C.
1 Oxford Rd
New Hartford, NY 13413-2650
(315)738-1795
FAX: (315)738-1798

Slocum-Dickson Medical Group, Pllc
1729 Burrstone Rd
New Hartford, NY 13413-1093
(315)798-1442
FAX: (315)624-2135

New Rochelle

Montefiore New Rochelle Hospital
16 Guion Pl
New Rochelle, NY 10801-5502
(914)365-4618
FAX: (914)365-5252

New Rochelle Radiology Associates, P.C.
175 Memorial Hwy, Ste Ll14 LL 14A
New Rochelle, NY 10801-5655
(914)633-7700
FAX: (914)576-8503

Westmed Medical Group
171 Huguenot St
New Rochelle, NY 10801-7760
(914)682-6430
FAX: (914)682-6462

White Plains Hospital Imaging At New Rochelle
1296 North Ave
New Rochelle, NY 10804-2603
(914)336-5900
FAX: (914)336-5980

New Windsor

Hudson Valley Imaging
575 Hudson Valley Ave Ste 101
New Windsor, NY 12553-4746
(845)220-2222
FAX: (845)220-2241

New York

Avon Foundation Breast Imaging Center
1130 Saint Nicholas Ave
New York, NY 10032-3802
(212)305-0519
FAX: (212)342-5385

Barbara Edelstein, MD Women's Radiology, Pc
1045 Park Ave
New York, NY 10028-1030
(212)860-7700
FAX: (212)860-7703

Beekman Radiology, Pllc
342 E 49th St, Ofc 1
New York, NY 10017-7315
(212)508-0045
FAX: (212)508-0047

Bellevue Hospital Center
462 1st Ave, Frnt 1 Rm 3W33
New York, NY 10016-9198
(212)562-6440
FAX: (212)263-7666

C. P. Advanced Imaging Pllc
155 Canal St
New York, NY 10013-4551
(212)431-9010
FAX: (212)219-9291

Canal Radiology Associatespc / Dba Community Radiology Ny
212 Canal St Rm 206
New York, NY 10013-4156
(212)349-5799
FAX: (212)349-6183

Chelsea Diagnostic Radiology P.C.
230 W 17th St
New York, NY 10011-5325
(212)989-8999
FAX: (212)989-1992

Clement M. Barone, M.D., P.C.
1440 York Ave Ofc P1
New York, NY 10075-2577
(212)988-1303
FAX: (212)628-9113

Columbiadoctors/Newyork-Presbyterian Imaging
51 W 51st St
New York, NY 10019-6113
(212)326-8517
FAX: (212)326-8528

East River Medical Imaging
430 E 59th St
New York, NY 10022-2396
(212)832-8320
FAX: (212)832-8322

Executive Health Exams
600 5th Ave, Fl 5 6th Fl
New York, NY 10020-2313
(212)332-5142
FAX: (646)665-4096

Executive Medical Services/Greenwich, Pc
255 Greenwich St, Rm 520
New York, NY 10007-5504
(212)935-8725
FAX: (212)349-2500

Gouverneur Healthcare Services
227 Madison St 4th Fl
New York, NY 10002-7537
(212)238-7510
FAX: (212)238-7526

Harlem Hospital Center
506 Malcolm X Blvd
New York, NY 10037-1889
(212)939-4294
FAX: (212)939-4987

Kathy Plesser MD Pllc
1440 York Ave Ofc P1
New York, NY 10075-2577
(212)744-2293
FAX: (212)744-6000

Laura And Isaac Perlmutter Cancer Center
160 E 34th St 3rd Fl
New York, NY 10016-4744
(212)731-5002
FAX: (212)731-5554

Laura Perlmutter Center For Women's Imaging
221 Lexington Ave
New York, NY 10016-4640
(646)754-1334
FAX: (646)754-1334

Lenox Hill Hospital
100 E 77th St
New York, NY 10075-1850
(212)434-6618
FAX: (212)434-2984

Lenox Hill Radiology
315 W 57th St Ste Ll4
New York, NY 10019-3149
(212)772-3111
FAX: (212)799-1289

Lenox Hill Radiology & Medical Imaging Assoc., Pc - Nypmi
525 Park Ave
New York, NY 10065-8141
(212)888-1000
FAX: (973)767-0259

Lenox Hill Radiology & Medical Imaging Associates P.C,
147 W 15th St
New York, NY 10011-6749
(212)473-2300
FAX: (212)473-4780

Lenox Hill Radiology & Medical Imaging Associates P.C.
144 4th Ave
New York, NY 10003-4901
(212)473-2300
FAX: (212)473-4780

Lenox Hill Radiology & Medical Imaging Associates P.C.-Nypmi
61 E 77th St
New York, NY 10075-1817
(212)772-3111
FAX: (212)288-1852

Lenox Hill Radiology & Medical Imaging Associates, P.C.
1790 Broadway 1790 Broadway 9th Floo
New York, NY 10019-1412
(212)590-2900
FAX: (212)590-5599

Lenox Hill Radiology & Medical Imaging Associates, Pc
4334 Broadway
New York, NY 10033-2412
(212)927-1717
FAX: (212)297-3453

Lenox Hill Radiology & Medical Imaging Associates, Pc
240 Madison Ave Fl 2
New York, NY 10016-2884
(212)772-3111
FAX: (212)490-3933

Lenox Hill Radiology - East 95th Street
215 E 95th St, Ste C
New York, NY 10128-4077
(646)680-2767
FAX: (212)423-3489

Lenox Hill Radiology - Harlem
215 W 125th St
New York, NY 10027-4426
(212)812-6569
FAX: (212)931-0619

Lenox Hill Radiology Pc - Washington Heights
4120 Broadway
New York, NY 10033-3703
(212)543-1800
FAX: (212)543-0591

Lenox Hill Radiology& Medical Imaging Associates P.C.
400 E 66th St
New York, NY 10065-9314
(646)253-7033
FAX: (973)767-0258

Madison Avenue Radiology Center
1820 Madison Ave
New York, NY 10035-3884
(212)860-3500
FAX: (212)860-3531

Madison Avenue Radiology Center - Washington Heights 152
3672 Broadway
New York, NY 10031-1536
(212)860-3500
FAX: (212)860-3531

Madison Avenue Radiology Center 190th Broadway
4448 Broadway
New York, NY 10040-2939
(212)860-3500
FAX: (212)860-3531

Maiden Lane Medical, Pllc
18 E 41st St, Bldg 2nd
New York, NY 10017-6222
(646)290-5960
FAX: (212)532-4362

Medical Imaging Of Manhattan, Llc.
106 E 61st St
New York, NY 10065-8102
(212)794-2500
FAX: (212)879-3846

Memorial Sloan-Kettering Cancer Diagnostic Imaging Dept
300 E 66th St
New York, NY 10065-6800
(646)227-3700
FAX: (646)888-5135

Metropolitan Hospital - Radiology Department
1901 1st Ave
New York, NY 10029-7494
(212)423-8341
FAX: (212)423-8398

Mount Sinai Downtown Chelsea Center
325 W 15th St
New York, NY 10011-5903
(212)604-6009
FAX: (212)367-1707

Mount Sinai Downtown Union Square
10 Union Sq E Ste 4L
New York, NY 10003-3314
(212)844-8776
FAX: (212)844-8795

Mount Sinai Hospital Cam Building
17 E 102nd St, Sixth Floor East Building
New York, NY 10029-5204
(212)824-7700
FAX: (212)824-2323

Mount Sinai Hospital Dubin Breast Center
1176 5th Ave Box 1160
New York, NY 10029-6503
(212)241-3300
FAX: (646)537-8611

Mount Sinai Mobile Mammography - Mobile
1 Gustave L Levy Pl, Box 1234
New York, NY 10029-6574
(844)396-2666
FAX: (212)824-2323

Mount Sinai Morningside
1111 Amsterdam Ave
New York, NY 10025-1716
(212)523-2467
FAX: (212)523-2888

Mount Sinai Radiology Associates West
425 W 59th St, Suite 6 B - C
New York, NY 10019-8022
(212)523-7049
FAX: (212)523-6019

Murray Hill Radiology & Mammography-Ny Private Medical Imag.
650 1st Ave, Second Floor
New York, NY 10016-3240
(212)686-4440
FAX: (212)683-3092

New York Hotel Trades Council Health Center
773 9th Ave 775
New York, NY 10019-6336
(212)586-1550
FAX: (212)586-6386

New York Medical Imaging Associates
165 E 84th St
New York, NY 10028-2049
(212)535-9770
FAX: (212)369-9826

New York Presbyterian Hospital Columbia Medical Ctr
161 Fort Washington Ave, Hip-10, Department Of Radiology
New York, NY 10032-3729
(212)305-0160
FAX: (212)342-5385

New York Radiology Associates
55 E 34th St
New York, NY 10016-4337
(212)252-6004
FAX: (212)252-6082

Newyork-Presbyterian/Lower Manhattan Hospital
170 William St
New York, NY 10038-2612
(212)312-5179
FAX: (212)312-5298

Northwell Health Imaging At Greenwich Village
200 W 13th St 5th Fl
New York, NY 10011-7702
(646)665-6700
FAX: (646)665-6740

Nyu Langone Women's Health Center
207 E 84th St, 3rd Fl
New York, NY 10028-2972
(646)754-3300
FAX: (917)829-2071

Project Renewal Scan Van - Mobile
200 Varick St, 9th Fl
New York, NY 10014-4810
(800)564-6868
FAX: (631)859-4904

Ralph Lauren Center For Cancer Care And Prevention
1919 Madison Ave, Frnt 2
New York, NY 10035-2745
(646)888-5357
FAX: (646)888-5333

Renaissance Health Care Network
264 W 118th St
New York, NY 10026-1620
(888)692-4692
FAX: (212)932-6599

Robert L. Bard, M.D., P.C.
121 E 60th St Apt 6A
New York, NY 10022-1198
(212)355-7017
FAX: (212)752-6192

Rosenbaum, Rosenfeld, M.D.'s
1421 3rd Ave, Frnt
New York, NY 10028-1900
(212)744-5538
FAX: (212)744-4767

Schaffer, Schonholz And Drossman, Llp
488 Madison Ave Fl 1220
New York, NY 10022-5715
(212)755-7656
FAX: (212)688-9474

Thomas Kolb MD Pc
106 E 61st St
New York, NY 10065-8102
(212)602-1168
FAX: (646)626-5591

Weill Cornell Imaging At New York Presbyterian
425 E 61st St Fl 9
New York, NY 10065-8722
(212)746-6000
FAX: (212)821-0671

Weill Cornell Imaging At New York-Presbyterian
53 Beekman St
New York, NY 10038-1510
(212)746-6000
FAX: (646)962-0122

Newark

Newark Wayne Community Hospital
PO Box 111, Driving Park Avenue
Newark, NY 14513-0111
(315)332-2241
FAX: (315)332-2454

Newburgh

Crystal Run Healthcare Llp
1200 Route 300 Ste E128, Crystal Run Healthcare Llp
Newburgh, NY 12550-5003
(845)796-5474
FAX: (845)796-5820

Orange Radiology Assoc., P.C.
320 Robinson Ave, Ste 1
Newburgh, NY 12550-3354
(845)565-3664
FAX: (845)863-0589

St Luke's Cornwall Hospital
70 Dubois St
Newburgh, NY 12550-4898
(845)458-4000
FAX: (845)458-4666

Niagara Falls

Summit Healthplex
6934 Williams Rd
Niagara Falls, NY 14304-3080
(716)298-5872
FAX: (716)298-5211

Niskayuna

Ellis Medicine Bellevue Women's Center
2210 Troy Schenectady Rd
Niskayuna, NY 12309-4797
(518)243-3333
FAX: (518)346-9545

North Babylon

Lenox Hill Radiology-Babylon
300 Bay Shore Rd
North Babylon, NY 11703-2823
(917)903-2617
FAX: (718)629-4493

North Syracuse

Associates For Womens Medicine
792 N Main St, Ste 200D
North Syracuse, NY 13212-1673
(901)752-4000
FAX: (877)352-5576

Norwich

Chenango Memorial Hospital, Inc
6 Newton Ave
Norwich, NY 13815-1153
(607)337-4999
FAX: (607)337-4205

Nyack

Montefiore Nyack
160 N Midland Ave
Nyack, NY 10960-1912
(845)348-8551
FAX: (845)348-8596

Oceanside

Mount Sinai South Nassau Center For Women's Imaging
440 Merrick Rd, Ste 3
Oceanside, NY 11572-1404
(516)255-8220
FAX: (516)255-8219

Ogdensburg

Claxton Hepburn Medical Center
214 King St, Radiology Department
Ogdensburg, NY 13669-1191
(315)713-5144
FAX: (315)393-8473

Olean

Olean General Hospital
515 Main St
Olean, NY 14760-1598
(716)375-6400
FAX: (716)375-6388

Olean Medical Group, Llp
535 Main St
Olean, NY 14760-1593
(716)376-2297
FAX: (716)376-2341

Oneida

Alice Gorman Imaging - Oneida Healthcare Center
139 Fields Dr
Oneida, NY 13421-2642
(315)361-2035
FAX: (315)361-2267

Oneonta

A. O. Fox Memorial Hospital
1 Norton Ave
Oneonta, NY 13820-2697
(607)431-5015
FAX: (607)431-5102

Foxcare Center Medical Imaging
1 Foxcare Dr Ste 400, Foxcare Center-Outpatient Testing
Oneonta, NY 13820-2473
(607)431-5015
FAX: (607)431-5102

Orchard Park

Buffalo Medical Group
3900 N Buffalo St
Orchard Park, NY 14127-1842
(716)630-1178
FAX: (716)995-1669

Great Lakes Medical Imaging
5959 Big Tree Rd, Ste 105
Orchard Park, NY 14127-2291
(716)256-1114
FAX: (716)256-1115

Mercy Ambulatory Care Center
3669 Southwestern Blvd
Orchard Park, NY 14127-1732
(716)828-2373
FAX: (716)828-3455

Oswego

Oswego Hospital
110 W 6th St
Oswego, NY 13126-2598
(315)349-5540
FAX: (315)349-5748

St Joseph's Imaging Associates
300 State Route 104, Ste 3
Oswego, NY 13126-2956
(315)216-6060
FAX: (316)216-6249

Owego

Guthrie Medical Group Owego
1246 State Route 38
Owego, NY 13827-3217
(607)687-6101
FAX: (607)687-5994

Ozone Park

Lenox Hill Radiology- Ozone Park
10234 Atlantic Ave
Ozone Park, NY 11416-1739
(347)726-8531
FAX: (718)425-9878

Patchogue

Lenox Hill Radiology & Medical Associates, P.C.
240 Patchogue Yaphank Rd, Sills Rd.
Patchogue, NY 11772-4868
(631)475-2639
FAX: (631)475-3369

Penfield

Highland Breast Imaging
2212 Penfield Rd Ste 500
Penfield, NY 14526-1770
(585)487-3300
FAX: (585)377-9746

Penn Yan

Soldiers And Sailors Memorial Hospital
418 N Main St
Penn Yan, NY 14527-1085
(315)531-2546
FAX: (315)531-2558

Perth

Perth Broadalbin Primary Care
4104 State Highway 30
Perth, NY 12010-6202
(518)883-8620
FAX: (518)883-2646

Plainview

Lenox Hill Radiology & Medical Associates, P.C.
146 Manetto Hill Rd
Plainview, NY 11803-1308
(516)822-3615
FAX: (516)822-0008

Prohealth Radiology Of Plainview
520 Old Country Rd
Plainview, NY 11803-6501
(516)495-5200
FAX: (516)495-5201

Zwanger - Pesiri Radiology Group
680 Old Country Rd
Plainview, NY 11803-4911
(516)681-8400
FAX: (516)433-7201

Plattsburgh

The University Of Vermont Health Network Cvph Womens Imaging
89 Plaza Blvd
Plattsburgh, NY 12901-6438
(518)562-1055
FAX: (518)562-1736

Port Jefferson

Fortunato Breast Health Ctr Mather Hospital Northwell Health
75 N Country Rd
Port Jefferson, NY 11777-2119
(631)686-2594
FAX: (631)476-2783

St. Charles Hospital
200 Belle Terre Rd
Port Jefferson, NY 11777-1968
(631)474-6163
FAX: (631)474-6883

Port Jefferson Station

Zwanger Pesiri Radiology
4 Medical Dr
Port Jefferson Station, NY 11776-1601
(631)225-7200
FAX: (631)870-8732

Port Jervis

Bon Secours Community Hospital
160 E Main St
Port Jervis, NY 12771-2114
(845)858-7050
FAX: (845)858-7432

Potsdam

Canton-Potsdam Hospital
50 Leroy St
Potsdam, NY 13676-1799
(315)265-3300
FAX: (315)261-6416

Poughkeepsie

Caremount Medical, P.C.
2507 South Rd Rte 9
Poughkeepsie, NY 12601-5458
(888)656-4723
FAX: (845)231-5616

Caremount Medical, P.C.
30 Columbia St
Poughkeepsie, NY 12601-3906
(888)656-4723
FAX: (845)231-5616

Medical Diagnostic Imaging, Pllc
14 Raymond Ave
Poughkeepsie, NY 12603-2312
(845)471-2848
FAX: (845)471-2919

Mid-Hudson Valley Division Of Westchester Medical Center
19 Baker Ave, Ste 101
Poughkeepsie, NY 12601-1379
(845)483-5274
FAX: (845)483-5797

Vassar Brothers Medical Center
21 Reade Pl, Ste 2000
Poughkeepsie, NY 12601-3968
(845)483-6563
FAX: (845)483-6566

Pulaski

Oswego Hospital Radiology Pulaski Health Center
61 Delano St, Pulaski Health Center
Pulaski, NY 13142-1400
(315)349-5540
FAX: (315)349-5748

Purchase

Westmed Medical Group
3030 Westchester Ave
Purchase, NY 10577-2574
(914)682-6430
FAX: (914)457-1474

Queensbury

Glens Falls Hospital - Breast Center At Baybrook
22 Willowbrook Rd
Queensbury, NY 12804-5876
(518)926-5333
FAX: (518)926-6628

Rego Park

Middle Village Radiology
6243 Woodhaven Blvd
Rego Park, NY 11374-3731
(718)507-4700
FAX: (718)397-0422

Nyu Langone Ambulatory Care Rego Park Imaging And Infusion
9777 Queens Blvd, First Floor
Rego Park, NY 11374-3335
(718)261-8686
FAX: (718)261-3803

Rensselaer

Northeast Health Imaging Center Albany Memorial Hosp
279 Troy Rd. Route 4, Rensselaer County Plaza
Rensselaer, NY 12144
(518)880-6304
FAX: (518)880-6337

Rhinebeck

Caremount Medical, P.C.
6734 Route 9
Rhinebeck, NY 12572-3724
(888)656-4723
FAX: (845)592-7713

Northern Dutchess Hospital
PO Box 5002, 6511 Springbrook Ave
Rhinebeck, NY 12572-5002
(845)871-3489
FAX: (845)871-3487

Richmond Hill

Jamaica Hospital Medical Ctr - Womens Health Ctr
13303 Jamaica Ave
Richmond Hill, NY 11418-2618
(718)206-6138
FAX: (718)206-6145

Richmond Hill Radiology
11614 Myrtle Ave
Richmond Hill, NY 11418-1748
(718)846-0606
FAX: (718)846-8684

Ridgewood

Allium Diagnostic Imaging
345 Saint Nicholas Ave
Ridgewood, NY 11385-2739
(718)408-5000
FAX: (718)381-2090

Lenox Hill Radiology- Ridgewood
5501 Myrtle Ave
Ridgewood, NY 11385-3550
(718)491-7750
FAX: (347)246-0656

Riverhead

Northwell Health Imaging At Northfork
1333 Heroes Way
Riverhead, NY 11901-2029
(631)727-2755
FAX: (631)727-4391

Stony Brook Medicine Advanced Imaging At Riverhead
350 Old Country Rd
Riverhead, NY 11901-2147
(631)638-2600
FAX: (631)216-7792

Rochester

Elizabeth Wende Breast Care Llc
3 Saredon Pl Ste 200
Rochester, NY 14606-4059
(585)442-2190
FAX: (585)758-7085

Elizabeth Wende Breast Care, Lcc
170 Sawgrass Dr
Rochester, NY 14620-4648
(585)442-2190
FAX: (585)758-7085

Highland Breast Imaging
500 Red Creek Dr Ste 130
Rochester, NY 14623-4284
(585)487-3300
FAX: (585)334-5519

Highland Breast Imaging At Anthony Jordan Health Center
82 Holland St Rm 101E
Rochester, NY 14605-2131
(585)487-3300
FAX: (585)334-5519

Highland Hospital Highland Breast Imaging
1000 South Ave
Rochester, NY 14620-2733
(585)341-6869
FAX: (585)341-8087

Ide Imaging Partners Inc Dba Borg & Ide Imaging Pc
2619 Culver Rd
Rochester, NY 14609-1738
(585)241-6400
FAX: (585)241-6715

Ide Imaging Partners Inc Dba Borg & Ide Imaging Pc
200 White Spruce Blvd, Ste 30
Rochester, NY 14623-1605
(585)241-6400
FAX: (585)475-1116

Ide Imaging Partners Inc Dba Borg And Ide Imaging
2655 Ridgeway Ave Ste 110
Rochester, NY 14626-4296
(585)241-6575
FAX: (585)241-6595

Ide Imaging Partners, Inc., Dba/Borg & Ide Imaging, Pc
995 Senator Keating Blvd, Bldg E Ste 100
Rochester, NY 14618-2775
(585)241-6400
FAX: (585)241-6630

Rgh Mobile Mammography Center
3495 Winton Pl, Ste D Suite 2
Rochester, NY 14623-2816
(585)922-9729
FAX: (585)336-5006

Rghs Imaging At Alexander Park
214 Alexander St Ste 1000
Rochester, NY 14607-4002
(585)922-9729
FAX: (585)336-5006

Rghs Imaging At Mob
1415 Portland Ave Ste 190
Rochester, NY 14621-3039
(585)922-9729
FAX: (585)336-5006

Riedman Health Center Imaging
1455 E Ridge Rd
Rochester, NY 14621-2006
(585)922-9729
FAX: (585)336-5006

Strong Memorial Hospital U Of R Medical Center
601 Elmwood Ave Box 648, Univ. Of Rochester Medical Center
Rochester, NY 14642-0001
(585)276-4517
FAX: (585)276-1067

Rock Hill

Crystal Run Healthcare Llp
61 Emerald Pl
Rock Hill, NY 12775-6049
(845)703-6167
FAX: (845)703-3793

Rockville Centre

Mercy Medical Center
PO Box 9024, 1000 N Village Ave
Rockville Centre, NY 11571-9024
(516)705-1300
FAX: (516)705-3028

Prohealth Radiology Rockville Centre
19 Morris Ave
Rockville Centre, NY 11570-5336
(516)766-1700
FAX: (516)763-2734

Rome

Mohawk Glen Radiology Associates Of Cny, Pllc
91 Perimeter Rd, Griffiss Technology Park
Rome, NY 13441-4018
(315)334-9729
FAX: (315)334-1185

Rome Memorial Hospital
1500 N James St, Radiology Department
Rome, NY 13440-2899
(315)338-7338
FAX: (315)338-7394

Ronkonkoma

Lenox Hill Radiology-Ronkonkoma
640 Hawkins Ave
Ronkonkoma, NY 11779-2324
(646)680-5634
FAX: (718)629-4493

Rye

The Westchester Medical Group, Pc Dba Westmed Medical Group
1 Theall Rd
Rye, NY 10580-1404
(914)682-6430
FAX: (914)719-5769

Rye Brook

Rye Radiology Associates, Llp
30 Rye Ridge Plz
Rye Brook, NY 10573-2830
(914)253-9200
FAX: (914)253-8827

White Plains Hospital Women's Imaging Ctr. At Rye Brook
90 S Ridge St
Rye Brook, NY 10573-2811
(914)935-0011
FAX: (914)935-9002

Saranac Lake

Adirondack Health At Saranac Lake
2233 State Rt 86
Saranac Lake, NY 12983
(518)891-4141
FAX: (518)897-2260

Saratoga Springs

Imagecare Saratoga
1 West Ave
Saratoga Springs, NY 12866-6045
(518)584-5000
FAX: (518)584-3387

Saratoga Imaging Center
3 Care Ln Ste 100
Saratoga Springs, NY 12866-8635
(518)587-7773
FAX: (518)583-4436

Wilton Medical Arts
3040 Route 50
Saratoga Springs, NY 12866-3073
(518)580-2273
FAX: (518)580-2234

Woman's Care Ob/Gyn
6 Carpenter Ln
Saratoga Springs, NY 12866-5521
(518)583-0020
FAX: (518)886-0040

Sayville

Zwanger Pesiri Radiology
5650 Sunrise Hwy
Sayville, NY 11782-1009
(631)265-9645
FAX: (631)870-8732

Schenectady

Carenet Medical Group
2123 River Rd
Schenectady, NY 12309-1135
(518)381-1121
FAX: (518)371-8102

Ellis Medicine McClellan Street Health Center
600 McClellan St
Schenectady, NY 12304-1009
(518)243-3333
FAX: (518)347-5498

Imagecare Balltown
2546 Balltown Rd Ste 100
Schenectady, NY 12309-1079
(518)372-1344
FAX: (518)372-9848

Imagecare Guilderland
3757 Carman Rd Ste 102
Schenectady, NY 12303-5438
(518)881-1188
FAX: (518)881-1192

Shirley

Zwanger-Pesiri Radiology
803 Montauk Hwy Unit F
Shirley, NY 11967-2124
(631)444-5544
FAX: (631)870-8732

Sidney

Chenango Memorial Hospital Sidney Clinic
44 Pearl St W
Sidney, NY 13838-1325
(607)561-2212
FAX: (607)563-7731

Sleepy Hollow

Phelps Memorial Breast Center
701 N Broadway, Radiology Department
Sleepy Hollow, NY 10591-1096
(914)366-3464
FAX: (914)366-1214

Smithtown

Northwell Health Imaging At Smithtown
226 E Main St
Smithtown, NY 11787-2918
(855)377-3456
FAX: (631)670-3497

St. Catherine Of Siena Medical Center
50 Route 25A
Smithtown, NY 11787-1398
(631)862-3222
FAX: (631)862-3619

Zwanger-Pesiri Radiology
987 W Jericho Tpke
Smithtown, NY 11787-3203
(631)265-5777
FAX: (631)265-5797

Southampton

University Hospital Stony Brook Southampton Hospital Campus
240 Meeting House Ln, Southampton Hospital
Southampton, NY 11968-5009
(631)726-8285
FAX: (631)726-8483

Springville

Bertrand Chaffee Hospital
224 E Main St
Springville, NY 14141-1497
(716)592-8169
FAX: (716)592-8117

Staten Island

Amboy Medical Practice
1161 Victory Blvd
Staten Island, NY 10301-3621
(718)818-1161
FAX: (718)273-2097

Gotham Health Vanderbilt
165 Vanderbilt Ave
Staten Island, NY 10304-2521
(718)616-0999
FAX: (718)616-0999

Lenox Hill Radiology-Annadale
4771 Hylan Blvd
Staten Island, NY 10312-6315
(646)680-5610
FAX: (718)777-4232

Lenox Hill Radiology-Clove Road
1050 Clove Rd
Staten Island, NY 10301-3627
(646)680-5610
FAX: (718)629-4493

Regional Management Service Organization,Llc
4849 Arthur Kill Rd
Staten Island, NY 10309-2630
(718)605-6500
FAX: (718)876-2012

Regional Management Service Organization,Llc
360 Bard Ave
Staten Island, NY 10310-1666
(718)605-6500
FAX: (718)876-2012

The Breast Imaging Ctr At Staten Island University Hosp.
256 Mason Ave B
Staten Island, NY 10305-3408
(718)226-1333
FAX: (718)226-6387

Stony Brook

Carol M. Baldwin Breast Care Ctr At Stony Brook Univ Med Ctr
3 Edmund D. Pellegrino Rd
Stony Brook, NY 11794-9460
(631)638-2121
FAX: (631)638-0623

Stony Brook Medicine Advanced Imaging
1320 Stony Brook Road
Stony Brook, NY 11794-0001
(631)638-2656
FAX: (631)638-2644

Stony Brook Medicine-Stony Brook University Hospital
Carol M. Baldwin Breast Care Center, 3 Edmund Pellegrino Rd
Stony Brook, NY 11794-9445
(833)638-4134
FAX: (631)638-0623

Zwanger - Pesiri Radiology
2500 Nesconset Hwy Bldg 15A
Stony Brook, NY 11790-2554
(631)225-7200
FAX: (631)870-8732

Suffern

Good Samaritan Hospital
255 Lafayette Ave
Suffern, NY 10901-4869
(866)596-8456
FAX: (845)368-5331

Ramapo Diagnostics Imaging
11 N Airmont Rd, Ste 6
Suffern, NY 10901-5103
(845)357-7245
FAX: (845)357-7457

Syosset

Northwell Health Imaging At Syosset
100 Lafayette Dr, Ste 1
Syosset, NY 11791-3941
(516)622-3456
FAX: (516)622-3450

Syracuse

Beth Houck MD
475 Irving Ave Ste 406
Syracuse, NY 13210-1535
(315)671-5310
FAX: (315)671-5304

Cny Diagnostic Imaging Associates, Llc
1000 E Genesee St Ste 100, The Hill Medical Center
Syracuse, NY 13210-1737
(315)472-8835
FAX: (315)476-3712

Dr.Hadley J. Falk Breast Health Center At Crouse Hospital
739 Irving Ave 1st Fl
Syracuse, NY 13210-1651
(315)470-5880
FAX: (315)470-1378

Loftus, Ryu, And Bartol Mds Pc
475 Irving Ave Ste 108
Syracuse, NY 13210-1691
(315)671-0070
FAX: (315)475-0620

Shane M. Sopp Md, Pc
4900 Broad Rd Ste 2V
Syracuse, NY 13215-2265
(315)492-5005
FAX: (315)492-5324

St. Joseph's Imaging Associates
104 Union Ave, Ste 905
Syracuse, NY 13203-1845
(315)703-5116
FAX: (315)703-5014

St. Joseph's Imaging Pc
109 Pine St
Syracuse, NY 13210-1215
(315)475-1669
FAX: (315)475-9518

Syracuse Community Health Center, Inc.
819 S Salina St, Radiology Department
Syracuse, NY 13202-3570
(315)471-4309
FAX: (315)234-5994

The Women's Health Network
550 Harrison St Ste D, The Women's Health Network, Breast Imagi
Syracuse, NY 13202-3188
(315)464-2588
FAX: (315)464-7411

Wellspring Breast Care Center Uuh At Community General
4900 Broad Rd
Syracuse, NY 13215-2265
(315)464-2588
FAX: (315)492-5299

Ticonderoga

Uvm Health Network/Elizabethtown Comm.Hosp./Moses Ludington
101 Adirondack Dr Ste 1
Ticonderoga, NY 12883-9334
(518)585-3758
FAX: (518)585-3845

Troy

Capital Region Women's Care
101 Jordan Rd, Ste 202
Troy, NY 12180-8337
(518)274-0476
FAX: (518)687-0003

St. Peter's Breast Center Troy
1300 Massachusetts Ave, 3rd Fl
Troy, NY 12180-1628
(518)268-5353
FAX: (518)268-5534

Tuckahoe

Hudson Valley Radiology Associates Of Westchester
115 Main St, Ste 201
Tuckahoe, NY 10707-2950
(914)793-1234
FAX: (914)793-4744

Uniondale

Memorial Sloan Kettering Nassau
1101 Hempstead Tpke
Uniondale, NY 11553-1112
(516)559-1157
FAX: (631)410-8379

Utica

Sister Rose Vincent Family Medicine Center
120 Hobart St
Utica, NY 13501-4308
(315)624-4600
FAX: (315)624-5790

The Imaging Center Of Faxton St. Luke's Healthcare
106 Business Park Dr
Utica, NY 13502-6301
(315)624-5374
FAX: (315)624-5781

Valatie

Valatie Medical Imaging Affiliate Of Columbia Memorial Hosp
1301 River St Ste 104
Valatie, NY 12184-9695
(518)758-7786
FAX: (518)758-7840

Valley Stream

Demeterio And Nejatheim Mds P.C.
265 E Merrick Rd Ste 103
Valley Stream, NY 11580-6004
(516)825-1667
FAX: (516)825-4006

Lenox Hill Radiology-Valley Stream
260 W Sunrise Hwy
Valley Stream, NY 11581-1011
(646)680-5635
FAX: (718)629-4493

Vestal

Uhs Breast Center
4417 Vestal Pkwy E
Vestal, NY 13850-3556
(607)240-2871
FAX: (607)240-2850

Women's Health Center Vestal
3101 Shippers Rd, Ste 106
Vestal, NY 13850-2081
(607)798-5723
FAX: (607)251-2005

Victor

Elizabeth Wende Breast Care Llc
7375 State Route 96 Ste 100
Victor, NY 14564-9662
(585)442-2190
FAX: (585)758-7085

Walton

Delaware Valley Hospital
1 Titus Pl
Walton, NY 13856-1498
(607)865-2126
FAX: (607)865-5457

Wappingers Falls

Medical Diagnostic Imaging, Pllc
1323 Route 9, Ste 107
Wappingers Falls, NY 12590-4977
(845)471-2848
FAX: (845)471-2919

Warrensburg

Hudson Headwaters Health Network
3767 Main St
Warrensburg, NY 12885-1837
(518)623-2844
FAX: (518)623-0012

Warsaw

Wyoming County Community Hospital
400 N Main St
Warsaw, NY 14569-1025
(585)786-8940
FAX: (585)786-1251

Warwick

Crystal Run Healthcare Llp
81 Ronald Reagan Blvd
Warwick, NY 10990-4105
(845)796-5474
FAX: (845)703-2023

St. Anthony Community Hospital - Women's Imaging Center
55 Ronald Reagan Blvd
Warwick, NY 10990-4105
(845)988-9905
FAX: (845)988-9911

Watertown

Northern Radiology Imaging
120 Washington St Ste 406
Watertown, NY 13601-3330
(315)786-5000
FAX: (315)786-5058

Smc-Women's Wellness And Breast Care
1575 Washington St
Watertown, NY 13601-9371
(315)785-4155
FAX: (315)779-5066

Webster

Elizabeth Wende Breast Care
55 Barrett Dr, Ste 300
Webster, NY 14580-4516
(585)442-2190
FAX: (585)758-7085

Rrh Baycreek Imaging Center
2000 Empire Blvd, Ste 120
Webster, NY 14580-1957
(585)922-2160
FAX: (585)671-4063

West Amherst

Windsong Radiology Group At Amherst
3950 E Robinson Rd
West Amherst, NY 14228-2041
(716)631-2500
FAX: (716)631-4051

West Harrison

Memorial Sloan Kettering Westchester
500 Westchester Ave
West Harrison, NY 10604-3200
(914)367-7000
FAX: (914)298-3405

West Islip

Good Samaritan Hospital Women's Imaging Center
735 Montauk Hwy
West Islip, NY 11795-4901
(631)376-3624
FAX: (631)669-7351

Lenox Hill Radiology West Islip
1161 Montauk Hwy
West Islip, NY 11795-4930
(631)277-4500
FAX: (631)669-1717

Zwanger-Pesiri Radiology Group
759 Montauk Hwy
West Islip, NY 11795-4999
(631)669-1103
FAX: (631)669-4824

West Nyack

Crystal Run Healthcare Llp
2 Centerock Rd
West Nyack, NY 10994-2215
(845)703-6366
FAX: (845)358-1948

Rockland Diagnostic Imaging
260 N Route 303
West Nyack, NY 10994-1608
(845)353-0400
FAX: (845)353-5563

West Point

Keller Army Community Hospital
900 Washington Rd, United States Military Academy
West Point, NY 10996-1197
(845)938-4840
FAX: (845)938-6399

West Seneca

Mercy Diagnostic And Treatment Center-West Seneca
550 Orchard Park Rd Ste C
West Seneca, NY 14224-2656
(716)828-2373
FAX: (716)677-5021

Southtowns Radiology Associates At Orchard Park
3050 Orchard Park Rd
West Seneca, NY 14224-4658
(716)558-5400
FAX: (716)558-5424

Westfield

Westfield Memorial Hospital
189 E Main St
Westfield, NY 14787-1195
(716)793-2221
FAX: (716)326-4986

White Plains

Westmed Medical Group
210 Westchester Ave, Radiology Department
White Plains, NY 10604-2901
(914)682-6430
FAX: (914)682-6462

White Plains Hospital Center
41 E Post Rd, Radiology Department
White Plains, NY 10601-4699
(914)681-2929
FAX: (914)681-2970

Williamsville

Buffalo Medical Group
295 Essjay Rd, X-Ray Department
Williamsville, NY 14221-5795
(716)630-1178
FAX: (716)631-0584

Dia Invision Health
100 College Pkwy Ste 180
Williamsville, NY 14221-6800
(716)636-1902
FAX: (716)636-1367

Great Lakes Medical Imaging Llc
199 Park Club Ln Ste 300
Williamsville, NY 14221-5269
(716)836-4646
FAX: (716)836-4696

Kaleida Health Millard Fillmore Suburban
1540 Maple Rd
Williamsville, NY 14221-3698
(716)568-6400
FAX: (716)568-6750

Roswell Park Comprehensive Cancer Center, Park Club Lane
199 Park Club Ln Ste 100
Williamsville, NY 14221-5269
(716)332-6384
FAX: (716)332-6856

Windsong Radiology Group At Williamsville
55 Spindrift Dr
Williamsville, NY 14221-7800
(716)631-2500
FAX: (716)631-4051

Windsong Radiology Group, Pc-Mobile
55 Spindrift Dr, Ste 200
Williamsville, NY 14221-7800
(716)631-2500
FAX: (716)631-4051

Wny Mri - Wny Womens Imaging
180 Park Club Ln
Williamsville, NY 14221-5263
(716)632-7465
FAX: (716)839-9832

Wnymri At Premier
8270 Wehrle Dr
Williamsville, NY 14221-7392
(716)631-8212
FAX: (716)631-8710

Woodbury

Nyu Langone-Nrad-Woodbury
105 Froehlich Farm Blvd
Woodbury, NY 11797-2906
(516)222-2022
FAX: (516)422-8444

Yonkers

Hvra Of Yonkers
984 N Broadway Ste Ll010
Yonkers, NY 10701-1308
(914)776-7700
FAX: (914)776-7789

Montefiore Medical Center
1010 Central Ave.
Yonkers, NY 10704
(914)964-4118
FAX: (914)375-0916

St. John's Riverside Hospital - Andrus Pavilion
967 N Broadway
Yonkers, NY 10701-1301
(914)964-4329
FAX: (914)798-8873

St. Joseph's Medical Center
127 S Broadway, Department Of Radiology
Yonkers, NY 10701-4080
(914)378-7683
FAX: (914)378-7167

Westmed Medical Group
1084 N Broadway
Yonkers, NY 10701-1107
(914)682-6430
FAX: (914)719-5769

Westmed Medical Group
73 Market St
Yonkers, NY 10710-7616
(914)682-6430
FAX: (914)682-6462

Yorktown Heights

Northern Westchester Hospital At Yorktown Imaging
1940 Commerce St Ste 101
Yorktown Heights, NY 10598-4447
(914)245-5200
FAX: (914)245-2930

NORTH CAROLINA

Ahoskie

Vidant Roanoke Chowan Hospital
PO Box 1385, 500 S Academy St
Ahoskie, NC 27910-1385
(252)209-3033
FAX: (252)209-3040

Albemarle

Atrium Health Stanly- The Breast Center
105 Yadkin St Ste 201
Albemarle, NC 28001-3455
(980)323-4259
FAX: (980)323-8239

Angier

Valley Radiology
169 Rawls Rd
Angier, NC 27501-8539
(919)331-2001
FAX: (919)331-2003

Arden

Adventhealth Imaging South Asheville
15 Skyland Inn Dr
Arden, NC 28704-7714
(828)681-2799
FAX: (828)681-2724

Asheboro

Randolph Hospital
364 White Oak St
Asheboro, NC 27203-5400
(336)625-5151
FAX: (336)328-4409

Asheville

Asheville Women's Diagnostic Center
143 Asheland Ave
Asheville, NC 28801-4013
(828)258-9191
FAX: (828)251-9048

Biltmore Ob Gyn
24 Medical Park Dr
Asheville, NC 28803-2493
(828)277-7727
FAX: (855)619-9998

Mission Breast Center
534 Biltmore Ave
Asheville, NC 28801-4610
(828)213-9729
FAX: (828)213-9329

Mission Breast Center - Biltmore Park
2 Town Square Blvd Ste 110
Asheville, NC 28803-5023
(828)213-9729
FAX: (828)213-9329

Mission Breast Center - Hope
100 Ridgefield Ct Ste C
Asheville, NC 28806-2246
(828)670-1876
FAX: (828)670-1438

Providence Imaging Center, Inc.-South Asheville
53 S French Broad Ave LL
Asheville, NC 28801-3272
(828)274-3717
FAX: (828)274-3720

Belmont

Caromont Imaging Services Belmont
1212 Spruce St, Ste 201
Belmont, NC 28012-3386
(704)671-5300
FAX: (704)829-7767

South Point Family Practice Caromont
1220 Spruce St
Belmont, NC 28012-3370
(980)834-5148
FAX: (704)825-1751

Benson

Eastern Carolina Medical Center
1 Medical Dr
Benson, NC 27504-1177
(919)894-5787
FAX: (919)207-0039

Bermuda Run

Davie Medical Center
329 Hwy 801 N
Bermuda Run, NC 27006
(336)716-7243
FAX: (336)713-4972

Bolivia

Novant Health Brunswick Medical Center
240 Hospital Dr NE
Bolivia, NC 28422-8346
(910)721-1485
FAX: (910)721-1264

Boone

Watauga Medical Center Outpatient Imaging And Lab Ctr
1200 State Farm Rd
Boone, NC 28607-4994
(828)268-9037
FAX: (828)266-2488

Brevard

Transylvania Regional Hospital
260 Hospital Dr
Brevard, NC 28712-3378
(828)883-5192
FAX: (828)883-5462

Bryson City

Dlp Swain County Hospital Llc
45 Plateau St, Ste 230
Bryson City, NC 28713-4518
(828)586-7950
FAX: (828)631-8738

Burlington

Cone Health/Alamance Regional Medical Center
1240 Huffman Mill Rd
Burlington, NC 27215-8700
(336)538-7577
FAX: (336)586-3754

Unc Hospitals Burlington Imaging & Breast Center
1225 Huffman Mill Rd Ste 101
Burlington, NC 27215-8789
(336)524-9989
FAX: (336)524-8323

Camp Lejeune

Naval Medical Center Camp Lejeune
100 Brewster Blvd
Camp Lejeune, NC 28547-2575
(910)450-3235
FAX: (910)450-4455

Cary

Cary Obgyn
550 New Waverly Pl, Ste 115
Cary, NC 27518-7412
(919)467-5941
FAX: (919)655-0532

Medical Park Of Cary Wakemed
210 Asheville Ave Ste 100
Cary, NC 27518
(919)350-2522
FAX: (919)350-2652

Raleigh Radiology- Cary
150 Parkway Office Ct Ste 100
Cary, NC 27518-0002
(919)781-1437
FAX: (919)787-4870

Triangle Physicians For Women
600 New Waverly Pl, Ste 310
Cary, NC 27518-7404
(919)678-6900
FAX: (919)678-6901

Wake Med Cary Hospital
1900 Kildaire Farm Rd
Cary, NC 27518-6616
(919)350-7000
FAX: (919)350-8959

Wake Radiology - Panther Creek
6715 McCrimmon Pkwy, Ste 101
Cary, NC 27519-1916
(919)232-4700
FAX: (919)232-2574

Wake Radiology Diagnostic Imaging
300 Ashville Ave Ste 260
Cary, NC 27518-8682
(919)854-2187
FAX: (919)852-4071

Cedar Point

Coastal Imaging And Vascular Associates
1165 Cedar Point Blvd, Ste I
Cedar Point, NC 28584-1030
(910)353-3759
FAX: (252)393-1076

Chapel Hill

Unc Hospitals Ambulatory Care Center
102 Mason Farm Rd, Ambulatory Care Center
Chapel Hill, NC 27599-6134
(984)974-8118
FAX: (984)974-2608

Unc Hospitals Imaging And Spine Center
1350 Raleigh Rd
Chapel Hill, NC 27517-4412
(984)974-8118
FAX: (984)974-2608

Unc Hospitals Nc Cancer Hospital
101 Manning Dr, Department Of Radiology
Attention: Mamm
Chapel Hill, NC 27514-4423
(984)974-8762
FAX: (984)974-2608

Wake Radiology Diagnostic Imaging
110 S Estes Dr
Chapel Hill, NC 27514-2867
(919)942-3196
FAX: (919)265-0008

Charlotte

Charlotte Radiology Breast Center - Ballentyne Office
12335 N Community House Rd, Ste B
Charlotte, NC 28277-1825
(704)684-8204
FAX: (704)944-1101

Charlotte Radiology Breast Center - Blakeney Office
8918 Blakeney Professional Dr, Ste 140
Charlotte, NC 28277-6691
(704)831-4221
FAX: (704)944-1084

Charlotte Radiology Breast Center - Medical Center Plaza
1001 Blythe Blvd Ste 103
Charlotte, NC 28203-5863
(704)355-6200
FAX: (704)831-3572

Charlotte Radiology Breast Center - Mobiles
8514 McAlpine Park Dr
Charlotte, NC 28211-6271
(980)579-6407
FAX: (704)414-7502

Charlotte Radiology Breast Center - Morehead Medical Plaza
1025 Morehead Medical Dr Ste 150
Charlotte, NC 28204-2973
(704)831-4200
FAX: (704)831-4210

Charlotte Radiology Breast Center - Pineville Office
10650 Park Rd Ste 280
Charlotte, NC 28210-0204
(704)540-9299
FAX: (704)831-3575

Charlotte Radiology Breast Center - Prosperity Crossing
5735 Prosperity Crossing Dr Ste 10
Charlotte, NC 28269-1360
(704)464-5727
FAX: (704)943-3005

Charlotte Radiology Breast Center - Randolph Road Office
1960 Randolph Rd Ste 200
Charlotte, NC 28207-1129
(704)332-0583
FAX: (704)831-3584

Charlotte Radiology Breast Center - Southpark Office
4525 Cameron Valley Pkwy, Ste 1000
Charlotte, NC 28211-4370
(704)365-0343
FAX: (704)364-5063

Charlotte Radiology Breast Center - University Office
101 E W T Harris Blvd Ste 2122A
Charlotte, NC 28262-3590
(704)863-6148
FAX: (704)831-3579

Charlotte Radiology Breast Center-Steele Creek Office
13425 Hoover Creek Blvd Ste 203
Charlotte, NC 28273-0170
(704)790-2990
FAX: (704)944-1100

Invision Diagnostics
11220 Elm Ln, Ste 200
Charlotte, NC 28277-0450
(704)257-0880
FAX: (704)935-4515

Invision Diagnostics
11220 Elm Ln Ste 200
Charlotte, NC 28277-0450
(877)318-1349
FAX: (704)966-2407

Novant Health Breast Center
1718 E 4th St Ste 103
Charlotte, NC 28204-3260
(704)384-4177
FAX: (704)417-1072

Novant Health Breast Center Mint Hill
8201 Healthcare Loop
Charlotte, NC 28215-7072
(704)384-7226
FAX: (704)384-5098

Novant Health Imaging Ballantyne
14215 Ballantyne Corporate Pl Ste 140
Charlotte, NC 28277-3671
(704)384-7226
FAX: (704)384-5083

Novant Health Imaging Center Steele Creek
13557 Steelecroft Pkwy Ste 1100
Charlotte, NC 28278-5002
(704)384-7226
FAX: (704)384-5098

Novant Health Imaging Museum
2900 Randolph Rd
Charlotte, NC 28211-1021
(704)384-7226
FAX: (704)417-1072

Novant Health Imaging South Park
6324 Fairview Rd Ste 120B
Charlotte, NC 28210-4162
(704)384-7226
FAX: (704)384-5083

Novant Health Imaging University
8401 Medical Plaza Dr Ste 110
Charlotte, NC 28262-9769
(704)384-7226
FAX: (704)384-5083

Cherokee

Cherokee Indian Hospital Authority
Usphs Hospital Rd, Caller Box C-268
Cherokee, NC 28719
(828)497-9163
FAX: (828)497-5073

Cherry Point

Naval Health Clinic - Cherry Point
Building 4389 Beaufort Rd, PSC Box 8023
Cherry Point, NC 28533
(252)466-0915
FAX: (252)466-0281

Clayton

Cardinal Points Imaging Clayton
166 Springbrook Ave Ste 103
Clayton, NC 27520-8520
(919)877-5400
FAX: (919)877-5480

Johnston Medical Center - Clayton
2138 Hwy 42 West
Clayton, NC 27520
(919)938-7191
FAX: (919)989-9795

Raleigh Radiology Clayton
11618 US 70 Business Hwy W, Ste 102
Clayton, NC 27520-2276
(919)781-1437
FAX: (919)787-4870

Clemmons

Breast Care Services At Medical Plaza Clemmons
2341 Lewisville Clemmons Rd
Clemmons, NC 27012-8905
(336)713-6721
FAX: (336)713-6747

Clinton

Sampson Regional Outpatient Diagnostic Center
233 Beaman St
Clinton, NC 28328-2905
(910)592-2689
FAX: (910)590-2568

Clyde

Dlp Haywood Regional Medical Center Outpatient Care Center
581 Leroy George Dr
Clyde, NC 28721-8084
(828)452-8999
FAX: (828)452-8349

Mission Imaging Services - Haywood
360 Hospital Dr Ste 104
Clyde, NC 28721-0107
(828)213-2222
FAX: (828)213-0889

Columbus

St. Luke's Hospital
101 Hospital Dr
Columbus, NC 28722-6418
(828)894-3311
FAX: (828)894-0609

Concord

Atrium Health-Cabarrus Breast Health Center
1045 NE Gateway Ct NE
Concord, NC 28025-2440
(704)403-1729
FAX: (704)403-3107

Atrium Health-Cabarrus Outreach Health Services-Mobile
920 Church St N
Concord, NC 28025-2927
(704)403-1729
FAX: (704)403-3107

Denver

Atrium Health Lincoln Imaging Denver
275 N Nc 16 Business Hwy Ste 201
Denver, NC 28037-3002
(980)212-1400
FAX: (980)212-1401

Dunn

Harnett Health Breast Care Ctr
700 Tilghman Dr Ste 714
Dunn, NC 28334-5519
(910)892-1000
FAX: (910)694-1308

Durham

Duke Cancer Center-Breast Imaging
20 Duke Medicine Cir, Cancer Center, Clinic 2-1
Durham, NC 27710-2000
(919)684-7999
FAX: (919)684-7144

Duke Health Center Imaging Center At Southpoint
6301 Herndon Rd
Durham, NC 27713-6315
(919)684-7999
FAX: (919)684-7144

Duke Radiology At Patterson Place
5324 McFarland Rd, Duke Medical Plaza Patterson Place
Durham, NC 27707-6865
(919)684-7999
FAX: (919)684-7144

Duke Regional Hospital
3643 N Roxboro St
Durham, NC 27704-2763
(919)470-5262
FAX: (919)470-5298

Durham Diagnostic Imaging, Llc
5107 Southpark Dr Ste 101
Durham, NC 27713-8400
(877)507-9729
FAX: (919)544-2621

Durham Diagnostic Imaging, Llc
4323 Ben Franklin Blvd
Durham, NC 27704-2177
(919)471-4840
FAX: (919)471-9345

Durham Womens Clinic
209 E Carver St
Durham, NC 27704-2133
(877)318-1349
FAX: (704)966-2407

Eden

Unc Rockingham Wright Imaging Center
618 S Pierce St
Eden, NC 27288-5863
(336)623-9711
FAX: (336)623-1923

Edenton

East Carolina Health-Chowan, Inc. Dba Vidant Chowan Hospital
211 Virginia Rd
Edenton, NC 27932-9668
(252)482-6245
FAX: (252)482-6398

Elizabeth City

Chesapeake Regional Breast Center
1138 N Road St
Elizabeth City, NC 27909-3353
(252)331-4104
FAX: (252)335-1495

Sentara Albemarle Medical Center
1144 N Road St
Elizabeth City, NC 27909-3473
(252)337-9220
FAX: (252)384-4385

Elizabethtown

Cape Fear Valley Bladen County Hospital
501 S Poplar St
Elizabethtown, NC 28337-9375
(910)862-5168
FAX: (910)862-1212

Elkin

Hugh Chatham Memorial Hospital
180 Parkwood Dr
Elkin, NC 28621-2430
(336)527-7398
FAX: (336)527-7175

Farmville

Physicians East Farmville
3681 North Main St
Farmville, NC 27828-1464
(252)753-7141
FAX: (252)753-2311

Fayetteville

Carolina Imaging, Llc Of Fayetteville
3628 Cape Center Dr
Fayetteville, NC 28304-4406
(910)483-1321
FAX: (910)323-5459

Diagnostic Center Of Cape Fear Valley Medical Center
524 Beaumont Rd
Fayetteville, NC 28304-4443
(910)615-5655
FAX: (910)615-5973

Medical Imaging Center Llc Dba Valley Reg Imaging
3186 Village Dr Ste 101
Fayetteville, NC 28304-3979
(910)323-2209
FAX: (910)323-9680

Women's Wellness Center Pa
2950 Village Dr, Ste 100
Fayetteville, NC 28304-4129
(910)323-3301
FAX: (910)323-4207

Fort Bragg

Department Of The Army-Womack Army Medical Center
2817 Reilly St
Fort Bragg, NC 28310-7301
(910)907-8266
FAX: (910)643-2480

Franklin

Angel Medical Center
120 Riverview St
Franklin, NC 28734-2612
(828)369-4259
FAX: (828)369-4453

Westcare Medical Park Of Franklin
55 Holly Springs Park Dr
Franklin, NC 28734-0719
(855)586-7950
FAX: (828)349-5050

Fuquay Varina

Raleigh Radiology Fuquay Varina
601 Attain St, Ste 100
Fuquay Varina, NC 27526-1972
(919)781-1437
FAX: (919)787-4870

Wake Radiology - Fuquay
7636 Purfoy Rd Ste 200
Fuquay Varina, NC 27526-2699
(919)346-5828
FAX: (919)577-9049

Garner

Wake Radiology Diagnostic Imaging
300 Health Park Dr Ste 100
Garner, NC 27529-4685
(919)662-9500
FAX: (919)662-2244

Gastonia

Caromont Imaging Services
620 Summit Crossing Pl Ste 106
Gastonia, NC 28054-2189
(704)671-5300
FAX: (704)671-7735

Courtview Gynecology
706 Summit Crossing Pl
Gastonia, NC 28054-2175
(704)854-9766
FAX: (704)854-3619

Goldsboro

Carolina Breast Imaging Specialists
204 N Spence Ave
Goldsboro, NC 27534-4318
(919)947-2021
FAX: (252)565-8958

Wayne Memorial Hospital, Inc.
2700 Wayne Memorial Dr
Goldsboro, NC 27534-9459
(919)587-4627
FAX: (919)587-4255

Wayne Radiologists, P.A.
2700 Medical Office Pl
Goldsboro, NC 27534-9402
(919)734-1866
FAX: (919)736-1804

Granite Falls

Laurel Park Women's Imaging
4355 Hickory Blvd
Granite Falls, NC 28630-2013
(828)757-5218
FAX: (828)757-5206

Greensboro

Central Carolina Ob/Gyn
3200 Northline Ave, Ste 130
Greensboro, NC 27408-7600
(336)286-6565
FAX: (336)286-6566

Green Valley Ob/Gyn
719 Green Valley Rd Ste 201
Greensboro, NC 27408-7025
(336)378-1110
FAX: (336)378-9986

Greensboro Ob/Gyn Associates
510 N Elam Ave, Ste 101
Greensboro, NC 27403-1135
(336)854-8800
FAX: (336)299-4308

Novant Health Breast Imaging Center Greensboro
3515 W Market St, Ste 320
Greensboro, NC 27403-4442
(336)660-5420
FAX: (336)660-5429

Physicians For Women Of Greensboro
802 Green Valley Rd, Ste 300
Greensboro, NC 27408-7099
(336)273-3661
FAX: (336)273-9438

Solis Mammography Of Greensboro, Llc
1126 N Church St Ste 200
Greensboro, NC 27401-1036
(336)379-0941
FAX: (336)379-7997

The Breast Center Of Greensboro Imaging
1002 N Church St Ste 401
Greensboro, NC 27401-1450
(336)271-4999
FAX: (336)387-3306

Wendover Ob/Gyn And Infertility, Inc
1908 Lendew St
Greensboro, NC 27408-7007
(336)273-2833
FAX: (877)526-1334

Greenville

Carolina Breast Imaging Specialists
990 Johns Hopkins Dr
Greenville, NC 27834-7224
(252)565-8951
FAX: (252)565-8958

Eastern Radiologists, Inc. Breast Imaging Center
2101 W Arlington Blvd, Ste 100
Greenville, NC 27834-5758
(252)752-5000
FAX: (252)931-7634

Physicians East P.A. Greenville Women's Clinic
2251 Stantonsburg Rd
Greenville, NC 27834-2841
(252)757-3131
FAX: (252)757-9600

Physicians East - Greenville Obstetrics And Gynecology
101 Bethesda Dr
Greenville, NC 27834-7201
(252)758-4181
FAX: (252)758-2603

Physicians East Diagnostic Center
1850 W Arlington Blvd
Greenville, NC 27834-5704
(252)413-6218
FAX: (252)413-5227

Vidant Medical Center
PO Box 6028, 2100 Stantonsburg Rd
Greenville, NC 27835-6028
(252)847-5260
FAX: (252)847-7553

Henderson

Maria Parham Health
566 Ruin Creek Rd
Henderson, NC 27536-5932
(252)436-1308
FAX: (252)436-1368

Hendersonville

Adventhealth Hendersonville
100 Hospital Dr
Hendersonville, NC 28792-5272
(828)681-2799
FAX: (828)681-2724

Margaret R. Pardee Outpatient Radiology Center
807 N Justice St
Hendersonville, NC 28791-3409
(828)698-7979
FAX: (828)696-4687

Providence Imaging Center, Inc.
2315 Asheville Hwy Ste 40
Hendersonville, NC 28791-1561
(828)692-6848
FAX: (828)693-7543

Hickory

A Woman's View
915 Tate Blvd SE, Ste 170
Hickory, NC 28602-4012
(828)345-0800
FAX: (828)485-5579

Blue Ridge Health Care Medical Group Dba Blue Ridge Radiolog
2134 14th Avenue Cir NW Ste D
Hickory, NC 28601-7358
(828)580-1247
FAX: (828)580-1992

Catawba Valley Imaging Center
1501 Tate Blvd SE Ste 101
Hickory, NC 28602-1385
(828)485-2766
FAX: (828)485-2768

Catawba Women's Center
1501 Tate Blvd SE Ste 201
Hickory, NC 28602-1385
(828)322-4140
FAX: (828)322-3767

Fryecare Mammography
1781 Tate Blvd SE Ste 101
Hickory, NC 28602-4252
(828)315-3390
FAX: (828)315-3203

High Point

Cone Health Medcenter High Point Imaging
2630 Willard Dairy Rd Ste A, Ste A
High Point, NC 27265-8354
(336)884-3600
FAX: (336)884-3601

High Point Regional Health Dba High Point Regional Hospital
601 N Elm St
High Point, NC 27262-4331
(336)878-6037
FAX: (336)878-6994

Piedmont Comprehensive Women's Center
1814 Westchester Dr Ste 200
High Point, NC 27262-7369
(336)702-2134
FAX: (336)802-2186

Premier Imaging
4515 Premier Dr, Ste 101
High Point, NC 27265-8356
(336)781-4299
FAX: (336)801-5855

Highlands

Highlands - Cashiers Hospital
190 Hospital Dr
Highlands, NC 28741-7600
(828)526-1450
FAX: (828)526-1468

Hillsborough

Unc Hospitals - Hillsborough Campus
430 Waterstone Dr
Hillsborough, NC 27278-9078
(984)974-1884
FAX: (984)974-2608

Holly Springs

Duke Health Holly Springs
401 Irving Pkwy, Ste 120
Holly Springs, NC 27540-5301
(919)385-3035
FAX: (919)385-1565

Wake Radiology - Holly Springs
781 Avent Ferry Rd
Holly Springs, NC 27540-7776
(919)232-4700
FAX: (919)235-3952

Huntersville

Charlotte Radiology Breast Center - Huntersville Office
16455 Statesville Rd Ste 110
Huntersville, NC 28078-7135
(704)895-3445
FAX: (704)895-4846

Novant Health Breast Center
10030 Gilead Rd Ste 330
Huntersville, NC 28078-7545
(704)384-7226
FAX: (704)389-5003

Jacksonville

Diagnostic Imaging Partners
2000 Brabham Ave, Ste 110
Jacksonville, NC 28546-0202
(910)939-3110
FAX: (910)332-5132

Onslow Imaging Ctr For Women-Onslow Memorial Hosp. Inc.
121 Memorial Dr
Jacksonville, NC 28546-6329
(910)577-2323
FAX: (910)577-2835

Onslow Radiology Center
299 Doctors Dr
Jacksonville, NC 28546-6373
(910)577-1171
FAX: (910)577-5112

Jefferson

Ashe Memorial Hospital
200 Hospital Ave, Imaging
Jefferson, NC 28640-9244
(336)846-0820
FAX: (336)846-0750

Kenansville

Vidant Duplin Hospital
401 N Main St
Kenansville, NC 28349-8801
(910)296-2665
FAX: (910)296-8826

Kernersville

Cone Health Imaging Center Medcenter Kernersville
1635 Hwy 66 South Ste. 110
Kernersville, NC 27284
(336)992-5950
FAX: (336)992-5951

Novant Health Kernersville Medical Center
1750 Kernersville Medical Pkwy
Kernersville, NC 27284-7146
(336)397-6704
FAX: (336)564-4699

Kings Mountain

Atriumhealth Kings Mtn, A Facility Of Atriumhealth Cleveland
706 W King St
Kings Mountain, NC 28086-2708
(980)487-5432
FAX: (980)487-5138

Kinston

Eastern Radiologists, Inc
701 Doctors Dr Ste M
Kinston, NC 28501-1584
(252)527-7077
FAX: (252)527-0565

Physicians East Pa Kinston
744 Airport Rd
Kinston, NC 28504-8800
(252)523-0026
FAX: (252)523-1855

Vidant Multi Speciality Clinic - Kinston
701 Doctors Dr Ste N
Kinston, NC 28501-1584
(252)559-2200
FAX: (252)559-5662

Knightdale

Raleigh Radiology Knightdale
1101 Great Falls Ct, Ste 100
Knightdale, NC 27545-7307
(919)781-1437
FAX: (919)787-4870

Wake Radiology - Knightdale
6602 Knightdale Blvd
Knightdale, NC 27545-6525
(919)232-4700
FAX: (919)235-3952

Laurinburg

Scotland Memorial Hospital Imaging Center
500 Lauchwood Dr
Laurinburg, NC 28352-5599
(910)291-7738
FAX: (910)291-6912

Leland

Novant Health Nhrmc - Brunswick Forest H & D
1333 S Dickinson Dr, Unit 100
Leland, NC 28451-6434
(910)452-8777
FAX: (910)815-5580

Wilmington Health , Leland Location
9101 Ocean Hwy E
Leland, NC 28451-7867
(910)815-6128
FAX: (910)341-3473

Lenoir

Caldwell Memorial Hospital
321 Mulberry St SW
Lenoir, NC 28645-5716
(828)757-5218
FAX: (828)757-5206

Laurel Park Women's Imaging
906 College Ave SW
Lenoir, NC 28645-5428
(828)757-5502
FAX: (828)757-5206

Lexington

Wake Forest Baptist Health Lexington Medical Center
250 Hospital Dr
Lexington, NC 27292-6792
(336)249-1515
FAX: (336)238-4817

Lillington

Central Harnett Hospital
215 Brightwater Dr
Lillington, NC 27546-5156
(910)892-1000
FAX: (910)984-3706

Lincolnton

Atrium Health Lincoln
433 McAlister Rd
Lincolnton, NC 28092-4147
(980)212-1400
FAX: (980)212-1401

Linville

Charles A.Cannon, Jr. Memorial Hospital
434 Hospital Drive
Linville, NC 28646
(828)737-7624
FAX: (828)737-7621

Locust

West Stanly Imaging
103 Stanly Pkwy Ste E
Locust, NC 28097-7711
(980)323-7000
FAX: (980)323-7001

Louisburg

Maria Parham Franklin
100 Hospital Dr
Louisburg, NC 27549-2256
(919)340-8755
FAX: (919)853-0168

Lumberton

Southeastern Radiology Associates
209 W 27th St
Lumberton, NC 28358-3016
(910)738-8222
FAX: (910)739-8175

Marion

Mission Hospital McDowell
430 Rankin Dr
Marion, NC 28752-6568
(828)659-5165
FAX: (828)659-5161

Mars Hill

Providence Imaging Center-Mars Hill
119 Mountain View Rd
Mars Hill, NC 28754-9500
(828)692-6848
FAX: (828)693-7543

Matthews

Charlotte Radiology Breast Center - Matthews Office
1401 Matthews Township Pkwy Ste 310
Matthews, NC 28105-5403
(704)844-9040
FAX: (704)831-3581

Novant Health Matthews Medical Center
1500 Matthews Township Pkwy
Matthews, NC 28105-4656
(704)384-6769
FAX: (704)384-6541

Mebane

Cone Health/Mebane Outpatient Center Alamance Regional
3940 Arrowhead Blvd Ste 120
Mebane, NC 27302-7637
(336)538-7012
FAX: (336)586-3760

Monroe

Charlotte Radiology Breast Center - Monroe Office
1550 Faulk St Ste 1200
Monroe, NC 28112-5087
(704)292-2272
FAX: (704)296-9082

Novant Health Imaging Monroe
2000 Wellness Blvd Ste 110, The Park At Monroe Imaging Center
Monroe, NC 28110-3354
(704)384-4177
FAX: (704)384-7226

Mooresville

Charlotte Radiology Breast Center - Mooresville Office
132 Gateway Blvd Ste A
Mooresville, NC 28117-5540
(704)235-6446
FAX: (704)943-3016

Iredell Mooresville
653 Bluefield Road
Mooresville, NC 28117
(704)360-6460
FAX: (704)746-0010

Lake Norman Imaging Center
146 Medical Park Rd
Mooresville, NC 28117-8528
(704)660-4920
FAX: (704)660-4981

Novant Health Imaging Center Langtree
106 Langtree Village Dr, Ste 200
Mooresville, NC 28117-7594
(704)384-4177
FAX: (704)417-1072

Piedmont Healthcare Mooresville Mammography
150 Fairview Rd Ste 200
Mooresville, NC 28117-9507
(704)235-6200
FAX: (704)658-0030

Morehead City

Carteret Obgyn Associates
3511 John Platt Dr
Morehead City, NC 28557-4389
(252)247-4297
FAX: (252)247-7383

Chc Imaging Center
3402 Arendell St
Morehead City, NC 28557-3205
(252)808-6551
FAX: (252)808-6548

Girltalk & Gynecology
4251 Arendell St
Morehead City, NC 28557-2869
(252)222-0660
FAX: (252)648-7219

Morganton

Burke Primary Care
103 Medical Heights Dr
Morganton, NC 28655-5197
(828)437-4211
FAX: (828)437-5017

Chs Blue Ridge Healthcare Hospital, Inc. Morganton
2201 S Sterling St
Morganton, NC 28655-4044
(828)580-5253
FAX: (828)580-6986

Morrisville

Duke Imaging Arringdon
5601 Arringdon Park Drive, Suite 110
Morrisville, NC 27560
(919)385-8707
FAX: (919)385-8725

Mount Airy

Northern Regional Hospital
830 Rockford St
Mount Airy, NC 27030-5365
(336)719-7135
FAX: (336)719-7132

Murphy

Erlanger Murphy Medical Center
3990 E US 64 Alt
Murphy, NC 28906-8707
(828)835-7540
FAX: (828)835-7546

Nags Head

The Outer Banks Hospital
4800 S Croatan Hwy
Nags Head, NC 27959-9704
(252)449-5927
FAX: (252)449-5916

New Bern

Carolinaeast Diagnostic Center
1302 Health Dr
New Bern, NC 28560-4370
(252)634-6400
FAX: (252)633-2808

Cchc Imaging
1030 Medical Park Ave
New Bern, NC 28562-5248
(252)637-5480
FAX: (252)637-2514

Eastern Carolina Women's Center
801 McCarthy Blvd
New Bern, NC 28562-5237
(252)633-3942
FAX: (252)637-3656

North Wilkesboro

Diagnostic Center Of Wilkes Regional
1900 W Park Dr
North Wilkesboro, NC 28659-3563
(336)651-8435
FAX: (336)903-7014

Oxford

Granville Medical Center
1010 College St
Oxford, NC 27565-2507
(919)690-3420
FAX: (919)690-0114

Pinehurst

Firsthealth Of The Carolinas - Moore Regional Hospital
155 Memorial Dr
Pinehurst, NC 28374-8710
(910)715-2778
FAX: (910)715-2266

Pinehurst Radiology Associates
30 Memorial Dr
Pinehurst, NC 28374-8707
(910)295-4400
FAX: (910)295-2810

Pinehurst Surgical Clinic
5 First Village Dr
Pinehurst, NC 28374-9495
(910)215-2641
FAX: (910)295-1018

Plymouth

Washington Regional Medical Center
958 US Highway 64 E
Plymouth, NC 27962-9216
(252)793-7655
FAX: (252)793-7740

Pollocksville

Carolinaeast Internal Medicine
137 Medical Ln
Pollocksville, NC 28573-8200
(252)635-3849
FAX: (252)224-1999

Raeford

Firsthealth Moore Regional Hospital-Hoke Campus
6408 Fayetteville Rd
Raeford, NC 28376-7977
(910)715-2778
FAX: (910)878-6635

Hoke Imaging, Llc
300 Medical Pavilion Dr Ste 210
Raeford, NC 28376-0018
(910)615-5116
FAX: (910)615-9754

Raleigh

Associates In Women's Healthcare, Pa
901 Ridgefield Dr
Raleigh, NC 27609-8504
(919)876-9797
FAX: (919)790-1254

Cardinal Points Imaging Brier Creek
8851 Ellstree Ln Ste 100
Raleigh, NC 27617-2046
(919)877-5400
FAX: (919)877-5480

Cardinal Points Imaging Midtown
1212 Cedarhurst Dr
Raleigh, NC 27609-5587
(919)877-5400
FAX: (919)877-5480

Carolina Breast Care Specialist, Pa
4414 Lake Boone Trl Ste 211
Raleigh, NC 27607-7520
(919)741-5966
FAX: (919)571-4330

Duke Cancer Center Macon Pond
4101 Macon Pond Rd
Raleigh, NC 27607-6319
(919)862-5209
FAX: (919)862-5213

Duke Raleigh Hospital
3400 Wake Forest Rd
Raleigh, NC 27609-7353
(919)862-5209
FAX: (919)862-5213

Duke Raleigh Hospital Outpatient Imaging Ctr
3480 Wake Forest Rd Ste 100
Raleigh, NC 27609-7379
(919)862-5277
FAX: (919)862-5213

Gynecology & Laparoscopic Surgeons, Pc
10941 Raven Ridge Rd, Ste 109
Raleigh, NC 27614-6487
(919)847-7475
FAX: (877)504-7361

North Carolina Correctional Institute For Women Hcf
1034 Bragg St
Raleigh, NC 27610-3846
(919)743-3607
FAX: (919)508-1660

Raleigh Radiology Oberlin
505 Oberlin Rd, Ste 110
Raleigh, NC 27605-1345
(919)781-1437
FAX: (919)787-4870

Raleigh Radiology-Blue Ridge
3200 Blue Ridge Rd, Ste 100
Raleigh, NC 27612-8087
(919)781-1437
FAX: (919)787-4870

Unc Rex Mobile Mammography-Mobile
2500 Blue Ridge Rd, Ste 219
Raleigh, NC 27607-7515
(919)784-4210
FAX: (919)784-4205

Wake Internal Medicine Consultants, Inc
3100 Blue Ridge Rd Ste 200
Raleigh, NC 27612-8035
(919)781-7500
FAX: (919)803-1742

Wake Med Raleigh Medical Park
23 Sunnybrook Rd Ste 110
Raleigh, NC 27610-7401
(919)350-7000
FAX: (919)350-9605

Wake Radiology
3821 Merton Dr
Raleigh, NC 27609-6693
(919)232-4700
FAX: (919)571-9583

Wake Radiology - Wakefield
11200 Governor Manly Way, Ste 106
Raleigh, NC 27614-7360
(919)232-4700
FAX: (919)235-3952

Wake Radiology - Breast Care Center
3100 Duraleigh Rd Ste 204
Raleigh, NC 27612-8104
(919)232-4700
FAX: (919)235-3952

Wakemed North Hospital
10000 Falls Of Neuse Rd, Ste 101
Raleigh, NC 27614-7838
(919)350-7000
FAX: (919)350-1515

Women's Hlth Alliance Mammography & Specialty Svcs
4414 Lake Boone Trl
Raleigh, NC 27607-7513
(919)615-2043
FAX: (877)640-9974

Reidsville

Annie Penn Hospital
618 S Main St
Reidsville, NC 27320-5094
(336)951-4443
FAX: (336)951-4553

Roanoke Rapids

Mammography Center
210 Smith Church Rd Ste E
Roanoke Rapids, NC 27870-4942
(252)535-3417
FAX: (252)535-8853

Robbinsville

Smoky Mountain Urgent Care
21 S Main St
Robbinsville, NC 28771-9054
(828)479-7682
FAX: (828)479-7683

Rockingham

First Health Richmond Memorial Hospital
925 S Long Dr
Rockingham, NC 28379-4835
(910)417-3766
FAX: (910)417-3380

Rocky Mount

Boice Willis Clinic, P.A.
901 N Winstead Ave
Rocky Mount, NC 27804-9345
(252)937-0482
FAX: (252)937-0272

Nash Breast Care Center
250 Nash Medical Arts Mall Ste B
Rocky Mount, NC 27804-1470
(252)962-6100
FAX: (252)962-6119

Opportunities Industrialization Center, Inc
260 Albemarle Avenue
Rocky Mount, NC 27801
(252)316-8215
FAX: (252)210-3115

Rocky Mount Family Medical Center
804 English Rd Ste 100
Rocky Mount, NC 27804-6027
(252)443-3133
FAX: (252)443-6726

Rocky Point

Pender Health And Diagnostics
7910 US Hwy 117 S Unit 100
Rocky Point, NC 28457-7409
(910)300-4325
FAX: (910)675-2032

Roxboro

Person Memorial Hospital
615 Ridge Rd
Roxboro, NC 27573-4659
(336)503-5788
FAX: (336)503-5648

Rutherfordton

The Mammography Place
175 Tryon Rd, Ste B
Rutherfordton, NC 28139-3088
(828)286-5380
FAX: (828)286-5672

Salisbury

Novant Health Imaging
514 Corporate Cir
Salisbury, NC 28147-8074
(704)210-7762
FAX: (704)210-6922

Sanford

Central Carolina Hospital
1135 Carthage St
Sanford, NC 27330-4162
(919)774-2157
FAX: (919)774-2399

Firsthealth Imaging Lee
2919 Beechtree Dr
Sanford, NC 27330-6934
(919)897-2265
FAX: (919)897-2266

Shelby

Atrium Health - Cleveland Imaging
315 Weathers St
Shelby, NC 28150-3951
(980)487-4810
FAX: (980)487-2721

Shelby Medical Associates, P.A.
711 N Dekalb St
Shelby, NC 28150-3911
(704)482-1482
FAX: (704)482-0811

Siler City

Chatham Hospital, Inc.
PO Box 649, 475 Progress Blvd
Siler City, NC 27344-0649
(919)799-4610
FAX: (919)799-4601

Smithfield

Ambulatory Imaging Center-Johnston Medical Center
514 N Brightleaf Blvd Ste 1302
Smithfield, NC 27577-4486
(919)938-7749
FAX: (919)989-4983

Wake Radiology Diagnostic Imaging
218 Venture Dr
Smithfield, NC 27577-4721
(919)662-9500
FAX: (919)662-3854

Snow Hill

Greene Co. Health Care - Snow Hill Medical Center
302 N Greene St
Snow Hill, NC 28580-1412
(252)747-2921
FAX: (252)747-4915

Southport

Dosher Memorial Hospital
924 N Howe St
Southport, NC 28461-3099
(910)457-3881
FAX: (910)457-3883

Sparta

Alleghany Memorial Hospital
233 Doctors St
Sparta, NC 28675-9247
(336)372-3210
FAX: (336)372-3288

Spruce Pine

Blue Ridge Regional Hospital
125 Hospital Dr
Spruce Pine, NC 28777-3035
(828)766-1630
FAX: (828)766-1631

Statesville

Davis Regional Medical Center
218 Old Mocksville Rd
Statesville, NC 28625-1930
(704)838-7390
FAX: (704)838-7413

Iredell Health System
557 Brookdale Dr
Statesville, NC 28677-4107
(704)878-4510
FAX: (704)878-7194

Iredell Memorial Hospital's Women's Health Center
735 Hartness Rd
Statesville, NC 28677-3424
(704)878-4551
FAX: (704)878-4553

Piedmont Healthcare Imaging Center
700 Sullivan Rd
Statesville, NC 28677-3440
(704)878-8623
FAX: (704)658-0030

Sylva

Harris Medical Park
98 Doctors Dr Ste 120, Outpt Imaging
Sylva, NC 28779-4503
(828)586-7950
FAX: (828)586-7779

Tarboro

Vidant Edgecombe Hospital
111 Hospital Dr
Tarboro, NC 27886-2011
(252)641-7777
FAX: (252)641-7472

Thomasville

Novant Health Thomasville Medical Center
207 Old Lexington Rd
Thomasville, NC 27360-3428
(336)476-2500
FAX: (336)476-2415

Troy

First Health Montgomery Memorial Hospital
520 Allen St
Troy, NC 27371-2802
(910)571-5240
FAX: (910)572-2472

Valdese

Chs Blue Ridge Mobile Mammography
720 Malcolm Blvd.
Valdese, NC 28690
(828)580-7524
FAX: (828)580-7612

Wadesboro

Atrium Health Anson
2301 US Highway 74 W
Wadesboro, NC 28170-7554
(704)994-4530
FAX: (704)994-4531

Wake Forest

Cardinal Points Imaging Wake Forest
839 Durham Rd Ste A
Wake Forest, NC 27587-8793
(919)877-5400
FAX: (919)877-5480

Duke Mammography At Heritage
3000 Rogers Rd Ste 120
Wake Forest, NC 27587-5745
(919)385-1570
FAX: (919)385-1565

Raleigh Radiology Wake Forest
11640 Northpark Dr, Ste 110
Wake Forest, NC 27587-5741
(919)781-1437
FAX: (919)787-4870

Wake Radiology
3150 Rogers Rd Ste 115
Wake Forest, NC 27587-4196
(919)232-4700
FAX: (919)235-3940

Washington

Eastern Radiologists Inc. - Washington, Nc
630 E 11th St
Washington, NC 27889-3700
(252)946-2137
FAX: (252)975-6117

Vidant Womens Care
1204 Brown St
Washington, NC 27889-4671
(252)975-4240
FAX: (252)948-4838

Whiteville

Columbus Regional Healthcare System
500 Jefferson St
Whiteville, NC 28472-3634
(910)642-9372
FAX: (910)641-3664

Williamston

Martin General Hospital
310 S McCaskey Rd
Williamston, NC 27892-2157
(252)809-6332
FAX: (252)809-6372

Wilmington

Delaney Radiologists
1025 Medical Center Dr
Wilmington, NC 28401-7354
(910)762-3882
FAX: (910)251-3115

Novant Health New Hanover Regional Medical Center
2131 S 17th St
Wilmington, NC 28401-7407
(910)667-8777
FAX: (910)815-5580

Novant Health Nhrmc - Military Cutoff H & D
1135 Military Cutoff Rd, Ste 101
Wilmington, NC 28405-3685
(910)452-8777
FAX: (910)256-7960

Novant Health Nhrmc Health & Diagnostic - North
151 Scotts Hill Medical Dr
Wilmington, NC 28411-7983
(910)667-8777
FAX: (910)815-5580

Novant Health Nhrmc-Medical Mall H & D
2243 S 17th St
Wilmington, NC 28401-7542
(910)667-8777
FAX: (910)667-6150

Wilmington Health
1202 Medical Center Dr
Wilmington, NC 28401-7394
(910)815-6128
FAX: (910)762-0849

Wilmington Health, Mayfaire
6727 Parker Farm Dr
Wilmington, NC 28405-3176
(910)815-6128
FAX: (910)762-0849

Wilson

Carolina Breast Imaging Specialists
2519 Airport Blvd NW Ste E
Wilson, NC 27896-9603
(252)561-7232
FAX: (252)565-8958

Nelms Family And Preventive Medicine, P.A.
2546 Ward Blvd
Wilson, NC 27893-1600
(252)399-0707
FAX: (252)291-7079

Vidant Healthplex, Wilson
3724 Raleigh Road Pkwy W
Wilson, NC 27896-9742
(252)246-8840
FAX: (252)246-8845

Wilson Medical Ctr OP Imaging
1711 Medical Park Dr W
Wilson, NC 27893-2788
(252)399-8900
FAX: (252)399-7443

Windsor

Vidant Bertie Hospital
1403 S King St
Windsor, NC 27983-9666
(252)794-6626
FAX: (252)794-6642

Winston Salem

Breast Screening & Diagnostic Center
Medical Center Blvd., Comprehensive Cancer Center
Winston Salem, NC 27157-0001
(336)713-6500
FAX: (336)713-6747

Hawthorne Obgyn Associates
4605 Country Club Rd
Winston Salem, NC 27104-3519
(336)768-3632
FAX: (336)768-4473

Lyndhurst Gynecologic Associates
111 Hanestown Ct, Ste 151
Winston Salem, NC 27103-1749
(336)765-9350
FAX: (336)760-4255

Novant Health Breast Center
2025 Frontis Plaza Blvd
Winston Salem, NC 27103-5663
(336)794-9729
FAX: (336)397-6149

Novant Health Breast Center-Mobile
2025 Frontis Plaza Blvd Ste 300
Winston Salem, NC 27103-5663
(336)794-9729
FAX: (336)397-6149

Piedmont Imaging
185 Kimel Park Dr Ste 100
Winston Salem, NC 27103-6973
(336)760-1880
FAX: (336)760-1807

Wake Forest Baptist Imaging
265 Executive Park Blvd
Winston Salem, NC 27103-1503
(336)765-5722
FAX: (336)765-5723

Wake Forest Baptist Imaging Kernersville
265 Executive Park Blvd
Winston Salem, NC 27103-1503
(336)765-5722
FAX: (336)765-5723

NORTH DAKOTA

Ashley

Ashley Medical Center
612 Center Ave N
Ashley, ND 58413-7013
(701)288-5278
FAX: (701)288-3937

Belcourt

Quentin N. Burdick Mem. Hlth Care Fac. - Phs Indian Hospital
PO Box 160, 1300 Hospital Loop
Belcourt, ND 58316-0160
(701)477-8412
FAX: (701)477-2530

Bismarck

Edith Sanford Breast Center Bismarck
222 N 7th St
Bismarck, ND 58501-4436
(701)323-5210
FAX: (701)323-5479

Mid Dakota Clinic - Center For Women
1000 E Rosser Ave
Bismarck, ND 58501-4414
(701)530-6014
FAX: (701)530-5989

Mid Dakota Clinic Pc
401 N 9th St
Bismarck, ND 58501-4506
(701)712-4501
FAX: (701)712-4084

St. Alexius Medical Center
900 E Broadway Ave, Radiology Department
Bismarck, ND 58501-4586
(701)530-5301
FAX: (701)530-5323

Bottineau

St. Andrew's Health Center
316 Ohmer St
Bottineau, ND 58318-1097
(707)228-9363
FAX: (701)228-9387

Bowman

Southwest Healthcare Services
802 2nd St NW, Ste 1
Bowman, ND 58623-4469
(701)523-5555
FAX: (701)523-2825

Cando

Towner County Medical Center
Hwy 281 N
Cando, ND 58324
(701)968-2541
FAX: (701)968-2516

Carrington

Carrington Health Center
800 4th St N
Carrington, ND 58421-1217
(701)652-7151
FAX: (701)652-7230

Devils Lake

Altru Clinic - Devils Lake
PO Box 1100, 1001 7th St NE
Devils Lake, ND 58301-1100
(701)662-2158
FAX: (701)665-5218

Dickinson

Chi St. Josephs Health
2500 Fairway St
Dickinson, ND 58601-2639
(701)456-4509
FAX: (701)456-4816

Sanford Health West Dickinson Clinic
2615 Fairway St
Dickinson, ND 58601-2590
(701)456-6160
FAX: (701)456-6102

Fargo

Dms Health Technologies-Mobile
1351 Page Dr S, Ste 300
Fargo, ND 58103-3536
(605)357-2612
FAX: (800)589-7405

Dms Imaging Inc - Mobile 10
1351 Page Dr S, Ste 300
Fargo, ND 58103-3536
(605)366-3358
FAX: (701)566-8286

Dms Imaging Inc - Mobile 4
1351 Page Dr S, Ste 300
Fargo, ND 58103-3536
(605)366-3358
FAX: (701)566-8286

Dms Imaging, Inc. - Mobile
1351 Page Dr S, Ste 300
Fargo, ND 58103-3536
(605)366-3358
FAX: (701)566-8286

Essentia Health
3000 32nd Ave S, Breast Imaging
Fargo, ND 58103-6132
(701)364-8200
FAX: (701)364-8241

Institute Of Diagnostic Imaging
2829 University Dr S Ste 102
Fargo, ND 58103-6050
(701)234-0112
FAX: (701)478-7903

Sanford Clinic Southpointe
2400 32nd Ave S
Fargo, ND 58103-5800
(701)234-7100
FAX: (701)234-7481

Sanford Medical Center Fargo
801 Broadway North
Fargo, ND 58122-0001
(701)234-7100
FAX: (701)234-7481

Sanford Southpointe-Mobile
2400 32nd Ave S
Fargo, ND 58103-5800
(701)234-7100
FAX: (701)234-7481

Fort Totten

Spirit Lake Health Center
PO Box 309, 3883 74th Ave NE
Fort Totten, ND 58335-0309
(701)766-1629
FAX: (701)766-1648

Garrison

Chi St. Alexius Garrison Memorial Hospital
407 3rd Ave SE
Garrison, ND 58540-7235
(701)463-2275
FAX: (701)463-6401

Grafton

Unity Medical Center
164 W 13th St
Grafton, ND 58237-1826
(701)379-3051
FAX: (701)352-9375

Grand Forks

Altru Health System
4440 S Washington St
Grand Forks, ND 58201-7245
(701)780-6157
FAX: (701)732-7592

Harvey

St. Aloisius Medical Center
325 Brewster St E
Harvey, ND 58341-1653
(701)324-5107
FAX: (701)324-4687

Hazen

Sakakawea Medical Center
510 8th Ave NE
Hazen, ND 58545-4600
(701)748-7278
FAX: (701)748-7298

Hettinger

West River Regional Medical Center
1000 Highway 12
Hettinger, ND 58639-7530
(701)567-6060
FAX: (701)567-6370

Jamestown

Jamestown Regional Medical Center
2422 20th St SW
Jamestown, ND 58401-6201
(701)952-4852
FAX: (701)952-3256

Sanford Health Jamestown Clinic
904 5th Ave NE
Jamestown, ND 58401-3437
(701)253-4016
FAX: (701)253-4053

Linton

Linton Hospital
518 N Broadway St
Linton, ND 58552-7308
(701)254-4531
FAX: (701)254-4318

Lisbon

Chi Lisbon Health
905 Main St
Lisbon, ND 58054-4334
(701)683-6454
FAX: (701)683-6411

Mandan

Edith Sanford Breast Center North Mandan Clinic
910 18th St NW
Mandan, ND 58554-1612
(701)667-5179
FAX: (701)667-5082

St Alexius Mandan Clinic North
2500 Sunset Dr
Mandan, ND 58554-1540
(701)667-4600
FAX: (701)667-3782

Minot

Chi St. Alexius Medical Plaza
2111 Landmark Cir NW
Minot, ND 58703-1967
(701)857-8081
FAX: (701)857-8023

Trinity Mammography - Hcma
400 Burdick Expy E
Minot, ND 58701-4768
(701)857-2640
FAX: (701)857-2660

New Town

Elbowoods Memorial Health Center
1058 College Dr
New Town, ND 58763-9112
(701)627-7680
FAX: (701)627-3050

Oakes

Oakes Community Hospital
1200 N 7th St
Oakes, ND 58474-2502
(701)742-3619
FAX: (701)742-3849

Rolla

Presentation Medical Center
213 2nd Ave NE
Rolla, ND 58367-7153
(701)477-1958
FAX: (701)477-5564

Rugby

Heart Of America Medical Center
800 S Main Ave
Rugby, ND 58368-2198
(701)776-5261
FAX: (701)776-7013

Stanley

Mountrail County Medical Center
PO Box 399, 615 6th St SE
Stanley, ND 58784-0399
(701)628-8629
FAX: (701)628-3074

Wahpeton

Essentia Health
275 11th St S
Wahpeton, ND 58075-4655
(701)642-2000
FAX: (701)671-4066

Watford City

McKenzie County Healthcare Systems Inc.
709 4th Ave NE
Watford City, ND 58854-7628
(701)842-3000
FAX: (701)842-2481

Williston

Chi St. Alexius Health Williston Medical Center
1301 15th Ave W
Williston, ND 58801-3821
(701)774-7435
FAX: (701)572-1668

Trinity Community Clinic - Western Dakota
1321 W Dakota Pkwy
Williston, ND 58801-3807
(701)774-0810
FAX: (701)774-0847

Williston Radiology Consultants Dba Fairlight Medical Center
3 4th St E
Williston, ND 58801-5350
(701)577-6337
FAX: (701)577-2838

Wishek

South Central Health
1007 4th Ave S
Wishek, ND 58495-7527
(701)452-2326
FAX: (701)452-2311

OHIO

Akron

Akron Gen. Reflections Breast Hlth Ctr - Akron
1 Akron General Ave
Akron, OH 44307-2432
(330)344-7757
FAX: (330)344-5842

Cleveland Clinic Akron General Reflections Brst Ctr- Bath
4125 Medina Rd Ste 100
Akron, OH 44333-4505
(330)344-5760
FAX: (330)665-8322

Summa Health Center At White Pond
1 Park West Blvd Ste 130
Akron, OH 44320-4230
(234)312-5800
FAX: (330)375-7668

Summa Health System Breast And Imaging Center
141 N Forge St Ste 500
Akron, OH 44304-1407
(234)312-5800
FAX: (330)375-7668

University Hospitals Fairlawn Health Center
3800 Embassy Pkwy
Akron, OH 44333-8387
(216)593-5680
FAX: (216)201-5325

Alliance

Alliance Community Hospital
200 E State St
Alliance, OH 44601-4936
(330)596-6000
FAX: (330)596-7795

Ashland

Samaritan Regional Health System
1025 Center St
Ashland, OH 44805-4097
(419)289-0491
FAX: (216)201-6658

Samaritan Womens Health Service
2212 Mifflin Ave Ste 210
Ashland, OH 44805-8846
(419)289-0491
FAX: (216)201-6658

Ashtabula

Ashtabula County Medical Center
2420 Lake Ave
Ashtabula, OH 44004-4970
(440)997-6590
FAX: (440)997-6493

Athens

Holzer
2131 E State St
Athens, OH 45701-2138
(740)589-3100
FAX: (740)566-4012

Ohiohealth O'Bleness Hospital
55 Hospital Dr, Mammography Department
Athens, OH 45701-2302
(740)592-9454
FAX: (740)566-4544

Austintown

Steward Imaging Center
20 Ohltown Rd, Ste 103
Austintown, OH 44515-2331
(330)841-1999
FAX: (330)884-2202

Avon

Cleveland Clinic Avon Hospital
33300 Cleveland Clinic Blvd
Avon, OH 44011-1172
(216)445-7050
FAX: (216)445-1654

University Hospitals Avon Health Center
1997 Healthway Dr Ste 101
Avon, OH 44011-2834
(440)988-6940
FAX: (440)988-6945

Barberton

Summa Health System - Summa Barberton Hospital
155 5th St NE
Barberton, OH 44203-3332
(234)312-5800
FAX: (330)375-7668

Barnesville

Barnesville Hospital
639 W Main St
Barnesville, OH 43713-1096
(740)425-5114
FAX: (740)425-5174

Batavia

Mercy Health Clermont Hospital
3000 Hospital Dr
Batavia, OH 45103-1998
(513)956-3729
FAX: (513)732-8686

Beachwood

Cleveland Clinic Foundation- Beachwood
26900 Cedar Rd 120
Beachwood, OH 44122-1191
(216)839-3200
FAX: (216)445-1654

Metrohealth Beachwood Health Center
3609 Park East Dr, N Bldg., Ste 300
Beachwood, OH 44122-4331
(216)957-9959
FAX: (216)778-4072

University Hospitals Ahuja Medical Center
3999 Richmond Rd
Beachwood, OH 44122-6046
(216)593-1649
FAX: (216)201-5325

Beavercreek

Kettering Breast Evaluation Center At Soin Medical Center
3535 Pentagon Blvd, Ste 230
Beavercreek, OH 45431-1705
(937)299-0099
FAX: (937)702-4011

Miami Valley Hospital Medical Imaging - Beavercreek
1244 Meadow Bridge Dr
Beavercreek, OH 45434-6388
(855)887-7364
FAX: (937)208-7657

Bedford

Uhhs Bedford Medical Center
44 Blaine Ave, Radiology Department
Bedford, OH 44146-2709
(440)735-3539
FAX: (440)735-3540

Bellefontaine

Mary Rutan Hospital Crawfis Imaging Center
120 Dowell Ave
Bellefontaine, OH 43311-2305
(937)592-1883
FAX: (937)593-3312

Bellevue

The Bellevue Hospital
1400 W Main St
Bellevue, OH 44811-9088
(419)483-4040
FAX: (419)484-5450

Belpre

Marietta Memorial Belpre Campus
807 Farson St Ste 120
Belpre, OH 45714-1068
(740)374-1750
FAX: (740)374-1746

Bluffton

Bluffton Hospital
139 Garau St, Radiology Department
Bluffton, OH 45817-1027
(419)423-5323
FAX: (419)369-4443

Boardman

Diagnostic Medical X-Ray & Imaging
8390 Tod Ave
Boardman, OH 44512-6366
(330)726-6010
FAX: (330)726-6017

Diagnostic Medical X-Ray & Imaging - Mobile
8390 Tod Ave
Boardman, OH 44512-6366
(330)726-6010
FAX: (330)726-6017

Mercyhealthyoungstown Llcd/B/Ast.Elizabethboardman Healthctr
8401 Market St
Boardman, OH 44512-6725
(330)729-3145
FAX: (330)729-3102

Southwoods Imaging
7623 Market St
Boardman, OH 44512-6054
(330)965-5100
FAX: (330)965-5197

Tiffany Breast Care Center At Advanced Womens Care
1111 Boardman Canfield Rd, Bldg B
Boardman, OH 44512-4068
(330)629-8624
FAX: (330)629-8625

Bowling Green

Wood County Hospital, Inc.
950 W Wooster St
Bowling Green, OH 43402-2699
(419)354-8743
FAX: (419)354-8745

Broadview Heights

Cleveland Clinic Medical Offices, Broadview Heights
2001 E Royalton Rd
Broadview Heights, OH 44147-2800
(216)636-8000
FAX: (216)445-1654

University Hospitals Broadview Heights Health Center
5901 E Royalton Rd, Ste 1200
Broadview Heights, OH 44147-3532
(440)792-9025
FAX: (440)792-9027

Brunswick

Brunswick Medical Center
4065 Center Rd
Brunswick, OH 44212-2918
(440)816-8605
FAX: (440)816-5565

Bryan

Parkview Phys Group Ohio McHa
442 W High St, Ste 3
Bryan, OH 43506-1681
(419)636-4517
FAX: (419)633-4098

Bucyrus

Avita Bucyrus Hospital
629 N Sandusky Ave
Bucyrus, OH 44820-1821
(419)563-9342
FAX: (419)562-1073

Cadiz

Harrison Community Hospital
951 E Market St
Cadiz, OH 43907-9749
(304)243-3032
FAX: (304)243-7170

Calcutta

Heritage Valley Health System - East Liverpool
48462 Bell School Rd Ste B
Calcutta, OH 43920-9625
(866)901-6266
FAX: (724)770-7929

Cambridge

Community Healthlink
1205 Clark St
Cambridge, OH 43725-9612
(740)432-5465
FAX: (740)432-4841

Southeastern Ohio Regional Medical Center
1341 Clark St
Cambridge, OH 43725-8911
(740)439-8930
FAX: (740)435-2909

Campbell

Mahoning Valley Imaging At Healthridge Medical Center
315 Struthers Liberty Rd
Campbell, OH 44405-1973
(330)750-6246
FAX: (330)750-6246

Canal Winchester

Diley Ridge Medical Center
7911 Diley Rd
Canal Winchester, OH 43110-9653
(614)838-7994
FAX: (614)838-7958

Canfield

The Center For Women
4139 Boardman Canfield Rd, Ste 1
Canfield, OH 44406-9034
(330)702-1281
FAX: (330)702-1287

Canton

Atrium Ob/Gyn Inc.
4151 Holiday St NW
Canton, OH 44718-2531
(330)492-8001
FAX: (330)639-2454

Aultman Hospital
2600 6th St SW, Breast Care Center
Canton, OH 44710-1702
(330)363-6285
FAX: (330)363-2282

Mercy Medical Center
1320 Mercy Dr NW
Canton, OH 44708-2641
(330)489-1493
FAX: (330)580-4776

Stark Womens Center
5000 Higbee Ave NW
Canton, OH 44718-2582
(330)244-8135
FAX: (330)493-1966

Carrollton

Aultman Carrollton Facility
1020 Trump Rd NW
Carrollton, OH 44615-8422
(330)627-0091
FAX: (330)627-4546

Centerville

Kettering Breast Evaluation Center
6438 Wilmington Pike, Ste 200
Centerville, OH 45459-7021
(937)299-0099
FAX: (937)299-0558

Miami Valley Hospital South
2400 Miami Valley Dr, Breast Center Ste. 200
Centerville, OH 45459-4774
(937)208-2080
FAX: (937)438-3794

Chagrin Falls

Cleveland Clinic Family Health Center Chagrin Falls
551 Washington St
Chagrin Falls, OH 44022-4403
(440)893-9393
FAX: (440)542-6840

Chardon

University Hospitals Geauga Medical Center
13207 Ravenna Rd
Chardon, OH 44024-7032
(440)285-6381
FAX: (216)201-5193

Chillicothe

Adena Health Center
272 Hospital Rd
Chillicothe, OH 45601-9031
(740)779-7711
FAX: (740)779-7406

Adena Health Center - Western Avenue
55 Centennial Blvd
Chillicothe, OH 45601-1187
(740)779-7711
FAX: (740)779-7406

Cincinnati

Good Samaritan Hospital
375 Dixmyth Ave, Breast Center - 5th Flr
Cincinnati, OH 45220-2489
(513)569-6777
FAX: (513)569-6617

Good Samaritan Outpatient Center
6350 Glenway Ave Ste 101
Cincinnati, OH 45211-6390
(513)569-6777
FAX: (513)389-7026

Good Samaritan Western Ridge
6949 Good Samaritan Dr
Cincinnati, OH 45247-5204
(513)569-6601
FAX: (513)569-6617

Jewish Hospital Llc
4700 E Galbraith Rd, Ste 100
Cincinnati, OH 45236-2754
(513)686-3300
FAX: (513)686-3302

Jewish Hospital Llc
4777 E Galbraith Rd, Ste 100
Cincinnati, OH 45236-2814
(513)559-7333
FAX: (513)559-7382

Mary Jo Cropper Breast Center
10506A Montgomery Rd
Cincinnati, OH 45242-4402
(513)569-6777
FAX: (513)865-1768

Mercy Health Anderson Hospital Women's Center
7502 State Rd, Stuite1100
Cincinnati, OH 45255
(513)956-3729
FAX: (513)624-4361

Mercy Health Eastgate Medical Center
601 Ivy Gtwy, Ste 2400
Cincinnati, OH 45245-2055
(513)782-9033
FAX: (513)782-9031

Mercy Health-West Hospital
3300 Mercy Health Blvd
Cincinnati, OH 45211-1103
(513)956-3729
FAX: (513)981-6108

Midtown Ambulatory Center
3590 Lucille Dr
Cincinnati, OH 45213-2674
(513)584-1500
FAX: (513)583-3633

Proscan Pink Ribbon Center Tri-County
11594 Springfield Pike, Ste 26
Cincinnati, OH 45246-3527
(513)772-7750
FAX: (513)527-7760

Proscan Women's Imaging
4850 Red Bank Rd
Cincinnati, OH 45227-1545
(513)527-7750
FAX: (513)527-7760

The Christ Hospital Comprehensive Breast Center - Montgomery
11150 Montgomery Rd, Ste 1100
Cincinnati, OH 45249-2300
(513)585-2668
FAX: (513)564-8596

The Christ Hospital Imaging Center
4440 Red Bank Rd Ste 100
Cincinnati, OH 45227-2177
(513)564-1340
FAX: (513)564-1370

The Christ Hospital Imaging Center Green Township
5885 Harrison Ave Ste 1100
Cincinnati, OH 45248-1720
(513)564-1350
FAX: (513)564-1370

The Christ Hospital OP Center
7545 Beechmont Ave Ste X
Cincinnati, OH 45255-4231
(513)585-2668
FAX: (513)232-8483

The Christ Hospital Womens Imaging Center
2123 Auburn Ave, Mob 324
Cincinnati, OH 45219-2906
(513)585-2668
FAX: (513)585-2702

Trihealth Anderson
7777 Beechmont Ave
Cincinnati, OH 45255-4209
(513)579-6602
FAX: (513)389-7026

Trihealth Kenwood
8240 Northcreek Dr
Cincinnati, OH 45236-2377
(513)569-6777
FAX: (513)569-6617

Trihealth Mobile Mammography
10494 Montgomery Rd
Cincinnati, OH 45242-5214
(513)569-6565
FAX: (513)865-1768

Uc Medical Center Breast Imaging Department
234 Goodman St, Ml 0772
Cincinnati, OH 45219-2364
(513)584-5678
FAX: (513)584-3633

Ucmc Screening Mammography Department
222 Piedmont Ave Ste 1400
Cincinnati, OH 45219-4231
(513)584-1500
FAX: (513)584-3633

Circleville

Ohiohealth Berger Hospital
600 N Pickaway St
Circleville, OH 43113-1499
(740)474-7701
FAX: (740)420-8697

Ohiohealth Imaging And Laboratory Services
1434 Circleville Plaza Dr
Circleville, OH 43113-2269
(740)474-7930
FAX: (740)420-8518

Cleveland

Fairview Breast Health Center
18200 Lorain Ave
Cleveland, OH 44111-5605
(216)476-9012
FAX: (216)476-6947

Langston Hughes Health Center
2390 E 79th St
Cleveland, OH 44104-2161
(216)361-1773
FAX: (216)445-1654

Lutheran Hospital
1730 W 25th St
Cleveland, OH 44113-3170
(216)363-2277
FAX: (216)696-7402

Metrohealth Broadway Health Center
6835 Broadway Ave
Cleveland, OH 44105-1313
(216)957-1500
FAX: (216)778-4072

Metrohealth Medical Center
2500 Metrohealth Dr, Breast Imaging Department
Cleveland, OH 44109-1900
(216)957-2778
FAX: (216)778-4072

Metrohealth West 150th Health & Surgery Center
4330 W 150th St
Cleveland, OH 44135-1316
(216)957-2778
FAX: (216)778-4072

Neon Hough Health Center
8300 Hough Ave
Cleveland, OH 44103-4247
(216)231-7700
FAX: (216)231-7920

St. Vincent Charity Medical Center
2351 E 22nd St
Cleveland, OH 44115-3197
(216)363-2592
FAX: (216)363-2764

The Cleveland Clinic Foundation
9500 Euclid Ave, Desk A-10 Mammograpy Dept
Cleveland, OH 44195-0002
(216)444-7509
FAX: (216)445-1654

Uhcmc Breen Breast Health Pavilion
11100 Euclid Ave B402, Mather Pavilion
Cleveland, OH 44106-1716
(216)844-3097
FAX: (216)201-7575

Cleveland Heights

Innovacare Llc
5 Severance Cir, Ste 108
Cleveland Heights, OH 44118-1513
(216)382-7165
FAX: (216)382-7166

Coldwater

Mercer County Community Hospital
800 W Main St
Coldwater, OH 45828-1698
(419)678-5111
FAX: (419)678-5237

Columbiana

Mercy Health Physicians Dba Joanie Abdu Mammo Columbiana
107 Royal Birkdale Dr
Columbiana, OH 44408-8493
(330)482-9350
FAX: (330)482-9402

Salem Community Hospital-Firestone Town Center Mammography
116 Carriage Dr, Town Center At Firestone Farms
Columbiana, OH 44408-8306
(330)332-7131
FAX: (330)332-7475

Columbus

Breast Health At The Bing Cancer Center
500 Thomas Ln, Ste 2A
Columbus, OH 43214-1419
(614)566-1111
FAX: (614)566-1953

Columbus Cancer Clinic Provided By Life Care Alliance
1699 W Mound St, Mammography Department
Columbus, OH 43223-1809
(614)437-2839
FAX: (614)263-5019

Columbus Obstetricians-Gynecologists, Inc.
150 Taylor Station Rd Ste 300
Columbus, OH 43213-4440
(614)434-2400
FAX: (614)324-0622

Jamescare Babe Zaharias Center
460 W 10th Ave, B120
Columbus, OH 43210-1240
(614)293-4455
FAX: (614)293-9662

Jamescare Mammography At Easton Town Center
4141 Brighton Rose Way
Columbus, OH 43219-6176
(614)293-4455
FAX: (614)293-9662

Jamescare Mobile Mammography- Hope
610 Ackerman Rd, Loading Dock
Columbus, OH 43202-4500
(614)293-4455
FAX: (614)296-9662

Jamescare Mobile Mammography-Mobile
610 Ackerman Rd Loading Dock
Columbus, OH 43202-4500
(614)293-4455
FAX: (614)293-9662

Katherine M. Cyran M.D. Breast Center
3360 Tremont Rd Ste 130
Columbus, OH 43221-2125
(614)459-1596
FAX: (614)459-1471

Lane Avenue Mammography
1315 W Lane Ave Ste D
Columbus, OH 43221-3544
(614)566-1111
FAX: (614)566-1953

Mammography At Carepoint East
543 Taylor Ave, Rm 1241
Columbus, OH 43203-1278
(614)293-4455
FAX: (614)293-9662

Ohio Health Jasonway Imaging Center
810 Jasonway Ave
Columbus, OH 43214-4359
(614)788-5212
FAX: (614)788-5225

Ohiohealth Corporation D/B/A Doctors Hospital
5131 Beacon Hill Rd Ste 180
Columbus, OH 43228-4442
(614)566-1111
FAX: (614)544-1760

Ohiohealth Mobile Mammography - Mobile
500 Thomas Ln Ste 2A
Columbus, OH 43214-1419
(614)566-1111
FAX: (614)566-1953

Ohiohealth Neighborhood Care Whitehall
4882 E Main St, Ste 100
Columbus, OH 43213-3189
(614)566-0900
FAX: (614)566-0947

Professionals For Women's Health
921 Jasonway Ave Ste B
Columbus, OH 43214-2456
(614)261-4214
FAX: (614)447-8876

Solis Women's Health At Columbus Mammography Ctr
974 Bethel Rd, Ste F
Columbus, OH 43214-2467
(614)791-9355
FAX: (614)362-5970

Stefanie Spielman Comprehensive Breast Center
1145 Olentangy River Rd
Columbus, OH 43212-3117
(614)293-4455
FAX: (614)293-9662

The Women's Health Center At Mt. Carmel East
5965 E Broad St Ste 100A
Columbus, OH 43213-1562
(614)234-7400
FAX: (614)234-8110

Wilkins Mob At Grant Medical Center
285 E State St, 3rd Fl. Ste. 320
Columbus, OH 43215-4354
(614)566-8340
FAX: (614)566-8167

Women's Health Center Mobile Services Unit - Mobile
775 W Broad St, Ste 260
Columbus, OH 43222-1471
(614)663-2936
FAX: (614)663-2913

Concord Township

University Hospitals Health System, Inc.
7590 Auburn Rd
Concord Township, OH 44077-9176
(440)375-8122
FAX: (440)375-8126

Concord Twp

University Hospital Concord Health Center
7500 Auburn Rd Ste 1350
Concord Twp, OH 44077-9612
(440)358-5490
FAX: (440)358-5413

Conneaut

Uh Conneaut Medical Center
158 W Main Rd
Conneaut, OH 44030-2039
(440)593-0150
FAX: (216)201-8017

Cortland

Stewardtrumbull Memorial Hospital, Inc. Center For Radiology
2586 State Route 5
Cortland, OH 44410-9353
(330)841-5911
FAX: (330)841-5916

Coshocton

Coshocton Regional Medical Center
1460 Orange St
Coshocton, OH 43812-2229
(740)623-4133
FAX: (740)623-4145

Cuyahoga Falls

Summa Health Center At Cuyahoga Falls
1860 State Rd Ste B
Cuyahoga Falls, OH 44223-1400
(234)312-5800
FAX: (330)375-7668

Dayton

Cornerstone Medical Imaging
7740 Washington Village Dr Ste 140
Dayton, OH 45459-3994
(937)439-7420
FAX: (937)439-7449

Grandview Hospital And Medical Center
405 W Grand Ave, Radiology Dept.
Dayton, OH 45405-4796
(937)723-3270
FAX: (937)723-3273

Miami Valley Hospital Breast Center
1 Wyoming St Ste 4120
Dayton, OH 45409-2711
(937)208-2080
FAX: (937)208-2829

Miami Valley Hospital North
9000 N Main St
Dayton, OH 45415-1180
(937)734-7768
FAX: (937)734-5851

Defiance

Mercy Health Defiance Hospital
1400 E 2nd St, Ste 200
Defiance, OH 43512-2440
(419)783-3239
FAX: (419)783-3204

Promedica Defiance Regional Hospital
1200 Ralston Ave
Defiance, OH 43512-1396
(419)783-6960
FAX: (419)782-6584

Delaware

Ohiohealth Breast Care At The Delaware Health Center
801 Ohio Health Blvd
Delaware, OH 43015-8900
(614)566-1111
FAX: (740)615-1118

Delphos

Mercy Health-Delphos Ambulatory Care Center
1800 E 5th St
Delphos, OH 45833-9180
(419)226-4500
FAX: (419)226-4501

Dennison

Trinity Hospital Twin City
819 N 1st St
Dennison, OH 44621-1098
(740)922-7450
FAX: (740)922-7457

Dover

Cleveland Clinic Union Hospital
659 Boulevard St
Dover, OH 44622-2026
(330)343-3311
FAX: (330)432-9777

Dublin

Avina Womens Care- Dublin
5150 Bradenton Ave, Ste A
Dublin, OH 43017-7589
(614)459-1000
FAX: (614)766-1335

Columbus Obstetricians-Gynecologists, Inc.
7450 Hospital Dr, Ste 280
Dublin, OH 43016-9641
(614)434-2400
FAX: (614)324-0622

Dublin Methodist Hospital
6700 Perimeter Dr, Ste 220
Dublin, OH 43016-8063
(614)566-1111
FAX: (614)544-8811

Solis Women's Health
5156 Blazer Pkwy Ste 120
Dublin, OH 43017-7318
(614)791-9355
FAX: (614)791-2970

The James Mammography Dublin
6790 Perimeter Dr Ste 300
Dublin, OH 43016-8068
(614)293-4455
FAX: (614)293-9662

East Cleveland

Stephanie Tubbs Jones Community Health Ctr
13944 Euclid Ave
East Cleveland, OH 44112-3804
(216)767-4236
FAX: (216)767-4275

East Liverpool

East Liverpool City Hospital
425 W 5th St
East Liverpool, OH 43920-2498
(330)386-2026
FAX: (330)386-2098

Eaton

Preble County Medical Center
450 Washington Jackson Rd
Eaton, OH 45320-8699
(937)456-8306
FAX: (937)456-8307

Elyria

Mercy Diagnostic Center North
1900 W River Rd N
Elyria, OH 44035-2778
(440)324-3226
FAX: (440)324-5936

Noms Premium Imaging
5319 Hoag Dr, Ste 130
Elyria, OH 44035-1495
(440)930-6020
FAX: (440)934-1082

The Cleveland Clinic Foundation Chestnut Commons
303 Chestnut Commons Dr
Elyria, OH 44035-9607
(216)445-5255
FAX: (216)445-1654

University Hospitals Elyria Medical Center
630 E River St, Radiology Dept.
Elyria, OH 44035-5902
(440)329-7576
FAX: (440)284-5509

Euclid

Cleveland Clinic Health System Euclid Hospital
18901 Lake Shore Blvd, Radiology Department
Euclid, OH 44119-1078
(216)636-8000
FAX: (216)445-1654

Fairfield

Mercy Health - Fairfield Hospital
3000 Mack Rd
Fairfield, OH 45014-5335
(513)870-7304
FAX: (513)603-8169

Findlay

Blanchard Valley Hospital-Eastern Woods
15900 Medical Dr S
Findlay, OH 45840-8894
(419)423-5323
FAX: (567)525-4336

Fostoria

Alma C. Kinn Mammo Ctr Promedica Fostoria Community Hospital
501 Van Buren St
Fostoria, OH 44830-1534
(419)436-6690
FAX: (419)436-6615

Fremont

Memorial Hospital Dba Promedica Memorial Hospital
715 S Taft Ave
Fremont, OH 43420-3237
(419)334-6605
FAX: (419)334-6638

Noms Fremont Imaging
1479 N River Rd, Ste 130
Fremont, OH 43420-9760
(419)559-2817
FAX: (419)559-2818

Gahanna

Mammography At Outpatient Care Gahanna
920 N Hamilton Rd
Gahanna, OH 43230-1757
(614)293-4455
FAX: (614)293-9662

Ohiohealth Neighborhood Care Of Gahanna
765 N Hamilton Rd
Gahanna, OH 43230-8703
(614)566-0525
FAX: (614)566-0537

Galion

Galion Hospital
269 Portland Way S
Galion, OH 44833-2399
(419)468-0773
FAX: (419)462-5212

Gallipolis

Holzer
100 Jackson Pike
Gallipolis, OH 45631-1563
(740)446-5289
FAX: (740)446-5697

Garfield Heights

Breast Care Center At Marymount
12300 McCracken Rd, Dept. Of Radiology
Garfield Heights, OH 44125-2914
(216)636-8200
FAX: (216)587-8894

Geneva

University Hospitals Geneva Medical Center
870 W Main St
Geneva, OH 44041-1295
(440)415-0162
FAX: (440)466-6970

Glandorf

Mercy Health-Putnam Medical Center
60L US 224
Glandorf, OH 45848
(419)226-4500
FAX: (419)226-4501

Grandview Heights

Columbus Obstetricians-Gynecologists, Inc.
1125 Yard St
Grandview Heights, OH 43212-3930
(614)434-2400
FAX: (614)324-0622

Greenville

Wayne Healthcare
835 Sweitzer St
Greenville, OH 45331-1007
(937)548-1141
FAX: (937)569-6920

Grove City

Mount Carmel Grove City
5300 N Meadows Dr, Ste 2900
Grove City, OH 43123-2546
(614)663-2936
FAX: (614)663-2913

Ohiohealth Grove City Health Center
2030 Stringtown Rd
Grove City, OH 43123-3993
(614)566-1111
FAX: (614)544-0021

The James Mammography Grove City
5775 N Meadows Dr Ste E
Grove City, OH 43123-7300
(614)293-4455
FAX: (614)293-9662

Women's Health Center At Mt. Carmel Medical Center
5300 N Meadows Dr
Grove City, OH 43123-2546
(614)234-2900
FAX: (614)234-2300

Hamilton

Bethesda Butler County
3075 Hamilton Mason Rd
Hamilton, OH 45011-8532
(513)569-6777
FAX: (513)569-6717

Fort Hamilton Hospital
630 Eaton Ave
Hamilton, OH 45013-2767
(513)867-2382
FAX: (513)867-2836

Hicksville

Community Memorial Hospital
208 Columbus St
Hicksville, OH 43526-1299
(419)542-5582
FAX: (419)542-6814

Hilliard

Columbus Obstetricians & Gynecologists, Inc.
3750 Ridge Mill Dr
Hilliard, OH 43026-9231
(614)434-2400
FAX: (614)324-0622

Ohiohealth Corporation - Hilliard Health Center
4343 All Seasons Dr Ste 260
Hilliard, OH 43026-1952
(614)544-1095
FAX: (614)566-1099

The James Mammography Mill Run
3641 Ridge Mill Dr
Hilliard, OH 43026-7752
(614)293-4455
FAX: (614)293-9662

Women's Health Center Mount Carmel Hilliard
4674 Britton Pkwy, Ste 1000
Hilliard, OH 43026-0044
(614)663-2936
FAX: (614)663-2913

Hillsboro

Highland District Hospital
1275 N High St
Hillsboro, OH 45133-5200
(937)393-6100
FAX: (937)840-6671

Huber Heights

Huber Health Center
8701 Troy Pike
Huber Heights, OH 45424-1063
(937)558-3320
FAX: (937)558-3322

Miami Valley Health Center-Huber Heights
6251 Miami Valley Way Ste 140
Huber Heights, OH 45424
(937)236-4780
FAX: (937)236-4855

Hudson

Summa Health Hudson Medical Center
5655 Hudson Dr Ste 200
Hudson, OH 44236-4454
(234)312-5800
FAX: (330)375-7668

Independence

Cleveland Clinic Foundation - Independence
5001 Rockside Rd, Ste 700
Independence, OH 44131-6803
(216)445-5255
FAX: (216)445-1654

Jackson

Holzer
280 Pattonsville Rd
Jackson, OH 45640-9452
(740)395-8766
FAX: (740)395-8893

Kent

University Hospitals Portage Medical Center Imaging At Kent
401 Devon Pl Ste 101
Kent, OH 44240-6481
(330)677-3434
FAX: (330)677-1345

Kenton

Hardin Memorial Hospital
921 E Franklin St
Kenton, OH 43326-2099
(419)675-8181
FAX: (419)675-3207

Kettering

Kettering Breast Evaluation Center
580 Lincoln Park Blvd Ste 200
Kettering, OH 45429-3493
(937)299-0099
FAX: (937)558-3727

Kettering Breast Evaluation Center
3700 Southern Blvd
Kettering, OH 45429-1265
(937)558-3711
FAX: (937)299-0558

Lakewood

Lakewood Family Health Center
14601 Detroit Ave
Lakewood, OH 44107-4205
(216)237-5500
FAX: (216)237-5705

Lancaster

Fairfield Medical Center - River Valley
2384 N Memorial Dr
Lancaster, OH 43130-1637
(740)687-8666
FAX: (740)687-8338

Lebanon

Bethesda Medical Center At Arrow Springs
100 Arrow Springs Blvd
Lebanon, OH 45036-7002
(513)569-6777
FAX: (513)282-7086

Lewis Center

Mammography At Outpatient Care Lewis Center
6515 Pullman Dr
Lewis Center, OH 43035-7380
(614)293-4455
FAX: (614)293-6560

Mount Carmel Fitness And Health Women's Health
7100 Graphics Way
Lewis Center, OH 43035-1123
(614)234-7400
FAX: (380)898-8524

Liberty Township

Mercy Health Center - Liberty Falls
6770 Cincinnati Dayton Rd Ste 107, Radiology
Liberty Township, OH 45044-9319
(513)981-4109
FAX: (513)981-4120

The Christ Hospital Medical Center Liberty Township
6939 Cox Rd
Liberty Township, OH 45069-7595
(513)585-2668
FAX: (513)585-1370

Lima

Lima Memorial Health System Medical Park Women
525 N Eastown Rd
Lima, OH 45807-2268
(419)998-4497
FAX: (419)998-4462

Mercy Health- St. Rita's Women's Wellness Center
770 W High St Ste 250
Lima, OH 45801-3993
(419)226-4500
FAX: (419)226-4501

Lodi

Lodi Community Hospital
225 Elyria St
Lodi, OH 44254-1096
(330)948-5531
FAX: (330)948-5539

Logan

Hocking Valley Community Hospital
PO Box 966
Logan, OH 43138-0966
(740)380-8204
FAX: (740)380-2343

London

Madison Health - Park Ave Medical Building
210 N Main St
London, OH 43140-1115
(740)845-7222
FAX: (740)845-7433

Lorain

Cleveland Clinic Foundation - Lorain Family Health Center
5700 Cooper Foster Park Rd W
Lorain, OH 44053-4152
(216)445-7050
FAX: (216)445-1654

Mercy Health Regional Medical Center, Llc
3700 Kolbe Rd, Mammography Department
Lorain, OH 44053-1611
(440)960-3522
FAX: (440)960-3753

Macedonia

Cleveland Clinic Express Outpatient Care
8210 Macedonia Commons Blvd Unit 40
Macedonia, OH 44056-1861
(216)444-7509
FAX: (216)445-1654

Madison

University Hospitals Health System, Inc.
6270 N Ridge Rd
Madison, OH 44057-2567
(440)354-1029
FAX: (440)354-8126

Mansfield

Ohiohealth Mansfield Women's Imaging Center
335 Glessner Ave
Mansfield, OH 44903-2269
(419)526-8559
FAX: (414)526-8298

Uh Samaritan Richland Health Center
1033 Ashland Rd
Mansfield, OH 44905-2156
(419)289-0491
FAX: (216)201-6658

Women's Care, Inc.
500 S Trimble Rd
Mansfield, OH 44906-4103
(419)756-6000
FAX: (419)756-7968

Marietta

Marietta Memorial Hospital Waynestreet Facility
802 Wayne St, Ste 101
Marietta, OH 45750-3374
(740)374-1750
FAX: (740)568-5203

Memorial Health System Mga- Campus
410 2nd St
Marietta, OH 45750-2115
(740)374-3622
FAX: (740)376-2668

Marion

Executive Imaging, Llc
1069 Delaware Ave Ste 104
Marion, OH 43302-6459
(740)751-6828
FAX: (740)751-6829

Marion General Hospital Inc
1050 Delaware Ave
Marion, OH 43302-6482
(740)383-7889
FAX: (740)375-6420

Martins Ferry

East Ohio Hospital, Llc.
90 N 4th St
Martins Ferry, OH 43935-1648
(740)633-4216
FAX: (740)633-4565

Marysville

Memorial Hospital
500 London Ave
Marysville, OH 43040-1594
(937)578-2377
FAX: (937)578-2809

Memorial Imaging At City Gate
120 Colemans Xing
Marysville, OH 43040-7115
(937)578-2377
FAX: (937)578-2809

Ohio Reformatory For Women
1479 Collins Ave
Marysville, OH 43040-9102
(937)642-1065
FAX: (937)642-1277

Mason

Jewish Hospital Llc
5075 Parkway Dr, Ste 106
Mason, OH 45040-9555
(513)686-5162
FAX: (513)686-3272

Massillon

Aultman Massillon Stark County Facility
2021 Wales Ave. NW
Massillon, OH 44646
(330)834-1111
FAX: (330)830-5454

Mercy Health Center At Jackson
7337 Caritas Cir NW Ste 100
Massillon, OH 44646-9127
(330)489-1493
FAX: (330)489-1298

Maumee

McLaren St. Lukes Medical Imaging-Fallen Timbers
5757 Monclova Rd Ste 31
Maumee, OH 43537-1863
(419)893-4856
FAX: (419)893-8978

St Luke's Hospital
5901 Monclova Rd
Maumee, OH 43537-1899
(419)897-8328
FAX: (419)891-8520

The Toledo Hospital Arrowhead Medical Center
660 Beaver Creek Cir Ste 120
Maumee, OH 43537-1746
(419)291-3000
FAX: (419)479-6060

Mayfield Heights

Hillcrest Hospital
6780 Mayfield Rd
Mayfield Heights, OH 44124-2294
(216)636-8000
FAX: (440)312-6420

Hillcrest Radiology
6803 Mayfield Rd Ste 206, Hillcrest Medical Bldg I
Mayfield Heights, OH 44124-2212
(216)636-8000
FAX: (440)312-1707

Medina

Medina Hospital
1000 E Washington St
Medina, OH 44256-2167
(330)721-5170
FAX: (330)721-5888

Summa Health Center At Lake Medina
3780 Medina Rd Ste 130
Medina, OH 44256-9312
(234)312-5800
FAX: (330)375-7668

Mentor

University Hospitals Health System, Inc.
9485 Mentor Ave Ste 4
Mentor, OH 44060-8711
(440)205-5473
FAX: (440)205-5426

Miamisburg

Kettering Breast Evaluation Center
4000 Miamisburg Centerville Rd, Ste 220
Miamisburg, OH 45342-7615
(937)299-0099
FAX: (937)558-3727

Middleburg Heights

Metro Health November Family Health Center
7800 Pearl Rd
Middleburg Heights, OH 44130-6552
(440)238-2124
FAX: (216)778-4072

Southwest Family Physicians, Inc.
7225 Old Oak Blvd, Ste A210
Middleburg Heights, OH 44130-3339
(440)816-5721
FAX: (440)816-5785

Southwest General Health Center
18697 Bagley Rd, Radiology Department
Middleburg Heights, OH 44130-3497
(440)816-8605
FAX: (440)816-2663

Middletown

Atrium Medical Center
1 Medical Center Dr
Middletown, OH 45005-1066
(513)420-5237
FAX: (513)420-5053

Kbec Middletown Health Center
6147 State Route 122
Middletown, OH 45005-5201
(937)299-0099
FAX: (937)558-3727

Milford

Mercy Health Milford - Imaging And Lab
201 Old Bank Rd Ste 101
Milford, OH 45150-2443
(513)831-4425
FAX: (513)831-4536

Millersburg

Pomerene Hospital
981 Wooster Rd
Millersburg, OH 44654-1094
(330)674-1015
FAX: (330)674-2914

Mount Gilead

Morrow County Hospital
651 W Marion Rd
Mount Gilead, OH 43338-1096
(419)949-3090
FAX: (419)949-3141

Mount Vernon

Knox Community Hospital
1330 Coshocton Ave
Mount Vernon, OH 43050-1495
(740)393-9937
FAX: (740)399-3145

Napoleon

Henry County Hospital, Inc.
1600 E Riverview Ave
Napoleon, OH 43545-9399
(419)591-3830
FAX: (419)591-3874

Nelsonville

Ohiohealth O'Bleness Hospital
11 John Lloyd Evans Memorial Dr
Nelsonville, OH 45764-2523
(740)591-8839
FAX: (740)592-9362

New Albany

Columbus Obstetricians-Gynecologists, Inc.
160 W Main St, Ste 220
New Albany, OH 43054-1189
(614)434-2400
FAX: (614)324-0622

Women's Health Center New Albany
7333 Smiths Mill Rd, Ste 1231
New Albany, OH 43054-9291
(614)234-7400
FAX: (380)898-8524

Newark

Licking Memorial Hospital
1320 W Main St
Newark, OH 43055-3699
(220)564-4722
FAX: (220)564-4740

Licking Memorial Womens Health
15 Messimer Dr
Newark, OH 43055-1841
(220)564-4684
FAX: (220)564-4690

North Canton

Aultman North Stark County Facility
6100 Whipple Ave NW
North Canton, OH 44720-7618
(330)305-6999
FAX: (330)305-6997

North Ridgeville

University Hospitals North Ridgeville Health Center
32800 Lorain Rd, Ste 1300
North Ridgeville, OH 44039-3430
(440)406-5380
FAX: (440)406-5382

Norwalk

Fisher-Titus Medical Center
272 Benedict Ave
Norwalk, OH 44857-2374
(419)668-8101
FAX: (419)660-2892

Oberlin

Mercy Health-Allen Hospital
200 W Lorain St
Oberlin, OH 44074-1026
(440)775-9120
FAX: (440)775-9184

Ontario

Avita Ontario
715 Richland Mall
Ontario, OH 44906-3802
(567)307-7742
FAX: (567)307-7745

Orange Village

University Hospitals Chagrin Highlands Breast Center
3909 Orange Pl, Ste 4400
Orange Village, OH 44122-4482
(216)292-1783
FAX: (216)292-7114

Oregon

Bay Park Community Hospital
2801 Bay Park Dr
Oregon, OH 43616-4925
(419)690-8600
FAX: (419)697-7741

Mercy Women's Care At St. Charles
2702 Navarre Ave Ste 101
Oregon, OH 43616-3224
(419)696-7900
FAX: (419)696-7431

Orrville

Aultman Orrville Hospital
832 S Main St
Orrville, OH 44667-2208
(330)684-4750
FAX: (330)684-4787

Ottawa

Ottawa Medical & Diagnostic Center
1740 N Perry St Ste D
Ottawa, OH 45875-1173
(419)523-3681
FAX: (419)523-3678

Oxford

McCullough - Hyde Memorial Hospital Trihealth
110 N Poplar St
Oxford, OH 45056-1204
(513)524-5361
FAX: (513)524-5364

Parma

Uh Parma Medical Center
6305 Powers Blvd
Parma, OH 44129-5468
(440)743-2054
FAX: (440)743-4054

Paulding

Paulding County Hospital
1035 W Wayne St
Paulding, OH 45879-9235
(419)399-1131
FAX: (419)399-2732

Perrysburg

Mercy Medical Center Perrysburg
12621 Eckel Junction Rd
Perrysburg, OH 43551-1304
(567)368-1027
FAX: (567)368-1073

Promedica Perrysburg
1601 Brigham Dr Ste 180
Perrysburg, OH 43551-7118
(419)291-3000
FAX: (419)479-6060

Pickerington

Ohiohealth Pickerington Medical Campus
1010 Refugee Rd
Pickerington, OH 43147-9653
(614)788-4150
FAX: (614)788-4255

The James Mammography Pickerington
1025 Refugee Rd, Ste 200
Pickerington, OH 43147-9861
(614)293-4455
FAX: (614)296-9662

Piqua

Outpatient Care Center North
280 Looney Rd Ste 103
Piqua, OH 45356-4199
(937)440-7111
FAX: (937)440-4381

Poland

Joanie Abdu Mammography, Poland
6615 Clingan Rd, Ste F
Poland, OH 44514-2196
(330)757-3643
FAX: (330)757-3893

Pomeroy

Holzer
88 E Memorial Dr
Pomeroy, OH 45769-9569
(740)992-0060
FAX: (740)446-5154

Port Clinton

H. B. Magruder Memorial Hospital
615 Fulton St
Port Clinton, OH 43452-2097
(419)734-3131
FAX: (419)732-4039

Portsmouth

King's Daughters Medical Center Ohio
1901 Argonne Rd
Portsmouth, OH 45662-2827
(606)408-2742
FAX: (606)408-6470

Southern Ohio Medical Center Cancer Center / Breast Center
1121 Kinneys Ln
Portsmouth, OH 45662-2806
(740)356-7490
FAX: (740)353-1377

Ravenna

University Hospitals Portage Medical Center
6847 N Chestnut St
Ravenna, OH 44266-3929
(330)297-2338
FAX: (330)297-2353

Richmond Heights

Uh Regional Hospitals Richmond Medical Center
27100 Chardon Rd
Richmond Heights, OH 44143-1116
(216)844-1700
FAX: (440)585-6179

Salem

Salem Regional Medical Center
1995 E State St
Salem, OH 44460-2423
(330)332-7131
FAX: (330)332-7475

Sandusky

Firelands Regional Medical Center The Center For Breast Care
703 Tyler St Ste 152
Sandusky, OH 44870-3392
(419)557-5239
FAX: (419)557-5233

Noms Imaging Sandusky
2500 W Strub Rd, Ste 220
Sandusky, OH 44870-5390
(419)502-5944
FAX: (419)502-5945

Seaman

Adams County Regional Medical Center
230 Medical Center Dr
Seaman, OH 45679-8002
(937)386-3400
FAX: (937)386-3489

Shelby

Ohiohealth Shelby Hospital
199 W Main St
Shelby, OH 44875-1490
(419)342-1749
FAX: (419)342-4203

Sidney

Wilson Health
915 Michigan St
Sidney, OH 45365-2401
(937)498-5533
FAX: (937)498-5437

Solon

Cleveland Clinic Foundation - Solon
29800 Bainbridge Rd
Solon, OH 44139-2202
(216)445-5255
FAX: (216)445-1654

South Euclid

University Hospitals Suburban Health Center
1611 S Green Rd Ste 16
South Euclid, OH 44121-4128
(216)382-2853
FAX: (216)201-5925

Springfield

Ohio Valley Imaging Center
140 W Main St, Ste 200
Springfield, OH 45502-1370
(937)521-4940
FAX: (937)521-4941

Springfield Regional Medical Center
1343 N Fountain Blvd
Springfield, OH 45504-1461
(937)523-9335
FAX: (937)342-5450

St Clairsville

St. Clairsville Health Center
51339 National Rd
St Clairsville, OH 43950-9107
(304)243-3176
FAX: (304)243-7170

Trinity Health System Medical Plaza
106 Plaza Dr Ste D, Radiology Dept. Nancy McFarland
St Clairsville, OH 43950-6700
(740)695-6917
FAX: (740)695-5738

St Marys

Joint Township District Memorial Hospital
200 Saint Clair Ave
St Marys, OH 45885-2494
(419)394-3387
FAX: (419)394-1146

Steubenville

Images - Trinity Health System
1 Ross Park Blvd
Steubenville, OH 43952-2681
(740)283-7848
FAX: (740)283-7398

Stow

Cleveland Clinic Akron General Reflections Breast Ctr-Stow
4300 Allen Rd
Stow, OH 44224-1032
(330)344-5760
FAX: (330)665-8322

Summa Health Stow Kent Medical Center
3825 Fishcreek Rd., Suite 130
Stow, OH 44224
(234)312-5800
FAX: (330)331-1929

Streetsboro

Uh Portage Medical Center Imaging At Streetsboro
9318 State Route 14
Streetsboro, OH 44241-5224
(330)297-2338
FAX: (330)297-2353

Strongsville

The Cleveland Clinic Foundation Strongsville
16761 Southpark Ctr
Strongsville, OH 44136-9302
(216)445-7050
FAX: (216)445-1654

University Hospitals Health System And Swghc
18181 Pearl Rd
Strongsville, OH 44136-6949
(440)816-4916
FAX: (440)816-4978

Sylvania

Mercy St Anne Outpatient Imaging
7640 Sylvania Ave Ste A-1
Sylvania, OH 43560-9263
(419)517-1700
FAX: (419)517-1711

Promedica Flower Hospital A Division Of Promedica Toledo Hos
5200 Harroun Rd
Sylvania, OH 43560-2168
(419)291-3000
FAX: (419)824-1728

The Toledo Hospital - Promedica Health And Wellness Center
5700 Monroe St Unit 108
Sylvania, OH 43560-2779
(419)291-3000
FAX: (419)479-6060

Tallmadge

Cleveland Clinic Akrongeneral Reflections Brst Ctr-Tallmadge
33 North Ave Ste 202
Tallmadge, OH 44278-1900
(330)344-5760
FAX: (330)665-8322

Summa Health Tallmadge Medical Center
60 North Ave
Tallmadge, OH 44278-2011
(234)312-5800
FAX: (330)375-7668

Tiffin

Mercy Health-Tiffin Hospital Llc
45 St Lawrence Dr
Tiffin, OH 44883-8310
(419)455-7870
FAX: (419)455-7413

Tipp City

Hyatt Imaging Center
450 N Hyatt St Ste 101
Tipp City, OH 45371-1433
(937)440-7111
FAX: (937)667-6977

Toledo

Mercy Women's Care At St. Anne
3404 W Sylvania Ave
Toledo, OH 43623-4467
(419)407-1770
FAX: (419)407-3862

Promedica Breast Care
2121 Hughes Dr
Toledo, OH 43606-3845
(419)291-3000
FAX: (419)479-6139

The Toledo Clinic, Inc
4126 N Holland Sylvania Rd, Ste 150
Toledo, OH 43623-3510
(419)517-7081
FAX: (419)517-9808

The Toledo Clinic, Inc.
4235 Secor Rd
Toledo, OH 43623-4299
(419)479-5935
FAX: (419)479-5501

The University Of Toledo Medical Center
3000 Arlington Ave
Toledo, OH 43614-2598
(419)383-3936
FAX: (419)383-4849

Troy

Troy Hospital Kettering Breast Evaluation Center
600 W Main St, Ste 240
Troy, OH 45373-3384
(937)299-0099
FAX: (937)558-3727

Upper Valley Medical Center
3130 N County Road 25A
Troy, OH 45373-1309
(937)440-7111
FAX: (937)641-2336

Twinsburg

Twinsburg Family Health Center
8701 Darrow Rd
Twinsburg, OH 44087-2105
(216)445-5255
FAX: (216)445-1654

Uniontown

Cleveland Clinic Akron General Reflections Brst Ctr-Green
1940 Town Park Blvd
Uniontown, OH 44685-7855
(330)344-5760
FAX: (330)665-8322

Summa Health Center At Green
3838 Massillon Rd Ste 300
Uniontown, OH 44685-7965
(234)312-5800
FAX: (330)375-7668

Upper Arlington

Mammography At Outpatient Care Upper Arlington
1800 Zollinger Rd
Upper Arlington, OH 43221-2849
(614)688-7284
FAX: (614)293-9662

Upper Sandusky

Wyandot Memorial Hospital
885 N Sandusky Ave
Upper Sandusky, OH 43351-1098
(419)294-4991
FAX: (419)294-6265

Urbana

Memorial Urbana Medical Center
1958 E US Highway 36
Urbana, OH 43078-9799
(937)578-2377
FAX: (937)578-2809

Mercy Health Urbana Hospital
904 Scioto St
Urbana, OH 43078-2200
(937)328-8100
FAX: (937)342-5450

Van Wert

Early Detection Imaging At Van Wert Family Physicians
1178 Professional Dr
Van Wert, OH 45891-2461
(419)860-3623
FAX: (419)232-2076

Van Wert County Hospital
140 Fox Rd Ste 106
Van Wert, OH 45891-2490
(419)238-8630
FAX: (419)238-8652

Vandalia

Dayton Medical Imaging - Vandalia
113 W National Rd
Vandalia, OH 45377-1934
(937)898-9729
FAX: (937)898-2995

Wadsworth

Summa Health Wadsworth-Rittman Medical Center
195 Wadsworth Rd
Wadsworth, OH 44281
(234)312-5800
FAX: (330)375-7083

Wapakoneta

Mercy Health-St. Rita's Mammography At Wapak
1100 Defiance St
Wapakoneta, OH 45895-1022
(419)996-5899
FAX: (419)941-1160

Warren

Mercy Health St. Jospeh Warren Hospital
667 Eastland Ave SE
Warren, OH 44484-4503
(330)841-4882
FAX: (330)841-4308

Steward Trumbull Memorial Hospital, Inc.
1350 E Market St
Warren, OH 44483-6628
(330)841-1999
FAX: (330)841-5675

Warrensville Heights

South Pointe Hospital
4110 Warrensville Center Rd, Radiology Department
Warrensville Heights, OH 44122-7099
(216)636-8000
FAX: (216)491-7575

Washington Court House

Adena Fayette Medical Center
1510 Columbus Ave Ste 110
Washington Court House, OH 43160-1986
(740)333-2743
FAX: (740)333-2937

Wauseon

Fulton County Health Center
725 S Shoop Ave
Wauseon, OH 43567-1701
(419)330-2651
FAX: (419)330-2652

Waverly

Adena Health Center - Waverly
12340 State Route 104
Waverly, OH 45690-8968
(740)779-8221
FAX: (740)779-7406

West Chester

Mobile Diagnostic University Of Cincinnati Medical Center
7700 University Dr
West Chester, OH 45069-2505
(513)584-5356
FAX: (513)584-3633

West Chester Hospital
7700 University Dr
West Chester, OH 45069-2505
(513)584-7465
FAX: (513)298-8950

West Union

Somc Family Health Center
90 Cic Blvd
West Union, OH 45693-8024
(740)356-8128
FAX: (937)544-5659

Westerville

Avina Womens Care
507 Executive Campus Dr, Ste 160
Westerville, OH 43082-9340
(614)459-1000
FAX: (614)918-9691

Mount Carmel St Anns Womens Health
477 Cooper Rd Ste 100
Westerville, OH 43081-8056
(614)234-7400
FAX: (380)898-8524

The James Mammography Westerville
465 N Cleveland Ave Ste 230
Westerville, OH 43082-8081
(614)293-4455
FAX: (614)293-9662

Westerville Medical Campus
300 Polaris Pkwy, Ste 1000
Westerville, OH 43082-7276
(614)566-1111
FAX: (614)533-3129

Westlake

Fairview Hospital Westlake Ptc-Women's Radiology Services
850 Columbia Rd Ste 320
Westlake, OH 44145-7214
(216)476-7200
FAX: (440)250-5740

Premier Physicians Center
25200 Center Ridge Rd, Ste 1500
Westlake, OH 44145-4142
(440)333-2246
FAX: (440)499-4283

St. John Medical Center
29000 Center Ridge Rd, Breast Health Center
Westlake, OH 44145-5219
(440)827-5668
FAX: (440)827-5480

University Hospitals Westlake Health Center
960 Clague Rd Ste 1300
Westlake, OH 44145-1585
(440)250-2093
FAX: (440)250-2091

Willard

Mercy Health-Willard Hospital Llc
1100 Neal Zick Rd
Willard, OH 44890-9287
(419)455-7870
FAX: (419)933-7173

Willoughby

University Hospitals Health System, Inc.
4176 State Route 306
Willoughby, OH 44094-9203
(440)918-4606
FAX: (440)918-4607

University Hospitals Health System, Inc.
36000 Euclid Ave
Willoughby, OH 44094-4625
(440)953-6040
FAX: (440)953-6124

Willoughby Hills

The Cleveland Clinic Foundation - Willoughby Hills
2550 Som Center Rd
Willoughby Hills, OH 44094-9655
(216)445-7050
FAX: (216)445-1654

Wilmington

Clinton Memorial Hospital
610 W Main St
Wilmington, OH 45177-2125
(937)382-9353
FAX: (937)382-9226

Wooster

Cleveland Clinic Wooster Specialty Center
721 E Milltown Rd
Wooster, OH 44691-1331
(330)287-4500
FAX: (330)287-4771

Wooster Community Hospital Women's Speciality Center
1761 Beall Ave
Wooster, OH 44691-2342
(330)263-8660
FAX: (330)263-8503

Worthington

James Mammography At Worthington Heights
160 W Wilson Bridge Rd
Worthington, OH 43085-2676
(614)293-4455
FAX: (614)293-6560

Wright Patterson Afb

88th Med. Group Dts/ Sgqq Wright Patterson Med. Ctr
4881 Sugar Maple Dr
Wright Patterson Afb, OH 45433-5529
(937)257-2168
FAX: (937)257-5229

Xenia

Greene Memorial Hospital, Inc.
1141 N Monroe Dr
Xenia, OH 45385-1600
(937)558-3717
FAX: (937)558-3727

Youngstown

Mahoning Valley Imaging At Millennia
1040 S Commons Pl
Youngstown, OH 44514-1959
(330)629-8624
FAX: (330)629-8625

Mahoning Valley Imaging At S W Run
800 E Western Reserve Rd
Youngstown, OH 44514-3359
(330)629-8624
FAX: (330)629-8625

Mercy Hllth Youngstown,Llc Dba Joanie Abdu Comp Brstcare Ctr
1044 Belmont Ave
Youngstown, OH 44504-1006
(330)480-2654
FAX: (330)480-2097

Tiffany Breast Care Center At Drs. Quirk And Haggerty
5533 Mahoning Ave
Youngstown, OH 44515-2366
(330)793-7966
FAX: (330)629-8625

Tiffany Breast Care Center At Mahoning Valley Imaging
7067 Tiffany Blvd
Youngstown, OH 44514-1993
(330)629-8624
FAX: (330)629-8625

Tiffany Breast Care Center Mobile 3
7067 Tiffany Blvd
Youngstown, OH 44514-1993
(330)629-8624
FAX: (330)629-8625

Zanesville

Genesis Healthcare System
2800 Maple Ave
Zanesville, OH 43701-1716
(740)586-6893
FAX: (740)586-6701

OKLAHOMA

Ada

Chickasaw Nation Medical Center
1921 Stonecipher Dr
Ada, OK 74820-3439
(580)272-1015
FAX: (580)272-1017

Mercy Hospital Ada
430 N Monte Vista St
Ada, OK 74820-4657
(580)421-6089
FAX: (580)421-6095

Altus

Jcmh Women's Imaging
1200 E Pecan St
Altus, OK 73521-6141
(580)379-5100
FAX: (580)379-5449

Alva

Share Medical Center
800 Share Dr
Alva, OK 73717-3618
(580)430-3300
FAX: (580)430-3350

Ardmore

Mercy Hospital Ardmore
1011 14th Ave NW
Ardmore, OK 73401-1828
(580)220-6162
FAX: (844)936-5798

The Chickasaw Nation Ardmore Health Clinic
2510 Chickasaw Blvd
Ardmore, OK 73401-1341
(580)226-8181
FAX: (580)222-2898

Bartlesville

Ascension St.John Jane Phillips
3500 E Frank Phillips Blvd
Bartlesville, OK 74006-2411
(918)331-1598
FAX: (918)331-1669

Ascension St.John Jane Phillips Imaging Center
2661 SE Washington Blvd
Bartlesville, OK 74006-7615
(918)331-3020
FAX: (918)331-3021

Broken Arrow

Saint Francis Broken Arrow Imaging Center
2950 S Elm Pl Ste 130
Broken Arrow, OK 74012-7816
(918)451-5141
FAX: (918)451-5103

St John Broken Arrow
1000 W Boise Cir
Broken Arrow, OK 74012-4900
(918)856-5789
FAX: (918)994-8029

Chickasha

Grady Memorial Hospital Womens Imaging Center
2220 W Iowa Ave
Chickasha, OK 73018-2700
(405)779-2195
FAX: (405)779-2364

Claremore

Claremore Indian Hospital
101 S Moore Ave
Claremore, OK 74017-5091
(918)342-6206
FAX: (918)342-6210

Hillcrest Hospital / Claremore
1202 N Muskogee Pl
Claremore, OK 74017-3058
(918)341-8316
FAX: (918)343-6938

Cleveland

Cleveland Area Hospital
1401 W Pawnee St
Cleveland, OK 74020-3019
(918)358-2501
FAX: (918)358-5798

Clinton

Alliancehealth Clinton
100 N 30th St
Clinton, OK 73601-3117
(580)323-8322
FAX: (580)331-1406

Usphs Clinton Indian Health Center
10321 N 2274 Rd
Clinton, OK 73601-7521
(580)331-3367
FAX: (580)331-3558

Coweta

Koweta Indian Health Facility
31870 E State Highway 51
Coweta, OK 74429-7900
(918)279-3311
FAX: (918)279-1097

Cushing

Hillcrest Hospital Cushing
1027 E Cherry St
Cushing, OK 74023-4101
(918)225-8220
FAX: (918)550-6706

Duncan

Drh Imaging
1414 Duncan Regional Loop
Duncan, OK 73533-1595
(580)251-6670
FAX: (580)251-6671

Durant

Alliance Health Durant
1800 W University Blvd, Radiology Dept.
Durant, OK 74701-3006
(580)931-2066
FAX: (580)920-8002

Choctaw Nation Regional Medical Clinic
1801 Chukka Hina
Durant, OK 74701-7117
(580)920-2100
FAX: (580)916-9197

Edmond

Breast Health Network - Edmond
2601 Kelley Pointe Pkwy Ste 101
Edmond, OK 73013-2996
(405)844-2601
FAX: (405)844-2610

Integris Health Edmond
4801 Integris Pkwy
Edmond, OK 73034-8864
(405)951-5000
FAX: (405)471-0008

Mercy Edmond I-35 Breast Services
2017 W I 35 Frontage Rd
Edmond, OK 73013-8550
(405)752-3500
FAX: (405)757-3496

Touchstone Imaging Of Oklahoma, Llc Dba Tmi Edmond
902 S Bryant Ave
Edmond, OK 73034-5742
(405)348-5252
FAX: (405)509-6803

Elk City

Great Plains Regional Medical Center
1801 W 3rd St
Elk City, OK 73644-5145
(580)225-2511
FAX: (580)821-5596

Enid

Baptist Healthcare Of Ok Dba Integris Bass Baptist Hlth Ctr
600 S Monroe St
Enid, OK 73701-7211
(580)548-1700
FAX: (580)548-1497

Women's Imaging- St Mary's Regional Medical Center
316 W Owen K Garriott Rd
Enid, OK 73701-5622
(580)249-3771
FAX: (580)237-1530

Fort Sill

Reynolds Army Health Clinic
4301 Wilson St
Fort Sill, OK 73503-4472
(580)558-2780
FAX: (580)558-2397

Glenpool

Saint Francis Glenpool
140 W 151st St S
Glenpool, OK 74033-4523
(918)321-7570
FAX: (918)321-7513

Grove

Integris Grove Hospital
1001 E 18th St
Grove, OK 74344-2907
(918)787-3750
FAX: (918)787-3747

Guthrie

Mercy Hospital Logan County
200 S Academy Rd
Guthrie, OK 73044-8727
(405)260-4201
FAX: (405)260-4202

Henryetta

Hillcrest Hospital Henryetta
2401 W Main B
Henryetta, OK 74437
(918)650-1327
FAX: (918)650-1394

Hobart

Elkview General Hospital
429 W Elm St
Hobart, OK 73651-1699
(580)726-1905
FAX: (580)726-1985

Hugo

Choctaw Memorial Hospital
1405 E Kirk St
Hugo, OK 74743-3603
(580)317-9540
FAX: (580)317-9603

Idabel

Choctaw Nation Health Clinic
902 E Lincoln Rd
Idabel, OK 74745-7337
(580)286-2600
FAX: (580)286-2011

McCurtain Memorial Hospital
1301 E Lincoln Rd
Idabel, OK 74745-7341
(580)208-3157
FAX: (580)208-3265

Kingfisher

Mercy Hospital Kingfisher
1000 Hospital Dr
Kingfisher, OK 73750-5029
(405)375-7821
FAX: (405)375-7932

Lawton

Comanche County Memorial Hospital
3401 W Gore Blvd, Mammography/Stacy Tucker
Lawton, OK 73505-6300
(580)250-5846
FAX: (580)585-5469

The Breast Center
5604 SW Lee Blvd Ste 150
Lawton, OK 73505-9674
(580)536-8000
FAX: (580)536-2584

Usph Lawton Indian Hospital
1515 NE Lawrie Tatum Rd
Lawton, OK 73507-3099
(580)354-5575
FAX: (580)354-5578

McAlester

Choctaw Nation Health Clinic
1127 S George Nigh Expy
McAlester, OK 74501-7143
(918)423-8440
FAX: (918)423-8442

McAlester Regional Imaging Center
10 S 3rd St
McAlester, OK 74501-5346
(918)421-8274
FAX: (918)421-8194

Warren Clinic McAlester Division
1401 E Van Buren Ave
McAlester, OK 74501-4245
(918)421-8491
FAX: (918)421-8741

Miami

Integris Miami Hospital
200 2nd Ave SW
Miami, OK 74354-6830
(918)540-7550
FAX: (918)540-7898

Northeastern Tribal Health System
7600 S Highway 69A
Miami, OK 74354-1016
(918)332-4475
FAX: (885)963-2537

Midwest City

Ssm Health St Anthony Hospital - Midwest
2825 Parklawn Dr, Radiology Department
Midwest City, OK 73110-4201
(405)610-8873
FAX: (405)610-8874

Moore

Norman Regional Hlth Sys. Dba Norman Regional Moore
700 S Telephone Rd, Ste 100
Moore, OK 73160-2549
(405)307-2605
FAX: (405)307-2625

Muskogee

Genesiscare USA Landmark, Llc
301 N 32nd St
Muskogee, OK 74401-2106
(918)683-2000
FAX: (918)686-0554

Saint Francis Hospital Muskogee Breast Care Center
101 Rockefeller Dr, Ste 101
Muskogee, OK 74401-5050
(918)684-5684
FAX: (918)684-2751

Three Rivers Health Center
1001 S 41st St E
Muskogee, OK 74403-6253
(918)781-6595
FAX: (918)682-1671

Mustang

Ssm Health St. Anthony Healthplex
201 S Sara Rd
Mustang, OK 73064-4306
(405)272-4226
FAX: (405)272-8407

Norman

Little Axe Health Center
15951 Little Axe Dr
Norman, OK 73026-9088
(405)447-0300
FAX: (405)701-7614

Norman Regional Breast Care Center
3440 Rc Luttrell Dr
Norman, OK 73072-9006
(405)307-2290
FAX: (405)307-2625

Okemah

Muscogee Creek Nation Community Hospital
1800 E Coplin St
Okemah, OK 74859-4642
(918)623-1424
FAX: (918)623-1896

Oklahoma City

Community Hospital North
9800 Broadway Ext
Oklahoma City, OK 73114-6303
(405)419-2988
FAX: (405)419-5925

Funnell & Strebel Inc.
4200 W Memorial Rd Ste 201
Oklahoma City, OK 73120-8305
(405)749-4200
FAX: (405)749-4218

Hospital For Special Surgery, Llc Dba Onecore-Cdi Location
5800 N Portland Ave
Oklahoma City, OK 73112-1661
(405)601-4500
FAX: (405)601-4525

Integris Comprehensive Breast Center
3525 NW 56th St Ste 100C
Oklahoma City, OK 73112-4549
(405)945-0512
FAX: (405)945-2254

Integris Southwest Breast Health & Imaging Center
4221 S Western Ave Ste 1000
Oklahoma City, OK 73109-3445
(405)636-7481
FAX: (405)644-6368

Lakeside Women's Hospital
10900 Hefner Pointe Dr, Ste 501
Oklahoma City, OK 73120-5080
(405)951-2603
FAX: (405)418-0310

Mercy Breast Center
4401 McAuley Blvd, Ste 1100
Oklahoma City, OK 73120-8533
(405)752-3500
FAX: (405)936-5217

Mercy Hospital Oklahoma City— South
5200 E-240 Service Rd.
Oklahoma City, OK 73135
(405)752-3500
FAX: (405)936-5217

Oklahoma City Indian Clinic
4913 W Reno Ave
Oklahoma City, OK 73127-6339
(405)948-4900
FAX: (405)348-0837

Ou Breast Health Network, Mobile 2
13401 N Macarthur Blvd
Oklahoma City, OK 73142-9109
(405)755-2273
FAX: (405)603-4103

Ou Breast Health Network, Northwest
13401 N Macarthur Blvd
Oklahoma City, OK 73142-9109
(405)755-2273
FAX: (405)603-4103

Ou Breast Health Network, Southwest
2607 SW 119th St
Oklahoma City, OK 73170-2637
(405)814-2273
FAX: (405)814-1010

Ou Breast Health Network- Mobile 1
13401 N Macarthur Blvd
Oklahoma City, OK 73142-9109
(405)755-2273
FAX: (405)603-4103

Ou Breast Institute
825 NE 10th St Ste 3E, Ou Physicians Building
Oklahoma City, OK 73104-5417
(405)271-4514
FAX: (405)271-3495

Ssm Health St Anthony Healthplex
13500 S Tulsa Dr
Oklahoma City, OK 73170-9719
(405)272-4226
FAX: (405)272-8407

Ssm Health St. Anthony Healthplex
3400 S Douglas Blvd
Oklahoma City, OK 73150-1001
(405)272-4226
FAX: (405)272-8407

Ssm Health St. Anthony Healthplex
13401 N Western Ave
Oklahoma City, OK 73114-1408
(405)272-4226
FAX: (405)272-8407

Ssm Health St. Anthony Hospital Oklahoma City
535 NW 9th St Ste 100
Oklahoma City, OK 73102-1071
(405)272-4226
FAX: (405)272-8407

Okmulgee

Muscogee Creek Nation Medical Center
1401 Morris Dr
Okmulgee, OK 74447-6429
(918)756-4500
FAX: (918)758-3037

Owasso

Bailey Medical Center
10502 N 110th East Ave, Ste 320
Owasso, OK 74055-6660
(918)376-8040
FAX: (918)550-6511

St. John Owasso
12451 E 100th St N
Owasso, OK 74055-4600
(918)274-5020
FAX: (918)274-5019

Pawhuska

Wahzhazhi Health Center
715 Grandview Ave
Pawhuska, OK 74056-3201
(918)287-9325
FAX: (918)287-6138

Pawnee

Pawnee Indian Health Center
1201 Heritage Cir
Pawnee, OK 74058-3744
(918)762-6685
FAX: (918)762-6687

Perry

Stillwater Medical - Perry
501 N 14th St
Perry, OK 73077-5021
(580)710-3166
FAX: (580)336-7222

Ponca City

Alliancehealth Ponca City
1908 N 14th St
Ponca City, OK 74601-2014
(580)765-0499
FAX: (580)765-0584

Poteau

Choctaw Nation Poteau Clinic
109 Kerr Ave
Poteau, OK 74953-5270
(918)649-1148
FAX: (918)649-1147

Eastern Oklahoma Medical Center
105 Wall St
Poteau, OK 74953-4433
(918)635-3590
FAX: (918)635-3231

Pryor

Ahs Pryor Hospital,Llc Dba Hillcrest Hospital Pryor
111 N Bailey St
Pryor, OK 74361-4201
(918)824-6450
FAX: (918)824-6333

Purcell

Chickasaw Nation Purcell Health Clinic
1438 Hardcastle Blvd
Purcell, OK 73080-8233
(405)527-4700
FAX: (405)767-8939

Salina

Cherokee Nation Amo Salina Health Center
900 N Owen Walters Blvd
Salina, OK 74365-5003
(918)434-8514
FAX: (918)434-1908

Sallisaw

Cherokee Nation Redbird Smith Health Center
301 S J T Stites St
Sallisaw, OK 74955-9302
(918)774-1420
FAX: (918)774-1451

Sequoyah County-City Of Sallisaw Hospital Authority
213 E Redwood Ave
Sallisaw, OK 74955-2811
(918)774-1100
FAX: (918)774-1142

Sapulpa

Ascension St John Sapulpa
1004 E Bryan Ave
Sapulpa, OK 74066-4513
(918)224-4280
FAX: (918)227-3906

Shattuck

Newman Memorial Hospital
905 S Main St
Shattuck, OK 73858-9208
(580)938-2551
FAX: (580)938-2928

Shawnee

Citizen Potawatomi Nation Health Services
781 Grand Casino Blvd
Shawnee, OK 74804-1005
(405)695-6003
FAX: (405)695-6030

Ssm Health Breast Care
3200 Medical Park Dr
Shawnee, OK 74804-5014
(405)395-5718
FAX: (405)395-5713

Ssm Health Medical Group Harrison - Shawnee
4651 N. Harrison Ave.
Shawnee, OK 74804
(405)395-5657
FAX: (405)395-5656

Spencer

Community Health Centers Of Oklahoma-Mary Mahoney Memorial
12716 NE 36th St
Spencer, OK 73084-9167
(405)769-3301
FAX: (405)769-3159

Stillwater

Women First Digital Breast Imaging
1411 W 7th Ave Ste C
Stillwater, OK 74074-4300
(405)742-5622
FAX: (405)742-5746

Stilwell

Adair County Health Center, Inc. Dba Physicians Clinic
1401 W Locust St Ste 102
Stilwell, OK 74960-3276
(918)696-4065
FAX: (918)696-3808

Wilma P. Mankiller Health Center
471688 Highway 51
Stilwell, OK 74960-4490
(918)696-8834
FAX: (918)696-8897

Tahlequah

Cherokee Nation Outpatient Health Center
19600 E Ross St
Tahlequah, OK 74464-0545
(539)234-1616
FAX: (539)234-1601

Northeastern Health Systems
1400 E Downing St
Tahlequah, OK 74464-3324
(918)458-2425
FAX: (918)458-2428

Talihina

Choctaw Nation Health Care Center - Radiology
1 Choctaw Way
Talihina, OK 74571-2022
(918)567-7000
FAX: (918)567-7043

Tishomingo

The Chickasaw Nation Tishomingo Health Clinic
817 E 6th St
Tishomingo, OK 73460-1800
(580)371-2392
FAX: (580)387-2727

Tulsa

Ascension St John Outpatient Radiology
8131 S Memorial Dr Ste 105
Tulsa, OK 74133-4348
(918)856-5789
FAX: (918)250-6448

Hillcrest Hospital South
8801 S 101st East Ave
Tulsa, OK 74133-5707
(918)294-4700
FAX: (918)294-4710

Hillcrest South Diagnostic Center
9001 S 101st East Ave
Tulsa, OK 74133-5708
(918)294-4700
FAX: (918)294-4710

Indian Health Care Resource Center Of Tulsa
550 S Peoria Ave
Tulsa, OK 74120-3820
(918)382-1283
FAX: (918)949-9487

Leta M. Chapman Breast Health Center
1120 S Utica Ave
Tulsa, OK 74104-4012
(918)579-8080
FAX: (918)579-8095

Morton Comprehensive Health Center
1334 N Lansing Ave
Tulsa, OK 74106-5907
(918)295-6137
FAX: (918)295-6190

Oklahoma State University Medical Center
744 W 9th St
Tulsa, OK 74127-9907
(918)599-4064
FAX: (918)599-1022

Oklahoma State University Outpatient Imaging
2345 Southwest Blvd Ste 100, Mammography Dept.
Tulsa, OK 74107-2705
(918)561-8577
FAX: (918)561-8574

Saint Francis Breast Health Services
6475 S Yale Ave Ste 410
Tulsa, OK 74136-7817
(918)494-9270
FAX: (918)494-9330

St. John Breast Center
1923 S Utica Ave, 8th Floor Siegfried Tower
Tulsa, OK 74104-6502
(918)744-3600
FAX: (918)744-3151

Vinita

Cherokee Nation Vinita Health Center
27371 S 4410 Rd
Vinita, OK 74301-7953
(918)256-4858
FAX: (918)256-9039

Saint Francis Hospital Vinita
735 N Foreman St
Vinita, OK 74301-1422
(918)256-0391
FAX: (918)256-8784

Wagoner

Wagoner Community Hospital
1200 W Cherokee St
Wagoner, OK 74467-4681
(918)485-1344
FAX: (918)485-1520

Weatherford

Weatherford Regional Hospital
3701 E Main St
Weatherford, OK 73096-3309
(580)772-5551
FAX: (580)774-4776

Wewoka

Wewoka Indian Health Clinic
PO Box 1475, 36640 Hwy 270 And Barking Water Rd
Wewoka, OK 74884-1475
(405)257-7509
FAX: (405)257-7529

Woodward

Alliance Health Woodward
900 17th St
Woodward, OK 73801-2448
(580)254-8402
FAX: (580)571-8056

Yukon

Integris Canadian Valley Regional Hospital
1201 Health Center Pkwy
Yukon, OK 73099-6392
(405)717-7812
FAX: (405)717-7992

Total Healthcare Partners
4400 Grant Blvd, Ste 100 Yukon
Yukon, OK 73099-0038
(405)787-8550
FAX: (405)652-0589

OREGON

Albany

Samaritan Valley Imaging Services
400 Hickory St NW
Albany, OR 97321-1700
(541)812-5200
FAX: (541)812-5201

Ashland

Asante Ashland Community Hospital, Llc
280 Maple St
Ashland, OR 97520-1593
(541)201-4380
FAX: (541)488-5385

Astoria

Columbia Memorial Hospital Health & Wellness Pavilion
2265 Exchange St, Radiology Dept.
Astoria, OR 97103-3331
(503)338-4025
FAX: (503)338-4527

Baker City

St Alphonsus Medical Center - Baker City
3325 Pocahontas Rd
Baker City, OR 97814-1464
(541)524-7812
FAX: (541)524-7929

Bandon

Southern Coos Hospital And Health Center
900 11th St SE
Bandon, OR 97411-9114
(541)329-1034
FAX: (541)347-0502

Beaverton

Beaverton Medical Office - Mammography
4855 SW Western Ave
Beaverton, OR 97005-3499
(503)571-5645
FAX: (503)571-8469

Epic Imaging, P.C.
8950 SW Nimbus Ave, Ste 100
Beaverton, OR 97008-7479
(503)253-1105
FAX: (503)535-8398

Epic Imaging, P.C. Bethany
1500 NW Bethany Blvd Ste 100
Beaverton, OR 97006-5233
(503)253-1105
FAX: (503)535-7080

Legacy Imaging Services At Cedar Hills
2725 SW Cedar Hills Blvd Ste 255
Beaverton, OR 97005-1469
(503)415-4150
FAX: (503)415-4151

The Portland Clinic - Beaverton
15950 SW Millikan Way
Beaverton, OR 97003-5170
(503)221-0161
FAX: (503)790-1053

Bend

Cascade Medical Imaging
1460 NE Medical Center Dr
Bend, OR 97701-6061
(541)382-9383
FAX: (541)382-6635

Cascade Medical Imaging - Southside
61270 SE Coombs Pl Ste 100
Bend, OR 97702-3739
(541)382-9383
FAX: (541)317-9348

Summit Medical Group Oregon/Bend Memorial Clinic
1501 NE Medical Center Dr
Bend, OR 97701-6051
(541)706-5329
FAX: (541)706-6489

Brookings

Curry Medical Center
500 5th St
Brookings, OR 97415-9702
(541)412-2050
FAX: (541)412-2084

Sutter Imaging At Brookings Harbor
555 5th St
Brookings, OR 97415-9730
(707)464-8966
FAX: (707)464-8967

Burns

Harney District Hospital
557 W Washington St
Burns, OR 97720-1497
(541)573-8359
FAX: (541)573-4186

Canby

Providence Canby Health Center
200 S Hazel Dell Way
Canby, OR 97013-7829
(503)650-6300
FAX: (503)650-6277

Clackamas

Epic Imaging P.C.
10121 SE Sunnyside Rd
Clackamas, OR 97015-5745
(503)253-1105
FAX: (503)372-1861

Kaiser Sunnyside Medical Center
10180 SE Sunnyside Rd
Clackamas, OR 97015-9303
(503)571-5645
FAX: (503)571-8469

Mt. Talbert
10100 SE Sunnyside Rd
Clackamas, OR 97015-8970
(503)571-5645
FAX: (503)571-8469

Coos Bay

Bay Area Hospital
1775 Thompson Rd
Coos Bay, OR 97420-2198
(541)269-8090
FAX: (541)269-8571

Bay Area Hospital Women's Imaging Ctr
2650 N 17th St
Coos Bay, OR 97420-2134
(541)269-8090
FAX: (541)269-8571

Coquille

Coquille Valley Hospital
940 E 5th St
Coquille, OR 97423-1699
(541)396-1056
FAX: (541)396-6942

Corvallis

Samaritan Corvallis Mammography
3615 NW Samaritan Dr Ste 102
Corvallis, OR 97330-3756
(541)768-5060
FAX: (541)768-5164

Cottage Grove

Peacehealth Cottage Grove Community Medical Center
1515 Village Dr
Cottage Grove, OR 97424-9700
(541)767-5332
FAX: (541)767-5245

Dallas

West Valley Hospital
525 SE Washington St
Dallas, OR 97338-2834
(503)917-2079
FAX: (503)917-2019

Enterprise

Wallowa Memorial Hospital
601 Medical Pkwy
Enterprise, OR 97828-5124
(541)426-5316
FAX: (541)426-1900

Eugene

Center For Womens Health
330 S Garden Way Ste 220
Eugene, OR 97401-8178
(541)242-4162
FAX: (541)345-2358

Kaiser Eugene Medical Office
360 S Garden Way
Eugene, OR 97401-8173
(503)571-5645
FAX: (503)571-8469

Oregon Imaging Centers
1200 Hilyard St Ste S330
Eugene, OR 97401-8133
(541)687-7134
FAX: (541)334-7564

The Cedar Clinic
600 Country Club Rd
Eugene, OR 97401-2240
(541)242-4162
FAX: (541)345-2358

Willamette Valley Mammography
2401 River Rd, Ste 4
Eugene, OR 97404-5412
(541)726-4694
FAX: (541)744-6069

Women's Care Imaging
590 Country Club Pkwy, Ste C
Eugene, OR 97401-6025
(541)686-2922
FAX: (541)683-1709

Florence

Peace Harbor Medical Center
400 9th St
Florence, OR 97439-7398
(541)997-2804
FAX: (541)997-1493

Gold Beach

Curry General Hospital
94220 4th St
Gold Beach, OR 97444-7772
(541)247-3970
FAX: (541)247-2435

Grants Pass

Asante Women's Imaging Asante Three Rivers Medical Ctr. Llc
1075 SW Grandview Ave Suite 100
Grants Pass, OR 97527
(541)955-5446
FAX: (541)955-5439

Gresham

Breast Health And Outpatient Imaging Center-Mount Hood
24988 SE Stark St Ste 100
Gresham, OR 97030-8323
(503)674-1233
FAX: (503)674-1860

Gresham Imaging Center
831 NW Council Dr, Ste 100
Gresham, OR 97030-3722
(503)251-6137
FAX: (503)489-2626

Hermiston

Good Shepherd Medical Center
610 NW 11th St
Hermiston, OR 97838-6601
(541)667-3520
FAX: (541)667-3519

Hillsboro

Center For Medical Imaging, Llc - Tanasbourne
180810 NE Cornell Rd Ste 100, Tanasbourne Medical Plaza
Hillsboro, OR 97124
(503)216-8403
FAX: (503)216-8410

Kaiser Westside Medical Center
2875 NW Stucki Ave.
Hillsboro, OR 97124
(503)571-5645
FAX: (503)571-8469

Tuality Healthcare
333 SE 7th Ave Ste 3200
Hillsboro, OR 97123-5193
(503)681-4015
FAX: (503)681-4023

Hood River

Providence Hood River Memorial Hospital
810 12th St
Hood River, OR 97031-1587
(541)387-8218
FAX: (541)387-6410

John Day

Blue Mountain Hospital
170 Ford Rd
John Day, OR 97845-2009
(541)575-4163
FAX: (541)575-3818

Klamath Falls

Sage Women's Imaging And Specialty Ultrasound
404 S 4th St
Klamath Falls, OR 97601-6168
(541)851-9395
FAX: (541)851-9399

Sky Lakes Outpatient Imaging
2900 Daggett Ave
Klamath Falls, OR 97601-7101
(541)274-3380
FAX: (541)274-6276

La Grande

Grande Ronde Hospital
900 Sunset Dr
La Grande, OR 97850-1387
(541)963-8421
FAX: (541)962-2561

Grande Ronde Hospital Regional Medical Plaza
710 Sunset Dr Ste E
La Grande, OR 97850-1200
(541)963-1452
FAX: (541)962-2561

Lake Oswego

Womens Imaging And Intervention Llc
17050 Pilkington Rd Ste 130
Lake Oswego, OR 97035-6308
(503)305-5432
FAX: (503)305-7294

Lakeview

Lake District Hospital
700 S J St
Lakeview, OR 97630-1623
(541)947-2114
FAX: (541)947-5575

Lebanon

Samaritan Lebanon Community Hospital
525 N Santiam Hwy
Lebanon, OR 97355-4363
(541)451-7191
FAX: (541)451-7105

Lincoln City

Samaritan North Lincoln Hospital
3043 NE 28th St
Lincoln City, OR 97367-4518
(541)996-7145
FAX: (541)996-7308

Madras

Cascade Medical Imaging Madras
470 NE A St
Madras, OR 97741-1844
(541)382-9382
FAX: (541)317-9348

McMinnville

Willamette Valley Medical Center
2700 SE Stratus Ave
McMinnville, OR 97128-6239
(503)435-6380
FAX: (503)435-4532

Medford

Asante Imaging
692 Murphy Rd
Medford, OR 97504-8310
(541)789-6150
FAX: (541)789-6152

Leila J. Eisenstein Breast Ctr. At Providence Medford Med
1698 E McAndrews Rd Ste 180
Medford, OR 97504-5590
(541)732-5082
FAX: (541)732-6120

Milwaukie

Providence Milwaukie Hospital
10150 SE 32nd Ave
Milwaukie, OR 97222-6516
(503)513-8350
FAX: (503)513-8309

Newberg

Providence Newberg Medical Center
1001 N Providence Dr
Newberg, OR 97132-7485
(503)537-1780
FAX: (503)537-5806

Newport

Samaritan Pacific Communities Hospital
930 SW Abbey St, Radiology Department
Newport, OR 97365-4820
(541)574-4710
FAX: (541)812-2083

Ontario

Saint Alphonsus Med Ctr Ontario
351 SW 9th St
Ontario, OR 97914-2639
(541)881-7474
FAX: (541)881-7039

Oregon City

Providence Willamette Falls Medical Center
1500 Division St, Diagnostic Imaging Department
Oregon City, OR 97045-1527
(503)650-6300
FAX: (503)650-6277

Women's Healthcare Associates, Llc
1508 Division St Ste 205
Oregon City, OR 97045-1585
(503)657-1071
FAX: (503)657-3321

Pendleton

Chi St. Anthony Hospital
2801 St Anthony Way
Pendleton, OR 97801-3800
(541)278-3228
FAX: (541)278-3219

Portland

Adventist Health Adventist Medical Center
10201 SE Main St Ste 24
Portland, OR 97216-2937
(503)251-6137
FAX: (503)261-6709

Broadway Medical Clinic
4212 NE Broadway
Portland, OR 97213-1422
(503)331-7646
FAX: (503)382-7703

Emanuel Outpatient Diagnostic Center
2801 N Gantenbein Ave
Portland, OR 97227-1674
(503)413-4517
FAX: (503)413-4402

Epic Imaging, P.C.
233 NE 102nd Ave
Portland, OR 97220-4106
(503)253-7080
FAX: (503)372-1861

Kaiser Interstate South Medical Office
3500 N Interstate Ave
Portland, OR 97227-1196
(503)571-5645
FAX: (503)571-8469

Kaiser Permanente Gateway Medical Office
1700 NE 102nd Ave
Portland, OR 97220-3804
(503)571-5645
FAX: (503)571-8469

Kaiser Rockwood Medical Office
19500 SE Stark St
Portland, OR 97233-5792
(503)571-5645
FAX: (503)571-8469

Legacy Good Samaritan Breast Health Center
1040 NW 22nd Ave Ste LL
Portland, OR 97210-3057
(503)413-8114
FAX: (503)413-8211

Northwest Gynecology Pk
9701 SW Barnes Rd Ste 150
Portland, OR 97225-6689
(503)296-7406
FAX: (503)416-2270

Northwest Gynecology-Lloyd District
700 NE Multnomah St Ste 1600
Portland, OR 97232-4111
(503)855-1492
FAX: (503)296-7406

Ohsu Center For Health & Healing Ll
3485 S Bond Ave
Portland, OR 97239-4503
(503)494-4673
FAX: (503)418-8980

Oregon Health And Science University
808 SW Campus Dr
Portland, OR 97239-3008
(503)494-4673
FAX: (503)418-8980

Providence Southeast Diagnostic Imaging
10538 SE Washington St
Portland, OR 97216-2809
(503)215-8900
FAX: (503)215-8930

Providence St.Vincent Medical Center
9205 SW Barnes Rd
Portland, OR 97225-6603
(503)216-4808
FAX: (503)216-4905

Safeway Foundation Breast Ctr, Providence Portland Med. Ctr
4805 NE Glisan St
Portland, OR 97213-2933
(503)215-6079
FAX: (503)215-6985

The Portland Clinic
800 SW 13th Ave
Portland, OR 97205-1999
(503)221-0161
FAX: (503)790-1053

Prineville

Cascade Medical Imaging Prineville
384 SE Combs Flat Rd
Prineville, OR 97754-2562
(541)382-9383
FAX: (541)382-6635

Redmond

Cascade Medical Imaging Redmond South
1523 NW Canal Blvd Ste 100
Redmond, OR 97756-1340
(541)382-9383
FAX: (541)317-9348

Cascade Medical Imaging, Llc
1531 NW Canal Blvd
Redmond, OR 97756-1341
(541)382-9383
FAX: (541)317-9348

Reedsport

Lower Umpqua Hospital
600 Ranch Rd
Reedsport, OR 97467-1795
(541)271-6326
FAX: (541)271-6358

Roseburg

Mercy Outpatient Imaging
1813 W Harvard Ave Ste 411
Roseburg, OR 97471-2752
(541)677-4418
FAX: (541)677-4518

Salem

Kaiser Skyline Medical Center
5125 Skyline Rd S
Salem, OR 97306-9427
(503)571-5645
FAX: (503)571-8469

North Lancaster Medical Office
2400 Lancaster Dr NE
Salem, OR 97305-1221
(503)571-5645
FAX: (503)571-8595

Salem Clinic, P.C.
2020 Capitol St NE
Salem, OR 97301-0698
(503)399-2484
FAX: (503)375-7541

Salem Hospital Women's Imaging
890 Oak St SE
Salem, OR 97301-3905
(503)814-1216
FAX: (503)814-1064

Salem Radiology Consultants, P.C.
2925 Ryan Dr SE
Salem, OR 97301-9687
(503)399-1262
FAX: (503)576-5906

Scappoose

Ohsu Family Medicine Scappoose
51377 SW Old Portland Rd
Scappoose, OR 97056-4023
(503)494-4673
FAX: (503)418-8980

Seaside

Providence Seaside Hospital
725 S Wahanna Rd
Seaside, OR 97138-7735
(503)717-7242
FAX: (503)717-7580

Silverton

Legacy Silverton Medical Center
342 Fairview St
Silverton, OR 97381-1917
(503)873-1750
FAX: (503)873-1734

Springfield

McKenzie Medical Imaging
960 16th St Ste 10
Springfield, OR 97477-4185
(541)726-4694
FAX: (541)744-6069

Oregon Imaging Center
3377 Riverbend Dr Ste 150
Springfield, OR 97477-8805
(541)334-7555
FAX: (541)687-7135

St Helens

Legacy Imaging Services At St. Helens
475 S Columbia River Hwy Ste 110
St Helens, OR 97051-2860
(503)397-1192
FAX: (503)366-3017

Stayton

Santiam Hospital
1401 N 10th Ave, Imaging Department
Stayton, OR 97383-1311
(503)769-9211
FAX: (503)769-1375

The Dalles

Mid-Columbia Medical Center - Mammography Services
1700 E 19th St
The Dalles, OR 97058-3398
(541)298-4000
FAX: (541)296-7622

Tigard

Center For Medical Imaging - Bridgeport
18040 SW Lower Boones Ferry Rd Ste 106
Tigard, OR 97224-7259
(503)216-0665
FAX: (503)216-0670

The Portland Clinic Tmc
9250 SW Hall Blvd
Tigard, OR 97223-6721
(503)221-0161
FAX: (503)790-1053

Tillamook

Adventist Health Tillamook
1000 3rd St
Tillamook, OR 97141-3430
(503)815-2292
FAX: (503)842-3062

Tualatin

Kaiser Tualatin Medical Office
19185 SW 90th Ave
Tualatin, OR 97062-7558
(503)571-5645
FAX: (503)571-8595

Legacy Meridian Park Medical Center
19300 SW 65th Ave
Tualatin, OR 97062-7706
(503)413-7800
FAX: (503)692-7720

Northwest Gynecology Tualatin
19250 SW 65th Ave Ste 325
Tualatin, OR 97062-7452
(503)855-1492
FAX: (503)734-3597

Woodburn

Legacy Woodburn Diagnostic Imaging
693 Glatt Cir Ste 1, Woodburn Diagnostic Imaging
Woodburn, OR 97071-9600
(503)982-4863
FAX: (503)982-4895

Woodburn Clinic
105 Arney Rd, Ste 130
Woodburn, OR 97071-9472
(503)902-3900
FAX: (503)902-3309

PENNSYLVANIA

Abington

Abington Memorial Hospital
1200 Old York Rd, Department Of Radiology
Abington, PA 19001-3788
(215)481-3926
FAX: (215)481-2183

Aliquippa

Heritage Valley Health System Women's Health Center
200 Pleasant Dr
Aliquippa, PA 15001-1321
(866)901-6266
FAX: (724)770-7929

Allentown

Breast Health Services
1240 S Cedar Crest Blvd Ste 203
Allentown, PA 18103-6218
(610)402-0691
FAX: (610)402-0695

Breast Health Services Mobile Mammography
1200 S Cedar Crest Blvd
Allentown, PA 18103-6202
(610)402-5846
FAX: (610)402-0695

Breast Health Services Seventeenth
1627 Chew St 1st Fl
Allentown, PA 18102-3648
(610)402-2791
FAX: (610)402-0695

Coordinated Health Lehigh Valleyhealth Network
1405 N Cedar Crest Blvd
Allentown, PA 18104-2308
(610)366-0444
FAX: (610)366-7988

Lanshe Breast Center
451 Chew St, Ste 210
Allentown, PA 18102-3414
(484)526-1000
FAX: (610)776-4711

Schuylkill Open Mri, Inc Dba Allentown Diagnostic Imaging
7450 Tilghman St, Ste 125
Allentown, PA 18106-9034
(610)774-0170
FAX: (610)774-0173

St. Luke's West End Womens Imaging Center
501 Cetronia Rd, Ste 130
Allentown, PA 18104-9569
(484)526-1000
FAX: (484)426-2572

Allison Park

Upmc Magee Womens Imaging Hampton
4490 Mount Royal Blvd Ste 3100
Allison Park, PA 15101-2685
(800)649-4077
FAX: (412)641-3390

Altoona

Upmc Altoona
1516 9th Ave
Altoona, PA 16602-2417
(814)889-4222
FAX: (814)889-3897

Annville

Upmc Pinnacle Lebanon Valley
1251 E Main St
Annville, PA 17003-1643
(717)230-3700
FAX: (717)724-6721

Bath

Health Center At Bath Breast Health Services
6649 Chrisphalt Dr, Ste 104
Bath, PA 18014-8500
(610)402-2791
FAX: (610)402-0695

Beaver Falls

Heritage Valley Diagnostic Center - Chippewa
2580 Constitution Blvd
Beaver Falls, PA 15010-1294
(866)901-6266
FAX: (724)770-7929

Bensalem

Holy Redeemer Healthcare At Bensalem
3300 Tillman Dr, 1st Fl
Bensalem, PA 19020-2071
(215)938-5700
FAX: (215)245-4140

Berwick

Berwick Hospital
701 E 16th St
Berwick, PA 18603-2397
(570)759-5131
FAX: (570)759-5170

Berwyn

Penn Medicine At Valley Forge
1001 Chesterbrook Blvd Ste 100
Berwyn, PA 19312-3800
(610)579-7550
FAX: (610)576-7551

Bethel Park

Jefferson Regional Medical Center
1010 Higbee Dr
Bethel Park, PA 15102-2806
(412)854-7100
FAX: (412)854-7120

Magee Womens Imaging-South
1300 Oxford Dr Ste 2100
Bethel Park, PA 15102-1896
(800)649-4077
FAX: (412)833-9152

St. Clair Memorial Hospital Breast Care Center
2000 Oxford Dr Ste 301
Bethel Park, PA 15102-1841
(412)942-8150
FAX: (412)942-7817

Bethlehem

Breast Health Services Bethlehem Township
2101 Emrick Blvd, Ste 101
Bethlehem, PA 18020-8040
(610)402-2791
FAX: (610)402-0695

Breast Health Services Muhlenberg
2597 Schoenersville Rd, Ste 202
Bethlehem, PA 18017-7330
(610)402-2791
FAX: (484)884-2949

Coordinated Health Lehigh Valleyhealth Network
2300 Highland Ave
Bethlehem, PA 18020-8920
(610)861-8080
FAX: (610)997-7173

Radiology And Mri Of Bethlehem
5325 Northgate Dr Ste 100
Bethlehem, PA 18017-9412
(610)691-8931
FAX: (610)691-8947

St. Luke's Hospital - North Breast Imaging Center
153 Brodhead Rd
Bethlehem, PA 18017-8931
(484)526-1000
FAX: (484)526-3297

Blairsville

Indiana At Chestnut Ridge
25 Colony Blvd, Ste 112
Blairsville, PA 15717-7971
(724)357-7075
FAX: (724)349-2407

Blandon

St. Joseph Health Network At Maidencreek
108 Plaza Dr Ste 101
Blandon, PA 19510-9476
(610)378-2100
FAX: (610)898-5969

Bloomsburg

Geisinger Bloomsburg Hospital
549 Fair St
Bloomsburg, PA 17815-1498
(570)387-2126
FAX: (570)387-2267

Susquehanna Valley Diagnostic Imaging Inc.
6850 Lowe Rd Ste 317
Bloomsburg, PA 17815-8708
(570)784-6243
FAX: (570)784-6242

Blue Bell

Abington Health Center At Blue Bell
721 Arbor Way
Blue Bell, PA 19422-1974
(215)481-3926
FAX: (215)481-5416

Chestnut Hill Hlth Sys. Women's Ctr At Blue Bell
1777 Sentry Pkwy W Ste 120
Blue Bell, PA 19422-2211
(215)248-8400
FAX: (215)646-7338

Solis Mammography Blue Bell Einstein Healthcare Network
676 Dekalb Pike Ste 200
Blue Bell, PA 19422-1223
(866)257-6884
FAX: (267)460-5353

Boyertown

Boyertown Imaging Pottstown Hospital
23 N Walnut St
Boyertown, PA 19512-1736
(610)367-8844
FAX: (610)367-1512

Bradford

Bradford Regional Medical Center
116 Interstate Pkwy
Bradford, PA 16701-1036
(814)362-8213
FAX: (814)362-8528

Bristol

Prime Health Care Services-Lower Bucks Hospital
501 Bath Rd
Bristol, PA 19007-3101
(215)785-9343
FAX: (215)785-9102

Brookville

Penn Highlands Brookville
100 Hospital Rd
Brookville, PA 15825-1367
(814)849-1870
FAX: (814)849-1452

Broomall

Broomall Imaging
30 Lawrence Rd
Broomall, PA 19008-3301
(484)446-3624
FAX: (484)446-3629

Main Line Health Radiology - Breast Diagnostic Center
1991 Sproul Rd Ste 400
Broomall, PA 19008-3517
(484)580-1800
FAX: (610)325-1449

Bryn Mawr

Barbara Brodsky Comprehensive Breast Ctr At Bryn Mawr Hosp.
101 S Bryn Mawr Ave, Susquehanna Bank Bldg - 1st Flr
Bryn Mawr, PA 19010-3120
(484)337-4400
FAX: (484)337-8709

Butler

Women's Imaging Center
129 Oneida Valley Rd Ste 210, Butler Health System-Crossroads Campus
Butler, PA 16001-2252
(724)284-4000
FAX: (724)477-3799

Camp Hill

Penn State Health Camp Hill Outpatient Center
875 Poplar Church Rd Ste 100, Imaging Services
Camp Hill, PA 17011-2203
(717)763-4900
FAX: (717)972-4601

Penn State Medical Group Camp Hill
3025 Market St
Camp Hill, PA 17011-4518
(717)531-3799
FAX: (717)531-0251

Upmc Imaging Camp Hill
240 Grandview Ave
Camp Hill, PA 17011-1706
(717)230-3700
FAX: (717)703-1111

Canonsburg

Canonsburg Hospital
L00 Medical Boulevard
Canonsburg, PA 15317
(724)873-5895
FAX: (724)746-6461

Carlisle

Dunham U.S. Army Health Clinic
450 Gibner Rd Ste 1, Carlisle Barracks
Carlisle, PA 17013-5086
(717)245-4799
FAX: (717)245-4988

Penn State Health Carlisle Outpatient Center
1211 Forge Rd
Carlisle, PA 17013-3183
(717)972-4900
FAX: (717)218-3901

Upmc Carlisle
361 Alexander Spring Rd
Carlisle, PA 17015-6940
(717)245-5244
FAX: (717)960-3571

Upmc Pinnacle Walnut Bottom
850 Walnut Bottom Rd
Carlisle, PA 17013-3615
(717)230-3700
FAX: (717)703-1111

Center Valley

St. Lukes Regional Breast Center
5848 Old Bethlehem Pike, Ste 103
Center Valley, PA 18034-9341
(484)526-1000
FAX: (484)499-1012

Chadds Ford

Christiana Care Imaging Services- Concord
161 Wilmington W Chester Pike
Chadds Ford, PA 19317-9041
(302)562-6451
FAX: (302)562-6451

Chalfont

Grand View Outpatient Center At Chalfont
700 Horizon Dr
Chalfont, PA 18914-3967
(215)453-4100
FAX: (215)453-4024

Chambersburg

Wellspan Rhonda Brake Shreiner Women's Center
12 St Paul Dr
Chambersburg, PA 17201-1035
(717)217-6750
FAX: (717)217-6959

Clairton

Jefferson Regional Medical Center
1200 Brooks Ln Ste G70
Clairton, PA 15025-3757
(412)460-8300
FAX: (412)460-8301

Clarion

Clarion Hospital
1 Hospital Dr
Clarion, PA 16214-8599
(814)226-9500
FAX: (814)226-1252

Clarion Hospital Mammography Services
Cricklewood Ctr
1008 S 5th Ave
Clarion, PA 16214-8676
(814)226-1247
FAX: (814)226-1252

Upmc Northwest Magee Womens Specialty-Clarion
1008 S 5th Ave
Clarion, PA 16214-8676
(814)677-7550
FAX: (814)676-7950

Clearfield

Clearfield Hospital
809 Turnpike Ave
Clearfield, PA 16830-1243
(814)768-2276
FAX: (814)768-2837

Coal Township

Geisinger Shamokin Area Community Hospital
4200 Hospital Rd
Coal Township, PA 17866-9697
(570)644-4341
FAX: (570)644-6179

Coaldale

St. Luke's Miners Memorial Hospital
360 W Ruddle St
Coaldale, PA 18218-1099
(484)526-1000
FAX: (570)645-8381

Coatesville

Brandywine Hospital
201 Reeceville Rd
Coatesville, PA 19320-1536
(610)383-8760
FAX: (610)383-8378

Collegeville

Mainline Health At Collegeville
599 Arcola Rd
Collegeville, PA 19426-3954
(484)565-1800
FAX: (484)565-1490

Columbia

Columbia Health Center-Lancaster General
306 N 7th St
Columbia, PA 17512-2137
(717)544-5941
FAX: (717)684-1539

Connellsville

Highlands Hospital
401 E Murphy Ave
Connellsville, PA 15425-2700
(724)626-2343
FAX: (724)626-2346

Coraopolis

West Hills Open Mri And Imaging Center
890 Beaver Grade Rd
Coraopolis, PA 15108-2653
(412)269-9995
FAX: (412)269-9525

Corry

Corry Memorial Hospital
965 Shamrock Ln
Corry, PA 16407-1196
(814)664-4641
FAX: (814)663-0719

Coudersport

Upmccole
1001 E 2nd St
Coudersport, PA 16915-8161
(814)274-8200
FAX: (814)260-5532

Cranberry Twp

Upmc Magee Womens Imaging Lemieux
8000 Cranberry Springs Dr Ste 100
Cranberry Twp, PA 16066-6687
(800)649-4077
FAX: (724)772-5477

Danville

Geisinger Medical Center
16 Woodbine Ln, Breast Imaging Third Floor
Danville, PA 17821-8029
(570)271-6309
FAX: (570)214-9495

Darby

Mercy Catholic Medical Center - Mercy Fitzgerald Campus
1503 Lansdowne Ave
Darby, PA 19023-1330
(610)237-2525
FAX: (610)237-2550

Dillsburg

Penn State Health Dillsburg Outpatient Center
126 W Church St, Imaging Services
Dillsburg, PA 17019-1280
(717)972-4900
FAX: (717)972-4601

Upmc Pinnacle Dillsburg
1 Trinity Dr E Ste 130
Dillsburg, PA 17019-8522
(717)230-3700
FAX: (717)703-1111

Dover

Dover Diagnostic Center
4020 Carlisle Rd
Dover, PA 17315-3508
(717)851-1901
FAX: (717)851-6499

Downingtown

Akumin Downingtown
150 E Pennsylvania Ave, Ste300
Downingtown, PA 19335-2632
(610)518-6300
FAX: (610)518-0600

Doylestown

Women's Diagnostic Center Of Doylestown Hospital
595 W State St
Doylestown, PA 18901-2554
(215)345-2274
FAX: (215)345-2591

Drexel Hill

Delaware County Memorial Hospital Womens Diagnostic Ctr
501 N Lansdowne Ave
Drexel Hill, PA 19026-1114
(610)284-8985
FAX: (610)394-1854

Dubois

Dubois Regional Medical Center
145 Hospital Ave Ste 115
Dubois, PA 15801-1463
(814)375-4075
FAX: (814)375-3749

Duncannon

Penn State Health Duncannon Outpatient Center
51 Business Campus Way Ste 100
Duncannon, PA 17020-9596
(717)834-8100
FAX: (717)972-4640

Dunmore

Advanced Imaging Specialists
1000 Meade St
Dunmore, PA 18512-3195
(570)504-2500
FAX: (570)504-2599

Lackawanna Mobile X-Ray, Inc. - Mobile
1229 Monroe Ave
Dunmore, PA 18509-2807
(570)344-1112
FAX: (570)344-7807

East Norriton

Jefferson Outpatient Imaging
1 W Germantown Pike
East Norriton, PA 19401-1513
(215)503-4900
FAX: (610)277-9640

Solis Mammography-A Dept Of Einstein Medical Ctr Montgomery
700 W Germantown Pike Fl 2, Suite 200
East Norriton, PA 19403-4273
(484)622-7750
FAX: (484)622-7776

East Stroudsburg

Dsp Health System
230 Independence Rd
East Stroudsburg, PA 18301-9447
(570)420-1955
FAX: (570)420-0707

Lehigh Valley Hospital -Pocono Radiology Services
447 Office Plaza, Bldg. 400, Ste. C, Route 447
East Stroudsburg, PA 18301
(272)762-2616
FAX: (570)420-2522

St. Luke's Pocono Women's Imaging Center
239 E Brown St
East Stroudsburg, PA 18301-3005
(800)801-7745
FAX: (484)503-8751

Easton

Breast Health Services Hecktown Oaks
3794 Hecktown Rd, Ste 230
Easton, PA 18045-2355
(610)402-2791
FAX: (610)402-0695

St Luke's Hospital Anderson Campus
1872 St Lukes Blvd
Easton, PA 18045-5669
(484)526-1000
FAX: (484)503-1351

Ebensburg

Dlp Conemaugh Mem. Med. Ctr Llc Dba Conemaugh Ebensburg
861 Hills Plz
Ebensburg, PA 15931-4211
(814)534-4444
FAX: (814)472-8854

Upmc Ebensburg
152 Zeman Dr
Ebensburg, PA 15931-4130
(814)471-2234
FAX: (814)472-9436

Edwardsville

Wilkes - Barre Hospital, Co Llc
468 Northampton St, Ste 1
Edwardsville, PA 18704-4566
(570)552-1701
FAX: (570)552-4565

Elizabethtown

Lancaster General Norlanco
424 Cloverleaf Rd
Elizabethtown, PA 17022-8833
(717)544-5941
FAX: (717)544-6318

Elkins Park

Solis Mammography At Einstein Medical Center Elkins Park
60 Township Line Rd
Elkins Park, PA 19027-2220
(484)622-7755
FAX: (484)622-7776

Ellwood City

Heritage Valley Ellwood City
271 Route 288, Franklin Plaza Shopping Center
Ellwood City, PA 16117-3055
(866)901-6266
FAX: (724)770-7929

Ephrata

Ephrata Community Hospital
169 Martin Ave
Ephrata, PA 17522-1755
(717)721-5870
FAX: (717)721-5770

Erie

Millcreek Community Hospital Imaging Center
5401 Peach St Ste 3200
Erie, PA 16509-2601
(814)868-7890
FAX: (814)868-2135

Ob/Gyn Associates Of Erie
2315 Myrtle St, Ste 220
Erie, PA 16502-4612
(814)454-8185
FAX: (814)454-3894

Obgyn Associates Of Erie
100 Peach St Ste 300
Erie, PA 16507-1423
(814)459-1851
FAX: (814)452-0026

Saint Vincent East Side Imaging Center
4950 Buffalo Rd, Ste 103
Erie, PA 16510-2304
(814)452-7564
FAX: (814)452-5773

Saint Vincent Imaging Center
4247 W Ridge Rd
Erie, PA 16506-1746
(814)452-5476
FAX: (814)452-7049

St Vincent Hospital-St Vincent Breast Imaging Center
2315 Myrtle St Ste 295
Erie, PA 16502-4609
(814)452-7804
FAX: (814)452-7049

Upmc Hamot Breast Imaging
300 State St, Ste 108
Erie, PA 16507-1427
(814)877-6123
FAX: (814)877-5561

Upmc Hamot Breast Imaging
3406 Peach St
Erie, PA 16508-2740
(814)877-6123
FAX: (814)864-3471

Upmc Hamot Breast Imaging At West Ridge
5050 W Ridge Rd, 3rd Fl
Erie, PA 16506-1216
(814)877-7608
FAX: (814)877-7601

Everett

Upmc Bedford Memorial
10455 Lincoln Hwy
Everett, PA 15537-7046
(814)623-3797
FAX: (814)623-3586

Exton

Chester County Hospital At Exton
700 W Lincoln Hwy
Exton, PA 19341-2547
(610)431-5131
FAX: (610)518-6695

Main Line Health At Exton Square
154 Exton Square Mall
Exton, PA 19341-2440
(484)565-1414
FAX: (484)565-1490

Feasterville

Holy Redeemer Healthcare At Feasterville
23 Bustleton Pike
Feasterville, PA 19053-6446
(215)938-5700
FAX: (215)396-3996

Fleetwood

Breast Health Services Moselem Springs
14351 Kutztown Rd
Fleetwood, PA 19522-9273
(610)402-2791
FAX: (610)402-0695

Franklin

Upmc Northwest Magee Womens Specialty-Franklin
1310 Liberty St
Franklin, PA 16323-1546
(814)432-3163
FAX: (814)676-7950

Gettysburg

Wellspan Adams Health Center
40 V Twin Dr Ste 110
Gettysburg, PA 17325-7878
(717)338-3281
FAX: (717)338-3276

Wellspan Washington Street Health Center
PO Box 3786, 450 S Washington St
Gettysburg, PA 17325-0786
(717)338-3281
FAX: (717)338-3276

Glen Mills

Brinton Lake Imaging
300 Evergreen Dr Ste 210
Glen Mills, PA 19342-1059
(610)579-3500
FAX: (610)579-3501

Mlh Breast Center In Concordville
1020 Baltimore Pike, Ste 100
Glen Mills, PA 19342-1365
(484)227-2828
FAX: (484)227-3791

Greencastle

Wellspan Greencastle Health Center
24 Antrim Commons Dr
Greencastle, PA 17225-1623
(717)267-7149
FAX: (717)765-5083

Greensburg

Ahn Hempfield Imaging
6321 State Route 30, Ste 200
Greensburg, PA 15601-9704
(724)671-1700
FAX: (724)523-7725

Excela Health Westmoreland Hospital
532 W Pittsburgh St, Westmoreland Hospital Breast Center
Greensburg, PA 15601-2282
(724)689-0100
FAX: (724)850-7971

Greenville

Upmc Horizon - Greenville
110 N Main St
Greenville, PA 16125-1726
(724)589-6166
FAX: (724)588-6366

Grove City

Grove City Medical Center
631 N Broad Street Ext
Grove City, PA 16127-4603
(724)450-7420
FAX: (724)450-7430

Hanover

Hillside Medical Center
250 Fame Ave Ste 104
Hanover, PA 17331-1587
(717)316-3500
FAX: (717)316-3550

Upmc Imaging Services At South Hanover
2201 Brunswick Dr, Ste 1100
Hanover, PA 17331-8350
(717)316-3500
FAX: (717)316-3550

Upmc Pinnacle Hanover
300 Highland Ave
Hanover, PA 17331-2297
(717)316-3437
FAX: (717)316-3550

Wellspan Health & Surgery Center
1227 Baltimore St
Hanover, PA 17331-4406
(717)338-3281
FAX: (717)338-3276

Harleysville

Grand View Hospitals Harleysville Outpatient Center
270 Main St
Harleysville, PA 19438-2400
(215)453-4100
FAX: (215)513-1806

Harrisburg

Penn State Health Medical Group Union Deposit Diagnostic Ce
4520 Union Deposit Rd
Harrisburg, PA 17111-2910
(717)484-9095
FAX: (717)484-9096

Penn State Health Progress Outpatient Center
20 Capital Dr
Harrisburg, PA 17110-9446
(717)972-4900
FAX: (717)731-9165

University Physicians Group
121 N Nyes Rd Ste B
Harrisburg, PA 17112-3248
(717)531-4698
FAX: (717)531-0322

Upmc Imaging Linglestown
2808 Old Post Rd, Linglestown Office
Harrisburg, PA 17110-3685
(717)230-3700
FAX: (717)737-4511

Upmc Imaging Union Deposit
4518 Union Deposit Rd
Harrisburg, PA 17111-2921
(717)230-3700
FAX: (717)652-9522

Upmc Pinnacle Community Osteopathic
4300 Londonderry Rd, Ste 203- Msp
Harrisburg, PA 17109-5317
(717)230-3700
FAX: (717)703-1111

Upmc Pinnacle Hamilton Health Center
110 S 17th St
Harrisburg, PA 17104-1123
(717)230-3700
FAX: (717)724-6721

Upmc Pinnacle Harrisburg
111 S Front St
Harrisburg, PA 17101-2010
(717)230-3700
FAX: (717)703-1111

Hastings

Dlp Conemaugh Miners Medical Center, Llc
290 Haida Ave
Hastings, PA 16646-5610
(814)247-3300
FAX: (814)247-3323

Haverford

Regional Women's Health Group, Llc - Haverford
355 W Lancaster Ave Bldg A Ste
Haverford, PA 19041-1547
(610)994-1136
FAX: (215)687-4775

Havertown

Akumin Haverford
600 E Township Line Rd
Havertown, PA 19083-5716
(610)446-1800
FAX: (610)446-3408

Hawley

Pike County Medical Center
750 Route 739
Hawley, PA 18428-6058
(570)775-4278
FAX: (570)775-4279

Hazleton

Imaging Associates Of Hazleton Pc
101 S Church St, Ste A
Hazleton, PA 18201-6279
(570)501-7226
FAX: (570)501-7232

Lehigh Valley Hosp At Health And Wellness Ctr Hazleton
50 Moisey Dr
Hazleton, PA 18202-9297
(570)501-6660
FAX: (570)501-6971

Hermitage

Sharon Regional Health System-Diagnostic & Imaging Center
2435 Garden Way
Hermitage, PA 16148-5211
(724)983-3945
FAX: (724)983-7332

Upmc Horizon Outpatient Center Hermitage
875 N Hermitage Rd
Hermitage, PA 16148-3278
(724)347-4844
FAX: (724)347-4654

Hershey

Penn State Milton S Hershey Medical Center
30 Hope Dr Ste 1800
Hershey, PA 17033-2036
(717)531-3799
FAX: (717)531-0251

Upmc Imaging Hershey
32 Northeast Dr Ste 101
Hershey, PA 17033-2760
(717)230-3700
FAX: (717)534-1307

Homestead

Jefferson Regional Medical Center
495 E Waterfront Dr Ste 100
Homestead, PA 15120-1151
(412)325-0990
FAX: (412)325-0991

Honesdale

Wayne Memorial Hospital
601 Park St, Dept. Of Radiology - Mammography Section
Honesdale, PA 18431-1498
(570)251-6689
FAX: (570)253-7336

Huntingdon

Penn Highlands Huntingdon
1225 Warm Springs Ave
Huntingdon, PA 16652-2350
(814)643-8624
FAX: (814)643-8765

Huntingdon Valley

Holy Redeemer Healthcare At 821
821 Huntingdon Pike Ste 110
Huntingdon Valley, PA 19006-8368
(215)938-5700
FAX: (215)214-0629

Indiana

Indiana Regional Medical Center
835 Hospital Rd, Radiology Department
Indiana, PA 15701-3629
(724)357-7075
FAX: (724)349-2407

Indiana Regional Medical Center-Mobile
835 Hospital Rd
Indiana, PA 15701-3629
(724)357-7075
FAX: (724)349-2407

Jefferson Hills

Jefferson Regional Medical Center
565 Coal Valley Rd
Jefferson Hills, PA 15025-3703
(412)469-5711
FAX: (412)469-7606

Jersey Shore

Geisinger Jersey Shore Hospital
1020 Thompson St, Radiology Department
Jersey Shore, PA 17740-1794
(570)398-5187
FAX: (570)398-4146

Johnstown

Dlp Conemaugh Mem. Med. Ctr Llc Dba Conemaugh Breast Imaging
1111 Franklin St, Ste 40
Johnstown, PA 15905-4330
(814)534-9186
FAX: (814)534-3455

Dlp Conemaugh Mem. Med. Ctr Llc Dba Conemaugh East Hills
1450 Scalp Ave
Johnstown, PA 15904-3321
(814)534-9166
FAX: (814)534-3242

Kane

Upmc Kane
4372 Route 6
Kane, PA 16735-3060
(814)837-4580
FAX: (814)837-4567

Kennett Square

Chester County Hospital Radiology At Kennett Square
402 McFarlan Rd Ste 204
Kennett Square, PA 19348-2453
(610)431-5335
FAX: (610)444-1939

King Of Prussia

Main Line Health King Of Prussia
120 Valley Green Ln
King Of Prussia, PA 19406-2079
(484)580-1309
FAX: (484)324-7691

Solis Mammography Kop-Dept Of Einstein Med Ctr Montgomery
210 Mall Blvd
King Of Prussia, PA 19406-3261
(484)622-7755
FAX: (484)622-7776

Kingston

Vision Imaging Of Kingston, Llc
517 Pierce St, Ste 1
Kingston, PA 18704-5757
(570)714-7226
FAX: (570)714-6288

Kittanning

Armstrong County Memorial Hospital
1 Nolte Dr
Kittanning, PA 16201-7111
(724)543-8131
FAX: (724)543-8652

Armstrong Out Patient Imaging Center
87 Glade Dr
Kittanning, PA 16201-7140
(724)543-8131
FAX: (724)543-8652

Lancaster

Lancaster General Health- Downtown Pavilion
540 N Duke St
Lancaster, PA 17602-2374
(717)544-5941
FAX: (717)544-5904

May-Grant Ob/Gyn
694 Good Dr, Ste 112
Lancaster, PA 17601-2433
(717)677-2417
FAX: (412)643-3851

Penn State Health Medical Group - Lime Spring
2221 Noll Dr, Ste 2000
Lancaster, PA 17603-7614
(717)531-3799
FAX: (717)531-0322

Suzanne H Arnold Center For Breast Health
2104 Harrisburg Pike Ste 100, Lg Health Pavilion
Lancaster, PA 17601-2644
(717)544-5941
FAX: (717)544-0320

Upmc Lititz-Lancaster Breast Imaging
2170 Noll Dr Ste 200
Lancaster, PA 17603-7609
(717)230-3700
FAX: (717)291-2151

Langhorne

Akumin Langhorne
825 Town Center Dr Ste 100
Langhorne, PA 19047-1757
(215)750-1760
FAX: (215)750-1615

Comprehensive Imaging And Diag
540 Woodbourne Rd
Langhorne, PA 19047-1835
(877)244-6266
FAX: (609)303-4134

Jefferson Bucks Hospital
380 N Oxford Valley Rd
Langhorne, PA 19047-8304
(215)612-4936
FAX: (215)612-4400

Regional Womens Health Group Llc - Langhorne
830 Town Center Dr
Langhorne, PA 19047-1748
(215)750-6611
FAX: (267)564-2120

St. Mary Imaging & Breast Ctr
1201 Langhorne Newtown Rd
Langhorne, PA 19047-1201
(215)710-5393
FAX: (215)710-2251

Lansdale

Abington Health Lansdale Hospital
100 Medical Campus Dr
Lansdale, PA 19446-1259
(215)361-4862
FAX: (215)361-4641

Grand View Hospital Outpatient Center At Lansdale
1019 S Broad St
Lansdale, PA 19446-5338
(215)453-4463
FAX: (215)453-4024

Latrobe

Excela Square At Latrobe
100 Excela Health Dr
Latrobe, PA 15650-9001
(724)689-0100
FAX: (724)804-1740

Lebanon

Lancaster General Health Center, Lebanon
1701 Cornwall Rd
Lebanon, PA 17042-7480
(717)675-1809
FAX: (717)675-1812

Wellspan Good Samaritan Hospital
4th And Walnut St.
Lebanon, PA 17042
(717)270-3845
FAX: (717)270-7648

Wellspan Gsh Outpatient Radiology Center
805 Helen Dr
Lebanon, PA 17042-7493
(717)273-9345
FAX: (717)274-7518

Leesport

The Reading Hospital Imaging Center At Leesport
5479 Pottsville Pike
Leesport, PA 19533-8650
(484)628-8611
FAX: (484)628-3111

Lehighton

Breast Health Services Lehighton
1205 Blakeslee Boulevard Dr E
Lehighton, PA 18235-2404
(610)402-0691
FAX: (610)402-0695

St. Luke's Hospital Gnaden Huetten Campus
211 N 12th St
Lehighton, PA 18235-1138
(610)377-7061
FAX: (484)464-4822

Lemoyne

Partners In Womens Healthcare Pc
1 Lemoyne Sq, Ste 102
Lemoyne, PA 17043-1230
(717)737-4511
FAX: (877)502-2231

Upmc Imaging Lemoyne
110 Lowther St
Lemoyne, PA 17043-2012
(717)230-3700
FAX: (717)703-1111

Lewisburg

Susquehanna Valley Imaging- A Service Of Geisinger Med Ctr
120 Hamm Dr
Lewisburg, PA 17837-7496
(570)551-6929
FAX: (570)522-9409

Thyra M Humphreys Center For Breast Health
1 Hospital Dr
Lewisburg, PA 17837-9350
(570)522-4200
FAX: (570)768-3985

Lewistown

Geisinger Clinic Lewistown
21 Geisinger Ln
Lewistown, PA 17044-3400
(717)242-4200
FAX: (717)242-4280

Geisinger-Lewistown Hospital
400 Highland Ave
Lewistown, PA 17044-1198
(717)242-7229
FAX: (717)242-7091

Limerick

Phoenixville Hospital Outpatient Center At Limerick
420 W Linfield Trappe Rd, Diagnostic Imaging
Limerick, PA 19468-4278
(610)495-3803
FAX: (610)495-2399

Regional Women's Health Group, Llc - Limerick
400 Enterprise Dr Ste 104
Limerick, PA 19468-1224
(610)416-7611
FAX: (215)687-4775

Lititz

Kissell Hill Outpatient Center
51 Peters Rd
Lititz, PA 17543-7685
(717)544-5941
FAX: (717)627-7025

Upmc Lititz
1500 Highlands Dr
Lititz, PA 17543-7694
(717)230-3700
FAX: (717)625-5519

Lock Haven

Upmc Lock Haven
24 Cree Dr
Lock Haven, PA 17745-2639
(570)893-5501
FAX: (570)893-5147

Mansfield

Susquehanna Health Imaging At Mansfield
416 S Main St, Ste 3
Mansfield, PA 16933-1510
(570)662-1910
FAX: (570)662-1941

Mc Kees Rocks

Allegheny Imaging Of Robinson
133 Church Hill Rd, Ste 2
Mc Kees Rocks, PA 15136-3279
(412)359-6034
FAX: (412)359-6799

McConnellsburg

Fulton County Medical Center
214 Peach Orchard Rd
McConnellsburg, PA 17233-1399
(717)485-3155
FAX: (717)485-6848

McKees Rocks

Heritage Valley Kennedy
25 Heckel Rd
McKees Rocks, PA 15136-1651
(866)901-6266
FAX: (724)770-7929

McKeesport

Magee-Womens Imaging At Upmc McKeesport
1500 5th Ave, Mammography Center
McKeesport, PA 15132-2422
(412)664-2273
FAX: (412)664-2271

McMurray

St. Clair Hospital Outpatient Center Peters
3928 Washington Rd
McMurray, PA 15317-2592
(412)942-8150
FAX: (412)942-7818

Washington Health System Peters Township
4198 Washington Rd, Suite201
McMurray, PA 15317-2560
(724)223-3313
FAX: (724)250-6023

Meadville

Meadville Medical Center-Vernon Place
11277 Vernon Pl, Ste 201
Meadville, PA 16335-3719
(814)333-5143
FAX: (814)373-3525

Mechanicsburg

Penn State Health Century Drive Outpatient Center
880 Century Dr
Mechanicsburg, PA 17055-4375
(717)972-4900
FAX: (717)972-4601

Penn State Health Silver Creek Outpatient Center
335 Lambs Gap Rd
Mechanicsburg, PA 17050-2784
(717)947-4900
FAX: (717)972-4601

Penn State Health Trindle Road Outpatient Center
4665 E Trindle Rd
Mechanicsburg, PA 17050-3640
(717)972-4900
FAX: (717)731-9165

Upmc Pinnacle Fredericksen Outpatient Center
2015 Technology Pkwy
Mechanicsburg, PA 17050-9414
(717)230-3700
FAX: (717)703-1111

Media

Comprehensive Breast Center At Riddle Hospital
1068 West Baltimore Pike, U.S. Route 1, Riddle Hospital
Media, PA 19063
(484)227-3010
FAX: (484)227-3791

Media Medical Imaging
200 E State St, Ste 200
Media, PA 19063-3434
(610)627-4360
FAX: (610)627-4361

Meyersdale

Dlp Conemaugh Meyersdale Medical Center, Llc
200 Hospital Dr
Meyersdale, PA 15552-1249
(814)634-5911
FAX: (814)634-0194

Mifflintown

Geisinger-Lewistown Hospital Outpatient Center - Jvm
27 Cjems Ln Ste 4
Mifflintown, PA 17059-8384
(717)436-6454
FAX: (717)436-2068

Millersburg

Upmc Pinnacle Millersburg
1000 Evelyn Dr
Millersburg, PA 17061-1258
(717)230-3700
FAX: (717)703-1111

Monongahela

Monongahela Valley Hospital, Inc.
1163 Country Club Rd
Monongahela, PA 15063-1095
(724)258-1685
FAX: (724)258-1290

Monroeville

Forbes Hospital
2580 Haymaker Rd, Ste 303
Monroeville, PA 15146-3500
(412)359-8366
FAX: (412)858-2955

Magee Womens Imaging-Monroeville
4075 Monroeville Blvd, Bldg 2 Suite 225
Monroeville, PA 15146-2525
(800)649-4077
FAX: (412)373-7351

Premier Medical Associates
3824 Northern Pike Ste 150, One Monroeville Center
Monroeville, PA 15146-2157
(412)373-6342
FAX: (412)373-6347

Montoursville

Geisinger Lycoming Clinic
780 Broad St
Montoursville, PA 17754-2419
(570)368-2870
FAX: (570)271-5976

Montrose

Endless Mountains Health System
100 Hospital Dr
Montrose, PA 18801-6402
(570)278-3801
FAX: (570)278-4973

Mount Pleasant

Excela Health Frick Hospital
508 S Church St
Mount Pleasant, PA 15666-1790
(724)689-0100
FAX: (724)850-8069

Mount Pocono

Geisinger Medical Group Mt. Pocono
126 Market Way
Mount Pocono, PA 18344-1039
(570)808-6136
FAX: (570)808-5994

Mountain Top

Wilkes - Barre Hospital Co
239 S Mountain Blvd
Mountain Top, PA 18707-1911
(570)552-1701
FAX: (570)552-1758

Muncy

Upmc Muncy
215 E Water St Fl 1
Muncy, PA 17756-8828
(570)321-2545
FAX: (570)546-4217

Natrona Heights

Akmc Dba Allegheny Valley Hospital, Radiological Imaging
2801 Freeport Rd
Natrona Heights, PA 15065-1968
(724)226-1840
FAX: (724)226-8440

Alle-Kiski Medical Center, Dba Allegheny Valley Hospital
1301 Carlisle St, Department Of Radiology
Natrona Heights, PA 15065-1152
(724)226-7300
FAX: (724)226-7386

New Castle

Upmc Jameson
26 Nesbitt Rd, Ste 300
New Castle, PA 16105-3418
(724)656-6036
FAX: (724)656-6008

New Freedom

Stonebridge Diagnostic Center
13515 Wolfe Rd, Ste B
New Freedom, PA 17349-9346
(717)851-1901
FAX: (717)812-2529

New Holland

Garden Spot Imaging
435 S Kinzer Ave Ste 4
New Holland, PA 17557-8706
(714)354-2424
FAX: (717)354-2440

New Kensington

Avh Outpatient Care Center-New Kensington
651 4th Ave, Department Of Radiology
New Kensington, PA 15068-6591
(724)226-7300
FAX: (724)226-7137

Newport

Upmc Pinnacle At Newport
300 Bretz Ct
Newport, PA 17074-8614
(717)230-3700
FAX: (717)703-1111

Newtown Square

Bryn Mawr Hospital Health Center
3855 West Chester Pike
Newtown Square, PA 19073-2304
(484)337-4400
FAX: (610)886-3957

The Diagnostic Breast Center
3475 West Chester Pike Ste 240
Newtown Square, PA 19073-4291
(610)356-9030
FAX: (610)356-9036

Norristown

Suburban Community Hospital
2701 Dekalb Pike
Norristown, PA 19401-1849
(610)278-2881
FAX: (610)270-8312

North Huntingdon

Excela Square At Norwin
8775 Norwin Ave
North Huntingdon, PA 15642-2718
(724)861-6306
FAX: (724)861-6316

Northampton

St. Luke's Sacred Heart Northampton Imaging Mammography Depa
602 E 21st St B
Northampton, PA 18067-1259
(484)526-1000
FAX: (610)262-6432

Orwigsburg

Geisinger St. Luke's
1165 Centre Tpke
Orwigsburg, PA 17961-9343
(484)526-1000
FAX: (484)499-1012

Palmyra

Wellspan Good Samaritan Hospital Ambulatory Services Center
1400 S Forge Rd, Ste 2
Palmyra, PA 17078-9519
(717)832-0960
FAX: (717)832-0971

Paoli

Breast Health Center At Paoli Hospital
255 W Lancaster Ave
Paoli, PA 19301-1763
(484)565-1414
FAX: (484)565-1490

Regional Women's Health Group,Llc-Paoli
4 Industrial Blvd Ste 130
Paoli, PA 19301-1605
(610)994-1136
FAX: (215)687-4775

Parkesburg

Penn Medicine Lancaster General Health Parkesburg
950 S Octorara Trl
Parkesburg, PA 19365-2100
(610)857-6624
FAX: (610)857-6619

Pen Argyl

Breast Health Services Bangor
1337 Blue Valley Dr, Ste 5
Pen Argyl, PA 18072-1815
(610)402-2791
FAX: (484)884-2949

Pennsburg

Pennsburg Outpatient Center Of Grand View Hospital
424 Pottstown Ave, Pennsburg Shopping Center, Building D
Pennsburg, PA 18073-1423
(215)453-4100
FAX: (215)679-0641

St Luke's Upper Perkiomen Out Patient Center
2793 Geryville Pike
Pennsburg, PA 18073-2306
(484)526-1000
FAX: (215)541-2984

Philadelphia

Akumin Northeast
8001 Roosevelt Blvd, Ste 104
Philadelphia, PA 19152-3037
(215)331-9100
FAX: (215)331-9102

Albert Einstein Med Ctr-Marion-Louise Saltzman Womens Ctr
5501 Old York Rd, Ste 1
Philadelphia, PA 19141-3018
(215)254-2700
FAX: (215)456-7578

Chestnut Hill Hospital Womens Center
8811 Germantown Ave
Philadelphia, PA 19118-2718
(215)248-8400
FAX: (215)248-6106

Einstein Center One Radiology
9880 Bustleton Ave, Ste 101
Philadelphia, PA 19115-2142
(215)951-8378
FAX: (215)827-1413

Fox Chase Cancer Center
333 Cottman Ave
Philadelphia, PA 19111-2497
(215)728-2646
FAX: (215)728-3134

Holy Redeemer Healthcare
7390 Bustleton Ave
Philadelphia, PA 19152-4311
(215)938-5700
FAX: (215)938-3479

Hospital Of University Of Pennsylvania-Perelman Ctr
3400 Civic Center Blvd, Perelman Center For Advanced Medicine- M
Philadelphia, PA 19104-5127
(215)662-3000
FAX: (215)662-7436

Independent Physicians Medical Center, Llc
9908 Roosevelt Blvd
Philadelphia, PA 19115-1705
(215)464-3300
FAX: (215)464-5403

Jeanes Hospital
7600 Central Ave
Philadelphia, PA 19111-2499
(215)728-3200
FAX: (215)728-2156

Jefferson Breast Imaging Navy Yard
3 Crescent Dr 2nd Fl
Philadelphia, PA 19112-1016
(215)955-2897
FAX: (215)923-7651

Jefferson Frankford Hospital
4900 Frankford Ave
Philadelphia, PA 19124-2695
(215)612-4936
FAX: (215)612-4400

Jefferson Outpatient Imaging North East
10106 Bustleton Avenue
Philadelphia, PA 19116
(215)503-4900
FAX: (215)827-0408

Jefferson Torresdale Hospital
Red Lion And Knights Rd Mob-Suite 104
Philadelphia, PA 19114
(215)612-4936
FAX: (215)612-4400

Methodist Hospital Division Of Jefferson Health System
2301 S Broad St
Philadelphia, PA 19148-3542
(215)952-1234
FAX: (215)952-1407

Nazareth Hospital
2601 Holme Ave
Philadelphia, PA 19152-2096
(215)335-6400
FAX: (215)335-7962

Pennsylvania Hospital Center For Breast Imaging
800 Spruce St
Philadelphia, PA 19107-6130
(215)829-6686
FAX: (215)829-5455

Phila. Dept. Of Health District 2
1720 S Broad St
Philadelphia, PA 19145-2315
(215)685-1603
FAX: (215)685-1541

Philadelphia Department Of Public Health, Health Center 10
2230 Cottman Ave
Philadelphia, PA 19149-1230
(215)685-0625
FAX: (215)685-6894

Philadelphia Department Of Public Health, Health Center 4
4400 Haverford Ave, District Health Center 4
Philadelphia, PA 19104-1361
(215)685-7611
FAX: (215)685-7337

Philadelphia Department Of Public Health, Health Center 5
1900 N 20th St
Philadelphia, PA 19121-2217
(215)685-2949
FAX: (215)685-4428

Prime Healthcare Services - Roxborough Memorial Hospital
5800 Ridge Ave
Philadelphia, PA 19128
(215)487-4502
FAX: (215)487-4384

Temple University Hospital
3401 N Broad St, Mammography Department
Philadelphia, PA 19140-5189
(215)707-9729
FAX: (215)707-7548

Temple University Hospital - Episcopal Campus
100 E Lehigh Ave
Philadelphia, PA 19125-1098
(215)707-4354
FAX: (215)707-7548

Thos Jefferson Univ Hosp Jefferson-Honickman Breast Imaging
1100 Walnut St - Mob, 3rd And 4th Fl
Philadelphia, PA 19107-5563
(215)955-5400
FAX: (215)923-7651

Tuh-Northeastern Campus
2301 E Allegheny Ave
Philadelphia, PA 19134-4499
(215)926-3631
FAX: (215)926-4302

Women's Imaging Center - Penn Medicine University City
3737 Market St, 7th Fl. Radiology
Philadelphia, PA 19104-5545
(215)349-5454
FAX: (215)222-8830

Philipsburg

Geisinger Medical Group - Philipsburg
210 Medical Center Dr
Philipsburg, PA 16866-1948
(717)242-7688
FAX: (717)242-7689

Moshannon Valley Community Medical Building
271 Railroad St
Philipsburg, PA 16866-2300
(814)768-2276
FAX: (814)768-2837

Phoenixville

Phoenixville Hospital
140 Nutt Rd, Diagnostic Imaging Department
Phoenixville, PA 19460-3900
(610)983-1100
FAX: (610)983-1138

Pittsburgh

Ahn Outpatient Center Waterworks
970 Freeport Rd
Pittsburgh, PA 15238-3100
(412)325-5007
FAX: (412)696-0381

Allegheny General Breast Care Center
320 E North Ave
Pittsburgh, PA 15212-4756
(412)359-6034
FAX: (412)359-6799

Heritage Valley Diagnostic Center Robinson
2201 Park Manor Blvd
Pittsburgh, PA 15205-4819
(866)901-6266
FAX: (412)749-6776

Jefferson Regional Medical Center
3722 Brownsville Rd Ste 3722
Pittsburgh, PA 15227-3520
(412)886-2700
FAX: (412)886-2710

Magee Womens Imaging McCandless
9100 Babcock Blvd
Pittsburgh, PA 15237-5815
(800)649-4077
FAX: (412)641-3390

Magee Womens Imaging-Hillman Cancer Center
5115 Centre Ave, 1st Floor Suite 140
Pittsburgh, PA 15232-1301
(800)649-4077
FAX: (412)641-3390

Magee- Womens Imaging- Oakland
300 Halket St, Breast Center- 3rd Floor
Pittsburgh, PA 15213-3108
(800)649-4077
FAX: (412)687-5451

Magee-Womens Imaging At Upmc St. Margaret
815 Freeport Rd Ste 2160, Mammography Department
Pittsburgh, PA 15215-3301
(800)649-4077
FAX: (412)784-7066

Upmc - Downtown Practice
339 6th Ave, Heinz 57 Ctr 5th Fl
Pittsburgh, PA 15222-2526
(412)560-8762
FAX: (412)281-7012

Weinstein Imaging Associates
1910 Cochran Rd, Ste 740
Pittsburgh, PA 15220-1213
(412)440-6999
FAX: (412)440-6998

Weinstein Imaging Associates
5500 Corporate Dr Ste 100
Pittsburgh, PA 15237-5863
(412)630-2649
FAX: (412)630-2676

Weinstein Imaging Associates, P.C.
5850 Centre Ave
Pittsburgh, PA 15206-3780
(412)441-1161
FAX: (412)441-9880

West Penn Hospital
4815 Liberty Ave Ste 143
Pittsburgh, PA 15224-2156
(412)578-1000
FAX: (412)578-5246

Pittston

Wilkes-Barre Hospital Co, Llc
1099 S Township Blvd
Pittston, PA 18640-3247
(570)552-1701
FAX: (570)552-1758

Port Matilda

Geisinger Gray's Woods Clinic
132 Abigail Ln
Port Matilda, PA 16870-7153
(814)272-7200
FAX: (814)272-6505

Pottstown

Pottstown Hospital
1600 E High St
Pottstown, PA 19464-5093
(610)327-7776
FAX: (610)970-3194

Pottsville

Geisinger Mobile Mammography-Mobile
529 Terry Reiley Way, Mobile Mammography Services
Pottsville, PA 17901-1774
(570)271-5555
FAX: (570)271-5976

Lehigh Valley Hospital-Schuylkill E. Norwegian St
700 E Norwegian St
Pottsville, PA 17901-2710
(570)621-5999
FAX: (570)621-4101

Lehigh Valley Schuylkill- Imaging Center
171 Red Horse Rd, Gordon Nagle Trail
Pottsville, PA 17901-9119
(570)621-5999
FAX: (570)621-4101

Punxsutawney

Punxsutawney Area Hospital
81 Hillcrest Dr
Punxsutawney, PA 15767-2616
(814)938-1835
FAX: (814)938-1834

Quakertown

Grand View Hospital OP Ctr At Quakertown
99 W End Blvd
Quakertown, PA 18951
(215)453-4100
FAX: (215)453-3210

St Luke's Quakertown Hosp Women's Imaging Ctr
121 SW 11th Street
Quakertown, PA 18951
(484)526-1000
FAX: (215)538-4950

Radnor

Penn Medicine At Radnor
145 King Of Prussia Rd
Radnor, PA 19087-4557
(610)902-4251
FAX: (610)902-1845

Reading

Reading Hospital Imaging Center At Exeter
2 Hearthstone Ct
Reading, PA 19606-3037
(484)628-8611
FAX: (484)628-3111

St. Joseph Health Network At Exeter
3970 Perkiomen Ave
Reading, PA 19606-2757
(610)378-2100
FAX: (610)898-5969

St. Joseph Medical Center Bern Township Campus
2500 Bernville Rd
Reading, PA 19605-9453
(610)378-2100
FAX: (610)898-5969

St. Joseph Medical Center Community Campus
145 N 6th St, Radiology Department
Reading, PA 19601-3096
(610)378-2100
FAX: (610)898-5969

Red Lion

Windsor Diagnostic Center
3065 Windsor Rd
Red Lion, PA 17356-8533
(717)851-1901
FAX: (717)851-1785

Richboro

St. Mary Imaging-Richboro
1059 2nd Street Pike
Richboro, PA 18954-1803
(215)710-7460
FAX: (215)710-2251

Roaring Spring

Nason Medical Center,Llcd/B/A Conemaugh Nason Medical Center
105 Nason Dr
Roaring Spring, PA 16673-1202
(814)224-6150
FAX: (814)224-6182

Rostraver Township

Monongahela Valley Hospital Inc. Healthplex Imaging
800 Plaza Dr Ste 170, Willow Pointe Plaza
Rostraver Township, PA 15012-4019
(724)379-1900
FAX: (724)379-1901

Sayre

Guthrie Robert Packer Hospital
1 Guthrie Sq
Sayre, PA 18840-1698
(570)887-4071
FAX: (570)887-6659

Scranton

Breast Care Center Of Delta Medix
300 Lackawanna Ave, Unit 200
Scranton, PA 18503-2001
(570)342-7864
FAX: (570)800-7514

Geisinger Mount Pleasant
531 Mt Pleasant Dr
Scranton, PA 18503-1987
(570)703-7495
FAX: (570)703-2084

Geisinger-Viewmont Imaging
435 Scranton Carbondale Hwy
Scranton, PA 18508-1115
(570)343-4334
FAX: (570)207-5492

Sellersville

Grand View Hospital Outpatient Center At Sellersville
915 Lawn Ave
Sellersville, PA 18960-1551
(215)453-4100
FAX: (215)453-3210

Seneca

Upmc Northwest
100 Fairfield Dr
Seneca, PA 16346-2130
(814)676-7130
FAX: (814)676-7950

Sewickley

Allegheny Clinic Radiology-Sewickley
301 Ohio River Blvd Ste 300
Sewickley, PA 15143-1300
(412)741-6800
FAX: (412)749-4454

Heritage Valley Edgeworth
100 Hazel Ln, Ste 104
Sewickley, PA 15143-1249
(866)901-6266
FAX: (724)770-7929

Magee-Womens Imaging - North
2599 Wexford Bayne Rd Ste 1000A
Sewickley, PA 15143-8769
(412)649-4077
FAX: (412)641-1414

Shippensburg

Wellspan Shippensburg Health
46 Walnut Bottom Rd
Shippensburg, PA 17257-8219
(717)530-5333
FAX: (717)262-4563

Slippery Rock

Bhs Outpatient Services Of Slippery Rock
100 Innovation Dr Ste 100
Slippery Rock, PA 16057-2468
(724)284-4000
FAX: (724)284-4465

Somerset

Upmc Somerset Hospital
225 S Center Ave
Somerset, PA 15501-2088
(814)443-5096
FAX: (814)443-5309

Southampton

Holy Redeemer Women's Healthcare At Southampton
45 2nd Street Pike
Southampton, PA 18966-3822
(215)938-5700
FAX: (215)396-3996

Springfield

Akumin Springfield
891 Baltimore Pike
Springfield, PA 19064-3954
(610)543-8860
FAX: (610)543-6237

Crozer Chester Medical Center - Springfield Division
190 W Sproul Rd
Springfield, PA 19064-2027
(610)328-8797
FAX: (610)328-8791

St Marys

Penn Highlands Elk
763 Johnsonburg Rd
St Marys, PA 15857-3498
(814)788-8000
FAX: (814)788-8168

State College

Mount Nittany Medical Center Breast Care Center
1850 E Park Ave Ste 105
State College, PA 16803-6706
(814)234-6752
FAX: (814)231-7351

Stroudsburg

Lehigh Valley Hospital Pocono Bartonsville Healthcare Center
600 Commerce Blvd
Stroudsburg, PA 18360-6214
(570)476-3500
FAX: (570)420-2522

St. Luke's Regional Breast Center, Monroe Campus
200 St Lukes Ln, Ste 301
Stroudsburg, PA 18360-6218
(484)526-1000
FAX: (484)499-1012

Titusville

Titusville Area Hospital
406 W Oak St
Titusville, PA 16354-1499
(814)827-1851
FAX: (814)827-3705

Towanda

Robert Packer Hospital Towanda Campus
91 Hospital Dr
Towanda, PA 18848-9702
(570)268-2240
FAX: (570)268-2286

Trexlertown

Breast Health Services - Trexlertown
6900 Hamilton Blvd
Trexlertown, PA 18087-9101
(610)402-2791
FAX: (610)402-0695

Troy

Troy Community Hospital
275 Guthrie Dr, Guthrie Healthcare System
Troy, PA 16947-1134
(570)297-9281
FAX: (570)297-3970

Tunkhannock

Geisinger Medical Group Tunkhannock
10 Trieble Dr Ste 3
Tunkhannock, PA 18657-7055
(570)808-6136
FAX: (570)808-5449

Tyler Memorial Hospital
5950 Sr 6
Tunkhannock, PA 18657-7905
(570)996-1494
FAX: (570)836-6341

Tyrone

Tyrone Hospital
187 Hospital Dr
Tyrone, PA 16686-1898
(814)684-6385
FAX: (814)682-1804

Uniontown

Cherry Tree Medical Associates, Inc
25 Highland Park Dr
Uniontown, PA 15401-8402
(724)438-3040
FAX: (724)438-3030

Wvu Medicine Uniontown Hospital
500 W Berkeley St
Uniontown, PA 15401-5514
(724)430-7277
FAX: (724)430-3358

Wvu Medicine Uniontown Hospital Outpatient Diagnostic Center
150 Wayland Smith Dr Ste B
Uniontown, PA 15401-2677
(724)430-7277
FAX: (724)430-3358

Upland

Crozer Chester Medical Center
1 Medical Center Blvd, Breast Center
Upland, PA 19013-3995
(610)447-2590
FAX: (610)447-6160

Warminster

Abington Health Center - Warminster Campus
215 Newtown Rd
Warminster, PA 18974-5221
(215)481-3926
FAX: (215)481-6916

Warren

Warren General Hospital
2 W Crescent Park
Warren, PA 16365-2199
(814)723-2677
FAX: (814)723-3062

Warrington

The Health & Wellness Ctr By Doylestown Hosp
847 Easton Rd Ste 2400
Warrington, PA 18976-2912
(215)345-2274
FAX: (215)345-2591

Washington

Washington Health System Women's Center
80 Landings Dr, Ste 201
Washington, PA 15301-9408
(724)223-3313
FAX: (724)250-6023

Waynesboro

Wellspan Waynesboro Hospital
501 E Main St
Waynesboro, PA 17268-2394
(717)765-3404
FAX: (717)765-3495

Waynesburg

Whs Greene
350 Bonar Ave
Waynesburg, PA 15370-1608
(724)627-2435
FAX: (724)627-2484

Wellsboro

Guthrie Medical Group Wellsboro
110 Plaza Ln
Wellsboro, PA 16901-1773
(570)724-4241
FAX: (570)724-5510

Upmc Wellsboro
32-36 Central Ave
Wellsboro, PA 16901-1840
(570)723-0165
FAX: (570)723-0188

West Chester

The Chester County Hospital At Fern Hill
915 Old Fern Hill Rd, Bldg D Ste 400
West Chester, PA 19380-3437
(610)431-5000
FAX: (610)738-2666

West Grove

Jennersville Hospital
1015 W Baltimore Pike
West Grove, PA 19390-9459
(610)869-1555
FAX: (610)869-1293

Penn Medicine Southern Chester County
455 Woodview Rd, Ste 120
West Grove, PA 19390-9229
(610)431-5131
FAX: (610)345-1972

West Mifflin

Magee- Womens Imaging - West Mifflin
275 Clairton Blvd Ste 600
West Mifflin, PA 15236-1426
(800)649-4077
FAX: (412)469-9311

Wexford

Health And Wellness Pavilion
12311 Perry Hwy
Wexford, PA 15090-8344
(878)332-4102
FAX: (878)332-4489

Wilkes Barre

Center For Women's Imaging Geisinger Wyoming Valley
1000 E Mountain Dr
Wilkes Barre, PA 18711-0027
(570)808-6136
FAX: (570)808-5449

Williamsport

Kathryn Candor Lundy Breast Health Center
1100 Grampian Blvd, 1st Fl
Williamsport, PA 17701-1907
(570)326-8200
FAX: (570)320-7540

Willow Grove

Abington Health - Mary T Sachs Breast Imaging Ctr
2701 Blair Mill Rd Ste 4, Schilling Campus
Willow Grove, PA 19090-1041
(215)481-3926
FAX: (215)481-5416

Willow Street

Lancaster General Medical Services At Willow Lakes
212 Willow Valley Lakes Dr Ste 101, Lancaster General Hospital
Willow Street, PA 17584-9668
(717)544-5941
FAX: (717)517-5327

Wind Gap

St. Luke's Wind Gap Women's Imaging
487 E Moorestown Rd, Ste 108
Wind Gap, PA 18091-9683
(484)526-1000
FAX: (484)526-7877

Windber

The Joyce Murtha Breast Care Center At Windber Hospital Inc.
600 Somerset Ave
Windber, PA 15963-1331
(814)467-3438
FAX: (814)467-3432

Wynnewood

Comprehensive Breast Center At Lankenau Medical Center
100 E Lancaster Ave, Ste 12 - 6th Flr Msb
Wynnewood, PA 19096-3400
(484)476-8119
FAX: (484)476-6792

Wyomissing

Reading Hospital At Spring Ridge, Breast Health Center
2603 Keiser Blvd, Ste 101
Wyomissing, PA 19610-3341
(484)628-8611
FAX: (484)628-3111

St. Joseph Regional Health Network At Spring Ridge
2607 Keiser Blvd
Wyomissing, PA 19610-3326
(610)378-2100
FAX: (610)898-5969

Yardley

University Of Pennsylvania
777 Township Line Rd Ste 150
Yardley, PA 19067-5567
(215)860-3360
FAX: (215)860-3362

York

East York Diagnostic Center
2250 E Market St
York, PA 17402-2857
(717)851-1901
FAX: (717)851-1860

Upmc Imaging At Acb
1703 Innovation Dr, Ste 300
York, PA 17408-8815
(717)815-2600
FAX: (171)815-2615

Upmc Memorial Breast Center
1600 6th Ave Ste 106
York, PA 17403-2626
(717)815-2601
FAX: (717)815-2616

Wellspan Hayshire Health Center
2775 N George St
York, PA 17406-3020
(717)851-1901
FAX: (717)812-3829

Women's Imaging At Apple Hill
35 Monument Rd Ste 201
York, PA 17403-5074
(717)851-1901
FAX: (717)812-3703

PUERTO RICO

Adjuntas

Diagnostic Imaging & Rad - Alberto M. Colon-Alvarado, MD
5516 Rd. Km 0.1
Adjuntas, PR 00601
(787)829-1626
FAX: (787)829-1665

Aguada

Aguada Medical Radiology
Carr. 115 Km. 24.5, Bo. Asomante
Aguada, PR 00602
(787)589-7433
FAX: (787)589-7434

Centro Radiologico Y Sonografico De Aguada
272 Calle Marina
Aguada, PR 00602-2956
(787)868-4593
FAX: (787)868-4593

Aguadilla

Bs Radiology And Women's Center
Carretera 2 Km 123.8 Barrio Caimital Al
Aguadilla, PR 00605
(787)658-0099
FAX: (787)658-0294

Hospital Buen Samaritano
Carr. 2, Km. 141.1, Avenue Kennedy 18
Aguadilla, PR 00603
(787)819-0883
FAX: (787)658-0294

Metro Pavia Clinic Aguadilla
Carr. 107 Km. 0.6 Barrio Camaseyes
Aguadilla, PR 00603
(787)296-9778
FAX: (787)882-0484

Aibonito

Menonite General Hospital, Inc.
PO Box 1379, Calle Jose C. Vazquez
Aibonito, PR 00705-1379
(787)735-8001
FAX: (787)954-8035

Arecibo

Arraiza Radiology Psc Dba Arecibo Radiology
Carr. 2 Km. 80.1 Bo. San Daniel, Edificio Arecibo Medical Center
Arecibo, PR 00612
(787)878-3000
FAX: (787)878-8106

Centro Radiologico Rolon Inc.
Carr 490 Km. 0.2 Hato Arriba
Arecibo, PR 00612
(787)879-0750
FAX: (787)879-0772

Hospital Metropolitano Dr. Susoni Inc.
55 Calle Palma
Arecibo, PR 00612-4526
(787)650-1030
FAX: (787)650-1036

Hospital Pavia Arecibo
San Luis Avenue, Carretera 129, Km 0.7
Arecibo, PR 00612
(787)650-7272
FAX: (787)650-7304

Instituto Radiologico De Arecibo
De Diego Ave 21
Arecibo, PR 00612
(787)878-6213
FAX: (787)878-4244

Metro Pavia Clinic Arecibo
PO Box 9976, Zona Industrial Victor Rojas 2 Carretera
Arecibo, PR 00613-9976
(787)650-0020
FAX: (787)650-0097

Arroyo

Centro De Salud Familiar Dr. Julio Palmieri Ferri, Inc.
PO Box 450
Arroyo, PR 00714-0450
(787)839-4150
FAX: (787)839-3989

Barceloneta

Atlantic Medical Center
Carr 2 Km 57.8 Cruce Davila
Barceloneta, PR 00617
(787)846-4412
FAX: (787)846-7410

Barranquitas

Barranquitas Ultrasound And Mammography Center
12 Calle Padre Berrios
Barranquitas, PR 00794-1840
(787)857-3989
FAX: (787)857-3900

Bayamon

Bayamon Medical Center
PO Box 306, 11.7 Road 2
Bayamon, PR 00960-0306
(787)620-8181
FAX: (787)622-8495

Bayamon Radiology Llc/ Dba Santa Juanita Radiology
Al26 Calle 30, Urb Santa Juanita
Bayamon, PR 00956-4706
(787)858-4300
FAX: (787)680-0835

C.T. Radiology Complex
1815 Carr 2, Ct Radiology Bldg.
Bayamon, PR 00959-7279
(787)780-9069
FAX: (787)780-2121

Cdt Grupo Medico San Pablo Inc.
B7 Calle Santa Cruz, Urb Santa Cruz
Bayamon, PR 00961-6902
(787)780-9196
FAX: (787)625-6124

Centro Imagenes Hima San Pablo
70 Calle Santa Cruz, Urb Santa Cruz
Bayamon, PR 00961-7052
(787)620-4323
FAX: (787)641-6796

Centro Imagenes Rio Hondo
Local 3 - R Suite 201, Plaza Rio Hondo
Bayamon, PR 00961
(787)261-2140
FAX: (787)261-3422

Clag Imaging Center Dba Salus
1 Ave Casa Linda Ste, RR 177 Los Filtros
Bayamon, PR 00959-9000
(787)789-1919
FAX: (787)272-8344

Doctors Center Hospital Bayamon
Calle Marginal Carrr. Numero 2, Esquina 3 - R Lote J - 4 Urb Hermanas Da
Bayamon, PR 00690
(787)622-5422
FAX: (787)625-2477

Galeria Radiologica Digital Llc
64 Calle Santa Cruz Ste 104, Galeria Medica
Bayamon, PR 00961-7001
(787)269-2250
FAX: (787)785-2229

Hato Tejas X Rays
Carr 862 Km 2.7 63 B, Hato Tejas
Bayamon, PR 00959
(787)787-1946
FAX: (787)787-1940

Metro Pavia Clinic Bayamon
8 & 9 Garcia St., Urb. Santa Cruz
Bayamon, PR 00954
(787)772-9850
FAX: (787)274-8895

Puerto Rico Imaging Center
Edificio Gallardo Towers, Carr 2 Int 167 First Floor
Bayamon, PR 00961
(787)785-8034
FAX: (787)787-8029

Rexville Radiology
Centro Comercial Bella Vista, Edificio 2
Bayamon, PR 00957
(787)730-4542
FAX: (787)730-8007

Sociedad Radiologica De Bayamon
73 Calle Santa Cruz Ste 103, Santa Cruz Medical Building
Bayamon, PR 00961-6911
(787)785-4620
FAX: (787)740-1399

Cabo Rojo

Hospital Metropolitano Cabo Rojo
108 Calle Munoz Rivera
Cabo Rojo, PR 00623-4060
(787)851-2025
FAX: (787)254-0235

Jesus A. Romero Perez Dba Advanced Radiology Center
87 Calle Carbonell
Cabo Rojo, PR 00623-3443
(787)335-0070
FAX: (787)255-0666

Caguas

Centro Ambulatorio Hima - San Pablo Caguas
Avenida Luis Munoz Rivera A-1
Caguas, PR 00725
(787)653-3434
FAX: (787)653-2218

Consolidated Radiology Complex, CSP
202 Gautier Benitez Ave. Office 105,205,, Consolidated Medical Plaz
Caguas, PR 00725
(787)746-8383
FAX: (787)746-5466

Degetau Ultrasound And X-Ray
F5 Ave Degetau, Urb Bonneville Terr
Caguas, PR 00725-5839
(787)743-7880
FAX: (787)747-0250

Hospital Hima San Pablo Caguas
Ave. Luis Munoz Marin Esquina Degetau, Mariolga
Caguas, PR 00725
(787)653-3434
FAX: (787)653-3105

Hospital Menonita Caguas
Carr 172, Urb Turabo Gardens
Caguas, PR 00725
(787)653-0550
FAX: (787)653-4540

Imagenes Radiology And Breast Diagnostic Center
Munoz Rivera Street, Suite 208-209, Professional Center Building
Caguas, PR 00725
(787)653-3434
FAX: (787)653-1534

Mediko Imaging Inc. Caguas
Ave. Jose Villares 23, Condado Viejo
Caguas, PR 00725
(787)743-1563
FAX: (787)745-9637

Radilogia Del Turabo, C.S.P. D/B/A Quadrangle Imaging Center
Quadrangle Medical Center, Ste. 208, Esq. San Andres
Caguas, PR 00725
(787)746-1688
FAX: (787)746-2292

Camuy

Centro Radiologico Rolon
152 Ave Munoz Rivera Oeste Ste 2
Camuy, PR 00627-2309
(787)820-2122
FAX: (787)879-0772

Canovanas

Insight Radiology Puerto Rico Canovanas
Carr 3 Km 19.9
Canovanas, PR 00729
(787)256-3222
FAX: (787)256-3220

Loiza Valley Mri & Ct Center
Local Aa-4 Loiza Valley Shopping Center, Calle Bahuinia
Canovanas, PR 00729
(787)954-9389
FAX: (786)364-1100

Carolina

Carolina Imaging Center
Fragoso Avenue 4A S4 Y5, Villa Fontana
Carolina, PR 00983
(787)757-0572
FAX: (787)757-6619

Clinica Las Americas Guaynabo,Dba Salus Carolina
Carr. 190, Km. 1.8, Bo. Sabana Abajo
Carolina, PR 00983
(787)789-1919
FAX: (787)706-2818

Country Club X-Ray Center
Avenida Campo Rico Gp-1
Carolina, PR 00982
(787)946-8100
FAX: (939)338-5770

Ctro. Radiodiagnostico Carolina - Carolina Breast Clinic
Local 0-23A 65th Inf. Ave., Carolina Shopping Court
Carolina, PR 00985
(787)257-0677
FAX: (787)257-3030

Doctor Center X-Ray, Inc.
Ave. Comandante Pq 24, Country Club
Carolina, PR 00982
(787)769-4905
FAX: (787)752-6011

Doctors Center Hospital San Fernando De La Carolina
Calle Fernandez Juncos Esquina Molinillo, Edificio Jesus T Pineiro
Carolina, PR 00985
(787)621-3322
FAX: (787)884-7604

Escorial Mri & Ct Imaging Center
1400 Ave De Diego Ste 170, Escorial Office Building One
Carolina, PR 00987-4708
(787)710-7385
FAX: (787)762-3623

Metro Pavia Clinic Carolina
Carr. 3, Km. 13.4 Int. Carr. 857
Carolina, PR 00987
(787)710-9860
FAX: (787)710-9871

Monserrate Imaging Center
Ave. Monserrate Ba 25, Valle Arriba Heights
Carolina, PR 00983
(787)762-3850
FAX: (787)257-3979

Premium Heath Group Clinic
10 Ave Laguna Ste 101A, Laguna Garden Shopp Ctr
Carolina, PR 00979-6420
(787)791-7287
FAX: (787)791-6273

Servicios Radiologicos Asociados Imaging Center
Ave Sanchez Osorios, Centro Comercial Villa Fontana Local A-5
Carolina, PR 00983
(787)276-6200
FAX: (787)710-7318

Cayey

Centro Medico Menonita De Cayey
Carretera 14K, K.M. 13.1 Bo. Rincon
Cayey, PR 00736
(787)535-1001
FAX: (787)535-1045

Mediko Imaging Cayey
56 Calle Jose Celso Barbosa S
Cayey, PR 00736-4727
(787)738-4592
FAX: (787)694-7039

Cidra

Centro Radiologico Sonografico De Cidra
Baldorioty St 18
Cidra, PR 00739
(787)739-4472
FAX: (787)739-9318

Centro Salud Familiar Dr. Luis Aramburu Hgm Inc
Ave Luis A. Santos Flores Carreteta 173
Cidra, PR 00739
(787)739-7911
FAX: (787)739-4421

Coamo

Centro Radiologico Hospital Menonita Coamo
Street Luis Munoz Rivera Numero 138
Coamo, PR 00769
(787)954-8001
FAX: (787)954-8035

Comerio

Salud Integral En La Montana, Comerio
18 Calle Georgetti
Comerio, PR 00782-2539
(787)568-3797
FAX: (787)875-4230

Corozal

Corporacion Ortiz Negron Centro Rad Sonog Digital De Corozal
14 Calle Gandara
Corozal, PR 00783-2057
(787)802-1259
FAX: (787)802-1795

Salud Integral De La Montana Corozal Pr
Carretera 891 Km 15.1, Bo. Pueblo
Corozal, PR 00783
(787)859-2560
FAX: (787)859-5390

Coto Laurel

Hospital San Cristobal
Pr 506, Km 1.0
Coto Laurel, PR 00780
(787)848-2100
FAX: (787)651-2295

Modern Radiology Psc
Primer Nivel 101 Km 75/Carr 506 Calle M, Legacy Office Park
Coto Laurel, PR 00780
(787)840-6322
FAX: (787)259-1177

Dorado

Dorado Breast & Radiology Center
604 Ave Jose Efron Ste 50
Dorado, PR 00646-4821
(787)965-2040
FAX: (787)998-6411

Dorado Xray Center
410 Calle Mendez Vigo, Ofc 206-207
Dorado, PR 00646-4800
(787)796-5425
FAX: (787)796-5316

Fajardo

Centro Senologia Dra Magda Costa II
B1 Ave El Conquistador Urb Veve Calzada
Fajardo, PR 00738-3715
(787)860-1642
FAX: (787)751-5685

Fajardo Imaging Inc.
316 Ave General Valero
Fajardo, PR 00738-4848
(787)860-3400
FAX: (787)863-2075

Hospital Hima San Pablo Fajardo
Ave General Valero Km 2.6 Carr. 194
Fajardo, PR 00738
(787)655-0505
FAX: (787)655-5018

Guayama

Cirt Guayama
Marginal Carretera Pr 54, Bo. Machete Solar A-3
Guayama, PR 00784
(787)686-0090
FAX: (787)686-0094

Hospital Menonita Guayama
Ave. Pedro Albizu Campo, Urb. La Hacienda
Guayama, PR 00785
(787)864-4300
FAX: (787)864-0054

Metro Pavia Clinic Guayama
300 Calle Arnaldo Bristol
Guayama, PR 00784-6935
(787)592-7180
FAX: (787)813-1144

Guaynabo

Dr Irma Colon Psc Radiologist
202 Ave Esmeralda, Urb Ponce De Leon
Guaynabo, PR 00969-4448
(787)272-5656
FAX: (787)720-3232

Guaynabo Medical Mall
140 Ave Las Cumbres
Guaynabo, PR 00969-5523
(787)789-2101
FAX: (800)921-7754

Plg Breast Imaging Services,Psc
100 Carr 165 Ste C107 Torre 1, Centro Internacional De Mercadeo
Guaynabo, PR 00968-8047
(787)999-5400
FAX: (787)999-5401

Gurabo

Tesla Radiology
8 Calle Marlin Carretera 189 Barri, Senderos De Gurabo
Gurabo, PR 00778-9824
(787)737-0707
FAX: (787)737-0708

Hatillo

Northshore Imaging Service
270 Marginal Carr 2 Km 86.1
Hatillo, PR 00659
(787)820-8200
FAX: (787)609-3071

Hato Rey

Hospital Auxilio Mutuo
PO Box 191227, 715 Ave Ponce De Leon Pda 37 1/2
Hato Rey, PR 00919-1227
(787)474-8878
FAX: (787)771-7445

Hospital Del Maestro
Avenida Domenech X-Ray Dept 1st Flr, Calle Sergio Bustanmante 550, Hosp Del M
Hato Rey, PR 00918
(787)523-2600
FAX: (787)474-7603

Hospital Pavia Hato Rey
435 Ave Ponce De Leon
Hato Rey, PR 00917-3424
(787)641-2323
FAX: (787)754-6876

Senos Puerto Rico
525 F.D. Roosevelt Ave, 4th Fl 403, La Torre De Plaza/Plaza Las Americas
Hato Rey, PR 00918
(787)756-7040
FAX: (787)523-1929

Humacao

Dr. Jose A. Nassar & Associates
63 Calle Cruz Ortiz Stella S
Humacao, PR 00791-3334
(787)852-0920
FAX: (787)852-6685

Hima-San Pablo Humacao
PO Box 639, 3 Calle Font Martelo St
Humacao, PR 00792-0639
(787)656-2424
FAX: (787)656-2444

Hospital Ryder Memorial
355 Calle Font Martelo
Humacao, PR 00791-3249
(787)852-0882
FAX: (787)852-0157

Humacao X-Ray Imaging Center
62 Calle Antonio Lopez S
Humacao, PR 00791-4272
(787)852-3540
FAX: (787)850-1141

Mediko Imaging Humacao
Barrio Tejas F12 Calle Victoria
Humacao, PR 00791
(787)403-4787
FAX: (787)745-9637

Juana Diaz

Juana Diaz Medical Imaging Center
107 Calle Comercio
Juana Diaz, PR 00795-1646
(787)837-3312
FAX: (787)837-3285

Lares

Centro De Salude De Lares Inc
Carretera 111 Km 1.9
Lares, PR 00669
(787)897-2727
FAX: (787)897-2725

Las Piedras

Cossma Inc.- Las Piedras
Parque Industrial Tejas Lote 8, Carr. 9922 Km. 0.3
Las Piedras, PR 00771
(787)739-8182
FAX: (787)739-8190

Loiza

Concilio De Salud Integral De Loiza, Inc.
Carretera 188, Int 187
Loiza, PR 00772
(787)876-2042
FAX: (787)256-1900

Luquillo

Insight Radiology Puerto Rico-Luquillo
26 Calle Fernandez Garcia
Luquillo, PR 00773-2236
(787)889-2483
FAX: (787)256-0437

Manati

Centro Imagenes Manati Yvf Psc
B1 Calle Marginal, Urb San Salvador
Manati, PR 00674-4906
(787)854-1818
FAX: (787)884-7301

Doctor's Center Hospital Inc.
St. Rd. 2, Km. 47.7
Manati, PR 00674
(787)621-3322
FAX: (787)884-7604

Manati Medical Center
Urbanizacion Atenas, Calle Hernandez Carrion
Manati, PR 00674
(787)621-3700
FAX: (787)621-3736

Mayaguez

Bioimagenes Medicas, C.S.P.
2638 Ave Hostos, Bioplaza Building, Suite 101
Mayaguez, PR 00682-6391
(787)805-2041
FAX: (787)986-0820

Centro Radiologico Clinica Yaguez, Inc.
Calle McKinley 114, Oficina 103-104 Plaza Yaguez
Mayaguez, PR 00680
(787)832-8444
FAX: (787)805-7440

Frontera, Colon & Suarez - Radiologos
1065 Ave Los Corazones, Edificio Medico Profesional
Mayaguez, PR 00680-7060
(787)831-5922
FAX: (787)831-5922

Frontera, Colon, And Suarez Radiologos
De Diego St 12
Mayaguez, PR 00680
(787)832-2312
FAX: (787)833-5433

Hospital Bella Vista Mamografia
Carretera 349 Kilometro 2.7, Cerro Las Mesas
Mayaguez, PR 00680
(787)652-6039
FAX: (787)832-3385

Hospital Perea-Clinica De La Mujer
Calle Dr. Basora 16 North
Mayaguez, PR 00680
(787)834-0101
FAX: (787)265-2120

Jesus A. Romero Perez Dba Adv Rad Ctrs
Mayaguez, Pr
5 Calle Pablo Maiz, Bo Barcelona
Mayaguez, PR 00680-4840
(787)832-3515
FAX: (787)832-3530

Mayaguez Medical Center
Ave Hostos 410 Carr 2, Bo Sabalos
Mayaguez, PR 00681
(787)652-9200
FAX: (787)652-1547

Policlinica Bella Vista
770 Ave Hostos, Edificio Professional Plaza
Radiology De
Mayaguez, PR 00682-1551
(787)834-6161
FAX: (787)831-1260

Ultrasonido Diagnostico Y Rayos X
57 Calle De Diego E
Mayaguez, PR 00680-4804
(787)833-4556
FAX: (787)265-3434

West Open Mri & Radiology Services
975 Ave. Hostos, Mayaguez Mall Ste. 2220
Mayaguez, PR 00680
(787)806-2900
FAX: (787)806-2226

Moca

Hospital San Carlos Borromeo
Calle Concepcion Vera Ayala 550 S
Moca, PR 00676
(787)877-8000
FAX: (787)877-1190

Radioimagenes Diagnosticas
Carr. 110 Km 12.5
Moca, PR 00676
(787)877-7705
FAX: (787)877-0454

Naranjito

Centro Radiologico De La Montana
Carretera 803 Km 10.1, Bo. Cedro Arriba
Naranjito, PR 00719
(787)869-2687
FAX: (787)869-0536

Patillas

Centro De Servicios Primarios De Salud De Patillas
Calle Guillermo Riefkhol 99
Patillas, PR 00723
(787)839-4320
FAX: (787)839-4355

Penuelas

Medcentro Penuelas
Cuebas Penuelas
Penuelas, PR 00624
(787)843-9393
FAX: (787)841-0077

Ponce

Caribbean Imaging & Radiation Treatment Center, Inc.
2225 Ponce Byp Ste 103, Edificio Parra
Ponce, PR 00717-1322
(787)842-2478
FAX: (787)842-2466

Centro Radiologico
1825 Calle Navarra, Ste 101
Ponce, PR 00716-4614
(787)774-3366
FAX: (787)789-2180

Centro Radiologico
8169 Calle Concordia Ste 1, Condominio San Vicente
Ponce, PR 00717-1555
(787)842-3073
FAX: (787)813-2779

Concordia Imaging Center
8159 Calle Concordia
Ponce, PR 00717-1551
(787)842-2313
FAX: (787)987-7171

Dr. Miguel A. Echevarria - Ponce Medical Imaging
1326 Calle Salud Ste 105, El Senorial Plaza
Ponce, PR 00717-1689
(787)840-3395
FAX: (787)844-2664

Hospital Episcopal San Lucas Ponce
917 Ave Tito Castro
Ponce, PR 00716-4717
(787)844-2080
FAX: (787)842-5105

Hospital Metropolitano Dr.Pila
2435 Blvd Luis A Ferre
Ponce, PR 00717-2112
(787)848-5600
FAX: (787)284-3421

Medcentro
1034 Ave Hostos
Ponce, PR 00716-1115
(787)843-9393
FAX: (787)841-0077

Medical X-Ray Center
509 Ave Tito Castro
Ponce, PR 00716-0207
(787)840-5090
FAX: (787)840-5090

Metro Pavia Clinic Ponce
Street Marina 38
Ponce, PR 00717
(787)844-8529
FAX: (787)813-1144

Modern Radiology, Psc.
9176 Calla Marina
Ponce, PR 00717
(787)843-1625
FAX: (787)843-1723

Quebradillas

Centro Radiologico Shalom Inc
Bo. Terranova Calle Marginal Del Parque, Carr 2 Km 101.6
Quebradillas, PR 00678
(787)501-5329
FAX: (787)952-6901

Rio Grande

Centro Radiologico Rio Grande
Ave. Agustin Perez Andino B- 30, Villas De Rio Grande
Rio Grande, PR 00745
(787)888-4545
FAX: (787)809-1606

Rio Piedras

Aid System Llc
A8 Ave 65 Infanteria, Urb San Agustin
Rio Piedras, PR 00926-1834
(787)740-3010
FAX: (787)740-3009

El Senorial Centro De Imagenes
1755 Calle Parana, Urb Crown Hls
Rio Piedras, PR 00926-6049
(787)764-9493
FAX: (787)759-3621

San Francisco Imaging
126 Ave De Diego Sein Medical Plaza, Reparto Metropolitan
Rio Piedras, PR 00921-3043
(787)751-1487
FAX: (787)774-7100

San German

Hospital De La Concepcion
Carretera 2, Km 173.4, Bo. Cain Alto
San German, PR 00683
(787)892-1860
FAX: (787)892-5803

Hospital Metropolitano - South West Health Corp.
8 Calle Javilla
San German, PR 00683-4102
(787)892-5300
FAX: (787)892-5504

San German X-Ray And Body Imaging Center
70 Calle Dr Santiago Veve
San German, PR 00683-4115
(787)892-5030
FAX: (787)264-7279

San Juan

Ashford Presbyterian Community Hospital
1451 Ave Ashford
San Juan, PR 00907-1511
(787)721-2160
FAX: (787)725-7564

Cardiovascular Radiology Institute Inc.
Pavia Medical Plaza, Suite 113, 611 Manuel Pavia Street
San Juan, PR 00910
(787)268-1015
FAX: (787)261-1788

Centro Mas Salud Dr. Gualberto Rabell Fernandez
Calle Cerra Final Esquina Hoare 900
San Juan, PR 00907
(787)480-3704
FAX: (787)724-4057

Clag- Mamo Hato Rey
400 Ave Fd Roosevelt, Ste 103
San Juan, PR 00918-2129
(787)789-1996
FAX: (787)272-8344

Demadi Psc Dba Pr Imaging Center
249 Ave Arterial Hostos, Avenida Chardon
San Juan, PR 00918-1534
(787)701-1180
FAX: (787)708-4635

Hato Rey X-Ray & Imaging Center
156 Ave Fd Roosevelt, Urb El Vedado
San Juan, PR 00918-2406
(787)754-1422
FAX: (787)754-8555

Health Image Diagnostics/Senos Puerto Rico
310 Ave Lomas Verdes Ste 209
San Juan, PR 00927-6638
(787)474-0820
FAX: (787)474-3655

Hospital Centro Comprensivo De Cancer Upr
Carr. Pr-21 Int. Pr-18, Bo. Monacillo Urbano
San Juan, PR 00927
(787)936-1477
FAX: (787)936-1491

Hospital Metropolitano
1785 Carr 21, Urb Las Lomas
San Juan, PR 00921-3399
(787)782-9999
FAX: (787)782-1442

Hospital San Francisco, Centro De Imagenes
371 Calle De Diego
San Juan, PR 00923-3002
(787)767-5100
FAX: (787)332-0017

Instituto Sonoradiologico Hostos
514 Ave Hostos, Urb Baldrich
San Juan, PR 00918-3260
(787)766-1575
FAX: (787)766-1574

Metro Santurce, Inc Dba Hospital Pavia Santurce
Calle Manuel Pavia 617 Santruce
San Juan, PR 00910
(787)641-1616
FAX: (787)268-2904

Modern Radiology, Psc San Juan, P.R.
Felisa Rincon 300 Suite 20, Las Vistas Shopping Village Ave.
San Juan, PR 00926
(787)709-4338
FAX: (787)843-1723

Montehiedra Ct & Mri Center
9484 Ave Los Romeros, Ste 205
San Juan, PR 00926-7009
(787)708-5000
FAX: (787)708-5010

Oncologic Hospital-I. Gonzalez Martinez Centro De Mamografia
PO Box 191811, Centro Medico - Rio Piedras
San Juan, PR 00919-1811
(787)763-4149
FAX: (787)763-4149

Servicios Radiologicos Asociados
390 Calle Manuel Domenech
San Juan, PR 00918-3716
(787)764-7328
FAX: (787)753-7675

San Lorenzo

Centro De Imagenes Sonograficas
Plaza Buxo 4B Carr 181 Int 183
San Lorenzo, PR 00754
(787)736-0980
FAX: (787)736-4226

San Sebastian

Centro De Medicina Y Cirugia Ambulatoria San Sebastian
PO Box 486, 3 Calle Jose Mendez Cardona
San Sebastian, PR 00685-0486
(787)896-1850
FAX: (787)280-1698

Pepino Health Group Inc.
126 Calle Pavia Fernandez
San Sebastian, PR 00685-2285
(787)280-1335
FAX: (787)280-4508

Servicios Preventivos Del Caribe - Mobile
3 Calle J Mendez Cardona
San Sebastian, PR 00685-2252
(787)896-1850
FAX: (787)280-1698

Santa Isabel

Centro De Imagenes San Cristobal Santa Isabel
Carr Pr 153, Bo Felicia 2
Santa Isabel, PR 00757
(787)848-2100
FAX: (787)651-2295

Centro Radiologico Santa Isabel
Munoz Rivera 60
Santa Isabel, PR 00757
(787)845-7700
FAX: (787)845-6218

Santurce

Hpm Foundation Inc Centro De Imagenes
2020 Ave Borinquen
Santurce, PR 00915-3822
(787)268-4171
FAX: (787)919-3656

Toa Alta

Toa Alta X-Ray And Ultrasound
9 Calle Antonio R Barcelo
Toa Alta, PR 00953-2444
(787)870-3245
FAX: (787)870-8300

Toa Baja

Centro De Servicios Medicos De Levittown
Hf16 Calle Lizzie Graham, Urb Levittown Lakes
Toa Baja, PR 00949-3634
(787)795-2935
FAX: (787)784-0680

Levittown Imaging Center Inc
1173 Ave Dos Palmas, Urb Levittown
Toa Baja, PR 00949-4102
(787)795-2055
FAX: (787)261-1788

Trujillo Alto

Rayos X Centro 4
Expreso Trujillo Alto, Entrada Saint Just
Trujillo Alto, PR 00976
(787)755-1075
FAX: (787)755-0265

Vega Alta

Vega Alta Radiology
1 Calle Marginal Ste 103
Vega Alta, PR 00692-6797
(787)270-0520
FAX: (787)270-0530

Vega Baja

Advanced Mri & Ct Institute
Road Pr-2 Marginal D-10, Urb, Villa Real
Vega Baja, PR 00693
(787)807-0900
FAX: (787)855-2729

Vega Baja Imaging Psc/Dba/ Vega Baja Radiology
3998 Carr 2 Ste 2
Vega Baja, PR 00693-4140
(787)855-2687
FAX: (787)858-8299

Yauco

Caribbean Imaging & Radiation Treatment Center
Calle Prolongacion 25 Julio 14
Yauco, PR 00698
(787)492-0260
FAX: (787)492-0265

Hospital Pavia Yauco
PO Box 5643, 1.0 Carr 128
Yauco, PR 00698-5643
(787)856-1000
FAX: (787)856-7714

Medical X-Ray Center
32 Calle Mattei Lluberas
Yauco, PR 00698-3753
(787)856-2157
FAX: (787)856-2157

RHODE ISLAND

Bristol

Medical Associates Of Rhode Island
1180 Hope St
Bristol, RI 02809-1126
(401)253-8900
FAX: (401)253-7547

Cranston

Rhode Island Medical Imaging
1301 Reservoir Ave
Cranston, RI 02920-6034
(401)490-0040
FAX: (401)490-0049

X-Ray Associates, Inc D/B/A Xra Medical Imaging
65 Sockanosset Cross Rd
Cranston, RI 02920-5536
(401)943-1454
FAX: (401)943-1140

East Greenwich

Rhode Island Medical Imaging, Inc.
1351 S County Trl Ste 105
East Greenwich, RI 02818-5079
(401)884-8125
FAX: (401)884-8290

South County Hospital Medical And Wellness Center
3461 S County Trl
East Greenwich, RI 02818-1465
(401)788-1486
FAX: (401)783-3943

Women & Infants Hospital - Eg East Greenwich Ri
1050 Main St
East Greenwich, RI 02818-3161
(401)274-1122
FAX: (401)453-7615

East Providence

Rhode Island Medical Imaging
450 Veterans Memorial Pkwy Ste 203
East Providence, RI 02914-5300
(401)435-3041
FAX: (401)435-3042

Hope Valley

Westerly Hospital - Wood River Health Services, Inc.
823 Main St
Hope Valley, RI 02832-1920
(401)539-2461
FAX: (401)539-8996

Johnston

Rhode Island Medical Imaging
1526 Atwood Ave Lowr Level
Johnston, RI 02919-3289
(401)331-0900
FAX: (401)455-0909

X-Ray Associates, Inc., D/B/A Xra Medical Imaging
1524 Atwood Ave Ste Ll5
Johnston, RI 02919-3228
(401)351-1570
FAX: (401)351-1371

Lincoln

Rhode Island Medical Imaging
6 Blackstone Valley Pl, Bldg 5 Ste 506
Lincoln, RI 02865-1179
(401)272-5500
FAX: (401)334-3697

Newport

Navy Medicine Readiness & Training Command New England
43 Smith Rd, Radiology Department
Newport, RI 02841-1006
(401)841-6840
FAX: (401)841-6193

Newport Hospital
11 Friendship St
Newport, RI 02840-2299
(401)845-1346
FAX: (401)848-6008

North Providence

Prospect Chartercare,Sjhsri,Llc Dba Our Lady Of Fatima Hosp
200 High Service Ave, Our Lady Of Fatima Hospital
North Providence, RI 02904-5113
(401)456-3507
FAX: (401)752-8176

Rhode Island Medical Imaging
1500 Mineral Spring Ave
North Providence, RI 02904-3130
(401)533-9300
FAX: (401)533-9309

Pawtucket

Kent Hospital - Acc
111 Brewster St
Pawtucket, RI 02860-4400
(401)737-7010
FAX: (401)736-1023

Rhode Island Medical Imaging, Inc.
333 School St Ste 105, Rhode Island Medical Imaging
Pawtucket, RI 02860-5335
(401)272-5500
FAX: (401)331-6461

Portsmouth

Portsmouth Imaging Center
69 Turnpike Ave
Portsmouth, RI 02871-1419
(401)845-1336
FAX: (401)848-6008

Providence

Anne C. Pappas Center For Breast Imaging
2 Dudley St Ste G85, Rhode Island Hospital
Providence, RI 02905-3209
(401)444-4491
FAX: (401)519-2903

Lifespan Medical Imaging At West River
146 W River St, Ste 11C
Providence, RI 02904-2609
(401)444-7770
FAX: (401)444-7779

Rhode Island Medical Imaging, Inc
1 Randall Sq Ste 103
Providence, RI 02904-2751
(401)432-2400
FAX: (401)331-6461

Roger Williams Medical Center
825 Chalkstone Ave
Providence, RI 02908-4735
(401)456-5701
FAX: (401)456-2220

Women & Infants Hospital
235 Plain St
Providence, RI 02905-3240
(401)274-1122
FAX: (401)453-7739

Women & Infants Hospital - Providence Ri
101 Dudley St, Diagnostic Imaging Level 0
Providence, RI 02905-2499
(401)430-1159
FAX: (401)453-7726

Riverside

Rhode Island Medical Imaging, Inc.
1525 Wampanoag Trl, Ste 101
Riverside, RI 02915-1091
(401)433-1166
FAX: (401)433-5279

Smithfield

X-Ray Associates, Inc. D/B/A Xra Medical Imaging
41 Sanderson Rd
Smithfield, RI 02917-2602
(401)949-0027
FAX: (401)949-0086

Wakefield

South County Hospital
100 Kenyon Ave
Wakefield, RI 02879-4299
(401)782-8020
FAX: (401)782-9894

X-Ray Associates, Inc., D/B/A Xra Medical Imaging
481 Kingstown Rd
Wakefield, RI 02879-3626
(401)792-9840
FAX: (401)792-9870

Warwick

Kent Hospital Women's Imaging Center
455 Toll Gate Rd
Warwick, RI 02886-2759
(401)736-1988
FAX: (401)736-1010

Rhode Island Medical Imaging
250 Toll Gate Rd
Warwick, RI 02886-4411
(401)921-2900
FAX: (401)921-2909

Tollgate Radiology Ii, Llc
300 Toll Gate Rd Ste 101A
Warwick, RI 02886-4447
(401)738-3100
FAX: (401)732-4236

Westerly

South County Health Medical And Wellness-Westerly
268 Post Rd
Westerly, RI 02891-6600
(401)782-8030
FAX: (401)783-3943

Westerly Hospital
25 Wells St
Westerly, RI 02891-2934
(401)348-3554
FAX: (401)348-3488

Woonsocket

Prime Healthcare Services-Landmark,Llc
115 Cass Ave
Woonsocket, RI 02895-4705
(401)769-4100
FAX: (401)767-1566

SOUTH CAROLINA

Abbeville

Abbeville Area Medical Center
420 Thomson Cir
Abbeville, SC 29620-5656
(864)366-3319
FAX: (864)366-3373

Aiken

Rhs-Clyburn Center For Primary Care
1000 Clyburn Pl
Aiken, SC 29801-4193
(803)380-7000
FAX: (803)508-4248

Southside Imaging Center
430 Society Hill Dr
Aiken, SC 29803-1731
(803)641-5803
FAX: (803)641-5810

Women's Breast Health & Imaging Center
400 Medical Park Dr
Aiken, SC 29801-6345
(803)641-5803
FAX: (803)641-5810

Women's Health Associates
121 Aurora Pl, Ste A
Aiken, SC 29801-5310
(803)648-0803
FAX: (803)648-8986

Anderson

Anderson Diagnostic Imaging, Inc.
2110 Highway 81 N
Anderson, SC 29621-1532
(864)225-6286
FAX: (864)231-6738

Anmed Health Women's & Children Hospital
2000 E Greenville St, Ste 4600
Anderson, SC 29621-1765
(864)512-6511
FAX: (864)512-4368

Beaufort

Beaufort Memorial Hosp. - Breast Health Center
989 Ribaut Rd Ste 110
Beaufort, SC 29902-5481
(843)522-5015
FAX: (843)522-5848

Beaufort Memorial Hospital
955 Ribaut Rd, Radiology Department
Beaufort, SC 29902-5454
(843)522-5015
FAX: (843)522-5848

Navy Medical Readiness & Training Command Beaufort
PO Box 6066B, 1 Pinckney Blvd
Beaufort, SC 29902-0225
(843)228-5440
FAX: (843)228-5177

Bluffton

Bluffton Medical Campus
75 Baylor Dr
Bluffton, SC 29910-8965
(843)836-1664
FAX: (843)705-7031

St Joseph Candler Imaging Of Bluffton
10 Oak Forest Rd Ste A
Bluffton, SC 29910-4974
(912)819-6800
FAX: (912)691-9290

Camden

Kershaw Hospital Llc
1315 Roberts St
Camden, SC 29020-3737
(803)713-6083
FAX: (803)713-6359

Chapin

Women's Imaging Ctr Chapin Lexington Med Ctr Chapin
557 Columbia Ave
Chapin, SC 29036-8324
(803)345-7555
FAX: (803)345-7554

Charleston

Hollings Cancer Center Breast Imaging Program
86 Jonathan Lucas St Ste 344
Charleston, SC 29425-8900
(843)792-8439
FAX: (843)876-0233

Roper Hospital
316 Calhoun St
Charleston, SC 29401-1125
(843)402-5000
FAX: (843)727-3379

St Francis Hospital Breast Care-Medical Plaza
2145 Henry Tecklenburg Dr Ste 130
Charleston, SC 29414-5894
(843)402-5000
FAX: (843)556-3924

Trident Medical Center—Trident Breast Care Center
9313 Medical Plaza Dr Ste 201
Charleston, SC 29406-9176
(843)847-3230
FAX: (843)847-4061

Cheraw

McLeod Health Cheraw
711 Chesterfield Hwy
Cheraw, SC 29520-7002
(843)777-2095
FAX: (843)537-8113

Chester

Musc Health Chester Medical Center
1 Medical Park Dr, Radiology Department
Chester, SC 29706-9769
(803)581-9413
FAX: (803)581-8898

Clinton

Prisma Health Laurens County Hospital
22725 Highway 76 E, PO Box Drawer 976
Clinton, SC 29325-7527
(864)833-9398
FAX: (864)938-1828

Columbia

Lexington Medical Center Irmo
7035 Saint Andrews Rd
Columbia, SC 29212-1177
(803)749-0894
FAX: (803)732-5380

Lexington Medical Center Northeast Women's Imaging
3016 Longtown Commons Dr
Columbia, SC 29229-7861
(803)791-2486
FAX: (803)791-2094

Lexington Women's Care Sandhills
233 Longtown Rd
Columbia, SC 29229-8550
(803)788-0268
FAX: (803)788-7384

Northeast Diagnostic Imaging
115 Blarney Dr Ste 206
Columbia, SC 29223-6291
(803)699-1847
FAX: (803)434-7676

Prisma Health Baptist Parkridge
400 Palmetto Health Pkwy, Imaging Dept, 1st Floor
Columbia, SC 29212-1760
(803)296-8888
FAX: (803)296-2969

Prisma Health Breast Center
1501 Sumter St
Columbia, SC 29201-2829
(803)296-8888
FAX: (803)296-3562

Prisma Health Richland Breast Center
1 Richland Medical Park Dr Ste 120
Columbia, SC 29203-6830
(803)296-8888
FAX: (803)434-7676

Providence Health
2435 Forest Dr, Radiology Department
Columbia, SC 29204-2098
(803)256-5351
FAX: (803)400-5094

Vista Women's Healthcare-Wic
700 Gervais St Ste 300
Columbia, SC 29201-3061
(803)254-3230
FAX: (803)540-1192

Womens Care At Image Care Llc
710 Rabon Rd Ste 101
Columbia, SC 29203-8903
(803)462-3680
FAX: (803)699-4060

Conway

Conway Medical Mammography Center-Mobile
300 Singleton Ridge Rd
Conway, SC 29526-9142
(843)234-6891
FAX: (843)347-8200

Outpatient Diagnostic Center Of Conway Medical Center
801 Farrar Dr
Conway, SC 29526-8747
(843)234-5474
FAX: (843)347-8200

Dillon

McLeod Medical Center - Dillon
301 E Jackson St
Dillon, SC 29536-2509
(843)774-1280
FAX: (843)487-1680

Easley

Prisma Health Baptist Easley Hospital
200 Fleetwood Dr
Easley, SC 29640-2022
(864)522-9729
FAX: (864)455-4500

Elgin

Kershaw Hospital Llc
40 Pinnacle Pkwy
Elgin, SC 29045-8390
(803)713-6083
FAX: (803)713-6359

Fairfax

Allendale County Hospital
1787 Allendale Fairfax Hwy
Fairfax, SC 29827-9133
(803)632-3311
FAX: (803)632-3567

Florence

McLeod Regional Medical Center Breast Imaging Center
555 E Cheves St, Breast Imaging Center
Florence, SC 29506-2617
(843)777-2095
FAX: (843)777-6333

Musc Health Florence Medical Center
805 Pamplico Hwy
Florence, SC 29505-6047
(843)674-4525
FAX: (843)674-4557

Musc Health Florence Women's Diagnostics Center
1590 Freedom Blvd
Florence, SC 29505-6071
(843)674-4525
FAX: (843)674-4678

Fort Jackson

Moncrief Army Health Clinic
4500 Stuart Ave, Department Of Radiology Imaging
Fort Jackson, SC 29207-5700
(803)751-2444
FAX: (803)751-0254

Fort Mill

Imaging Center At Baxter Village
509 6th Baxter Xing
Fort Mill, SC 29708-6428
(802)329-6878
FAX: (803)329-6812

Gaffney

Bearden-Josey Center For Breast Health - Cherokee
1530 N Limestone St
Gaffney, SC 29340-4742
(864)487-1556
FAX: (864)206-6228

Georgetown

Georgetown Memorial Hospital
606 Black River Rd
Georgetown, SC 29440-3368
(843)527-7446
FAX: (843)520-8118

Goose Creek

Naval Health Clinic Charleston
110 Nnptc Cir
Goose Creek, SC 29445-6314
(843)794-6250
FAX: (843)794-6027

Greenville

Bon Secours Diagnostic Imaging Llc, Dba Innervision Medical
1 Marcus Dr
Greenville, SC 29615-4818
(864)751-2051
FAX: (864)751-2050

Bon Secours Diagnostic Imaging Llc,Dba St.Francis Millennium
2 Innovation Drive, Suite 350
Greenville, SC 29607
(864)242-4011
FAX: (864)232-6085

Bon Secours Diagnostic Imaging, Llc Dba Innervision-Grove
1 Cannon Dr
Greenville, SC 29605-4201
(864)242-4011
FAX: (864)232-6085

Pearlie Harris Center For Breast Health
131 Commonwealth Dr Ste 220
Greenville, SC 29615-4887
(864)675-4101
FAX: (864)675-4895

Prisma Health Outpatient Radiology
1210 W Faris Rd
Greenville, SC 29605-4444
(864)522-9729
FAX: (864)220-8847

Prisma Health Patewood Medical Campus
200 Patewood Dr Ste A16
Greenville, SC 29615-3544
(864)454-1000
FAX: (864)454-1048

Greenwood

The Imaging Center Of Self Regional Healthcare
102 Academy Ave
Greenwood, SC 29646-3808
(864)725-5000
FAX: (864)725-7183

Greer

Bearden-Josey Center For Breast Health Pelham
2755 S Highway 14 Ste 1575
Greer, SC 29650-4902
(864)612-9076
FAX: (864)560-1953

Prisma Health Greer Memorial Hospital
830 S Buncombe Rd
Greer, SC 29650-2400
(864)522-9729
FAX: (864)797-8099

Hardeeville

Coastal Carolina Hospital
1000 Medical Center Dr
Hardeeville, SC 29927-3446
(843)784-8230
FAX: (843)784-8028

Donald E. Gatch Medical Center
552 Stiney Rd
Hardeeville, SC 29927-5228
(843)987-7508
FAX: (843)987-7515

Hartsville

Carolina Pines Regional Medical Center
1304 W Bobo Newsom Hwy
Hartsville, SC 29550-4710
(843)339-4500
FAX: (843)339-4791

Hilton Head

Island Imaging, Llc
40 Palmetto Pkwy
Hilton Head, SC 29926-3759
(843)681-1999
FAX: (843)681-5999

Hilton Head Island

Hilton Head Hospital
25 Hospital Center Blvd, Radiology Dept
Hilton Head Island, SC 29926-2793
(843)836-1664
FAX: (843)689-8489

Kingstree

Williamsburg Regional Hospital
500 Nelson Blvd
Kingstree, SC 29556-4027
(843)355-0341
FAX: (843)355-0349

Lake City

Lake City Community Hospital
258 N Ron McNair Blvd
Lake City, SC 29560-2462
(843)374-6147
FAX: (843)374-6133

Lancaster

Musc Health Lancaster Imaging Center
1037 W Meeting St
Lancaster, SC 29720-2205
(803)313-3170
FAX: (803)313-3195

Musc Health Lancaster Medical Center
800 W Meeting St
Lancaster, SC 29720-2202
(803)286-1764
FAX: (803)286-1370

Lexington

Lexington Medical Center - Lexington Women's Imaging
811 W Main St
Lexington, SC 29072-2507
(803)358-6170
FAX: (803)358-6155

Little River

Little River Medical Center
4303 Live Oak Dr
Little River, SC 29566-9138
(843)663-8000
FAX: (843)663-8121

McLeod/Seacoast Medical Center
4000 Highway 9 E
Little River, SC 29566-7833
(843)390-8265
FAX: (843)390-8170

Loris

McLeod Loris Community Hosp
3655 Mitchell St
Loris, SC 29569-2844
(843)716-7512
FAX: (843)716-7542

Manning

McLeod Health Clarendon
10 E Hospital St
Manning, SC 29102-3153
(803)435-3121
FAX: (803)435-3124

Moncks Corner

Roper Hospital Diagnostics & Er-Berkeley
730 Stony Landing Rd, Radiology Department
Moncks Corner, SC 29461-2904
(843)402-5000
FAX: (843)899-7130

Trident Medical Center, Llc Moncks Corner Medical Ctr.
401 N Live Oak Dr
Moncks Corner, SC 29461-5603
(843)847-3230
FAX: (843)847-4061

Mount Pleasant

Musc Health East Cooper
1600 Midtown Ave
Mount Pleasant, SC 29464-3771
(843)876-8282
FAX: (843)876-8181

Mt Pleasant

East Cooper Medical Center
2000 Hospital Dr
Mt Pleasant, SC 29464-3764
(843)416-6067
FAX: (843)416-6857

Imaging Specialists Of Charleston
1241 Woodland Ave
Mt Pleasant, SC 29464-3288
(843)881-4020
FAX: (843)881-7515

Mount Pleasant Hospital Breast Care - Medical Offices
3510 N Highway 17 Ste 205
Mt Pleasant, SC 29466-8229
(843)402-5000
FAX: (843)606-7927

Mullins

Musc Health - Marion Medical Center
2829 E Highway 76
Mullins, SC 29574-6035
(843)431-2668
FAX: (843)431-2692

Murrells Inlet

The Imaging Center At Waccamaw Medical Park
4181 Highway 17
Murrells Inlet, SC 29576-5019
(843)652-8000
FAX: (843)652-0045

Waccamaw Women's Imaging
4017 Highway 17 Ste 101
Murrells Inlet, SC 29576-5032
(843)652-8040
FAX: (843)652-8044

Myrtle Beach

Carolina Forest Imaging Center
199 Village Center Blvd Ste 110
Myrtle Beach, SC 29579-3589
(843)236-7878
FAX: (843)903-8637

Parkway Medical Center - Women's Diagnostic Center
945 82nd Pkwy
Myrtle Beach, SC 29572-4612
(888)858-9936
FAX: (843)692-1981

Tidelands Health Market Common Llc
2200 Crow Ln
Myrtle Beach, SC 29577-1663
(843)652-8014
FAX: (843)652-0045

Newberry

Newberry County Memorial Hospital
PO Box 497, 2669 Kinard St
Newberry, SC 29108-0497
(803)405-7122
FAX: (803)405-7536

North Charleston

Musc Health North Charleston
8992 University Blvd Ste 100
North Charleston, SC 29406-8104
(843)876-8146
FAX: (843)553-9864

Okatie

Beaufort Memorial Okatie Medical Pavilion
122 Okatie Center Blvd N
Okatie, SC 29909-3781
(843)706-8851
FAX: (843)706-8681

Orangeburg

Inmed Diagnostics Services Of Sc Llc
1728 Village Park Dr
Orangeburg, SC 29118-2426
(803)536-1106
FAX: (803)535-6033

The Regional Medical Center
3000 Saint Matthews Rd
Orangeburg, SC 29118-1498
(803)395-2841
FAX: (803)395-4722

Pickens

Cannon Memorial Hospital
123 Wg Acker Dr
Pickens, SC 29671-2739
(864)898-1169
FAX: (864)898-1050

Port Royal

Port Royal Medical Center
1320 Ribaut Rd
Port Royal, SC 29935-1118
(843)986-1849
FAX: (843)322-1834

Rock Hill

Charlotte Radiology Breast Center - Rock Hill Office
1656 Riverchase Blvd, Ste 1200
Rock Hill, SC 29732-0270
(803)327-9934
FAX: (704)831-3574

Women's Diagnostic Center - Piedmont Medical Center
218 Herlong Ave S
Rock Hill, SC 29732-1158
(803)329-6878
FAX: (803)327-2480

Seneca

Mountainview Medical Imaging
1059 By Pass 123
Seneca, SC 29678-4762
(864)885-0551
FAX: (864)885-1822

Prisma Health - Oconee Memorial Hospital
298 Memorial Dr
Seneca, SC 29672-9499
(864)885-7424
FAX: (864)885-7304

Simpsonville

Prisma Health Hillcrest Hospital
729 SE Main St
Simpsonville, SC 29681-3280
(864)454-6584
FAX: (864)454-6585

Spartanburg

Bearden Josey Center For Breast Health
101 E Wood St
Spartanburg, SC 29303-3040
(864)560-6186
FAX: (864)560-7354

Bearden Josey Center For Breast Health - North Grove
1330 Boiling Springs Rd Ste 1000
Spartanburg, SC 29303-4202
(864)560-6186
FAX: (864)560-1955

Bearden Josey Center For Breast Health Westside
8311 Warren H Abernathy Hwy
Spartanburg, SC 29301-1249
(864)560-6186
FAX: (864)560-1953

Bearden Josey Center For Breast Health-Mary Black
1650 Skylyn Dr Ste 130
Spartanburg, SC 29307-1069
(864)573-3245
FAX: (864)573-3446

Bearden Josey Ctr For Breast Health Heywood
475 Heywood Ave
Spartanburg, SC 29307-1726
(864)560-6186
FAX: (864)560-7354

Summerville

Roper St. Francis Hospital - Berkeley
100 Callen Blvd
Summerville, SC 29486-2807
(843)402-5000
FAX: (854)529-3085

Summerville Breast Center
77 Springview Ln
Summerville, SC 29485-8154
(843)970-5050
FAX: (843)832-5028

Sumter

Prisma Health Breast Center
115 N Sumter St Ste 210
Sumter, SC 29150-4968
(803)774-9188
FAX: (803)774-9399

Surfside Beach

South Strand Medical Center
5050 Hwy 17 Bypass
Surfside Beach, SC 29575
(888)839-6051
FAX: (843)839-2051

Travelers Rest

Prisma Health North Greenville Hospital
807 N Main St
Travelers Rest, SC 29690-1598
(864)522-9729
FAX: (864)455-9208

Union

Bearden-Josey Center For Breast Health - Union
407 W South St
Union, SC 29379-2771
(864)560-6186
FAX: (864)560-1955

Varnville

Hampton Regional Medical Center
595 W Carolina Ave
Varnville, SC 29944-4735
(803)943-1246
FAX: (803)943-1247

Walterboro

Colleton Medical Center
501 Robertson Blvd
Walterboro, SC 29488-2787
(843)782-2545
FAX: (843)782-3317

West Columbia

Lexington Medical Center Women's Imaging
2728 Sunset Blvd Ste 1, Lexington Medical Park
West Columbia, SC 29169-4838
(803)791-2486
FAX: (803)791-2094

Sc Obgyn Associates
2728 Sunset Blvd, Lexington Medical Park One Suite 201
West Columbia, SC 29169-4840
(803)254-1300
FAX: (803)771-7597

Women's Imaging Ctr-Mobile Lexington Med. Ctr. - Mobile
2728 Sunset Blvd, Ste 401
West Columbia, SC 29169-4839
(803)791-2486
FAX: (803)791-2094

SOUTH DAKOTA

Aberdeen

Avera Breast Center
620 3rd Ave SE
Aberdeen, SD 57401-4554
(605)622-5556
FAX: (605)622-2551

Sanford Clinic Aberdeen
3015 3rd Ave SE, Ste 100
Aberdeen, SD 57401-5539
(605)226-5539
FAX: (605)226-5507

Brookings

Avera Medical Group Brookings
400 22nd Ave
Brookings, SD 57006-2450
(605)697-9500
FAX: (605)697-9541

Chamberlain

Sanford Chamberlain
300 S Byron Blvd
Chamberlain, SD 57325-9741
(605)234-7169
FAX: (605)234-7298

Custer

Monument Health Custer Hospital
1220 Montgomery St
Custer, SD 57730-1705
(605)673-9434
FAX: (605)673-9567

Dakota Dunes

Mercyone Dakota Dunes Breast Center
330 Dakota Dunes Blvd, Ste 200
Dakota Dunes, SD 57049-5462
(605)232-6200
FAX: (605)235-0004

Deadwood

Monument Health Lead-Deadwood
61 Charles St
Deadwood, SD 57732-1303
(605)717-6113
FAX: (605)717-6138

Dell Rapids

Avera Dells Area Hospital
909 N Iowa Ave
Dell Rapids, SD 57022-1231
(605)428-2431
FAX: (605)428-2473

Eagle Butte

Cheyenne River Health Center
24276 166th St Airport Rd
Eagle Butte, SD 57625
(605)964-0556
FAX: (605)964-1176

Freeman

Freeman Regional Health Services
510 E 8th St
Freeman, SD 57029-2086
(605)925-2105
FAX: (605)925-2132

Gregory

Avera Gregory Hospital
400 Park Ave
Gregory, SD 57533-1302
(605)835-5180
FAX: (605)835-8101

Huron

Huron Regional Medical Center
172 4th St SE
Huron, SD 57350-2590
(605)353-6246
FAX: (605)353-6317

Madison

Madison Regional Health System
323 SW 10th St
Madison, SD 57042-3200
(605)256-8638
FAX: (605)256-8983

Milbank

Milbank Area Hospital-Avera Health
301 Flynn Dr
Milbank, SD 57252-1508
(605)432-3350
FAX: (605)432-5220

Mitchell

Avera Breast Center - Mitchell
525 N Foster St
Mitchell, SD 57301-2999
(605)995-2280
FAX: (605)995-6349

Mobridge

Mobridge Regional Hospital
1401 10th Ave W
Mobridge, SD 57601-1106
(605)845-8175
FAX: (605)845-8248

Parkston

Avera St. Benedict
401 W Glynn Dr
Parkston, SD 57366-9605
(605)928-3311
FAX: (605)928-4416

Pierre

Avera St. Mary's Hospital
801 E Sioux Ave
Pierre, SD 57501-3323
(605)224-3190
FAX: (605)224-3417

Pine Ridge

Pine Ridge Reservation Comprehensive Health Care Ctr
East Hwy. 18
Pine Ridge, SD 57770
(605)867-3083
FAX: (605)867-3364

Platte

Platte Health Center Avera
601 E 7th St
Platte, SD 57369-2123
(605)337-1508
FAX: (605)337-3599

Rapid City

Dakota Women's Imaging
2929 5th St Ste 100
Rapid City, SD 57701-7355
(605)342-2852
FAX: (605)721-8805

Gptlhb-Oyate Health Center
3200 Canyon Lake Dr, Ste 1
Rapid City, SD 57702-8114
(605)355-2232
FAX: (605)355-2446

Monument Health Rapid City Clinic, Flormann Street
640 Flormann St
Rapid City, SD 57701-4679
(605)755-3300
FAX: (605)755-3145

Rapid City Medical Center, Llp
2820 Mount Rushmore Rd
Rapid City, SD 57701-5474
(605)721-8160
FAX: (605)721-8450

Rosebud

Rosebud Ihs Hospital
400 Soldier Creek Dr
Rosebud, SD 57570-8502
(605)747-0512
FAX: (605)747-0693

Sioux Falls

Avera Breast Center
1000 E 23rd St, Ste 330
Sioux Falls, SD 57105-2134
(605)322-7465
FAX: (605)322-3835

Avera Breast Center - Mobile
1000 E 23rd St
Sioux Falls, SD 57105-2108
(605)322-7465
FAX: (605)322-3835

Avera Breast Center West
2100 S Marion Rd Ste 300
Sioux Falls, SD 57106-3650
(605)322-7465
FAX: (605)322-3835

Avera Medical Group McGreevy 69th And Western
1910 W 69th St
Sioux Falls, SD 57108-5612
(605)322-5273
FAX: (605)322-5237

Avera Medical Group McGreevy 69th And Cliff
6215 S Cliff Ave, Ste 115
Sioux Falls, SD 57108-8596
(605)322-3300
FAX: (605)322-3301

Avera Medical Group McGreevy 7th Avenue
1200 S 7th Ave
Sioux Falls, SD 57105-0998
(605)336-2140
FAX: (605)782-8326

Dms Imaging Inc - Mobile 3
109 S Petro Ave
Sioux Falls, SD 57107-0577
(605)366-3358
FAX: (701)566-8286

Edith Sanford Breast Center
1309 W 17th St Ste G01
Sioux Falls, SD 57104-4664
(605)312-3455
FAX: (605)312-3453

Edith Sanford Breast Center-Plaza
5019 S Western Ave Ste 200
Sioux Falls, SD 57108-5155
(605)312-3455
FAX: (605)312-3453

Sisseton

Coteau Des Prairies Healthcare System
205 Orchard Dr
Sisseton, SD 57262-2398
(605)698-4638
FAX: (605)698-4637

Woodrow Wilson Keeble Memorial Health Care Center
100 Lake Traverse Dr
Sisseton, SD 57262-7046
(605)742-3771
FAX: (605)698-3607

Spearfish

Monument Health Spearfish Hospital
1440 N Main St
Spearfish, SD 57783-1505
(605)644-4056
FAX: (605)644-4058

Regional Health Medical Clinic-Dpt Reg Health Spearfish Hosp
1420 N 10th St
Spearfish, SD 57783-1532
(605)717-8595
FAX: (605)717-8465

Sturgis

Monument Health Sturgis Hospital
2140 Junction Ave
Sturgis, SD 57785-2358
(605)720-2510
FAX: (605)720-0339

Tyndall

St. Michael's Hospital
410 W 16th Ave
Tyndall, SD 57066-2318
(605)589-2100
FAX: (605)589-2115

Vermillion

Sanford Vermillion Hospital
20 S Plum St
Vermillion, SD 57069-3346
(605)677-3500
FAX: (605)677-3511

Vermillion Medical Clinic
101 S Plum St
Vermillion, SD 57069-3306
(605)624-8643
FAX: (605)624-2362

Watertown

Brown Clinic Pllp
506 1st Ave SE
Watertown, SD 57201-4499
(605)886-8482
FAX: (605)884-4508

Sanford Clinic Watertown Breast Health Institute
901 4th St NW
Watertown, SD 57201-1558
(605)886-1587
FAX: (605)882-8629

Webster

Sanford Hospital Webster
1401 W 1st St
Webster, SD 57274-1054
(605)345-3336
FAX: (605)345-2462

Winner

Winner Regional Health Care Center
745 E 8th St
Winner, SD 57580-2677
(605)842-7139
FAX: (605)842-7300

Yankton

Avera Sacred Heart Hospital
501 Summit St
Yankton, SD 57078-3855
(605)668-8150
FAX: (605)668-8153

Yankton Medical Clinic
1104 W 8th St
Yankton, SD 57078-3306
(605)664-2742
FAX: (605)665-6978

TENNESSEE

Antioch

Premier Radiology Antioch
3754 Murfreesboro Pike, Ste 102
Antioch, TN 37013-3878
(615)467-4642
FAX: (615)467-4643

Athens

Starr Regional Breast Center
711 Cook Dr Ste 240
Athens, TN 37303-3486
(423)744-3372
FAX: (423)744-0648

Bartlett

Memphis Ob/Gyn Association, P.C. Wolfchase
8110 N Brother Blvd
Bartlett, TN 38133-2760
(901)373-9221
FAX: (901)202-5995

Saint Francis Hospital - Bartlett
2986 Kate Bond Rd
Bartlett, TN 38133-4003
(901)820-7575
FAX: (901)820-7601

Bolivar

West Tennessee Healthcare Bolivar Hospital
650 Nuckolls Rd
Bolivar, TN 38008-1532
(731)659-0243
FAX: (731)659-0257

Brentwood

Heritage Medical Associates
1622 Westgate Cir
Brentwood, TN 37027-8019
(629)255-3300
FAX: (629)255-3978

Premier Radiology Brentwood
789 Old Hickory Blvd
Brentwood, TN 37027-4504
(615)832-9551
FAX: (615)234-1509

Bristol

Outpatient Diagnostic Center At Sapling Grove
240 Medical Park Blvd, Ste 1100
Bristol, TN 37620-7347
(423)990-2440
FAX: (423)990-2441

Volunteer Parkway Imaging
1230 Volunteer Pkwy
Bristol, TN 37620-4628
(423)844-5600
FAX: (423)844-2335

Wellmont Bristol Regional Medical Center
Leonard Breast Cent
1 Medical Park Blvd, Rear
Bristol, TN 37620-7495
(423)844-4585
FAX: (423)844-5609

Camden

Camden General Hospital
175 Hospital Dr
Camden, TN 38320-1617
(731)593-6305
FAX: (731)593-6177

Carthage

Riverview Regional Medical Center
158 Hospital Dr
Carthage, TN 37030-1083
(615)735-5300
FAX: (615)735-5243

Chattanooga

Chattanooga Imaging - East
1710 Gunbarrel Rd
Chattanooga, TN 37421-3127
(423)553-1234
FAX: (423)553-1248

Chattanooga Imaging Downtown
440 N Holtzclaw Ave
Chattanooga, TN 37404-1916
(423)602-5323
FAX: (423)493-9576

Erlanger East Breast Center
1635 Gunbarrel Rd Ste 200
Chattanooga, TN 37421-4985
(423)680-8690
FAX: (423)778-9185

Erlanger Imaging Mammography Center
979 E 3rd St
Chattanooga, TN 37403-2136
(423)778-6494
FAX: (423)778-2902

Erlanger North Breast Center
632 Morrison Springs Rd
Chattanooga, TN 37415-3498
(423)778-3399
FAX: (423)778-3372

Mary Ellen Locher Breast Center At Memorial Hospital
605 Glenwood Dr, Ste 100
Chattanooga, TN 37404-1122
(423)495-4040
FAX: (423)495-4646

Parkridge Medical Center, Inc. Dba Parkridge Medical Center
2333 McCallie Ave
Chattanooga, TN 37404-3258
(423)493-6703
FAX: (423)697-4033

Prime Imaging And Vein Center
1604 Gunbarrel Rd
Chattanooga, TN 37421-3125
(423)893-7226
FAX: (423)893-7398

Prime Imaging Chattanooga Outpatient Ctr.
1301 McCallie Ave
Chattanooga, TN 37404-2934
(423)622-4700
FAX: (423)624-1557

Women's Health Services, Chattanooga, P.C.
6229 Vance Rd Ste 119
Chattanooga, TN 37421-0311
(423)296-8171
FAX: (423)826-2205

Clarksville

Premier Medical Group, P.C.
490 Dunlop Ln
Clarksville, TN 37040-5007
(931)245-7000
FAX: (931)245-8663

Tennova Healthcare-Clarksville
651 Dunlop Ln, Bhc
Clarksville, TN 37040-5015
(931)502-1180
FAX: (931)502-1515

Cleveland

Cleveland Imaging
2253 Chambliss Ave NW Ste 102
Cleveland, TN 37311-3963
(423)553-1234
FAX: (423)478-0105

Tennova Healthcare-Cleveland
2800 Westside Dr NW
Cleveland, TN 37312-3501
(423)339-4281
FAX: (423)478-2396

Tennova Primary Care-Peerless
1060 Peerless Xing NW Ste 200
Cleveland, TN 37312-3785
(423)479-4165
FAX: (423)648-5473

Collierville

Baptist Collierville
1500 W Poplar Ave
Collierville, TN 38017-0601
(901)861-8807
FAX: (901)861-8804

Columbia

Maury Regional Women's Center
1220 Trotwood Ave, Ste 401
Columbia, TN 38401-6416
(931)381-1111
FAX: (931)540-4313

Cookeville

Cookeville Regional Medical Ctr Out Patient Imaging Ctr
251 W 3rd St
Cookeville, TN 38501-2463
(931)783-2468
FAX: (931)783-2806

Premier Diagnostic Imaging, L.L.C.
315 N Washington Ave Ste 103
Cookeville, TN 38501-2623
(931)528-1800
FAX: (931)528-8112

Covington

Baptist Memorial Hospital - Tipton
1995 Highway 51 S
Covington, TN 38019-3635
(901)475-5333
FAX: (901)475-5459

Crossville

Cmc Medical Arts Building At Fairfield Glade
132 Stonehenge Dr
Crossville, TN 38558-6279
(931)459-7040
FAX: (931)210-5089

Cumberland Medical Center
421 S Main St
Crossville, TN 38555-5031
(931)459-7368
FAX: (931)210-5024

Dayton

Rhea Medical Center
9400 Rhea County Hwy Ste 1
Dayton, TN 37321-7922
(423)775-8636
FAX: (423)843-4593

Dickson

Dickson Medical Associates
127 Crestview Park Dr, Ste 104
Dickson, TN 37055-2854
(615)441-4550
FAX: (615)441-4561

Horizon Medical Center Dba Natchez Imaging Center
101 Natchez Park Dr
Dickson, TN 37055-9013
(615)326-2910
FAX: (615)326-2932

Dyersburg

West Tennessee Healthcare Dyersburg Hospital
400 E Tickle St
Dyersburg, TN 38024-3120
(731)287-3668
FAX: (731)287-2187

East Ridge

Parkridge East Hospital
941 Spring Creek Rd
East Ridge, TN 37412-3909
(423)493-1271
FAX: (423)493-1794

Elizabethton

Ballad Health Dba Sycamore Shoals Hospital
1501 W Elk Ave
Elizabethton, TN 37643-2854
(423)542-1289
FAX: (423)542-1293

Medical Care Pllc
1500 W Elk Ave, Ste 101
Elizabethton, TN 37643-2655
(426)929-2584
FAX: (423)722-2060

Erwin

Unicoi County Hospital
2030 Temple Hill Rd
Erwin, TN 37650-8721
(423)735-4761
FAX: (423)735-4745

Fayetteville

Lincoln Medical Center
106 Medical Center Blvd
Fayetteville, TN 37334-2684
(931)438-7492
FAX: (931)438-7497

Franklin

Premier Radiology Cool Springs
3310 Aspen Grove Dr Ste 101
Franklin, TN 37067-2851
(615)771-0171
FAX: (615)234-1501

Vanderbilt Franklin Womens Ctr
4155 Carothers Pkwy
Franklin, TN 37067-5905
(615)322-2064
FAX: (615)343-0746

Williamson Imaging Llc Dba Cool Springs Imaging
2009 Mallory Ln Ste 150
Franklin, TN 37067-2872
(615)771-8668
FAX: (615)771-9298

Williamson Medical Ctr OP Imaging
4601 Carothers Pkwy
Franklin, TN 37067-5976
(615)435-5022
FAX: (615)595-4590

Gallatin

Imaging For Women At Sumner Station A Dept Of Srmc
225 Big Station Camp Blvd
Gallatin, TN 37066-8464
(615)328-6500
FAX: (615)328-6525

Premier Radiology Gallatin
110 Saint Blaise Rd Ste 102
Gallatin, TN 37066-4442
(615)467-4640
FAX: (615)467-4641

Germantown

Diagnostic Ultrasound Consultants, P.C.
2120 S Germantown Rd
Germantown, TN 38138-3804
(901)755-5562
FAX: (901)755-5143

Margaret West Comprehensive Breast Center
7945 Wolf River Blvd Ste 170
Germantown, TN 38138-1762
(901)683-0055
FAX: (901)682-9600

McDonald Murrmann Center For Wellness And Health
7205 Wolf River Blvd Ste 150
Germantown, TN 38138-1776
(901)752-4000
FAX: (877)208-9036

Memphis Obgyn Association, P.C.
7705 Poplar Ave, Ste 340
Germantown, TN 38138-3930
(901)755-8696
FAX: (901)755-7232

Methodist Comprehensive Breast Center
1381 S Germantown Rd
Germantown, TN 38138-2225
(901)516-9000
FAX: (901)922-6797

Women's Health Specialists Pllc
7800 Wolf Trail Cv
Germantown, TN 38138-1753
(901)682-9222
FAX: (901)682-9505

Greeneville

Greeneville Community Hospital-East Campus
1420 Tusculum Blvd
Greeneville, TN 37745-4279
(423)787-5123
FAX: (423)787-5141

Harriman

Roane Medical Center
8045 Roane Medical Center Dr
Harriman, TN 37748-8333
(865)316-2304
FAX: (865)316-3727

Hendersonville

Premier Radiology Hendersonville
262 New Shackle Island Rd Ste 206
Hendersonville, TN 37075-2489
(615)986-6050
FAX: (615)234-1529

Tristar Women's Imaging At Hendersonville
201 N Anderson Ln Ste 100
Hendersonville, TN 37075-6939
(615)338-1486
FAX: (615)338-1481

Hermitage

Heritage Medical Associates
5653 Frist Blvd, Ste 630
Hermitage, TN 37076-2094
(629)255-3303
FAX: (629)255-3978

Premier Radiology Hermitage
5045 Old Hickory Blvd Ste 101
Hermitage, TN 37076-2581
(615)884-7674
FAX: (615)234-1507

Tristar Summit Medical Center - Women's Imaging
3901 Central Pike Ste 154
Hermitage, TN 37076-3485
(615)695-7229
FAX: (615)316-3905

Hixson

Chattanooga Imaging Hixson
2070 Hamill Rd
Hixson, TN 37343-4027
(423)553-1234
FAX: (423)643-4712

Maryellen Locher Breast Center Hixson
5022 Old Godsey Ln, Ste 8
Hixson, TN 37343-6604
(423)495-4040
FAX: (423)495-4646

Prime Imaging Hixson
5441 Highway 153 Ste 103
Hixson, TN 37343-3702
(423)591-7226
FAX: (423)591-7227

Hohenwald

Lewis Health Center
617 W Main St
Hohenwald, TN 38462-1355
(931)796-6222
FAX: (931)796-6264

Huntingdon

Baptist Memorial Hospital - Carroll County
631 Rb Wilson Dr, Radiology Department
Huntingdon, TN 38344-1727
(731)986-7252
FAX: (731)986-7064

Jackson

Pink Ribbon Mammography Woman's Clinic
244 Coatsland Dr
Jackson, TN 38301-3948
(731)422-4642
FAX: (731)422-2277

The Jackson Clinic North
2863 Highway 45 Byp
Jackson, TN 38305-3618
(731)422-0213
FAX: (731)422-0329

West Tennessee Healthcare North Hospital
367 Hospital Blvd, Radiology Department
Jackson, TN 38305-2080
(731)661-2140
FAX: (731)661-2457

West Tennessee Imaging Center
300 Coatsland Dr
Jackson, TN 38301-3908
(731)541-8301
FAX: (731)541-8667

Jasper

Parkridge West Hospital
1000 Highway 28
Jasper, TN 37347-3638
(423)837-9445
FAX: (423)837-3469

Jefferson City

Jefferson County Hma, Llc
110 Hospital Dr
Jefferson City, TN 37760-5281
(865)471-2650
FAX: (865)471-2484

Johnson City

Johnson City Community Health Center
2151 Century Ln
Johnson City, TN 37604-4469
(423)929-6937
FAX: (423)926-5999

Medical Care, Pllc
401 E Main St, Ste 1
Johnson City, TN 37601-4891
(423)431-0315
FAX: (423)722-2060

Outpatient Diagnostic Center At Johnson City Center
3019 Peoples St
Johnson City, TN 37604-1977
(423)461-2150
FAX: (423)461-2151

State Of Franklin Healthcare Assocs Comprehensive Breast Ctr
818 Sunset Dr, Ste 100
Johnson City, TN 37604-8310
(423)202-6347
FAX: (423)232-8575

Women's Health & Imaging Center
200 Med Tech Pkwy Ste 10
Johnson City, TN 37604-2278
(423)979-3888
FAX: (423)979-3864

Kingsport

Ballad Health Coach - Mobile
1905 American Way
Kingsport, TN 37660-5882
(423)723-6877
FAX: (423)230-8179

Comprehensive Breast Center At Balladhealth Hv OP Center
103 W Stone Dr
Kingsport, TN 37660-3220
(423)224-5312
FAX: (423)224-5747

Outpatient Diagnostic Center At Meadowview Lane
2033 Meadowview Ln, Outpatient Diagnostic Center
Kingsport, TN 37660-7569
(423)857-2800
FAX: (423)857-2801

Women's Diagnostic Center At Indian Path Hospital
2002 Brookside Dr Ste 100
Kingsport, TN 37660-4634
(423)431-1709
FAX: (423)857-6069

Knoxville

Abercrombie Radiological Consultants
1112 E Weisgarber Rd
Knoxville, TN 37909-2620
(865)584-3444
FAX: (865)824-0038

Fort Sanders Obstetrical & Gynecological Group Pc
501 19th St Ste 509
Knoxville, TN 37916-1874
(865)524-3208
FAX: (877)441-7836

Ft Sanders West Diag Ctr Div Of Ft Sanders Regional Med Ctr
210 Fort Sanders West Blvd, Bldg 3 Suite 100
Knoxville, TN 37922-3355
(865)531-5400
FAX: (865)531-5043

Knoxville Comprehensive Breast Ctr.
1400 Dowell Springs Blvd Ste 200
Knoxville, TN 37909-2457
(865)584-0291
FAX: (865)584-4426

Knoxville West Center For Breast Health
9330 Park West Blvd Ste 302
Knoxville, TN 37923-4311
(865)531-5878
FAX: (865)531-5856

Parkwest Comprehensive Breast Center
9330 Park West Blvd, Ste 103
Knoxville, TN 37923-4309
(865)373-7010
FAX: (865)373-7021

Summit Diagnostic Imaging Center - Cedar Bluff
9333 Park West Blvd Ste 102
Knoxville, TN 37923-4305
(865)531-9457
FAX: (865)694-0846

Summit Diagnostic Imaging Center - Ft. City
103 Midlake Dr, Lower Level
Knoxville, TN 37918-3002
(865)688-8993
FAX: (865)688-7858

Summit Diagnostic Imaging Center - Wellington
7211 Wellington Dr, Lowr Level Ste 101
Knoxville, TN 37919-5968
(865)588-8005
FAX: (865)588-5305

Tennova Ambulatory Care Center South
7323 Chapman Hwy Ste 190
Knoxville, TN 37920-6757
(865)545-7771
FAX: (865)859-7301

Tennova Women's Imaging Ctr. At Turkey Creek Med. Ctr.
10820 Parkside Dr
Knoxville, TN 37934-1956
(865)545-7771
FAX: (865)218-6040

Thompson Comprehensive Breast Center
1915 White Ave, Dept. Of Fort Sanders Regional Medical C
Knoxville, TN 37916-2300
(865)331-1624
FAX: (865)331-1001

University Breast Center
1926 Alcoa Hwy Ste 120, Medical Bldg F
Knoxville, TN 37920-1558
(865)305-9729
FAX: (865)305-8869

University Breast Center - Mobile
1926 Alcoa Hwy Bldg F Ste 120
Knoxville, TN 37920-1545
(865)305-8850
FAX: (865)305-8869

University Breast Center At Northshore Town Center
1975 Town Center Blvd Ste 201
Knoxville, TN 37922-6669
(865)305-9069
FAX: (865)305-8869

Lafayette

Macon Community Hospital
305 W Locust St
Lafayette, TN 37083-1712
(615)688-7909
FAX: (615)666-2109

Lafollette

Campbell County Hma, Llc D/B/A Tennova Healthcare-Lafollette
923 E Central Ave
Lafollette, TN 37766-2768
(423)907-1200
FAX: (423)907-1536

Lawrenceburg

Southern Tennessee Regional Health System Lawrenceburg
1607 S Locust Ave, US Highway 43 South
Lawrenceburg, TN 38464-4011
(931)766-3100
FAX: (931)766-3348

Lebanon

Summit Imaging At Lebanon
100 Physicians Way Ste 100
Lebanon, TN 37090-8107
(615)695-7229
FAX: (615)316-3905

Vanderbilt Wilson County Hospital
1411 W Baddour Pkwy
Lebanon, TN 37087-2513
(615)449-8621
FAX: (615)443-2549

Lenoir City

Fort Loudoun Medical Center
550 Fort Loudoun Medical Center Dr
Lenoir City, TN 37772-5686
(865)271-6070
FAX: (865)271-6208

Lewisburg

Marshall Medical Center
1080 N Ellington Pkwy
Lewisburg, TN 37091-2227
(931)359-6241
FAX: (931)270-3613

Lexington

Henderson Co Community Hosp Lexington Tennessee
200 W Church St
Lexington, TN 38351-2038
(731)968-3646
FAX: (731)968-1898

Livingston

Livingston Regional Hospital
315 Oak St
Livingston, TN 38570-1734
(931)403-2333
FAX: (931)403-2343

Madison

Premier Radiology Briarville
1210 Briarville Rd, Bldg F Suite 602
Madison, TN 37115-5136
(615)884-7674
FAX: (615)234-1507

Manchester

Unity Medical Center
482 Interstate Dr
Manchester, TN 37355-3485
(931)450-1105
FAX: (931)728-3601

Martin

Wth Volunteer Hospital
161 Mount Pelia Rd
Martin, TN 38237-3811
(731)588-3224
FAX: (731)588-3239

Maryville

Blount Breast Health Center Blount Memorial Hospital
907 E Lamar Alexander Pkwy
Maryville, TN 37804-5015
(865)977-5590
FAX: (865)980-4950

Tennessee Breast Center, Inc
1111 E Lamar Alexander Pkwy
Maryville, TN 37804-5130
(865)984-9282
FAX: (865)981-1716

Mc Kenzie

Baptist Memorial Hospital Carroll County, OP Diagnostic Cent
205A Hospital Dr
Mc Kenzie, TN 38201-1649
(731)393-7044
FAX: (731)352-6668

McMinnville

Saint Thomas River Park Hospital
1559 Sparta St
McMinnville, TN 37110-1316
(931)815-4485
FAX: (931)815-4491

Memphis

Baptist Memorial Hospital For Women - Mobile
50 Humphreys Center Dr Ste 23
Memphis, TN 38120-2369
(901)227-7465
FAX: (901)226-0835

Baptist Womens Health Center
50 Humphreys Center Dr Ste 23
Memphis, TN 38120-2369
(901)227-7465
FAX: (901)226-0835

Diagnostic Imaging, P.C.
6401 Poplar Ave Ste 100
Memphis, TN 38119-4840
(901)387-2340
FAX: (901)680-1928

Diagnostic Ultrasound Consultants, P.C.
1325 Eastmoreland Ave Ste 545
Memphis, TN 38104-7510
(901)516-8970
FAX: (901)274-6600

Diagnostic Ultrasound Consultants, P.C.
4274 Faronia Rd
Memphis, TN 38116-6500
(901)346-3058
FAX: (901)346-3057

Lifesigns Prevention Group
1727 Kirby Pkwy Ste 100
Memphis, TN 38120-4335
(901)685-5520
FAX: (901)685-0782

Memphis Health Center, Inc.
360 E Eh Crump Blvd
Memphis, TN 38126-5394
(901)261-2000
FAX: (901)853-7881

Memphis Ob-Gyn Associates Pc
6215 Humphreys Blvd Ste 401
Memphis, TN 38120-2382
(901)767-8442
FAX: (901)684-6260

Methodist Diagnostic Center
1801 Union Ave
Memphis, TN 38104-3942
(901)516-9000
FAX: (901)722-3125

Methodist Hospital - South
1300 Wesley Dr
Memphis, TN 38116-6499
(901)516-3805
FAX: (901)516-3183

Methodist Hospital North Radiology
3960 New Covington Pike, Department Of Radiology
Memphis, TN 38128-2589
(901)516-9000
FAX: (901)516-5581

Mroz-Baier Breast Care Clinic
6005 Park Ave, 700 Loewenberg Building
Memphis, TN 38119-5202
(901)527-3391
FAX: (901)578-3969

Park Avenue Diagnostic Center
5190 Park Ave
Memphis, TN 38119-3544
(901)767-0505
FAX: (901)761-1335

Regional One Health
877 Jefferson Ave
Memphis, TN 38103-2807
(901)545-7228
FAX: (901)545-8806

Regional One Health East
6555 Quince Rd
Memphis, TN 38119-8202
(901)515-3610
FAX: (901)515-3637

St. Francis Hospital Women Center
5959 Park Ave
Memphis, TN 38119-5198
(901)765-3279
FAX: (901)765-3241

Women's Care Center Of Memphis
6215 Humphreys Blvd Ste 501
Memphis, TN 38120-2384
(901)763-2212
FAX: (901)685-9273

Milan

Milan General Hospital
4039 Highland St
Milan, TN 38358-3493
(731)723-1379
FAX: (731)723-3464

Morristown

Healthstar Physicians, P.C.
420 W Morris Blvd Ste 400-H
Morristown, TN 37813-2283
(423)586-4545
FAX: (423)587-8899

Mhhs Dba Morristown Regional Diagnostic Center
901 W 4th North St
Morristown, TN 37814-3814
(423)492-9001
FAX: (423)492-6501

Mountain City

Johnson County Community Hospital
1901 S Shady St
Mountain City, TN 37683-2021
(423)727-1101
FAX: (423)727-1125

Mt Juliet

Premier Radiology Mt Juliet
5002 Crossings Cir Ste 140
Mt Juliet, TN 37122-8498
(615)773-7237
FAX: (615)773-1250

Summit Imaging Center In Mt. Juliet
660 S Mount Juliet Rd, Ste 110
Mt Juliet, TN 37122-3968
(615)514-6460
FAX: (615)514-6509

Murfreesboro

Center For Diagnostic Imaging
1001 N Highland Ave
Murfreesboro, TN 37130-2450
(615)890-8999
FAX: (615)890-6053

Middle Tennessee Imaging - Murfreesboro
1840 Medical Center Pkwy Ste 101
Murfreesboro, TN 37129-3237
(615)896-1234
FAX: (615)896-7171

Murfreesboro Medical Clinic & Surgicenter
1272 Garrison Dr, Ste 303
Murfreesboro, TN 37129-0053
(615)867-8150
FAX: (615)867-8168

Premier Radiology New Salem
2723 New Salem Hwy
Murfreesboro, TN 37128-5253
(615)986-6055
FAX: (615)234-1508

Sanitas Medical Center Of Tennessee - Murfreesboro
1648 Memorial Blvd
Murfreesboro, TN 37129-2104
(615)527-4568
FAX: (877)592-0884

Nashville

Hca Health Srv Of Tn Inc Dba Tristar Centennial Med Ctr
330 23rd Ave N Ste 200
Nashville, TN 37203-1536
(615)342-5006
FAX: (615)342-5009

Heritage Medical Associates
222 22nd Ave N, Ste 100
Nashville, TN 37203-1870
(629)255-3303
FAX: (615)284-2257

Matthew Walker Comprehensive Health Center
1035 14th Ave N
Nashville, TN 37208-3050
(615)340-1285
FAX: (615)320-9437

Meharry Med. College Ctr For Women's Hlth Research
1005 Dr Db Todd Jr Blvd, Meharry Medical College
Nashville, TN 37208-3501
(615)963-3133
FAX: (615)963-3129

Nashville General Hospital At Meharry
1818 Albion St
Nashville, TN 37208-2918
(615)341-4181
FAX: (615)341-4439

One Hundred Oaks Imaging North
719 Thompson Ln, Ste 20920
Nashville, TN 37204-3609
(615)936-3606
FAX: (615)322-0433

Outpatient Diagnostic Center Of Nashville
337 22nd Ave N
Nashville, TN 37203-1840
(615)327-1500
FAX: (615)327-1421

Premier Radiology Belle Meade
28 White Bridge Pike, Ste 111
Nashville, TN 37205-1466
(615)356-3999
FAX: (615)353-0462

Premier Radiology Bellevue
5700 Temple Rd, Ste 102
Nashville, TN 37221-4224
(615)986-5993
FAX: (615)234-1522

Premier Radiology Lenox Village
6130 Nolensville Pike, Ste 102
Nashville, TN 37211-6813
(615)986-7026
FAX: (615)234-1510

Premier Radiology Nashville
1800 Charlotte Ave
Nashville, TN 37203-2105
(615)329-4840
FAX: (615)986-6407

Solis Mammography At Skyline Medical Center, Llc
3443 Dickerson Pike, Ste 260
Nashville, TN 37207-2534
(615)760-0511
FAX: (615)769-2484

St Thomas Medical Partners - Our Mission In Motion Mobile
460 Metroplex Dr, Ste 115
Nashville, TN 37211-3136
(615)284-6266
FAX: (615)333-3661

St. Thomas West Hospital Center For Breast Health
4220 Harding Pike
Nashville, TN 37205-2005
(615)222-3456
FAX: (615)222-6273

St.Thomas Midtown Hospital Center For Breast Health
2004 Hayes St Ste 150 Suite
Nashville, TN 37203-2652
(615)284-5000
FAX: (615)284-5980

Tristar Southern Hills Medical Center
510 Recovery Rd Ste 101
Nashville, TN 37211-4874
(615)695-7226
FAX: (866)578-9720

Vanderbilt Breast Center At Tvc
1301 Medical Center Dr Ste 1638B
Nashville, TN 37232-0028
(615)322-8651
FAX: (615)936-2590

Vanderbilt Health One Hundred Oaks Breast Center
719 Thompson Ln Ste 25000
Nashville, TN 37204-4683
(615)322-2064
FAX: (615)343-0746

Newport

Newport Medical Center
435 2nd St
Newport, TN 37821-3703
(423)625-2191
FAX: (423)625-2184

Oak Ridge

Oak Ridge Breast Ctr A Div Of Methodist Med Ctr
944 Oak Ridge Tpke Ste 300
Oak Ridge, TN 37830-6960
(865)835-3760
FAX: (865)835-3761

Ooltewah

Chattanooga Imaging Ooltewah
9368 Bradmore Ln
Ooltewah, TN 37363-4445
(423)553-1234
FAX: (423)553-1235

Maryellen Locher Breast Imaging Ctr Memorial Ooltewah
6400 Mountain View Rd Ste 100
Ooltewah, TN 37363
(423)495-4040
FAX: (423)495-4646

Paris

Henry County Diagnostic Center
302 Tyson Ave Ste A
Paris, TN 38242-4555
(731)644-8486
FAX: (731)644-8488

Pikeville

Erlanger Bledsoe Hospital
71 Wheelertown Ave
Pikeville, TN 37367-5246
(423)447-5311
FAX: (423)447-5284

Powell

Tennova Women's Ctr North Knoxville Med Ctr
7551 Dannaher Dr
Powell, TN 37849-4029
(865)859-7089
FAX: (865)859-7303

Pulaski

Southern Tennessee Regional Health System Pulaski
1265 E College St, Mammography Department
Pulaski, TN 38478-4541
(931)363-9314
FAX: (931)363-9398

Rogersville

Ballad Health
851 Locust St
Rogersville, TN 37857-2407
(423)921-7240
FAX: (423)921-7179

Savannah

Hardin Medical Center
935 Wayne Rd
Savannah, TN 38372-1904
(731)926-8161
FAX: (731)926-8320

Selmer

Prime Care Medical Center
270 E Court Ave
Selmer, TN 38375-2304
(731)645-7932
FAX: (731)645-5195

Sevierville

Leconte Medical Center
742 Middle Creek Rd
Sevierville, TN 37862-5019
(865)446-8000
FAX: (865)446-8014

Shelbyville

Vanderbilt Bedford Hospital
2835 Highway 231 N
Shelbyville, TN 37160-7327
(931)685-8305
FAX: (931)685-8306

Smithville

Saint Thomas Dekalb Hospital
520 W Main St
Smithville, TN 37166-1138
(615)215-5530
FAX: (615)215-5613

Smyrna

Center For Diagnostic Imaging
537 Stonecrest Pkwy Ste 102
Smyrna, TN 37167-6887
(615)890-8999
FAX: (615)890-6053

Premier Radiology Smyrna
741 President Pl Ste 100
Smyrna, TN 37167-6808
(615)220-0674
FAX: (615)355-4348

Solis Mammography At Stonecrest Medical Center, Llc
537 Stonecrest Pkwy Ste 202
Smyrna, TN 37167-6896
(615)768-2368
FAX: (615)625-0058

Sparta

Saint Thomas Highlands Hospital
401 Sewell Dr, Radiology Department
Sparta, TN 38583-1223
(931)738-4173
FAX: (931)738-9224

Spring Hill

Spring Hill Imaging Center, Llc
5421 Main St, Ste 3 Ste C
Spring Hill, TN 37174-4411
(931)486-3425
FAX: (931)489-5844

Springfield

Northcrest Medical Center
100 Northcrest Dr
Springfield, TN 37172-3961
(615)382-6068
FAX: (615)382-3888

Sweetwater

Sweetwater Hospital Association
304 Church St
Sweetwater, TN 37874-2897
(865)213-8547
FAX: (865)213-8482

Tazewell

Claiborne Medical Center
1850 Old Knoxville Rd
Tazewell, TN 37879-3601
(423)526-2370
FAX: (423)626-8080

Tullahoma

Tullahoma Imaging D/B/A Cumberland Radiation Assoc., Llc
2114 N Jackson St, Ste B
Tullahoma, TN 37388-2208
(931)454-9002
FAX: (931)454-9690

Vanderbilt Coffee Hospital, Llc
1801 N Jackson St
Tullahoma, TN 37388-8259
(931)461-4800
FAX: (931)461-4900

Union City

Baptist Memorial Hospital - Union City
1201 Bishop St, Radiology Dept.
Union City, TN 38261-5403
(731)884-8550
FAX: (731)884-8785

Waverly

Three Rivers Hospital
PO Box 437, 451 Highway 13 S
Waverly, TN 37185-0437
(931)296-0298
FAX: (931)296-9074

Waynesboro

Wayne Medical Center
103 Jv Mangubat Dr, Highway 64 E
Waynesboro, TN 38485-2440
(931)722-2060
FAX: (931)722-2015

Winchester

Woman's Center Of Strhs-Winchester
183 Hospital Rd Ste C, A.R. Fite Professional Bldg
Winchester, TN 37398-2471
(931)967-8258
FAX: (931)967-8219

Woodbury

Saint Thomas Stones River Hospital
324 Doolittle Rd
Woodbury, TN 37190-1139
(615)563-7229
FAX: (615)563-7283

TEXAS

Abilene

Hendrick Medical Center
6250 US Highway 83, 6250 Hwy 83-84
Abilene, TX 79606-5215
(325)428-1380
FAX: (325)428-1399

Hendrick Medical Center
1850 Hickory St, Ste 203
Abilene, TX 79601-2305
(325)670-2600
FAX: (325)670-2637

Alice

Radiology Associates, L.L.P.
2000 Dr N W Atkinson Blvd, Ste 801
Alice, TX 78332-4241
(361)887-7000
FAX: (361)561-3185

Allen

North Star Mri, Lp
997 Raintree Cir, Ste 110
Allen, TX 75013-4952
(972)649-6460
FAX: (972)649-6461

Texas Health Presbyterian Hospital Allen
1105 Central Expy N Ste 210
Allen, TX 75013-6102
(972)747-6000
FAX: (972)747-6002

Amarillo

Bsa Hospital, Llc
1310 Wallace Blvd, Dba Harrington Breast Center
Amarillo, TX 79106-1745
(806)356-1905
FAX: (806)352-9240

Northwest Texas Healthcare Systems, Inc.
1501 S Coulter St
Amarillo, TX 79106-1770
(806)351-6266
FAX: (806)351-6269

Panhandle Obstetrics And Gynecology, Pllc
7620 Wallace Blvd
Amarillo, TX 79124-2154
(806)359-5468
FAX: (806)358-1162

Texas Oncology, P.A. Dba Texas Breast Specialists
1000 S Coulter St
Amarillo, TX 79106-1781
(806)457-2060
FAX: (806)457-2061

Womens Healthcare Associates Pllc
1301 S Coulter St, Ste 205
Amarillo, TX 79106-1765
(806)355-6330
FAX: (806)457-2262

Andrews

Permian Regional Medical Center
720 Hospital Dr
Andrews, TX 79714-3617
(432)464-2152
FAX: (432)523-2609

Angleton

University Of Texas Medical Branch
132 E Hospital Dr, Dba Utmb Health Angleton Danbury Campus
Angleton, TX 77515-4112
(979)848-9160
FAX: (979)849-1292

Anna

Uhs Of Texoma
2710 W Hackberry Ln
Anna, TX 75409-2573
(214)831-2630
FAX: (214)831-2631

Arlington

Btdi Jv, Llp Dba Touchstone Imaging Arlington Breast Center
4501 Matlock Rd Ste 101
Arlington, TX 76018-1004
(817)472-0801
FAX: (817)472-0840

Envision Imaging Of North Arlington
801 Road To Six Flags W Ste 106
Arlington, TX 76012-2615
(817)265-1099
FAX: (817)317-7062

Envision Imaging Of South Arlington
4601 Matlock Rd
Arlington, TX 76018-1005
(817)375-3170
FAX: (817)375-3185

Medical Clinic Of North Texas, Pllc
811 W Interstate 20, Ste 218 Ste G40
Arlington, TX 76017-5873
(817)505-1777
FAX: (817)419-4471

Solis Mammography At Medical Center Of Arlington
515 W Mayfield Rd Ste 100
Arlington, TX 76014-2084
(817)375-9357
FAX: (817)375-0467

Texas Health Arlington Memorial Hospital
810 W Randol Mill Rd, Mammography Center
Arlington, TX 76012-2504
(817)960-6564
FAX: (817)960-6353

Athens

Athens Hospital, Llc
2000 S Palestine St, Dba Ut Health East Texas Athens Hospital
Athens, TX 75751-5610
(903)676-2165
FAX: (903)676-5462

Lakeland Medical Associates
117 Medical Cir
Athens, TX 75751-9003
(903)676-3200
FAX: (903)676-3211

Atlanta

Christus St Michael Hospital - Atlanta
1007 S William St
Atlanta, TX 75551-3245
(903)799-3108
FAX: (903)799-3188

Austin

Ara/St. David's Imaging, L.P.
1701 W Ben White Blvd Ste 170
Austin, TX 78704-7669
(512)453-6100
FAX: (512)836-8869

Ara/St. David's Imaging, L.P.
2501 W William Cannon Dr Bldg 5
Austin, TX 78745-5281
(512)453-6100
FAX: (512)836-8869

Ascension Seton
1201 W 38th St, Dba Ascension Seton Medical Center
Austin, TX 78705-1006
(512)324-1000
FAX: (512)324-1093

Austin Area Breast Imaging Llc
12200 Renfert Way Ste 100
Austin, TX 78758-5654
(512)451-8211
FAX: (512)832-6331

Austin Breast Imaging, Llc
12319 N Mo Pac Expy, Bldg C Ste 320
Austin, TX 78758-2414
(512)776-1000
FAX: (512)399-6360

Austin Breast Imaging, Llc
5815 W William Cannon Dr, Ste 101
Austin, TX 78749-1966
(512)776-1000
FAX: (512)339-6360

Austin Radiological Association
5656 Bee Caves Rd Ste H200
Austin, TX 78746-5236
(512)453-6100
FAX: (572)836-8869

Austin Radiological Association
11714 Wilson Parke Ave Ste 175
Austin, TX 78726-0002
(512)453-6100
FAX: (512)836-8869

Austin Radiological Association
4515 Seton Center Pkwy Ste 105
Austin, TX 78759-5268
(512)453-6100
FAX: (512)836-8869

Austin Radiological Association
6818 Austin Center Blvd, Ste 101
Austin, TX 78731-3199
(512)453-6100
FAX: (512)836-8869

Austin Radiological Association
5625 Eiger Rd Ste 165
Austin, TX 78735-8980
(512)453-6100
FAX: (512)836-8869

Austin Regional Clinic, Pa
3828 S 1st St
Austin, TX 78704-7048
(512)346-6611
FAX: (512)406-7315

Austin Regional Clinic, Pa
6835 Austin Center Blvd
Austin, TX 78731-3189
(512)346-6611
FAX: (512)465-1607

Bsw Medical Centers-Capitol Area, Dba Bsw Medical Ctr-Austin
5245 US Hwy 290
Austin, TX 78735
(512)654-2122
FAX: (254)724-1589

Central Texas Community Health Centers
1210 W Braker Ln, Dba Community Care
Austin, TX 78758-3801
(512)978-9300
FAX: (512)901-9737

Central Texas Community Health Centers
2901 Montopolis Dr, Ste 100
Austin, TX 78741-6411
(512)978-9901
FAX: (512)901-9765

Renaissance Austin Breast Imaging, Llc
12201 Renfert Way, Ste 205
Austin, TX 78758-5392
(512)339-6626
FAX: (512)339-6360

St David's Hlthcare Partnership Lp Llp Dba S Austin Med Ctr
901 W Ben White Blvd
Austin, TX 78704-6903
(512)816-6367
FAX: (512)816-7435

St Davids Healthcare Partnership Lp Llp North Austin Med Ctr
12221 N Mo Pac Expy
Austin, TX 78758-2401
(512)901-8729
FAX: (512)901-3930

St. David's Hlthcare Partnership Llp Dba St David's Med Ctr
900 E 30th St Ste 111
Austin, TX 78705-3378
(512)544-8800
FAX: (512)544-8888

Toga Austin Breast Imaging, Llc
1301 W 38th St, Ste 300
Austin, TX 78705-1013
(512)776-1000
FAX: (512)339-6360

Ut Health Austin
1601 Trinity St, Stop Z0200
Austin, TX 78712-1850
(512)495-5300
FAX: (512)495-5680

Women Partners Austin Breast Imaging, Llc
1305 W 34th St Ste 201, Ste 201
Austin, TX 78705-1923
(512)459-8082
FAX: (512)339-6360

Azle

Texas Health Harris Methodist Hospital Azle
108 Denver Trl, Radiology Department
Azle, TX 76020-3614
(817)444-8640
FAX: (817)444-8738

Ballinger

Ballinger Memorial Hospital District
608 Avenue B
Ballinger, TX 76821-2406
(325)365-4957
FAX: (325)365-3953

Bastrop

Ascension Seton
Dba Ascension Seton Bastrop, 630 Hwy 71 W
Bastrop, TX 78602
(512)304-0334
FAX: (830)693-8734

Bay City

Matagorda Co Hosp District Dba Matagorda Reg Med Ctr
600 Hospital Cir
Bay City, TX 77414-4771
(979)241-5966
FAX: (979)241-5965

Baytown

Altus Women's Center Of Baytown, Lp
1626 W Baker Rd
Baytown, TX 77521-2271
(281)837-7600
FAX: (281)837-7601

Jacinto Mri And Diagnostic Center
2800 Garth Rd
Baytown, TX 77521-3947
(281)427-3700
FAX: (281)425-3899

San Jacinto Methodist Dba Houston Methodist Baytown Hosp
1677 W Baker Rd
Baytown, TX 77521-2422
(346)292-7465
FAX: (346)292-1061

Beaumont

Baptist Hospitals Of Southeast Texas
740 Hospital Dr Ste 140
Beaumont, TX 77701-4670
(409)212-7950
FAX: (409)212-7951

Baptist Hospitals Of Southeast Texas
3282 College St
Beaumont, TX 77701-4610
(409)212-5000

Christus Health Southeast Tx Dba Christus Hosp St. Elizabeth
755 N 11th St Ste 1091
Beaumont, TX 77702-1500
(409)236-7500
FAX: (409)236-8182

Diagnostic Health, Beaumont
3220 Medical Center Dr
Beaumont, TX 77701-4627
(409)838-0033
FAX: (409)951-2472

Winnie Community Hospital, Llp
3405 College St
Beaumont, TX 77701-4613
(409)832-2211
FAX: (409)434-4635

Bedford

Solis Mammography
1615 Hospital Pkwy Ste 108
Bedford, TX 76022-5935
(817)857-2800
FAX: (817)952-1755

Bellaire

The Rose Galleria
6575 West Loop S, Ste 200
Bellaire, TX 77401-3513
(281)484-4708
FAX: (713)668-3173

Bellville

Bellville Medical Center
44 N Cummings St
Bellville, TX 77418-1347
(979)413-7260
FAX: (979)413-7193

Big Spring

Steward Texas Hospital Holdings, Llc
1501 W 11th Pl, Dba scenicmtn medcntr
Asteward family hosp
Big Spring, TX 79720-4119
(432)268-4880
FAX: (432)263-0005

Boerne

Avestee Women's Imaging Center Of Boerne
112 Herff Rd, Ste 350
Boerne, TX 78006-2752
(210)826-2666
FAX: (210)314-7545

South Texas Radiology Imaging Centers
134 Menger Spgs Ste 1110
Boerne, TX 78006-7219
(210)617-9000
FAX: (210)617-9516

Bonham

Fannin County Hospital Authority Dba Tmc Bonham Hopsital
504 Lipscomb St
Bonham, TX 75418-4028
(903)583-8585
FAX: (903)640-7601

Borger

Gpch Llc
100 Medical Dr, Dba Golden Plains Community Hospital
Borger, TX 79007-7579
(806)467-5700
FAX: (806)467-5704

Brady

Heart Of Texas Healthcare System
2008 Nine Rd
Brady, TX 76825-7210
(325)792-3535
FAX: (325)597-2981

Breckenridge

Stephens Memorial Hospital District
200 S Geneva St, Dba Stephens Memorial Hospital
Breckenridge, TX 76424-4799
(254)559-2241
FAX: (254)559-7265

Brenham

Scott & White Clinic Dba Baylor Scott & White - The Brenham
693 N Market St
Brenham, TX 77833-2770
(979)337-5800
FAX: (979)337-5962

Brownsville

Baaxten, Llc
3819 N Expressway, Ste 3 77/83
Brownsville, TX 78520-9510
(956)435-9948
FAX: (956)621-1697

Heart Institute Of Brownsville, Llp
213 Heart Dr
Brownsville, TX 78520-3602
(956)504-3278
FAX: (956)504-3287

McAllen Advanced Medical Imaging, Llc
1260 W Price Rd Bldg B
Brownsville, TX 78520-8655
(956)544-2264
FAX: (956)554-7939

South Texas Neurosurgery Associates
3475 W Alton Gloor Blvd
Brownsville, TX 78520-4474
(956)541-6725
FAX: (956)541-2070

Valley Baptist Medical Center-Brownsville
1040 W Jefferson St
Brownsville, TX 78520-6338
(956)698-5412
FAX: (956)546-3643

Valley Regional Medical Center
100 E Alton Gloor Blvd, Ste 100A A
Brownsville, TX 78526-3354
(956)350-7525
FAX: (956)350-7526

Brownwood

Hendrick Medical Center Brownwood
105 Streckert Dr
Brownwood, TX 76801-5956
(325)641-9498
FAX: (325)641-8290

Bryan

Chi St. Joseph Health Regional Hospital
2722 Osler Blvd
Bryan, TX 77802-2517
(979)485-5004
FAX: (979)704-3336

Burleson

Btdi Jv, Llp Dba Touchstone Imaging Burleson
665 NE Alsbury Blvd
Burleson, TX 76028-2660
(817)447-3443
FAX: (817)447-9094

Solis Women's Health
12500 South Fwy Ste 202
Burleson, TX 76028-7129
(866)717-2551
FAX: (866)366-5798

Texas Health Harris Methodist Hospital Ft Worth
2750 SW Wilshire Blvd, Dba tx health neighborcare
Burleson, TX 76028-8338
(817)782-8020
FAX: (817)782-8035

Texas Health Huguley Inc.
12001 South Fwy Ste 100
Burleson, TX 76028-7214
(817)568-5460
FAX: (817)568-5462

Canton

Mf Hosp Reg Hc Ctr/Dba Christus Mother Frances Hosp. Tyler
18780 I-20
Canton, TX 75103
(903)606-5433
FAX: (903)510-1160

Carrizo Springs

Dimmit Regional Hospital
302 S 5th St, 704 Hospital Dr.
Carrizo Springs, TX 78834-3802
(830)876-2424
FAX: (830)876-3160

Carrollton

Sana Healthcare Carrollton, Llc
4525 N Josey Ln, Dba Carrollton Regional Medical Center
Carrollton, TX 75010-4607
(972)394-3657
FAX: (972)394-5520

Cedar Hill

Solis Mammography Of Cedar Hill, Llc
617 Uptown Blvd Ste 103
Cedar Hill, TX 75104-3510
(214)294-9070
FAX: (469)382-2525

Cedar Park

Austin Radiological Association
12800 W Parmer Ln Ste 200
Cedar Park, TX 78613-7721
(512)453-6100
FAX: (512)836-8869

Cedar Park Health System Lp
1401 Medical Pkwy, Dba Cedar Park Regional Medical Center
Cedar Park, TX 78613-7763
(512)528-7130
FAX: (512)528-7044

Scott & White Hospital - Round Rock
910 E Whitestone Blvd
Cedar Park, TX 78613-9093
(512)260-6154
FAX: (512)260-6115

Childress

Childress County Hospital District
901 US Highway 83 N, Dba Childress Regional Medical Center
Childress, TX 79201-2320
(940)937-9114
FAX: (940)937-9144

Cleburne

Texas Health Harris Methodist Hospital Cleburne
201 Walls Dr, Radiology Dept.
Cleburne, TX 76033-4007
(817)556-5400
FAX: (817)556-4303

Clifton

Bosque County Hospital District
101 Posey Ave, Dba Goodall-Witcher Hospital
Clifton, TX 76634-1289
(254)675-8322
FAX: (254)675-7935

College Station

Baylor Scott & White Medical Center - College Station
800 Scott And White Dr
College Station, TX 77845-6440
(979)207-4281
FAX: (979)207-4283

St. Joseph Regional Health Center
1602 Rock Prairie Rd Ste 2400, Dbachi St. Joseph-Collegestationhospital
College Station, TX 77845-0001
(979)764-5100
FAX: (979)776-2550

The Breast And Imaging Center L.L.C
1602 Rock Prairie Rd, West Bldg Suite 220
College Station, TX 77845-8306
(979)776-5602
FAX: (979)703-1300

Columbus

Columbus Community Hospital
110 Shult Dr
Columbus, TX 78934-3010
(979)493-7604
FAX: (979)732-9242

Comanche

Comanche County Medical Center Company
Dba Comanche County Medical Center, 10201
Highway 16 North
Comanche, TX 76442
(254)879-4900
FAX: (254)879-4989

Conroe

Solis Mammography At Conroe Regional Medical Center
500 Medical Center Blvd, Ste 175
Conroe, TX 77304-2899
(866)717-2551
FAX: (866)366-5798

University Of Texas MD Anderson Cancer Center - Woodlands
100 Fellowship Dr
Conroe, TX 77384-4797
(832)750-2703
FAX: (936)446-5266

Corpus Christi

Bay Area Healthcare Group, Ltd.
7121 S Padre Island Dr, Ste 110
Corpus Christi, TX 78412-4939
(361)761-3430
FAX: (361)761-3764

Naval Health Clinic Corpus Christi
10651 E St
Corpus Christi, TX 78419-5131
(361)961-6101
FAX: (361)961-3468

Ob-Gyn Associates Of Corpus Christi, Llp
5920 Saratoga Blvd Ste 200
Corpus Christi, TX 78414-4105
(361)994-5459
FAX: (361)985-0233

Radiology & Imaging Of South Texas
3226 S Alameda St
Corpus Christi, TX 78404-2508
(361)888-6684
FAX: (361)991-7733

Radiology & Imaging Of South Texas
2825 Spohn Dr S
Corpus Christi, TX 78414-4176
(361)888-8875
FAX: (361)991-9494

Radiology Associates Llp
5742 Spohn Dr
Corpus Christi, TX 78414-4116
(361)887-7000
FAX: (361)561-3185

Radiology Associates, L.L.P.
1812 S Alameda St
Corpus Christi, TX 78404-2933
(361)887-7000
FAX: (361)561-3185

Radiology Associates, Llp
3929 River East Dr
Corpus Christi, TX 78410-5101
(361)561-3000
FAX: (361)767-3427

Corsicana

Navarro Hospital Lp
3201 W State Highway 22, Ste 100
Corsicana, TX 75110-2450
(817)908-4144
FAX: (903)329-9928

Crockett

Crockett Medical Center
1100 E Loop 304
Crockett, TX 75835-1810
(936)545-4616
FAX: (936)545-4550

Cuero

Dewitt Medical District Dba Cuero Regional Hospital
2550 N Esplanade St
Cuero, TX 77954-4736
(361)275-6191
FAX: (361)275-0553

Cypress

Memorial Hermann Health System
27700 Highway 290, Ste 140
Cypress, TX 77433-6767
(346)231-6800
FAX: (346)231-6801

Solis Mammography Of North Cypress, Llc
21216 Northwest Fwy, Ste 220
Cypress, TX 77429-4778
(866)717-2551
FAX: (866)366-5798

Solis Mammography Of Towne Lake
9818 Fry Rd, Ste 100
Cypress, TX 77433-5369
(866)717-2551
FAX: (866)366-5798

Tmh Physician Associates, Pllc
18121 Tuckerton Rd Ste 180
Cypress, TX 77433-7105
(281)737-1830
FAX: (281)737-1831

Dallas

Baylor University Medical Center
3900 Junius St, Dba darlenegcass women imagingcntr junius
Dallas, TX 75246-1629
(214)820-2430
FAX: (214)818-9300

Baylor University Medical Center
9101 N Central Expy, Dba darlenegcass womens imagingcntr-Ndallas
Dallas, TX 75231-5945
(214)820-2430
FAX: (214)818-9300

Btdi Jv, Llp Dba Touchstone Imaging Forest Lane
11617 N Central Expy, Ste 132
Dallas, TX 75243-3853
(214)369-3795
FAX: (866)225-8389

Cooper Medical Imaging, Llp
12200 Preston Rd
Dallas, TX 75230-2223
(972)560-2651
FAX: (972)560-2681

Dallas Medical Center
7 Medical Pkwy
Dallas, TX 75234-7823
(972)406-0266
FAX: (972)888-7292

Envision Imaging Of Dallas
12201 Merit Dr, Ste 100
Dallas, TX 75251-2122
(214)276-0050
FAX: (214)276-0057

Healthtexas Provider Network
3417 Gaston Ave, Ste 660
Dallas, TX 75246-2030
(469)800-9240
FAX: (469)800-9250

Methodist Charlton Medical Center
3500 W Wheatland Rd
Dallas, TX 75237-3460
(214)947-5490
FAX: (214)947-5499

Methodist Hospitals Of Dallas
1441 N Beckley Ave
Dallas, TX 75203-1201
(214)947-2913
FAX: (214)947-2980

North Texas Imaging/Hampton Center Ii, Ltd.
2301 S Hampton Rd, Ste 100
Dallas, TX 75224-1653
(214)333-3600
FAX: (214)333-0300

Parkland Moody Center For Breast Health
5151 Maple Ave., Suite 1A
Dallas, TX 75235
(214)266-3300
FAX: (214)266-3302

Pipeline East Dallas, Llc
9440 Poppy Dr, Ste 100
Dallas, TX 75218-3652
(214)324-6155
FAX: (214)324-6051

Solis Mammography At Medical City Dallas, Llc
7777 Forest Ln Ste C236
Dallas, TX 75230-7514
(866)717-2551
FAX: (866)366-5798

Solis Mammography Of Dallas
6805 W Northwest Hwy, Ste A
Dallas, TX 75225-4202
(972)596-4033
FAX: (469)467-7678

Southeast Dallas Health Center
9202 Elam Rd
Dallas, TX 75217-4199
(214)266-3318
FAX: (214)266-3302

Southwest Diagnostic Imaging Center
8230 Walnut Hill Ln Ste 102
Dallas, TX 75231-4407
(214)345-6905
FAX: (214)345-6230

Texas Health Presbyterian Hospital Dallas
8160 Walnut Hill Ln Ste 108
Dallas, TX 75231-4442
(214)345-1800
FAX: (214)345-1200

Ut Southwestern Medical University Hospital Breast Imaging
2201 Inwood Rd
Dallas, TX 75235-7320
(214)645-9729
FAX: (214)645-2596

Decatur

Decatur Hospital Authority
2000 Ben Merritt Dr, Ste A
Decatur, TX 76234-3848
(940)626-1329
FAX: (940)626-1794

Del Rio

Val Verde Regional Medical Center
801 N Bedell Ave
Del Rio, TX 78840-4112
(830)703-1743
FAX: (830)774-4599

Denison

Uhs Of Texoma Inc.
5004 Pool Rd
Denison, TX 75020-4595
(903)416-3730
FAX: (903)416-4297

Denton

Medical City Obgyn, Pllc
2805 S Mayhill Rd, Dba Caring For Women
Denton, TX 76208-5910
(940)999-5500
FAX: (940)999-5501

Solis Mammography
2660 Scripture St, Ste 220
Denton, TX 76201-4344
(940)999-2269
FAX: (940)483-9550

Solis Mammography At Denton Regional Medical Center
3537 S. I35E, Ste 211
Denton, TX 76210
(866)257-6884
FAX: (940)382-5477

Texas Health Presbyterian Hospital Denton
3000 N Interstate 35
Denton, TX 76201-5199
(940)898-7378
FAX: (940)323-7917

Desoto

Methodist-Cdi D/B/A Center For Diagnostic Imaging
1750 N Hampton Rd
Desoto, TX 75115-2306
(214)420-5400
FAX: (214)420-5401

Dripping Springs

Austin Radiological Association
170 Benney Ln Ste 101
Dripping Springs, TX 78620-5566
(512)453-6100
FAX: (512)776-1170

Dumas

Moore County Hospital District
224 E 2nd St, Radiology Department
Dumas, TX 79029-3808
(806)935-7171
FAX: (806)934-0094

Eagle Lake

Cahrmc, Llc
600 S Austin Rd, Dba Rice Medical Center
Eagle Lake, TX 77434-3202
(979)232-7027
FAX: (979)234-5942

Eagle Pass

Fort Duncan Medical Center, Inc
3333 N Foster Maldonado Blvd
Eagle Pass, TX 78852-5148
(800)465-5585
FAX: (830)872-2868

Eastland

Eastland Memorial Hospital District
304 S Daugherty Ave, Dba Eastland Memorial Hospital
Eastland, TX 76448-2609
(254)629-2601
FAX: (254)629-2825

Edinburg

South Texas Health System Edinburg
1102 W Trenton Rd
Edinburg, TX 78539-9105
(956)388-6730
FAX: (956)388-6030

Weslaco Advanced Medical Imaging, Llc
2616 Cornerstone Blvd
Edinburg, TX 78539-9122
(956)994-1752
FAX: (956)994-8745

Edna

Jackson County Hospital District
1013 S Wells St
Edna, TX 77957-4098
(361)782-7836
FAX: (361)782-5905

El Campo

El Campo Memorial Hospital
303 Sandy Corner Rd
El Campo, TX 77437-9844
(979)543-6251
FAX: (979)578-5245

El Paso

Akumin Imaging Texas, Llc
10501 Gateway Blvd W, Ste 150A
El Paso, TX 79925-7900
(915)544-7300
FAX: (915)544-7301

Akumin Imaging Texas, Llc
2204 Joe Battle Blvd, Ste 107
El Paso, TX 79938-4660
(915)544-7300
FAX: (915)544-7301

Akumin Imaging Texas, Llc
4930 Osborne Dr, Ste H
El Paso, TX 79922-1043
(915)544-7300
FAX: (915)544-7301

Akumin Imaging Texas, Llc
9870 Gateway Blvd N, Ste E
El Paso, TX 79924-4425
(915)544-7300
FAX: (915)544-7301

Desert Imaging Services L.P.
4855 N Mesa St, Ste 130
El Paso, TX 79912-5939
(915)577-0100
FAX: (888)263-4112

Desert Imaging Services, Lp
3080 Joe Battle Blvd
El Paso, TX 79938-2653
(915)577-0100
FAX: (915)532-3876

Desert Imaging Services, Lp
1727 N Lee Trevino Dr
El Paso, TX 79936-4521
(915)577-0100
FAX: (915)532-3876

Desert Imaging Services, Lp
116 W Castellano Dr
El Paso, TX 79912-6170
(915)577-0100
FAX: (915)532-3876

Diagnostic Outpatient Imaging Partnership, Ltd.
1426 George Dieter Dr, Dba Diagnostic Outpatient Imaging Ltd
El Paso, TX 79936-7601
(915)881-1900
FAX: (915)771-9345

Diagnostic Outpatient Imaging Partnership, Ltd.
6065 Montana Ave, Ste A6
El Paso, TX 79925-1837
(915)881-1900
FAX: (915)771-9345

El Paso County Hosp Dist Dba University Med Ctr El Paso/East
1521 Joe Battle Blvd.
El Paso, TX 79936
(915)521-2255
FAX: (915)521-7108

El Paso County Hosp Dist Dba University Med Ctr El Paso/West
6600 Nort Desert Blvd
El Paso, TX 79912
(915)521-2255
FAX: (915)521-7108

El Paso Healthcare System Ltd.
1700 N Oregon St Ste G30, Dba Las Palmas Medical Center
El Paso, TX 79902-3545
(915)521-1183
FAX: (915)599-4069

Professional Radiology, Pllc
10501 Gateway Blvd W, Ste 101
El Paso, TX 79925-7929
(915)225-2480
FAX: (915)315-2481

Salud Y Vida
6974 Gateway Blvd E, Ste F
El Paso, TX 79915-1115
(915)591-2704
FAX: (915)225-0413

Tenet Hospitals Limited
3270 Joe Battle Blvd, Dba the hosp providence breast&Womens
El Paso, TX 79938-2639
(915)832-2874
FAX: (915)832-2557

Tenet Hospitals Ltd Dba Thop Imaging Center Trawood
2400 Trawood Dr, Ste 100
El Paso, TX 79936-4122
(915)577-7777
FAX: (915)577-8081

Thop - Imaging Center West
601 Sunland Park Dr
El Paso, TX 79912-5131
(915)577-8400
FAX: (915)577-8465

University Medical Center Of El Paso
4801 Alberta Ave
El Paso, TX 79905-2707
(915)521-2255
FAX: (915)521-7108

University Medical Center Of El Paso
9839 Kenworthy St
El Paso, TX 79924-4402
(915)521-2255
FAX: (915)521-7108

William Beaumont Army Medical Center
5005 North Piedras St
El Paso, TX 79920
(915)742-1735
FAX: (915)742-1003

Ennis

Prhc - Ennis, Lp Dba Ennis Regional Medical Ctr
2201 W Lampasas St
Ennis, TX 75119-5644
(469)256-2410
FAX: (469)256-2485

Fairfield

Fairfield Hospital District
125 Newman St, Dba Freestone Medical Center
Fairfield, TX 75840-1419
(903)389-1625
FAX: (903)389-1635

Floresville

Connally Memorial Medical Center
499 10th St
Floresville, TX 78114-3175
(830)393-1317
FAX: (830)393-1336

Flower Mound

Flower Mound Hospital Partners, Llc
2560 Central Park Ave, Dba Tx Health Presby Hosp Flower Mound
Flower Mound, TX 75028-1555
(469)322-7744
FAX: (469)322-7858

North Star Fm, Lp
4951 Long Prairie Rd, Ste 105
Flower Mound, TX 75028-2709
(972)649-6460
FAX: (972)649-6461

Solis Mammography Of Flower Mound, Llc
4001 Long Prairie Rd, Ste 115
Flower Mound, TX 75028-1528
(866)717-2551
FAX: (469)630-3984

Forney

Lake Pointe Operating Company L.L.C.
763 E US Highway 80, Ste 120
Forney, TX 75126-8679
(972)520-9002
FAX: (972)520-9520

Fort Hood

Carl R. Darnall Army Medical Center
36065 Santa Fe Ave, Radiology Dept, Mammo Box 145
Fort Hood, TX 76544-5060
(254)553-1448
FAX: (254)287-0515

Fort Worth

Btdi Jv, Llp Dba Touchstone Imaging Fossil Creek
5455 Basswood Blvd Ste 550
Fort Worth, TX 76137-4478
(817)428-5002
FAX: (817)428-8101

Comprehensive Breast Care Ctr Of Tx Dba Solis Womens Health
1250 8th Ave Ste 130
Fort Worth, TX 76104-4156
(866)257-6884
FAX: (817)924-9349

Envision Imaging At Pennsylvania
815 Pennsylvania Ave
Fort Worth, TX 76104-2224
(817)321-0300
FAX: (817)321-0399

Federal Medical Center Carswell
PO Box 27066 J Street, Building 3000
Fort Worth, TX 76127-0066
(817)782-4256
FAX: (817)782-4460

Solis Mammography At Medical Center Of Alliance
3025 N Tarrant Pkwy, Ste 250
Fort Worth, TX 76177-8626
(866)717-2551
FAX: (817)349-6915

Tarrant County Hospital District
1201 S Main St Ste J, Dba Jps Health Network
Fort Worth, TX 76104-4804
(817)702-7484

Texas Health Harris Meth Hosp Fort Worth
1300 W Terrell Ave, Kupferle Breast Center
Fort Worth, TX 76104-2820
(817)820-4800
FAX: (817)820-1896

Touchstone Imaging Downtown Ft. Worth
1701 W Rosedale St
Fort Worth, TX 76104-7425
(817)922-7780
FAX: (817)922-7864

Tx Health Harris Methodist Hosp Alliance
10840 Texas Health Trl, Dba Tx Health Harris Methodist Hospital
Fort Worth, TX 76244-6847
(682)212-5301
FAX: (682)212-9210

Tx Health Harris Methodist Hosp Southwest Ft Worth
6100 Harris Pkwy, Dba Virginia Clay Dorman Breast Carecntr
Fort Worth, TX 76132-4101
(817)433-1780
FAX: (817)433-1796

University Hospital Breast Imaging Services
400 W Magnolia Ave
Fort Worth, TX 76104-7617
(214)645-9729
FAX: (817)924-1182

Usmd - Imaging Center At Clearfork
5450 Clearfork Main St, Ste 110
Fort Worth, TX 76109-3580
(817)505-1777
FAX: (817)510-3690

Fredericksburg

Hill Country Memorial Hospital
808 Reuben St
Fredericksburg, TX 78624-4484
(830)990-6181
FAX: (830)990-2825

Friendswood

Care Connectors Medical Group Associates
1704 Sunmeadow Blvd, Dba Care Connectors Medical Group
Friendswood, TX 77546-6018
(310)927-0919
FAX: (949)402-0042

Frisco

Envision Imaging Of Frisco
3211 Internet Blvd, Ste 120
Frisco, TX 75034-1948
(972)334-0908
FAX: (972)335-0375

North Star Mri Of Frisco, Lp
8501 Wade Blvd, Ste 220
Frisco, TX 75034-5895
(972)649-6460
FAX: (972)649-6461

Solis Mammography
PO Box 1 Suite 220, 5575 Warren Pkwy
Frisco, TX 75034-0001
(214)618-6892
FAX: (214)705-9240

Solis Mammography Of Frisco, Llc
5757 Main St, Ste 102
Frisco, TX 75034-3238
(972)941-4802
FAX: (469)252-1310

Ft Worth

Assured Imaging Women's Wellness Of Southern Arizona- Mobile
5801 Oakbend Trl
Ft Worth, TX 76132-3912
(520)403-3341
FAX: (520)572-7138

Gainesville

Gainesville Community Hospital, Inc.
1900 Hospital Blvd, Dba North Texas Medical Center
Gainesville, TX 76240-3599
(940)665-1751
FAX: (940)612-8241

Galveston

University Of Texas Medical Branch @ Galveston
301 University Blvd
Galveston, TX 77555-5302
(409)772-9179
FAX: (409)772-7120

Garland

Btdi Jv, Llp Dba Touchstone Imaging North Garland
7217 Telecom Pkwy Ste 150
Garland, TX 75044-2204
(972)495-1837
FAX: (972)495-7756

Solis Mammography Of Garland, Llc
4430 Lavon Dr Ste 326
Garland, TX 75040-2974
(972)596-4033
FAX: (972)530-0110

Gatesville

Coryell County Memorial Hospital Authority
1507 W Main St, Dba Coryell Health
Gatesville, TX 76528-1024
(254)248-8251
FAX: (254)248-6210

Utmb / Tdcj Managed Care
1401 State School Rd, Dba Gatesville Unit Breast Imaging Cntr
Gatesville, TX 76599-0001
(254)865-8431
FAX: (254)248-1071

Georgetown

Ara - St. David's Imaging, Lp
3201 S Austin Ave Ste 105
Georgetown, TX 78626-7547
(512)453-6100
FAX: (512)836-8869

Lone Star Circle Of Care
2423 Williams Dr, Ste 109
Georgetown, TX 78628-3269
(512)686-0207
FAX: (512)861-2368

Scott & White Hospital - Round Rock
4945 Williams Dr
Georgetown, TX 78633-2008
(512)819-0500
FAX: (512)819-0504

St. David's Healthcare Partnership, L.P., L.L.P
2000 Scenic Dr
Georgetown, TX 78626-7726
(512)942-4575
FAX: (512)942-4465

Glen Rose

Somervell County Hospital District
1021 Holden St
Glen Rose, TX 76043-4937
(254)897-1432
FAX: (254)897-1412

Gonzales

Gonzales Healthcare Systems
1110 N Sarah Dewitt Dr
Gonzales, TX 78629-3311
(830)672-8499
FAX: (830)672-8479

Graham

Graham Hospital District
1301 Montgomery Rd
Graham, TX 76450-4240
(940)521-5430
FAX: (940)521-5179

Granbury

Lake Granbury Medical Center
1310B Paluxy Rd
Granbury, TX 76048-5655
(866)717-2551
FAX: (866)366-5798

Grand Prairie

Btdi Jv, Llp Dba Touchstone Imaging At Grand Prairie
2740 N State Highway 360 Ste 200
Grand Prairie, TX 75050-6405
(972)579-4480
FAX: (972)579-3909

Solis Mammography Of Grand Prairie, Llc
4927 Lake Ridge Pkwy Ste 150
Grand Prairie, TX 75052-3069
(866)257-6884
FAX: (469)430-4314

Grapevine

Baylor Regional Medical Center At Grapevine
1631 Lancaster Dr, Dbabaylors women imaging cntr grapevine
Grapevine, TX 76051-3586
(817)305-5014
FAX: (817)305-5019

Greenville

Hunt Memorial Hospital District
4215 Joe Ramsey Blvd E, Dba Hunt Regional Medical Center
Greenville, TX 75401-7852
(903)408-5000
FAX: (903)408-5002

Lake Pointe Operating Company, Llc
4400 Interstate Highway 30 W, Dba Baylor S&W Imaging Center Greenville
Greenville, TX 75402-4642
(903)259-3128
FAX: (903)454-3040

Gun Barrel City

Athens Hospital, Llc
100 Municipal Dr, Dba Ut Health East Texas Athens Hospital
Gun Barrel City, TX 75156-3702
(903)713-1520
FAX: (903)713-1529

Hallettsville

Lavaca Hospital District
1400 N Texana St, Dba Lavaca Medical Center
Hallettsville, TX 77964-2021
(361)798-3671
FAX: (361)798-5649

Hamilton

Hamilton County Hospital District
400 N Brown St
Hamilton, TX 76531-1518
(254)386-1536
FAX: (254)386-5012

Harker Heights

Hh / Killeen Health System, Llc
850 W Central Texas Expy, Dba Seton Med Cntr Harker Heights
Harker Heights, TX 76548-1890
(254)680-6201
FAX: (254)680-6380

Harlingen

Baaxten, Llc
2302 S 77 Sunshine Strip, Ste 101
Harlingen, TX 78550-8371
(956)412-2121
FAX: (956)412-2125

Harlingen Medical Center L.P.
5501 S Expressway 77, Dba Harlingen Medical Center
Harlingen, TX 78550-3213
(956)365-1099
FAX: (956)365-1098

Valley Women's Clinic
601 E Sesame Dr
Harlingen, TX 78550-0234
(956)423-4030
FAX: (956)423-9188

Vhs Harlingen Hosp Comp Dba Valley Baptist Med Ctr Harlingen
2101 Pease St
Harlingen, TX 78550-8307
(956)389-6709
FAX: (956)389-6704

Henderson

Henderson Hospital,Llc
300 Wilson St, Dba Ut Health East Tx Henderson Hospital
Henderson, TX 75652-5956
(903)655-6535
FAX: (903)655-3892

Hillsboro

Nhci Of Hillsboro Inc., Dba Hill Regional Hospital
101 Circle Dr
Hillsboro, TX 76645-2670
(254)580-8815
FAX: (254)580-8830

Hondo

Medina Regional Hospital
3100 Avenue E
Hondo, TX 78861-3599
(830)426-7719
FAX: (830)426-7904

Houston

Ad Hospital East, Llc
12890 East Fwy, Dba Advanced Imaging & Breast Center
Houston, TX 77015-5708
(713)848-4790

Ad Hospital East, Llc
4200 Twelve Oaks Dr, Dba River Oakes Hospital And Clinics
Houston, TX 77027-6812
(713)980-7900
FAX: (713)600-1786

Baylor St. Luke's Medical Center
7200 Cambridge St Ste 7A
Houston, TX 77030-4202
(713)798-2181
FAX: (713)798-8717

Chi St. Luke's Health Baylor College Of Medicine Med Center
6624 Fannin, Oquinn Medical Towers, Women's Center 10th Floor
Houston, TX 77030
(832)355-8000
FAX: (832)355-7612

Doctors Hospital 1997, Lp
16750 Red Oak Dr, Dba united memorial medcenter North Hosp
Houston, TX 77090-2543
(281)453-7822
FAX: (832)666-7982

East Side Imaging, Inc.
10912 East Fwy
Houston, TX 77029-1912
(713)451-2900
FAX: (713)451-2103

Gulf Coast Cancer & Diagnostic Center @ South East, Inc.
12811 Beamer Rd
Houston, TX 77089-6140
(713)474-1414
FAX: (713)474-8477

Harris County Hospital District
2525 Holly Hall St A, Dba Ben Taub General Hospital
Houston, TX 77054-4108
(713)566-3474
FAX: (713)566-3476

Harris County Hospital District
4755 Aldine Mail Route Rd, Dba Aldine Health Center
Houston, TX 77039-5934
(281)985-7759
FAX: (832)487-2473

Harris County Hospital District
8901 Boone Rd, Dba El Franco Lee Health Center
Houston, TX 77099-1659
(281)454-0982
FAX: (281)454-0980

Harris County Hospital District
2525 Holly Hall St A, Dba Smith Clinic
Houston, TX 77054-4108
(713)566-3475
FAX: (713)566-3476

Harris County Hospital District
3550 Swingle Rd, Dba Martin Luther King Jr Health Center
Houston, TX 77047-3763
(713)547-1181

Harris County Hospital District
6630 De Moss Dr, Vallbona Health Center
Houston, TX 77074-5004
(713)547-1181

Harris County Hospital District
5656 Kelley St, Dba Lyndon Baines Johnson Hospital
Houston, TX 77026-1967
(713)566-6119
FAX: (713)566-6140

Houston Medical Imaging
9230 Katy Fwy Ste 440
Houston, TX 77055-7468
(713)797-1919
FAX: (713)383-9933

Houston Medical Imaging, Llc.
427 W 20th St, Ste 401
Houston, TX 77008-2430
(713)869-6296
FAX: (713)869-5612

Houston Methodist Clear Lake Hospital
18100 Houston Methodist Dr, Ste 125
Houston, TX 77058-4603
(281)523-3432
FAX: (281)523-2062

Houston Methodist Hospital
6550 Fannin St, Ste 447
Houston, TX 77030-2718
(713)441-7465
FAX: (713)790-3124

Houston Methodist Hospital
2615 Southwest Fwy Ste 110
Houston, TX 77098-4609
(713)441-9740
FAX: (713)790-3119

Houston Methodist West Hospital
18300 Katy Fwy, Ste 125
Houston, TX 77094-1520
(832)522-1234
FAX: (832)522-1031

Houston Methodist Willowbrook Hospital
18220 State Highway 249, Houston Methodist Willowbrook Hospital
Houston, TX 77070-4349
(281)737-1929
FAX: (281)737-4656

Kelsey - Seybold Medical Group, Pllc
1200 McKinney St Ste 473, Radiology Department
Houston, TX 77010-2004
(713)442-1161
FAX: (713)442-2410

Kelsey-Seybold Medical Group, Pllc
15655 Cypress Wood Medical Dr, Ste 100
Houston, TX 77014-1487
(713)442-1161
FAX: (713)442-1176

Kelsey-Seybold Medical Group, Pllc
1111 Augusta Dr
Houston, TX 77057-2209
(713)442-1161
FAX: (713)442-2410

Kelsey-Seybold Medical Group, Pllc
7900 Fannin St Ste 2100
Houston, TX 77054-2935
(713)442-1161
FAX: (713)442-3931

Kelsey-Seybold Medical Group, Pllc
2727 W Holcombe Blvd, 2nd Fl Mammography
Houston, TX 77025-1669
(713)442-0000
FAX: (713)442-3653

Kelsey-Seybold Medical Group, Pllc
10701 Vintage Preserve Pkwy
Houston, TX 77070-2158
(713)442-1589
FAX: (713)442-1557

Kelsey-Seybold Medical Group, Pllc Dba Kelsey-Seybold Clinic
13105 Wortham Center Dr
Houston, TX 77065-5611
(713)442-1589
FAX: (713)442-1551

Life Extension Institute, Inc.
5555 San Felipe St, Ste 800
Houston, TX 77056-2738
(713)622-9900
FAX: (713)622-9931

Medical Clinic Of Houston Llp
1701 Sunset Blvd
Houston, TX 77005-1798
(713)526-5511
FAX: (713)520-4728

Medical Imaging Associates Of America, Pa
1351 Clear Lake City Blvd, Dba Community Imaging At Clear Lake
Houston, TX 77062-2372
(713)344-1514
FAX: (713)344-1433

Memorial Hermann Health System
925 Gessner Rd, Dba Memorial hermann memorial city hospital
Houston, TX 77024-2521
(713)242-3480
FAX: (713)242-2056

Memorial Hermann Health System
6400 Fannin St, Dba Mem Hermann-Hermann Out Pt Img Ctrs
Houston, TX 77030-1521
(713)704-9536
FAX: (713)704-9072

Memorial Hermann Health System
1635 North Loop W, Dba Memorial Hermann Greater Heightshosp
Houston, TX 77008-1532
(713)867-2543
FAX: (713)867-2548

Memorial Hermann Health System
7600 Beechnut St, Dba Memorial Hermann Southwest Hospital
Houston, TX 77074-4302
(713)456-5150
FAX: (713)456-5599

Memorial Hermann Health System
13114 Fm 1960 Rd W, Ste 104
Houston, TX 77065-4296
(281)897-1712
FAX: (281)897-1710

Memorial Hermann Health System
Dba Memorial Hermann Imaging Centers,
11476 Space Center Blvd
Houston, TX 77059
(832)658-5121
FAX: (832)658-5130

Memorial Hermann Health System
2900 Richmond Ave, Dba Memorial Hermann Imaging Centers
Houston, TX 77098-3106
(713)363-2471
FAX: (713)807-7039

Memorial Hermann Hlth Sys Dba Memorial Hermann Se Hospital
11800 Astoria Blvd
Houston, TX 77089-6041
(281)929-4478
FAX: (281)929-6340

Memorial Mri & Diagnostic, Llc
9434 Katy Fwy Ste 408
Houston, TX 77055-6309
(713)461-3399

One Step Diagnostic Iv, Lp
2051 Greenhouse Rd, Ste 100
Houston, TX 77084-7858
(281)492-2400
FAX: (281)492-2427

SJ Medical Ctr Llc Dba St Joseph Medical Center
1401 St Joseph Pkwy
Houston, TX 77002-8301
(713)757-7416
FAX: (713)757-7559

Solis Mammography At The Woman's Hospital Of Texas, Llc
7400 Fannin St
Houston, TX 77054-1920
(866)717-2551
FAX: (281)947-2490

Solis Mammography At West Houston Medical Center
12606 West Houston Center Blvd Ste 330
Houston, TX 77082-2788
(786)290-8724
FAX: (281)596-5979

Solis Mammography Of Cyfair
11307 Fm 1960 Rd W Ste 340
Houston, TX 77065-4917
(281)897-3405
FAX: (866)366-5798

Solis Mammography Of Houston Nw
800 Peakwood Dr Ste 1F
Houston, TX 77090-2913
(866)717-2551
FAX: (866)366-5798

Solis Mammography Of Louetta/249 Llc
20326 State Highway 249, Ste 225
Houston, TX 77070-2790
(866)717-2551
FAX: (866)366-5798

Solis Mammography Of Memorial Villages
8731 Katy Fwy, Ste 100
Houston, TX 77024-1735
(866)717-2551
FAX: (866)366-5798

Solis Mammography Of North Loop, Llc
1900 North Loop W, Ste 350
Houston, TX 77018-8136
(866)717-2551
FAX: (832)930-5930

St. Luke's Hospital At The Vintage
20171 Chasewood Park Dr, Mammography
Houston, TX 77070-1437
(832)534-5180
FAX: (713)852-2274

Steeplechase Diagnostic Center, Inc.
10694 Jones Rd, Ste 150
Houston, TX 77065-4260
(281)955-0440
FAX: (281)995-0755

The Breast And Imaging Center, Llc
7900 Fannin St Ste 1500
Houston, TX 77054-2950
(713)512-7651
FAX: (713)512-7637

The Rose
12700 N Featherwood Dr, Ste 260
Houston, TX 77034-4494
(281)484-4708
FAX: (281)484-5626

The Ut Mdacc Diagnostic Imaging-West Houston
15021 Katy Fwy Ste 100
Houston, TX 77094-1915
(281)994-0700
FAX: (281)994-0800

Tops Speciality Hospital Ltd.
17030 Red Oak Dr
Houston, TX 77090-2602
(281)580-6171
FAX: (281)765-4650

Tops Specialty Hospital, Ltd
13215 Dotson Rd, Ste 220
Houston, TX 77070-4535
(281)580-6171
FAX: (281)765-4650

Ut M.D. Anderson Cancer Center
PO Box 301439, 1515 Holcombe Blvd
Houston, TX 77230-1439
(713)745-5170
FAX: (713)745-3262

Ut MD Anderson Cancer Center Mobile
PO Box 301439, 1515 Holcombe Ave
Houston, TX 77230-1439
(713)745-4000
FAX: (713)745-4055

Woman's Clinic Pllc
2424 W Holcombe Blvd, Ste 102
Houston, TX 77030-1933
(832)804-8119
FAX: (832)804-8120

Humble

Kelsey Seybold Medical Group Pllc
8233 N Sam Houston Pkwy E
Humble, TX 77396-2922
(713)442-2043
FAX: (713)442-2137

Memorial Hermann Hlth System
Dba Memorial Hermann Northeast, 18955 Memorial Hermann North
Humble, TX 77338
(281)540-7390
FAX: (281)913-3492

Huntsville

Huntsville Community Hospital,Dba Huntsville Memorial Hosp.
123 Medical Park Ln Ste B
Huntsville, TX 77340-4981
(936)435-7577
FAX: (936)293-4694

Hurst

Btdi Jv, Llp Dba Touchstone Imaging Hurst
1717 Precinct Line Rd Ste 103
Hurst, TX 76054-3169
(817)498-6575
FAX: (817)498-8854

Irving

Baylor Medical Center At Irving
Dba Bs&W Women's Imaging Cntr Lascolinas, 440 West I-635
Irving, TX 75063
(972)990-5650
FAX: (972)990-5695

Baylor Medical Center At Irving
2001 N Macarthur Blvd Ste 250, Dba Baylor S&W Women imagingcntr irving
Irving, TX 75061-2284
(972)579-4270
FAX: (972)579-4259

Solis Mammography At Las Colinas Medical Center
6750 N Macarthur Blvd Ste 153, Plaza 1
Irving, TX 75039-2833
(866)717-2551
FAX: (972)556-2939

Jacksonville

Jacksonville Hospital, Llc
203 Nacogdoches St, Dba Ut Health East Tx Jacksonville Hosp
Jacksonville, TX 75766-2462
(903)541-5192
FAX: (903)541-5010

Mf Hosp-Jacksonville/Dba Christus Mf Hospital Jacksonville
2026 S Jackson St
Jacksonville, TX 75766-5822
(903)531-5433
FAX: (903)510-1160

Jasper

Christus Health Southeast Texas
1275 Marvin Hancock Dr, Dba Christus Jasper Memorial Hospital
Jasper, TX 75951-4935
(409)384-1924
FAX: (409)384-1883

Jbsa Ft Sam Houston

Brooke Army Medical Ctr - Department Of Radiology
3551 Roger Brooke Dr
Jbsa Ft Sam Houston, TX 78234-4504
(210)916-4229
FAX: (210)916-1072

Jbsa Lackland

Wilford Hall Ambulatory Surgical Center
1100 Wilford Hall Loop
Jbsa Lackland, TX 78236-5638
(210)292-4279
FAX: (210)292-6156

Jourdanton

Methodist Healthcare Sys Sa Ltd Llp Dba Methodist Hosp South
1905 E State Highway 97
Jourdanton, TX 78026-1504
(830)769-5258
FAX: (830)769-5228

Katy

Ag Radiology Imaging Center, Llc
601 Park Grove Dr
Katy, TX 77450-5542
(832)321-3434
FAX: (832)321-5031

Kelsey-Seybold Medical Group, Pllc
2510 W Grand Pkwy N
Katy, TX 77449-2853
(713)442-1161
FAX: (713)442-1176

Memorial Hermann Health System
23920 Katy Fwy, Dba Memorial Hermann Katy Hospital
Katy, TX 77494-1341
(281)455-2008
FAX: (281)337-9736

Memorial Mri & Diagnostic, Llc
21820 Katy Fwy, Ste 100
Katy, TX 77449-7901
(713)461-3399
FAX: (713)554-1402

Solis Mammography Of Katy, Llc
1331 W Grand Pkwy N, Ste 240
Katy, TX 77493-2711
(866)717-2551
FAX: (866)717-5798

Kaufman

Texas Health Presbyterian Hosp Kaufman
850 Ed Hall Dr
Kaufman, TX 75142-1861
(972)932-7390
FAX: (972)932-5579

Keller

Btdi Jv Llp Dba Touchstone Imaging Keller
601 S Main St, Ste 100
Keller, TX 76248-7027
(817)482-2000
FAX: (682)224-7121

Kenedy

Karnes County Hospital District
3349 S Highway 181, Dba Otto Kaiser Memorial Hospital
Kenedy, TX 78119-5247
(830)583-3401
FAX: (830)583-4566

Kerrville

Medical Arts Imaging Inc.
212 Wesley Dr
Kerrville, TX 78028-5809
(830)257-4777
FAX: (830)896-6767

Sid Peterson Memorial Hospital
260 Cully Dr, Dba Peterson Health
Kerrville, TX 78028-5950
(830)258-7200
FAX: (830)258-7084

Killeen

Adventhealth Central Texas
2201 Clear Creek Rd
Killeen, TX 76549-4110
(254)519-8537
FAX: (254)519-8413

Scott & White Mem Hosp Dba Baylor S&W Clinic - Killeen
3801 Scott And White Dr
Killeen, TX 76543-5252
(254)680-1179
FAX: (254)680-1387

Kingsville

Christus Spohn Hospital Kleberg
1311 E General Cavazos Blvd
Kingsville, TX 78363-7130
(361)595-9764
FAX: (361)595-9896

Kingwood

Memorial Hermann Health System
4533 Kingwood Dr, Dba Memorial Hermann convenient care cntr
Kingwood, TX 77345-2608
(281)359-4442
FAX: (281)913-3492

Solis Mammography At Kingwood Medical Center
22999 Highway 59 N Ste 240
Kingwood, TX 77339-4440
(281)348-8091
FAX: (281)348-8092

Tops Specialty Hospital Ltd.
350 Kingwood Medical Dr, Ste 110
Kingwood, TX 77339-6406
(281)580-6171
FAX: (281)754-4486

Kyle

Ascension Seton
6001 Kyle Pkwy, Dba Ascension Seton Hays
Kyle, TX 78640-6112
(512)504-5000
FAX: (512)324-7488

Austin Radiological Association
4211 Benner Ste 100
Kyle, TX 78640-2140
(512)453-6100
FAX: (512)275-0036

Seton Family Of Doctors
5103 Kyle Center Dr, Ste 108
Kyle, TX 78640-6164
(512)504-8099
FAX: (855)629-2832

La Grange

St. Mark's Medical Center
1 Saint Marks Pl, Imaging Department
La Grange, TX 78945-1250
(979)242-2230
FAX: (979)242-5140

Lake Jackson

Chi St. Lukes Health Brazosport
100 Medical Dr
Lake Jackson, TX 77566-5674
(979)299-2888
FAX: (979)297-3688

Lakeway

Scott & White Hospital - Round Rock
100 Medical Pkwy, Dba Baylor S&W Medical Center Lakeway
Lakeway, TX 78738-5621
(512)571-5152
FAX: (512)571-5157

Lampasas

Adventhealth Rollins Brook
608 N Key Ave, Mammography Dept
Lampasas, TX 76550-1106
(512)556-3682
FAX: (512)564-2283

Laredo

Doctors Hospital Of Laredo
230 Calle Del Norte
Laredo, TX 78041-5957
(956)693-5040
FAX: (956)693-5047

Laredo Medical Center
1700 E Saunders St
Laredo, TX 78041-5474
(956)796-3729
FAX: (956)796-4408

Laredo Regional Medical Center
10700 McPherson Rd, Dba Doctors Hospital Of Laredo
Laredo, TX 78045-6268
(956)523-2088
FAX: (956)523-2840

Laredo Texas Hospital Company Lp Dba Lmc North
7210 McPherson Rd
Laredo, TX 78041-6507
(956)796-3729
FAX: (956)796-4760

Lmc - South
4151 Jaime Zapata Memorial Hwy Ste 101
Laredo, TX 78043-4741
(956)796-3729
FAX: (956)796-4760

Radiology Clinics Of Laredo
5401 Springfield Ave
Laredo, TX 78041-3296
(956)718-0092
FAX: (956)726-9735

League City

Memorial Hermann Health System
2555 Gulf Fwy S, Dba mem hermann victory womens imaging ctr
League City, TX 77573-6742
(281)337-9730
FAX: (281)337-9737

University Of Texas MD Anderson Cancer Center League City
2280 Gulf Fwy S
League City, TX 77573-5143
(713)792-7171
FAX: (713)745-2022

Utmb League City Campus
2240 Gulf Fwy S, Dba Utmb Health League City Campus
League City, TX 77573-5143
(832)505-1700
FAX: (281)309-0147

Levelland

Methodist Hospital Levelland Inc.
1900 College Ave, Dba Covenant Hospital Levelland
Levelland, TX 79336-6508
(806)894-4963
FAX: (806)894-7047

Lewisville

Solis Mammography At Medical Center Of Lewisville Llc
500 W Main St Ste 300
Lewisville, TX 75057-3640
(866)717-2551
FAX: (972)221-2491

Touchstone Imaging Lewisville
190 Civic Cir, Ste 110
Lewisville, TX 75067-3635
(972)434-6737
FAX: (972)434-6739

Lindale

Mf Hosp Reg Hc Ctr/Dba Christus Mother Frances Hosp Tyler
3203 S Main St
Lindale, TX 75771-7727
(903)606-5433
FAX: (903)606-1160

Live Oak

Radiation Oncology Of The South Plains, Pa
12705 Toepperwein Rd
Live Oak, TX 78233-3257
(210)247-0888
FAX: (210)558-0758

Livingston

Memorial Hospital Of Polk County
1717 US Hwy 59 Bypass
Livingston, TX 77351
(936)329-8570
FAX: (936)329-8262

Longview

Associated Clinicians Of East Texas, Pllc Dba: Dcol
707 Hollybrook Dr, 2nd Fl
Longview, TX 75605-2410
(903)291-6230
FAX: (903)232-8581

Christus Good Shepherd Medical Center
705 E Marshall Ave Ste 1003
Longview, TX 75601-5660
(903)315-2130
FAX: (903)315-5310

Longview Medical Center Lp
709 Hollybrook Dr Ste 5604
Longview, TX 75605-2411
(903)232-8596
FAX: (903)232-8294

Lubbock

Lubbock County Hospital District
4004 82nd St, Ste 100
Lubbock, TX 79423-2063
(806)722-4674
FAX: (806)775-8442

Lubbock Heritage Hospital, Llc
4515 Marsha Sharp Fwy, Dba Grace Medical Center
Lubbock, TX 79407-2520
(806)744-7223
FAX: (806)740-3302

Lubbock Radiology L.P.
3707 21st St
Lubbock, TX 79410-1219
(806)792-2354
FAX: (806)771-3367

Methodist Childrens Hosp Dba Arrington Comprehensive Brstctr
4102 24th St
Lubbock, TX 79410-1806
(806)725-7908
FAX: (806)723-6034

Methodist Diagnostic Imaging
3525 19th St, Dba Covenant Diagnostic Imaging
Lubbock, TX 79410-1202
(806)792-4444
FAX: (806)791-6733

Radiation Oncology Of The South Plains Pa
4009 19th St, Ste E
Lubbock, TX 79410-1003
(806)799-9355
FAX: (806)771-4077

University Medical Center
808 Joliet Ave Unit 320, Umc Breast Imaging Center
Lubbock, TX 79415-1153
(806)775-8660
FAX: (806)775-8661

Lufkin

Chi St Luke's Health Memorial
1105 W Frank Ave, Ste 100
Lufkin, TX 75904-3366
(936)631-3014
FAX: (936)639-3083

Pineywoods Healthcare System, Lp
125 Gaslight Medical Pkwy, Dba Woodland Heights Medical Center
Lufkin, TX 75904-3150
(936)631-8491
FAX: (936)631-8484

Luling

Ascension Seton
130 Hays St, Dba Ascension Seton Edgar B. Davis
Luling, TX 78648-3207
(830)875-7000
FAX: (830)875-7084

Manor

Austin Radiological Association
12700 Lexington St, Bldg C Suite 300
Manor, TX 78653-2011
(512)453-6100
FAX: (512)836-8869

Mansfield

Methodist Mansfield Medical Center
2700 E Broad St
Mansfield, TX 76063-5899
(682)662-2724
FAX: (682)622-7250

Solis Mammography Of Mansfield
3141 E Broad St, Ste 331
Mansfield, TX 76063-6445
(972)965-0708
FAX: (469)382-2525

Texas Health Hospital Mansfield
2302 Lone Star Rd
Mansfield, TX 76063-8765
(682)341-5053
FAX: (682)341-5052

Marble Falls

Ascension Seton
1800 Mormon Mill Rd
Marble Falls, TX 78654-4192
(830)693-8733
FAX: (830)693-8734

Scott & White Hospital - Marble Falls
810 W Highway 71
Marble Falls, TX 78654-8602
(830)201-8130
FAX: (830)201-8137

Marshall

Christus Good Shepherd Medical Center
811 S Washington Ave
Marshall, TX 75670-5336
(903)927-6785
FAX: (903)927-6110

McAllen

Advanced Medical Imaging
1200 S Col Rowe Blvd Ste B2
McAllen, TX 78501-2954
(956)686-8422
FAX: (956)661-2135

Columbia Rio Grande Hlthcare Lp Dba Rio Grande Reg Hosp
101 E Ridge Rd Ste B
McAllen, TX 78503-1848
(956)632-6700
FAX: (956)686-3048

Comfort Image 2 Ltd.
4900 N 10th St, Ste F1
McAllen, TX 78504-2781
(956)668-8282
FAX: (956)668-8181

Doctors Hospital At Renaissance
300 Lindberg Ave
McAllen, TX 78501-2943
(956)362-7503
FAX: (956)362-3760

Doctors Hospital At Renaissance
1100 E Dove Ave Ste 100
McAllen, TX 78504-4680
(956)362-8600
FAX: (956)362-8609

McAllen Hospitals,Lp Dba South Texas Health System Mcallen
301 W Expressway 83
McAllen, TX 78503-3045
(956)388-2190
FAX: (956)971-5744

Optimum Diagnostic Imaging Center, Llc
500 S Bicentennial Blvd, Ste 100-B
McAllen, TX 78501-7995
(956)585-8700
FAX: (956)215-7511

McKinney

Andrew Shimer, M.D., P.A.
7900 Henneman Way, Ste 200
McKinney, TX 75070-3125
(214)544-6600
FAX: (214)544-7700

Baylor Medical Centers At Garland And McKinney
5236 W University Dr Ste 2500, Dbabaylors women imaging center mckinney
McKinney, TX 75071-8114
(469)764-7001
FAX: (469)764-7026

Methodist - Cdi Dba Methodist Center For Diagnostic Imaging
7300 Eldorado Pkwy, Ste 170
McKinney, TX 75070-7895
(972)920-0120
FAX: (214)592-0035

Solis Mammography At The Medical Center Of McKinney, Llc
4201 Medical Center Dr, Ste 100A
McKinney, TX 75069-1766
(972)596-4033
FAX: (469)467-7678

Mesquite

Btdi Jv, Llp Dba Touchstone Imaging- Mesquite
1425 Gross Rd Ste 130
Mesquite, TX 75149-1362
(972)289-5558
FAX: (972)289-5786

Genesiscare USA Landmark, Llc
1645 N Town East Blvd, Ste 503
Mesquite, TX 75150-4147
(972)686-3901

Memorial Mri & Diagnostic Llc
3400 Interstate 30, Ste 100
Mesquite, TX 75150-2601
(713)461-3399
FAX: (713)554-1402

Prime Healthcare Services - Mesquite, Llc
1011 N Galloway Ave, Dba Dallas Regional Medical Center
Mesquite, TX 75149-2433
(214)320-7008
FAX: (214)320-7656

Solis Mammography Of Mesquite, Llc
1515 N Town East Blvd Ste 141
Mesquite, TX 75150-4196
(866)257-6884
FAX: (469)609-0909

Mexia

Mexia Principal Healthcare, L.P.
600 S Bonham St, Dba Parkview Regional Hospital
Mexia, TX 76667-3603
(254)562-5332
FAX: (254)562-2392

Midland

Midland Women's Clinic
2500 W Illinois Ave, Ste 100
Midland, TX 79701-6339
(432)699-2370
FAX: (432)697-3524

The Breast Center Midland Health
5615 Deauville Ste 100
Midland, TX 79706-2708
(432)221-3627
FAX: (432)221-3004

Midlothian

Methodist Hospitals Of Dallas
Dba Methodist Midlothian Medical Center, 1201 E US Hwy 287
Midlothian, TX 76065
(469)846-2079
FAX: (469)846-2066

Mineral Wells

Palo Pinto County Hosp District Dba Palo Pinto General Hosp
400 SW 25th Ave
Mineral Wells, TX 76067-8246
(940)325-7891
FAX: (940)328-6489

Mission

Mission Hospital Inc.
910 S Bryan Rd Ste 102, Dba Mission Regional Medical Center
Mission, TX 78572-6615
(956)323-1700
FAX: (956)323-1705

Optimum Diagnostic Imaging Center, Llc
1300 S Bryan Rd, Ste 104
Mission, TX 78572-6688
(956)583-0004
FAX: (956)583-5790

Sths Er At Mission
900 E Interstate Highway 2
Mission, TX 78572-5756
(956)388-2190
FAX: (956)388-6030

Montgomery

Solis Mammography Of Montgomery Llc.
20042 Eva St, Ste 104
Montgomery, TX 77356-2042
(866)717-2551
FAX: (866)366-5798

Mt Pleasant

Titus County Memorial Hospital
2015 Mulberry Ave Ste 340, Radiology Department
Mt Pleasant, TX 75455-2318
(903)434-8045
FAX: (903)434-8049

Nacogdoches

Nacogdoches Cnty Hosp District Mem Hosp Dba Women's Wellness
1018 N Mound St Ste 103
Nacogdoches, TX 75961-4434
(936)564-1895
FAX: (936)569-4677

Nacogdoches Medical Center
4920 NE Stallings Dr
Nacogdoches, TX 75965-1254
(936)568-3450
FAX: (936)568-3316

New Braunfels

Baptist M&S Imaging New Braunfels
1763 Medical Way
New Braunfels, TX 78132-4521
(830)327-1878
FAX: (210)651-7325

Christus Santa Rosa Health Care Corporation
600 N Union Ave
New Braunfels, TX 78130-4194
(830)643-6162
FAX: (830)643-6165

Resolute Health Hospital
555 Creekside Xing
New Braunfels, TX 78130-2594
(830)500-6618
FAX: (830)500-7069

River City Imaging Centers, Llc
1750 E Common St, Ste 1101
New Braunfels, TX 78130-6869
(830)302-4355
FAX: (830)312-7677

North Richland Hills

Columbia North Hills Hospital Subsidiary L.P.
4375 Booth Calloway Rd, Dba Medical City North Hills
North Richland Hills, TX 76180-8359
(817)255-1880
FAX: (817)255-1871

Odessa

Odessa Regional Hospital L.P.
420 E 6th St, Ste 206
Odessa, TX 79761-4572
(432)582-8000
FAX: (432)582-8945

The Ctr For Women's Imaging At Medical Center Hospital
318 N Alleghaney Ave Ste 101
Odessa, TX 79761-5027
(432)640-2255
FAX: (432)640-4218

Orange

Baptist Beaumont Hospital
608 Strickland Dr
Orange, TX 77630-4717
(409)883-1377
FAX: (409)883-1374

Palestine

Christus Trinity Clinic Dba: Christus Trinity Clinic
3201 S Loop 256 Ste 900
Palestine, TX 75801-6901
(903)661-7167
FAX: (903)723-0460

Palestine Regional Medical Center
2900 S Loop 256
Palestine, TX 75801-6958
(903)731-1081
FAX: (903)731-1077

Pampa

Prime Healthcare Services - Pampa, Llc
1 Medical Plz, Dba Pampa Regional Medical Center
Pampa, TX 79065-3525
(806)663-5770
FAX: (806)663-5777

Paris

Paris Regional Medical Center
865 Deshong Dr
Paris, TX 75460-9313
(903)737-3900
FAX: (903)737-1544

Solis Mammography Of Paris, Llc.
3160 Clarksville St
Paris, TX 75460-8015
(903)784-2571
FAX: (903)783-0624

Pasadena

Harris County Hospital District
927 Shaw Ave, Dba Strawberry Health Center
Pasadena, TX 77506-1430
(713)982-5989

Kelsey-Seybold Medical Group, Pllc
5001 E Sam Houston Pkwy S
Pasadena, TX 77505-3965
(713)442-4327
FAX: (713)442-4325

Pmc Hospital, Llc
4600 E Sam Houston Pkwy S, Dba St Luke's Patients Medical Center
Pasadena, TX 77505-3948
(713)948-7000
FAX: (713)948-7124

Solis Mammography At Bayshore Medical Center, Llc
3801 Vista Rd Ste 200
Pasadena, TX 77504-2139
(866)717-2551
FAX: (866)366-5798

Pearland

Kelsey-Seybold Medical Group, Pllc
2515 Business Center Dr
Pearland, TX 77584-2294
(713)442-4327
FAX: (713)442-4325

Memorial Hermann Health System
10905 Memorial Hermann Dr, Dba memoria hermann pearland imaging svce
Pearland, TX 77584-3490
(713)383-4933
FAX: (713)383-4926

Pearland Mri & Imaging Center
8633 Broadway St Ste 109
Pearland, TX 77584-8497
(682)208-6417
FAX: (281)485-5712

Sky Mri & Diagnostics, Llc
11711 Shadow Creek Pkwy, Ste 147
Pearland, TX 77584-7234
(832)288-5550
FAX: (281)741-3500

Solis Mammography At Pearland Medical Center
10970 Shadow Creek Pkwy Ste 190
Pearland, TX 77584-0117
(866)717-2551
FAX: (866)366-5798

Pearsall

Frio Regional Hospital
200 S Interstate 35
Pearsall, TX 78061-6601
(830)334-3617
FAX: (830)334-9804

Pecos

Reeves County Hospital District
2323 Texas St
Pecos, TX 79772-7338
(432)447-3551
FAX: (432)447-4861

Perryton

Ochiltree County Hospital District
3101 Garrett Dr, Dba Ochiltree General Hospital
Perryton, TX 79070-5323
(806)648-7121
FAX: (806)435-6039

Pflugerville

Baylor Scott & White Medical Centers-Capitol Area
2600 E Pflugerville Pkwy
Pflugerville, TX 78660-5998
(512)654-6113
FAX: (512)654-6112

Plainview

Methodist Hospital Plainview Dba Covenant Hospital Plainview
2601 Dimmitt Rd, Radiology Dept.
Plainview, TX 79072-1833
(806)291-3331
FAX: (806)296-4293

Plainview Radiology, Llc
2404 Yonkers St Ste 4, Dba Garvish Radiology
Plainview, TX 79072-1820
(806)293-4231
FAX: (806)293-7346

Plano

Baylor Regional Medical Center At Plano
4716 Alliance Blvd Ste 100, Dba Baylor S&W Womens Imaging Cntr Plano
Plano, TX 75093-5376
(469)814-4401
FAX: (469)814-2022

Genesiscare USA Landmark, Llc
6957 W Plano Pkwy, Ste 1400
Plano, TX 75093-1627
(972)820-1480

Methodist - Cdi
5425 W Spring Creek Pkwy, Ste 110
Plano, TX 75024-4244
(972)920-0100
FAX: (214)778-0102

Methodist-Cdi Dba Center For Diagnostic Imaging
8080 Independence Pkwy, Ste 105
Plano, TX 75025-4003
(972)920-0120
FAX: (972)592-0035

Ob/Gyn North Dallas
6124 W Parker Rd, Ste 134
Plano, TX 75093-8124
(972)981-7777
FAX: (972)981-7761

Sandra Oneal Institute
5072 W Plano Pkwy Ste 190
Plano, TX 75093-4469
(972)733-3531
FAX: (972)346-6564

Solis Mammography At The Medical Center Of Plano, Llc
3801 W 15th St, Ste 150A
Plano, TX 75075-4737
(972)596-4033
FAX: (469)241-8775

Solis Mammography Of West Plano, Llc
5920 W Parker Rd Ste 200
Plano, TX 75093-6413
(866)717-2551
FAX: (972)805-8870

Texas Health Presbyterian Hospital Plano
6020 W Parker Rd Ste 110
Plano, TX 75093-8165
(972)981-4070
FAX: (972)981-3903

Womens Specialists Of Plano Pllc
3801 W 15th St, Bldg B Suite 200
Plano, TX 75075-4737
(972)379-2416
FAX: (972)867-1018

Port Arthur

Christus Health Southeast Texas Dba Christus Outpatient Cent
8801 9th Ave
Port Arthur, TX 77642-8013
(409)899-7500
FAX: (409)899-8182

Riceland Diagnostic Health
3445 Regional Dr
Port Arthur, TX 77642-8063
(409)626-3648
FAX: (409)729-0082

The Medical Center Of Southeast Texas
2555 Jimmy Johnson Blvd
Port Arthur, TX 77640-2007
(409)853-5836
FAX: (409)853-5833

Port Lavaca

Memorial Medical Center
815 N Virginia St
Port Lavaca, TX 77979-3025
(361)552-0250
FAX: (361)552-0418

Porter

Kelsey-Seybold Medical Group, Pllc
25553 Highway 59, Kelsey-Seybold Clinic
Porter, TX 77365-6154
(713)442-2137
FAX: (713)442-2114

Portland

Radiology Associates Llp
1776 Billy G Webb
Portland, TX 78374-3706
(361)561-3199
FAX: (361)643-5945

Prosper

Solis Mammography Of Prosper Llc
1000 N Preston Rd Ste 30
Prosper, TX 75078-8892
(972)941-4802
FAX: (214)705-9240

Texas Health Presbyterian Hospital Plano
1970 W University Dr, Dba tx health neighborhood care&Wellness
Prosper, TX 75078-8133
(469)329-7720
FAX: (469)329-7882

Randolph Afb

Randolph Air Force Base 359th Med Group
221 3rd St W, 359th Medical Group
Randolph Afb, TX 78150-4800
(210)652-0311
FAX: (210)652-3344

Red Oak

Btdi Jv, Llp Dba Touchstone Imaging At Red Oak
305 E Ovilla Rd
Red Oak, TX 75154-3833
(972)617-7731
FAX: (682)224-7121

Solis Mammography Of Red Oak
317 E Ovilla Rd Ste 300
Red Oak, TX 75154-3878
(469)240-8592
FAX: (469)505-0535

Richardson

Baylor Regional Medical Center At Plano
3301 E Renner Rd Ste 100, Dba Baylo S&W Ejekotmd Wic Richardson
Richardson, TX 75082-1802
(214)442-7050
FAX: (469)814-2022

Methodist Hospitals Of Dallas - Methodist Richardson Med Ctr
2831 E President George Bush Hwy, Center For Womens Health
Richardson, TX 75082-3561
(469)204-2140
FAX: (214)947-8572

Richmond

Kelsey - Seybold Medical Group, Pllc
22121 Fm 1093 Rd
Richmond, TX 77407-2140
(713)442-1161
FAX: (713)442-2410

Oakbend Medical Center
1705 Jackson St
Richmond, TX 77469-3246
(281)341-4817
FAX: (281)238-7855

Rio Grande City

Starr County Hospital District
128 N Fm 3167, Dba Starr County Memorial Hospital
Rio Grande City, TX 78582-6211
(956)487-9035
FAX: (956)487-4087

Rockwall

Lake Pointe Operating Company, Llc
1005 W Ralph Hall Pkwy, Dba Baylor S&W Imaging Center Rockwall
Rockwall, TX 75032-6663
(469)698-8555
FAX: (469)698-8551

Rockwall Regional Hospital Llc
3136 Horizon Rd, Dba Tx Health Presbyterian Hosp Rockwall
Rockwall, TX 75032-7821
(469)698-1334
FAX: (972)772-2811

Round Rock

Ara/St. David's Imaging, L.P.
2120 N Mays St Ste 220
Round Rock, TX 78664-2108
(512)453-6100
FAX: (512)836-8869

Oakwood Austin Breast Imaging
511 Oakwood Blvd, Ste 301
Round Rock, TX 78681-4068
(512)776-1000
FAX: (512)399-6390

Scott & White Hospital- Round Rock
300A University Blvd
Round Rock, TX 78665-1032
(512)509-9100
FAX: (512)509-9136

St David's Round Rock Medical Center
2400 Round Rock Ave, Radiology Department
Round Rock, TX 78681-4004
(512)341-6440
FAX: (512)255-6706

Rowlett

Lake Pointe Operating Company, Llc
6800 Scenic Dr, Dba Baylor S&W Medical Center Lakepointe
Rowlett, TX 75088-4552
(972)412-3380
FAX: (972)412-7457

San Angelo

Shannon Medical Center
3301 S Bryant Blvd
San Angelo, TX 76903-9305
(325)481-2339
FAX: (325)482-0841

Shannon Medical Center South
3501 Knickerbocker Rd
San Angelo, TX 76904-7610
(325)947-6691
FAX: (325)947-6770

San Antonio

Avestee Women's Imaging Center Of Alamo Heights
303 W Sunset Rd Ste 200
San Antonio, TX 78209-1744
(210)826-2666
FAX: (210)314-7545

Avestee Women's Imaging Center Of Westover Hills
9842 Westover Hills Blvd Ste 101
San Antonio, TX 78251-4321
(210)826-2666
FAX: (210)314-7545

Baptist Breast Center
502 Madison Oak Dr, Ste 450
San Antonio, TX 78258-4806
(210)228-9729
FAX: (210)730-9690

Baptist Breast Center At Westover Hills
3903 Wiseman Blvd Ste 321
San Antonio, TX 78251-4401
(210)521-2989
FAX: (210)520-0491

Baptist Breast Center Downtown
215 E Quincy St Ste 100
San Antonio, TX 78215-2032
(210)228-9729
FAX: (210)351-0720

Baptist M & S Imaging - Mission Trail
3327 Research Plz Ste 108
San Antonio, TX 78235-5156
(210)423-3950
FAX: (210)423-3957

Baptist M&S Imaging - Legacy Oaks
5368 Fredericksburg Rd Ste 305
San Antonio, TX 78229-6108
(210)228-9729
FAX: (210)692-3472

Bexar County Hosp. District Dba University Health System
903 W Martin St
San Antonio, TX 78207-0903
(210)644-8850
FAX: (210)743-4303

Bexar County Hospital District Dba University Health Sys
4502 Medical Dr
San Antonio, TX 78229-4402
(210)644-8850
FAX: (210)702-4303

Bexar County Hospital District Dba University Hlth System
7979 Wurzbach Rd, Ste Z500
San Antonio, TX 78229-4427
(210)644-8850
FAX: (210)702-4303

Bexar Imaging Center Llc
25 NE Loop 410, Ste 121
San Antonio, TX 78216-8404
(210)384-8439
FAX: (210)348-1913

Btdi Jv, Llp Dba Touchstone Imaging Stone Oak
18802 Meisner Dr
San Antonio, TX 78258-4251
(210)614-0600
FAX: (210)614-1611

Christus Santa Rosa Health Care Corporation
11212 State Highway 151
San Antonio, TX 78251-4498
(210)703-8108
FAX: (210)703-8180

Christus Santa Rosa Imaging Center-Alamo Heights
423 Treeline Park Ste 100
San Antonio, TX 78209-2068
(210)704-0030
FAX: (210)704-0001

Gmg Health Systems Ltd.
7219 Culebra Rd, Dba Gonzaba Medical Group
San Antonio, TX 78251-1305
(210)395-3550
FAX: (210)921-3873

Gmg Health Systems, Ltd.
720 Pleasanton Rd, Dba Gonzaba Medical Group
San Antonio, TX 78214-1306
(210)921-3800
FAX: (210)921-3873

Ifwh Austin Breast Imaging, Llc
222 W Cypress St
San Antonio, TX 78212-5509
(210)226-9705
FAX: (210)223-4555

South Texas Radiology Imaging Centers
155 E Sonterra Blvd Ste 100
San Antonio, TX 78258-3988
(210)617-9000
FAX: (210)617-9516

South Texas Radiology Imaging Centers
9150 Huebner Rd Ste 195
San Antonio, TX 78240-1599
(210)617-9000
FAX: (210)617-9516

South Texas Radiology Imaging Centers
4458 Medical Dr Ste 345
San Antonio, TX 78229-3748
(210)617-9000
FAX: (210)617-9516

South Texas Radiology Imaging Centers
18707 Hardy Oak Blvd Ste 110
San Antonio, TX 78258-4791
(210)617-9000
FAX: (210)617-9516

South Texas Radiology Imaging Centers
7333 Barlite Blvd, Ste 200
San Antonio, TX 78224-1322
(210)617-9000
FAX: (210)617-9516

South Texas Radiology Imaging Centers
1200 Brooklyn Ave Ste 100
San Antonio, TX 78212-4810
(210)617-9000
FAX: (210)617-9516

South Texas Radiology Imaging Centers
5510B Presidio Pkwy, Ste 2201
San Antonio, TX 78249-2988
(210)617-9000
FAX: (210)617-9516

South Texas Radiology Imaging Centers
12709 Toepperwein Rd Ste 106
San Antonio, TX 78233-3260
(210)617-9000
FAX: (210)617-9516

South Texas Radiology Imaging Centers
11923 Culebra Rd Ste 201, Building 2
San Antonio, TX 78253-6781
(210)617-9000
FAX: (210)617-9516

South Texas Radiology Imaging Centers
4383 Medical Dr Ste 150
San Antonio, TX 78229-3307
(210)617-9000
FAX: (210)617-9516

South Texas Radiology Imaging Centers
1888 Nacogdoches Rd
San Antonio, TX 78209-2216
(210)617-9000
FAX: (210)617-9516

South Texas Radiology Imaging Centers
7950 Floyd Curl Dr Ste 200
San Antonio, TX 78229-3933
(210)617-9000
FAX: (210)617-9516

San Augustine

Memorial Medical Center San Augustine
511 E Hospital St
San Augustine, TX 75972-2121
(936)275-3446
FAX: (936)275-2621

San Marcos

Austin Radiological Association
1348 N State Highway 123 Ste B
San Marcos, TX 78666-7848
(512)453-6100
FAX: (512)836-8869

Christus Santa Rosa Health Care Corporation
1301 Wonder World Dr, Dba Christus santarosa hospital San Marcos
San Marcos, TX 78666-7533
(512)353-8979
FAX: (512)753-3598

Schertz

Baptist M&S Imaging Schertz
16977 Interstate 35 N Ste 220
Schertz, TX 78154-1472
(210)339-9401
FAX: (210)651-7325

South Texas Radiology Imaging Centers
5000 Schertz Pkwy Ste 500
Schertz, TX 78154-1457
(210)617-9000
FAX: (210)617-9516

Seguin

Guadalupe Regional Medical Center
1215 E Court St
Seguin, TX 78155-5129
(830)401-7850
FAX: (830)401-7512

Seminole

Seminole Hospital District Of Gaines County
209 NW 8th St, Dba Memorial Hospital
Seminole, TX 79360-3447
(432)758-5811
FAX: (432)758-4882

Shenandoah

Kelsey-Seybold Medical Group, Pllc
106 Vision Park Blvd
Shenandoah, TX 77384-3000
(713)442-1589
FAX: (713)442-1577

Sherman

Sherman Grayson Hospital, Llc
300 N Highland Ave, Dba Wilson N Jones Regional Medical Ctnr
Sherman, TX 75092-7388
(903)891-2237
FAX: (903)891-2240

Smithville

Ascension Seton
1201 Hill Rd, Dba Ascension Seton Smithville
Smithville, TX 78957-9533
(512)237-5733
FAX: (512)504-5548

Snyder

Scurry County Hospital District
1700 Cogdell Blvd, Dba D.M. Cogdell Memorial Hospital
Snyder, TX 79549-6162
(325)574-7441
FAX: (325)574-7229

Sonora

Sutton County Hospital District
308 Hudspeth St, Dba Lillian M Hudspeth Memorial Hospital
Sonora, TX 76950-8003
(325)387-2521
FAX: (325)387-2396

Southlake

Envision Imaging At Southlake
525 E Southlake Blvd
Southlake, TX 76092-6235
(817)424-5872
FAX: (817)424-3022

Medx Imaging, Llc
630 E State Highway 114, Dba Eve's Breast Center
Southlake, TX 76092-4410
(817)329-8910
FAX: (817)329-8911

Solis Mammography
1545 E Southlake Blvd, Ste 200
Southlake, TX 76092-6465
(817)749-2000
FAX: (817)751-2060

Spring

Memorial Hermann Health System
7474 N Grand Pkwy W, Dba Memorial hermann convenient care centr
Spring, TX 77379-1570
(713)897-4194
FAX: (713)897-2040

St Luke's The Woodlands Hospital
2255 E Mossy Oaks Rd
Spring, TX 77389-1811
(936)266-3250
FAX: (936)266-2388

Stephenville

Stephenville Medical & Surgical Clinic, Pa
150 River North Blvd
Stephenville, TX 76401-1879
(254)968-6051
FAX: (254)968-6954

Texas Health Harris Methodist Hospital Stephenville
411 N Belknap St
Stephenville, TX 76401-3415
(254)965-1524
FAX: (254)965-8478

Sugar Land

Fort Bend Imaging, Inc.
14835 Southwest Fwy
Sugar Land, TX 77478-5016
(281)242-5800
FAX: (281)207-8955

Global Imaging Llp
1435 Highway 6
Sugar Land, TX 77478-4908
(281)313-1700
FAX: (281)313-1705

Houston Methodist Sugar Land Hospital
16655 Southwest Fwy
Sugar Land, TX 77479-2329
(281)274-1726
FAX: (281)274-0180

Kelsey-Seybold Medical Group, Pllc
11555 University Blvd
Sugar Land, TX 77478-3889
(713)442-1161
FAX: (713)442-6376

Memorial Hermann Health System
17510 W Grand Pkwy S, Dba Memorial Hermann Sugar Land Hospital
Sugar Land, TX 77479-2646
(281)725-5319
FAX: (281)725-5919

Memorial Mri & Diagnostic Llc
11211 S Highway 6, Ste B
Sugar Land, TX 77498-4994
(713)461-3399
FAX: (713)461-1969

One Step Diagnostic Vii Lp
6921 Brisbane Ct, Ste 110
Sugar Land, TX 77479-7094
(281)313-1414
FAX: (281)313-1415

Solis Mammography Of Sugar Land, Llc
1111 Highway 6, Ste 260
Sugar Land, TX 77478-4913
(866)717-2551
FAX: (281)947-2490

St. Luke's Sugar Land Hospital
1317 Lake Pointe Pkwy
Sugar Land, TX 77478-3997
(281)637-7001
FAX: (281)637-7907

Sulphur Springs

Christus Mother Frances Hospital- Sulphur Springs
115 Airport Rd
Sulphur Springs, TX 75482-2105
(903)439-4040
FAX: (903)438-4711

Sunnyvale

Texas Regional Medical Center, Llc
231 S Collins Rd, Dba baylor scott&White medcntr-Sunnyvale
Sunnyvale, TX 75182-4624
(972)892-3000
FAX: (972)892-4771

Sweeny

Sweeny Hospital District
305 N McKinney St, Dba Sweeny Community Hospital
Sweeny, TX 77480-2895
(979)548-1500
FAX: (979)548-1575

Sweetwater

Nolan County Hospital District
200 E Arizona Ave, Dba Rolling Plains Memorial Hospital
Sweetwater, TX 79556-7120
(325)235-1701
FAX: (325)235-4129

Taylor

Baylor Scott & White Medical Center - Taylor
305 Mallard Ln
Taylor, TX 76574-1208
(512)509-9100
FAX: (512)509-9136

Temple

Scott & White Memorial Hosp Dba Baylor S&W Med Ctr - Temple
2401 S 31st St
Temple, TX 76508-0001
(254)724-7038
FAX: (254)724-7937

Seton Family Of Doctors
1905 SW H K Dodgen Loop, Ste 107
Temple, TX 76502-1814
(254)298-2530
FAX: (254)773-9742

Texarkana

Brim Healthcare Of Texas Llc Dba Wadley Regional Medical Ctr
1000 Pine St
Texarkana, TX 75501-5100
(903)798-7207
FAX: (903)798-8740

Christus St. Michael Health System
2500 Saint Michael Dr
Texarkana, TX 75503-5218
(903)614-2273
FAX: (903)614-7020

Collom & Carney Clinic
5002 Cowhorn Creek Dr.
Texarkana, TX 75503
(903)614-3093
FAX: (903)614-3512

The Woodlands

Houston Methodist The Woodlands Hospital
17183 Interstate 45 S Ste 310
The Woodlands, TX 77385-3313
(936)270-3600
FAX: (936)270-3602

Memorial Hermann Health System
9200 Pinecroft Dr, Dba memorial hermann the woodlands hosp
The Woodlands, TX 77380-3279
(281)897-2794
FAX: (281)897-2060

St. Luke's The Woodlands Hospital
17200 St Lukes Way
The Woodlands, TX 77384-8007
(936)266-3250
FAX: (936)266-2388

The Breast And Imaging Center L.L.C.
4840 W Panther Creek Dr, Ste 107
The Woodlands, TX 77381-3528
(281)292-1192
FAX: (713)512-7713

Tops Specialty Hospital Ltd.
111 Vision Park Blvd, Ste 230
The Woodlands, TX 77384-3006
(281)580-6171
FAX: (281)765-4650

Tomball

David P. Ellent, Pllc
24721 State Highway 249, Dba Venus Mri And Women's Center
Tomball, TX 77375-7727
(346)336-7700
FAX: (281)205-0339

Solis Mammography At Hca Houston Tomball, Llc
13426 Medical Complex Dr, Ste 100
Tomball, TX 77375-6453
(866)717-2551
FAX: (866)366-5798

Tomball Mri Inc. Dba Tomball Medical Imaging Inc.
425 Holderrieth Blvd Ste 206
Tomball, TX 77375-4552
(281)207-8800
FAX: (281)207-8999

Tyler

Mf Hosp Reg Hc Ctr/Dba Christus Mother Frances Hosp Tyler
8288 S Broadway Ave Ste 1000
Tyler, TX 75703-5273
(903)606-5433
FAX: (903)606-1160

Mf Hosp Reg Hc Ctr/Dba Christus Mother Frances Hosp. Tyler
910 E Houston St Ste 650
Tyler, TX 75702-8370
(903)606-5433
FAX: (903)606-1160

University Health Clinic
3310 Patriot Dr
Tyler, TX 75701-6606
(903)939-7870
FAX: (903)939-7879

University Of Texas Health Science Center At Tyler
11937 US Highway 271
Tyler, TX 75708-3154
(903)877-7777
FAX: (903)877-2846

Ut Health East Texas Tyler Regional Hospital
700 Olympic Plaza Cir Ste 101
Tyler, TX 75701-1952
(903)596-3164
FAX: (903)596-3168

Uvalde

Uvalde Memorial Hospital
1025 Garner Field Rd
Uvalde, TX 78801-4895
(830)278-6251
FAX: (830)278-7145

Vernon

Wilbarger County Hospital District
920 Hillcrest Dr, Dba Wilbarger General Hospital
Vernon, TX 76384-3132
(940)552-9351
FAX: (940)553-2864

Victoria

Citizens Medical Center
2701 Hospital Dr
Victoria, TX 77901-5749
(361)570-7277
FAX: (361)572-5091

O'Sullivan Radiology
6915 N Main St
Victoria, TX 77904-2930
(361)572-3139
FAX: (361)572-8610

Victoria Of Texas, L.P. Dba Detar Healthcare System
115 Medical Dr Ste 107
Victoria, TX 77904-3105
(361)788-2512
FAX: (361)788-2649

Vinton

El Paso / Vinton Diagnostic Pa
7930 Doniphan Dr
Vinton, TX 79821-7613
(915)886-4488
FAX: (915)886-4688

Waco

Ascension Providence
6600 Fish Pond Rd
Waco, TX 76710-2582
(254)537-1715
FAX: (254)537-1798

Hillcrest Baptist Medical Center
50 Hillcrest Medical Blvd, Dba Baylor Scott&White Medcntr-Hillcrest
Waco, TX 76712-8953
(254)202-4220
FAX: (254)202-4299

Scott & White Memorial Hospital Dba Baylor S&W Clinic-Waco
7700 Fish Pond Rd
Waco, TX 76710-1031
(254)761-4407
FAX: (254)761-4597

Waxahachie

Baylor Medical Center At Waxahachie
2400 N Interstate Highway 35 E, Dba Baylor S&W Medical Center Waxahachie
Waxahachie, TX 75165-5240
(469)843-5160
FAX: (469)843-5163

Weatherford

Medical City Weatherford
914 Foster Ln
Weatherford, TX 76086-5714
(817)594-8239
FAX: (817)594-7326

Webster

Kelsey-Seybold Medical Group, Pllc
1010 S Ponds Dr
Webster, TX 77598-1409
(713)442-4327
FAX: (713)442-4325

Solis Mammography At Clearlake
400 W Medical Center Blvd, Ste 100
Webster, TX 77598-4223
(866)717-2551
FAX: (281)526-6845

University Of Texas Medical Branch At Galveston
250 Blossom St Ste 160, Dba Utmb Health Clear Lake Campus
Webster, TX 77598-4204
(409)772-9202

Weslaco

Doctors Hospital At Renaissance
1121 James St
Weslaco, TX 78596-6656
(956)362-3660
FAX: (956)362-3642

Knapp Medical Center
1401 E 8th St
Weslaco, TX 78596-6640
(956)969-5175
FAX: (956)973-5538

Sths Er At Weslaco
330 W Expressway 83
Weslaco, TX 78599-4332
(956)388-2190
FAX: (956)388-6030

Wichita Falls

Clinics Of North Texas L.L.P.
501 Midwestern Pkwy E
Wichita Falls, TX 76302-2302
(940)766-3551
FAX: (940)766-8793

Solis Mammography
5500 Kell Blvd, Ste 110
Wichita Falls, TX 76310-1612
(866)717-2551
FAX: (940)696-3706

Texoma Womens Clinic P.A.
6 Burnside, Dba The Womens Clinic
Wichita Falls, TX 76310-1128
(940)723-8151
FAX: (940)687-8243

United Regional Health Care System Inc.
1600 11th St
Wichita Falls, TX 76301-4388
(940)764-6014
FAX: (940)764-6147

Willow Park

Texas Health Harris Methodist Hosp Ft Worth
101 Crown Pointe Blvd, Dba tx health neighborhood care
Willow Park, TX 76087-1191
(817)757-1520
FAX: (817)757-1530

Wylie

Lake Pointe Operating Company, Llc
2300 W Fm 544, Ste 110
Wylie, TX 75098-4935
(972)366-3450
FAX: (972)442-8317

Yoakum

Yoakum Community Hospital
1200 Carl Ramert Dr
Yoakum, TX 77995-4868
(361)293-2321
FAX: (361)741-2298

UTAH

American Fork

American Fork Hospital
170 N 1100 E
American Fork, UT 84003-2961
(801)855-3350
FAX: (801)855-3384

Revere Health Imaging, American Fork
1175 E 50 S Ste 141
American Fork, UT 84003-2845
(801)492-5996
FAX: (801)812-4699

Blanding

Blue Mountain Hospital
802 S 200 W
Blanding, UT 84511-3910
(435)678-4820
FAX: (435)678-4691

Bountiful

Bountiful Health Center
390 N Main St
Bountiful, UT 84010-6046
(801)397-6392
FAX: (801)397-6399

Lakeview Hospital
630 Medical Dr
Bountiful, UT 84010-4908
(801)299-3822
FAX: (801)299-3823

Brigham City

Brigham City Community Hospital
950 Medical Dr, Lbby
Brigham City, UT 84302-3090
(435)734-4214
FAX: (435)734-4189

Cedar City

Cedar City Imaging Center
1333 N Main St Ste 7
Cedar City, UT 84721-5332
(435)868-5584
FAX: (435)868-5287

Delta

Delta Community Hospital
126 White Sage Ave
Delta, UT 84624-8937
(435)864-1535
FAX: (435)864-1932

Draper

Lone Peak Hospital
11925 S State St
Draper, UT 84020-7735
(801)545-8129
FAX: (801)545-8009

Farmington

Farmington Health Center
165 N University Ave
Farmington, UT 84025-2990
(801)581-5496
FAX: (801)587-9282

Fillmore

Fillmore Community Hospital
674 S Highway 99
Fillmore, UT 84631-5013
(435)743-1531
FAX: (435)743-6312

Gunnison

Gunnison Valley Hospital
PO Box 759, 64 E 100 N
Gunnison, UT 84634-0759
(435)528-2125
FAX: (435)528-3895

Heber

Heber Valley Hospital
454 E Medical Way
Heber, UT 84032-1391
(435)657-4397
FAX: (435)657-4387

Hurricane

Intermountain Hurricane Clinic
75 N 2260 W
Hurricane, UT 84737-2034
(435)251-1777
FAX: (435)688-6406

Layton

Davis Hospital And Medical Center
2132 N Robins Dr Ste B100
Layton, UT 84041-7058
(801)807-7120
FAX: (801)807-7650

Intermountain Layton Clinic
2075 University Park Blvd
Layton, UT 84041-1611
(801)525-5700
FAX: (801)779-6202

Tanner Clinic Mammography
1756 W Antelope Dr
Layton, UT 84041-1143
(801)773-4840
FAX: (801)773-3458

Lehi

Mountain Point Medical Center
3000 N Triumph Blvd
Lehi, UT 84043-4999
(385)345-3512
FAX: (385)345-3163

Logan

Women's Imaging & Mammography Center At Logan Hospital
1400 N 500 E, Women's Center - Logan Regional Hospital
Logan, UT 84341-2455
(435)716-5307
FAX: (435)716-2522

Midvale

University Of Utah Hospitals & Clinics Greenwood Health Ctr
7495 S State St
Midvale, UT 84047-2013
(801)213-9640
FAX: (801)213-9644

Moab

Moab Regional Hospital
450 Williams Way
Moab, UT 84532-2185
(435)719-3794
FAX: (435)719-3769

Montezuma Creek

Montezuma Creek Health Center
1478 East Highway 162
Montezuma Creek, UT 84534
(435)651-3751
FAX: (435)678-0499

Mt Pleasant

Sanpete Valley Hospital
1100 S Medical Dr
Mt Pleasant, UT 84647-2222
(435)462-4136
FAX: (435)462-4609

Murray

Intermountain Healthcare Mobile Mammography-Mobile
5063 S Cottonwood St
Murray, UT 84107-6766
(833)626-4666
FAX: (801)507-7899

Intermountain Medical Center
5121 S Cottonwood St
Murray, UT 84107-5701
(801)507-7835
FAX: (801)507-7898

Mountain Medical Imaging Llc Mobile
5323 S Woodrow St Ste 100
Murray, UT 84107-5842
(801)713-0600
FAX: (801)713-0601

Nephi

Central Valley Medical Center
48 W 1500 N
Nephi, UT 84648-8900
(435)623-3165
FAX: (435)623-3062

North Logan

Cache Valley Hospital
2380 N 400 E, Bldg Main
North Logan, UT 84341-1749
(435)713-9700
FAX: (435)753-8018

North Ogden

Intermountain North Ogden Clinic
2400 N 400 E
North Ogden, UT 84414-7233
(801)786-7500
FAX: (801)786-7563

Ogden

McKay - Dee Hospital Center
4401 Harrison Blvd, Women's Imaging 4th Fl
Ogden, UT 84403-3195
(801)387-4633
FAX: (801)387-4631

Ogden Clinic
4650 Harrison Blvd
Ogden, UT 84403-4303
(801)475-3800
FAX: (801)475-3838

Ogden Regional Medical Center
5475 S 500 E
Ogden, UT 84405-6905
(801)479-2470
FAX: (801)479-2969

Orem

Orem Community Hospital
331 N 400 W
Orem, UT 84057-1999
(801)714-3332
FAX: (801)714-3337

Timpanogos Regional Hospital
750 W 800 N
Orem, UT 84057-3660
(801)714-6280
FAX: (801)714-6283

Panguitch

Garfield Memorial Hosp Mobile Mammo Unit Mobile
200 N 400 E
Panguitch, UT 84759-7803
(435)676-1267
FAX: (435)676-1540

Park City

Park City Hospital
900 Round Valley Dr
Park City, UT 84060-7552
(435)658-7051
FAX: (435)658-7054

Redstone Mammography Center
1743 Redstone Center Dr, Ste 115
Park City, UT 84098-7930
(801)581-5496
FAX: (801)587-9282

Payson

Mountain View Hospital
1000 E 100 N
Payson, UT 84651-1600
(801)465-7300
FAX: (801)465-7145

Price

Castleview Hospital
300 N Hospital Dr, Radiology Department
Price, UT 84501-4200
(435)636-4844
FAX: (435)636-4877

Provo

Revere Health Imaging, Provo
1055 N 500 W Ste 112
Provo, UT 84604-3305
(801)812-4624
FAX: (801)812-4699

Riverwoods Advanced Diagnostic Imaging Center
3152 N University Ave Ste 100
Provo, UT 84604-4746
(801)229-2002
FAX: (801)229-1003

Utah Valley Hospital
1034 N 500 W
Provo, UT 84604-3337
(801)357-3165
FAX: (801)357-3101

Richfield

Sevier Valley Medical Center
1000 N Main St
Richfield, UT 84701-2061
(435)893-0262
FAX: (435)893-0260

Riverton

Riverton Hospital
3741 W 12600 S
Riverton, UT 84065-7215
(801)507-7840
FAX: (801)507-7899

Roosevelt

Uintah Basin Medical Center Women's Health Ctr
250 W 300 N 75-2
Roosevelt, UT 84066-2351
(435)725-2081
FAX: (435)725-2082

Roy

Davis Hospital & Medical Center Weber Campus
3451 W 5600 S
Roy, UT 84067-9112
(801)807-7120
FAX: (801)807-7650

Salem

Revere Health Imaging, Salem
555 W 2000 N Suite 107
Salem, UT 84653
(801)812-4624
FAX: (801)812-4699

Salt Lake City

Huntsman Comprehensive Breast Care Center
1950 Circle Of Hope Dr
Salt Lake City, UT 84112-5500
(801)581-5496
FAX: (801)587-9282

Intermountain Salt Lake Clinic Imaging Svcs
389 S 900 E
Salt Lake City, UT 84102-2310
(385)282-2205
FAX: (385)282-2206

Lds Hospital
8th Avenue & C St
Salt Lake City, UT 84143-0001
(801)507-7840
FAX: (801)507-7899

Redwood Health Center
1525 W 2100 S
Salt Lake City, UT 84119-1407
(801)581-5496
FAX: (801)587-9282

Salt Lake Regional Medical Center Breast Care Center
1050 E South Temple
Salt Lake City, UT 84102-1507
(801)350-4451
FAX: (801)961-9299

St Mark's Hospital - Women's Diagnostic Center
1140 E 3900 S
Salt Lake City, UT 84124-1228
(801)268-7900
FAX: (801)743-6512

Sugar House Health Center
1280 E Stringham Ave
Salt Lake City, UT 84106-2490
(801)581-5496
FAX: (801)587-9282

Sandy

Alta View Hospital
9660 S 1300 E
Sandy, UT 84094-3793
(801)507-7835
FAX: (801)507-7897

Optum Mobile Clinic Utah
1403 E Sego Lily Dr Ste 100
Sandy, UT 84092-4350
(801)941-4808
FAX: (385)274-3970

South Jordan

South Jordan Health Center
5126 W Daybreak Pkwy
South Jordan, UT 84009-5994
(801)581-5496
FAX: (801)587-9282

Spanish Fork

Spanish Fork Hospital
765 E Market Place Dr
Spanish Fork, UT 84660-1396
(385)344-5822
FAX: (385)344-5815

St George

Intermountain St. George Women's Imaging Center
1380 E Medical Center Dr
St George, UT 84790-2123
(435)251-5110
FAX: (435)251-5101

Revere Health Imaging St. George
2825 E Mall Dr
St George, UT 84790-1954
(435)986-2238
FAX: (435)986-2237

Tooele

Mountain West Medical Center
2055 N Main St
Tooele, UT 84074-9819
(435)843-3600
FAX: (435)843-3676

Tremonton

Unr Bear River Hospital
905 N 1000 W
Tremonton, UT 84337-2497
(435)207-4545
FAX: (435)207-4560

Vernal

Ashley Regional Medical Center
150 W 100 N
Vernal, UT 84078-2036
(435)781-6822
FAX: (435)781-6884

West Jordan

Breast Care Center At Jordan Valley
3580 W 9000 S
West Jordan, UT 84088-8812
(801)562-3171
FAX: (801)562-3191

West Valley City

Jordan Valley Medical Center- West Valley Campus
3460 S Pioneer Pkwy
West Valley City, UT 84120-2049
(801)964-3888
FAX: (801)964-3292

VERMONT

Barre

Central Vermont Medical Center
PO Box 547, Fisher Pond Rd
Barre, VT 05641-0547
(802)371-4249
FAX: (802)371-5352

Bennington

Southwestern Vermont Medical Center
100 Hospital Dr
Bennington, VT 05201-5013
(802)442-6361
FAX: (802)447-5108

Brattleboro

Brattleboro Memorial Hospital
17 Belmont Ave
Brattleboro, VT 05301-3498
(802)251-8451
FAX: (802)251-8432

Burlington

University Of Vermont Medical Ctr.- Main Campus
111 Colchester Ave, Main Pavilion, Level 2, Breast Care Cent
Burlington, VT 05401-1473
(802)847-2446
FAX: (802)847-8493

Uvm Medical Ctr.- South Prospect St. Campus
1 S Prospect St
Burlington, VT 05401-3456
(802)847-2446
FAX: (802)847-8493

Colchester

University Of Vermont Medical Ctr. - Fanny Allen Campus
790 College Pkwy, Radiology Department
Colchester, VT 05446-3007
(802)847-2446
FAX: (802)847-1387

Middlebury

Uvmhn/Porter Medical Center
115 Porter Dr
Middlebury, VT 05753-8629
(802)388-4757
FAX: (802)388-8821

Morrisville

Copley Hospital
528 Washington Hwy
Morrisville, VT 05661-8973
(802)888-8358
FAX: (802)888-8394

Newport

North Country Hospital
189 Prouty Dr
Newport, VT 05855-9820
(802)334-3210
FAX: (802)334-4174

Randolph

Gifford Medical Center
44 S Main St
Randolph, VT 05060-1381
(802)728-2214
FAX: (802)728-2112

Rutland

Rutland Regional Medical Center
160 Allen St, Mammography Dpt.
Rutland, VT 05701-4595
(802)775-7111
FAX: (802)772-1937

Springfield

Springfield Hospital
25 Ridgewood Rd
Springfield, VT 05156-3057
(802)885-7069
FAX: (802)885-7312

St Albans

Northwestern Medical Center
133 Fairfield St
St Albans, VT 05478-1726
(802)524-1058
FAX: (802)524-1289

St Johnsbury

Northeastern Vermont Regional Hospital
1315 Hospital Dr
St Johnsbury, VT 05819-9758
(802)748-7567
FAX: (802)748-7549

Windsor

Mt. Ascutney Hospital & Health Center
289 County Rd
Windsor, VT 05089-9000
(802)674-7276
FAX: (802)674-7099

VIRGINIA

Abingdon

The Women's Center At Johnston Memorial Hospital
16000 Johnston Memorial Dr, Suite 201 Medical Plaza
Abingdon, VA 24211-7664
(276)258-4520
FAX: (276)258-2705

Alexandria

Association Of Alexandria Radiologists
Alexandria Va
4660 Kenmore Ave Ste 525
Alexandria, VA 22304-1314
(703)824-3260
FAX: (703)370-3889

Inova Diagnostic Imaging Center
6355 Walker Ln
Alexandria, VA 22310-3238
(571)423-5400
FAX: (571)423-4477

Inova Imaging Center - Mark Center
1800 N Beauregard St Ste 150
Alexandria, VA 22311-1730
(703)933-2591
FAX: (703)379-7606

Inova Mount Vernon Hospital
2501 Parkers Ln, Radiology Department
Alexandria, VA 22306-3282
(571)423-5400
FAX: (703)664-8311

Kaiser Permanente Alexandria Medical Center
3000 Potomac Ave
Alexandria, VA 22305-3084
(877)390-0033
FAX: (301)548-5849

Sentara Ultrasound Associates Womens Imaging Center
5055 Seminary Rd Ste 104, Monticello Bldg.
Alexandria, VA 22311-2026
(703)820-8295
FAX: (703)820-8366

Arlington

Ifrc,Llc Dba Fairfax Radiology Center Of Ballston
3833 Fairfax Dr Ste 110
Arlington, VA 22203-1773
(703)788-8420
FAX: (571)665-6691

Virginia Hospital Center
1625 N George Mason Dr
Arlington, VA 22205-3683
(703)558-8500
FAX: (703)558-2488

Washington Radiology
1005 N Glebe Rd, Ste 110
Arlington, VA 22201-4751
(703)698-8800
FAX: (703)573-2318

Ashburn

Loudoun Imaging Center
20905 Professional Plz Ste 100
Ashburn, VA 20147-3409
(571)223-0230
FAX: (571)223-0330

Bedford

Centra Bedford Memorial Hospital
1613 Oakwood St
Bedford, VA 24523-1213
(540)587-7806
FAX: (540)586-0317

Big Stone Gap

Ballad Health Lonesome Pine Hospital
1990 Holton Ave E
Big Stone Gap, VA 24219-3350
(276)523-8617
FAX: (276)523-8671

Blacksburg

Carilion Clinic, Blacksburg Screening Mammography
901 Plantation Rd
Blacksburg, VA 24060-3880
(540)951-5860
FAX: (540)557-1237

Lewisgale Hospital Montgomery
813 Davis St
Blacksburg, VA 24060-7013
(540)443-9919
FAX: (540)443-9928

Bluefield

Community Radiology Of Virginia, Inc.
2000 Leatherwood Ln
Bluefield, VA 24605-2020
(304)327-7177
FAX: (304)327-5850

Surgical Care Of The Virginias, Llc
100B Westwood Cmn, Westwood Medical Park
Bluefield, VA 24605-2031
(276)322-2322
FAX: (276)322-2325

Carrollton

Sentara St. Luke's
20209 Sentara Way Ste 108
Carrollton, VA 23314-3573
(758)934-4542
FAX: (757)542-1201

Centreville

Ifrc,Llc Dba Fairfax Radiology Center Of Centreville
6211 Centreville Rd Ste 400
Centreville, VA 20121-2641
(703)698-4488
FAX: (703)961-8312

Charlottesville

Eccc Screening Mammograpphy
1240 Lee St
Charlottesville, VA 22908-0817
(434)243-1805
FAX: (434)924-5672

Jefferson Obstetrics And Gynecology
600 Peter Jefferson Pkwy, Ste 130
Charlottesville, VA 22911-8835
(434)977-4488
FAX: (888)397-4581

Sentara Martha Jefferson Comprehensive Breast Center
595 Martha Jefferson Dr Ste 380
Charlottesville, VA 22911-4669
(434)654-7130
FAX: (434)654-4593

Sentara Martha Jefferson Occ At Proffit Road
3263 Proffit Rd
Charlottesville, VA 22911-5639
(434)654-7130
FAX: (434)654-4593

The University Of Virginia Breast Care Center
PO Box 800743, 652 Peter Jefferson Pkwy
Charlottesville, VA 22908-0743
(434)243-1805
FAX: (434)924-5672

Virginia Mammography Center
2955 Ivy Rd Ste 102
Charlottesville, VA 22903-9353
(434)243-4704
FAX: (434)924-5672

Chatham

Chatham Diagnostic Imaging Center
19144 US Highway 29 Ste C
Chatham, VA 24531-5548
(434)799-3883
FAX: (434)773-6837

Chesapeake

Diagnostic Center Of Chesapeake
844 Battlefield Blvd N
Chesapeake, VA 23320-4802
(757)312-6137
FAX: (757)312-6668

Mid-Atlantic Imaging Centers
300 Medical Pkwy Ste 302
Chesapeake, VA 23320-4985
(757)312-8403
FAX: (757)312-8314

Sentara Greenbrier Healthplex At Advanced Imaging Ctr
713 Volvo Pkwy Ste 105
Chesapeake, VA 23320-1614
(757)282-4011
FAX: (757)410-3655

Tricare Prime Clinic Chesapeake
1400 Crossways Blvd, Ste 114 Ste 1232
Chesapeake, VA 23320-0207
(757)953-6335
FAX: (757)953-6329

Christiansburg

Carilion New River Valley Medical Center
2900 Lamb Cir
Christiansburg, VA 24073-6344
(540)731-2720
FAX: (540)731-2526

Colonial Heights

Appomattox Imaging Center
930 South Ave Ste 1
Colonial Heights, VA 23834-3620
(804)524-2340
FAX: (855)720-4159

Bon Secours Medical Group Richmond Specialty Care, Llc
439 Jennick Dr
Colonial Heights, VA 23834-4901
(804)765-5206
FAX: (804)765-5809

Culpeper

Outpatient Imaging Culpeper
509 Main Street
Culpeper, VA 22701
(540)321-3190
FAX: (540)321-3191

Daleville

Carilion Clinic Daleville Imaging
150 Market Ridge Ln
Daleville, VA 24083-3258
(540)966-0454
FAX: (540)591-5346

Lewis-Gale Imaging Center Daleville
65 Shenandoah Ave
Daleville, VA 24083-3201
(540)776-4983
FAX: (540)966-6659

Danville

Danville Diagnostic Imaging Center
125 Executive Dr Ste D
Danville, VA 24541-4155
(434)799-3883
FAX: (434)799-0202

Danville Women's Care, Pc
927 S Main St
Danville, VA 24541-4001
(434)797-4620
FAX: (434)793-8992

Ob-Gyn Associates Of Danville, Inc.
101 Holbrook St
Danville, VA 24541-1759
(434)792-7765
FAX: (434)793-4061

Dulles

Stonesprings Hospital Center
24440 Stone Springs Blvd
Dulles, VA 20166-2247
(571)349-4737
FAX: (571)349-4040

Dumfries

Dumfries Health Center
3700 Fettler Park Dr, Ste 101
Dumfries, VA 22025-2051
(703)441-7543
FAX: (703)441-7697

Emporia

Southern Virginia Regional Medical Center
727 N Main St
Emporia, VA 23847-1274
(434)348-4821
FAX: (434)348-4945

Fairfax

Fair Oaks Imaging Center
4001 Fair Ridge Dr, Ste 103
Fairfax, VA 22033-2917
(703)385-5203
FAX: (703)385-3058

Fairfax Health Center
4375 Fair Lakes Ct
Fairfax, VA 22033-4234
(571)432-2717
FAX: (571)432-2794

Ifrc, Llc Dba Fairfax Radiology Center Of Fairfax City
3801 University Dr Ste 120
Fairfax, VA 22030-2503
(703)698-4488
FAX: (703)788-8422

Ifrc,Llc Dba Fairfax Radiology Breast Center Of Fairfax
8260 Willow Oaks Corporate Dr, Ste 200
Fairfax, VA 22031-4515
(703)698-4488
FAX: (703)205-9884

Inova Fair Oaks Hospital
3600 Joseph Siewick Dr, Radiology Department
Fairfax, VA 22033-1798
(703)391-3500
FAX: (703)391-3900

Inova Schar Cancer Institute- Diagnostic Imaging Center
8081 Innovation Park Dr, Imaging- 2nd Floor Pavilion
Fairfax, VA 22031-4867
(571)423-5400
FAX: (571)472-1639

Kaiser Permanente - Fair Oaks
12255 Fair Lakes Pkwy
Fairfax, VA 22033-3952
(877)390-0333
FAX: (301)548-5849

Washington Radiology
3022 Williams Dr Ste 204
Fairfax, VA 22031-4600
(703)280-9800
FAX: (703)573-2318

Falls Church

Kaiser Permanente - Falls Church Center
201 N Washington St, Dept. Of Radiology
Falls Church, VA 22046-4518
(703)359-7878
FAX: (240)632-4451

Farmville

Centra Southside Community Hospital
800 Oak St, Radiolog/Mammography Departm
Farmville, VA 23901-1199
(434)315-2779
FAX: (434)315-2769

Fishersville

Augusta Health
78 Medical Center Dr
Fishersville, VA 22939-2332
(540)932-4486
FAX: (540)932-5387

Fort Belvoir

Ft Belvoir Community Hospital
9300 Dewitt Loop, Sunrise Bldg Si 233
Fort Belvoir, VA 22060-5285
(571)231-3224
FAX: (571)231-6657

Fort Eustis

McDonald Army Health Center
576 Jefferson Ave Bldg, Hsxh-Rad-Mammo
Fort Eustis, VA 23604-5548
(757)314-7745
FAX: (757)314-7994

Fort Lee

Kenner Army Health Clinic
700 24th St Bldg 8130, Radiology Department
Fort Lee, VA 23801-1716
(804)734-9118
FAX: (804)734-9008

Franklin

Southampton Memorial Hospital
100 Fairview Dr
Franklin, VA 23851-1238
(757)569-6100
FAX: (757)516-1109

Fredericksburg

Kaiser Permanente Fredericksburg
1201 Hospital Dr
Fredericksburg, VA 22401-8428
(703)359-7878
FAX: (301)548-5849

Medical Imaging Of Fredericksburg At Lee's Hill
10401 Spotsylvania Ave Ste 101
Fredericksburg, VA 22408-8606
(540)741-9729
FAX: (540)741-1981

Spotsylvania Regional Medical Center
4600 Spotsylvania Pkwy
Fredericksburg, VA 22408-7762
(540)498-4000
FAX: (540)498-4769

The Imaging Center For Women
1300 Hospital Dr Ste 100
Fredericksburg, VA 22401-8451
(540)741-9729
FAX: (540)741-1981

Front Royal

Warren Memorial Hospital, Inc.
351 Valley Health Way
Front Royal, VA 22630-6480
(855)724-3384
FAX: (540)636-0414

Gainesville

Inova Fairfax Hospital Outpatient Imaging Center Gainesville
13575 Heathcote Blvd, Ste 200
Gainesville, VA 20155-6700
(703)468-2609
FAX: (703)468-2601

Galax

Twin County Regional Hospital
200 Hospital Dr
Galax, VA 24333-2227
(276)236-1680
FAX: (276)238-3579

Glen Allen

Bon Secours Imaging Center At Innsbrook
4900 Cox Rd Ste 100
Glen Allen, VA 23060-6508
(804)923-1417
FAX: (804)346-1686

Paredes Institute For Women's Imaging
4480 Cox Rd Ste 100
Glen Allen, VA 23060-6751
(804)523-2303
FAX: (804)523-3210

Gloucester

Riverside Walter Reed Hospital
7519 Hospital Dr
Gloucester, VA 23061-4178
(804)693-8853
FAX: (804)693-8857

Sentara Gloucester Imaging Ctr
5659 Parkway Dr Ste 130
Gloucester, VA 23061-3792
(804)210-1070
FAX: (804)210-1074

Gordonsville

Sentara Spring Creek Family Medicine
29 Jefferson Ct
Gordonsville, VA 22942-9602
(434)654-7130
FAX: (434)654-4593

Gretna

Centra Gretna Medical Center
291 McBride Ln
Gretna, VA 24557-2773
(434)200-4048
FAX: (434)200-5546

Grundy

Buchanan General Hospital
1535 Slate Creek Rd
Grundy, VA 24614-6974
(276)935-1133
FAX: (276)935-1392

Hampton

Riverside Diagnostic Center Hampton
850 Enterprise Pkwy Ste 1500
Hampton, VA 23666-6251
(757)989-8830
FAX: (757)251-7842

Sentara Careplex Hospital
3000 Coliseum Dr
Hampton, VA 23666-5963
(757)594-1899
FAX: (757)594-1901

The Breast Center Of Tpmg Hampton
2205 Executive Dr Ste B
Hampton, VA 23666-2948
(757)873-0848
FAX: (757)223-7760

USAF Hospital Langley
633 Sgcs/Sgox, 77 Nealy Avenue
Hampton, VA 23665
(757)764-6947
FAX: (757)764-1942

Harrisonburg

Harrisonburg Obgyn
2291 Evelyn Byrd Ave
Harrisonburg, VA 22801-5424
(540)434-3831
FAX: (877)202-2032

Sentara Rmh Funkhouser Women's Center
2275 Health Campus Dr
Harrisonburg, VA 22801-8809
(540)689-6800
FAX: (540)689-6801

Shenandoah Womens Healthcare
240 Lucy Dr
Harrisonburg, VA 22801-8036
(540)438-1314
FAX: (877)336-4701

Haymarket

Kaiser Permanente Haymarket Medical Center
15040 Heathcote Blvd
Haymarket, VA 20169-6251
(877)390-0033
FAX: (301)548-5849

Novant Health Uva Health System Haymarket Medical Center
15225 Heathcote Blvd
Haymarket, VA 20169-6264
(703)369-8073
FAX: (703)369-8675

Herndon

Ifrc, Llc Dba Fairfax Radiology Breast Center Of Reston/Hern
106 Elden St Ste 16
Herndon, VA 20170-4826
(703)698-4488
FAX: (703)796-1103

Hopewell

Hca John Randolph Medical Center
411 W Randolph Rd
Hopewell, VA 23860-2938
(804)458-2400
FAX: (804)452-3388

Hot Springs

Bath Community Hospital
106 Park Dr
Hot Springs, VA 24445-2921
(540)839-7037
FAX: (540)839-7134

Kilmarnock

Bon Secours Rappahannock Gen Hosp Women's Imaging Center
101 Harris Rd
Kilmarnock, VA 22482-3880
(804)435-8325
FAX: (804)435-8040

King George

Medical Imaging Of King George
11131 Journal Pkwy
King George, VA 22485-3468
(540)741-9729
FAX: (540)741-1981

Lake Ridge

Sentara Lake Ridge Advanced Imaging Center
12825 Minnieville Rd, Ste 100
Lake Ridge, VA 22192-3601
(703)523-1560
FAX: (571)492-6014

Lansdowne

Ifrc, Llc Dba Fairfax Radiology Breast Center Of Loudoun
19465 Deerfield Ave Ste 105
Lansdowne, VA 20176-1702
(703)698-4488
FAX: (703)724-0600

Lebanon

Msha Dba Russel County Hospital
58 Carroll St
Lebanon, VA 24266
(276)883-8157
FAX: (276)883-8150

Leesburg

Inova Loudoun Diagnostic Imaging Ctr At Leesburg
224 Cornwall St NW, Outpatient Imaging Dept
Leesburg, VA 20176-2701
(703)858-6470
FAX: (703)737-7555

Lexington

Carilion Stonewall Jackson Hospital
1 Health Cir
Lexington, VA 24450-2492
(540)458-3321
FAX: (540)458-3334

Lorton

Inova Healthplex - Lorton
9321 Sanger St
Lorton, VA 22079-2720
(703)982-8293
FAX: (703)982-8356

Sentara Lorton Station Women's Imaging Center
8986 Lorton Station Blvd Ste 200
Lorton, VA 22079-4755
(703)523-8844
FAX: (703)372-1570

Low Moor

Lewisgale Hospital Alleghany
1 Arh Lane
Low Moor, VA 24457
(540)862-6811
FAX: (540)862-6462

Luray

Page Memorial Hospital
200 Memorial Dr
Luray, VA 22835-1000
(540)743-8103
FAX: (540)843-0861

Lynchburg

Centra Breast Imaging Center
3300 Rivermont Ave
Lynchburg, VA 24503-2030
(434)200-4048
FAX: (434)200-5546

Centra Health Mobile Mammography-Mobile
20293 Timberlake Rd
Lynchburg, VA 24502-7202
(434)200-4048
FAX: (434)200-3645

Centra Mammography Center - Tate Springs
1900 Tate Springs Rd, Ste 15
Lynchburg, VA 24501-1115
(434)200-4048
FAX: (434)200-7766

Timberlake Mammography Center
20293 Timberlake Rd
Lynchburg, VA 24502-7202
(434)200-4048
FAX: (434)200-3645

Women's Health Breast Imaging Center
114 Nationwide Dr
Lynchburg, VA 24502-4271
(434)239-7890
FAX: (434)237-9222

Manassas

Kaiser Permanente Manassas
10701 Rosemary Dr
Manassas, VA 20109-7282
(703)359-7878
FAX: (301)548-5849

Novant Health Uva Health System Prince William Medical Ctr
8700 Sudley Rd
Manassas, VA 20110-4418
(703)369-8073
FAX: (703)369-8675

Marion

Smyth County Community Hospital
245 Medical Park Dr
Marion, VA 24354-1100
(276)378-1300
FAX: (276)378-1315

Martinsville

Julius Hermes Breast Care Center Sovah Health Martinsville
320 Hospital Dr
Martinsville, VA 24112-1900
(276)666-7561
FAX: (276)666-7653

McLean

Kaiser Permanente - Tysons Corner
8008 Westpark Dr
McLean, VA 22102-3109
(703)899-2287
FAX: (301)548-5849

Mechanicsville

Hanover Imaging Center
9275 Chamberlayne Rd
Mechanicsville, VA 23116-2800
(804)327-8702
FAX: (804)730-1491

Memorial Regional Medical Center
8260 Atlee Rd, Mammography Dept
Mechanicsville, VA 23116-1844
(804)764-6513
FAX: (804)764-6039

Virginia Women's Center
7515 Right Flank Rd
Mechanicsville, VA 23116-3818
(804)545-6858
FAX: (804)559-2046

Midlothian

Bon Secours Richmond Ob - Gyn
13700 St Francis Blvd Ste 305
Midlothian, VA 23114-3222
(804)320-2483
FAX: (804)419-1860

Bon Secours St. Francis Medical Center
13710 St Francis Blvd
Midlothian, VA 23114-3267
(804)627-5660
FAX: (804)627-5658

Bon Secours Westchester Women's Imaging Center
601 Watkins Centre Pkwy Ste 230
Midlothian, VA 23114-4412
(804)627-5660
FAX: (804)794-7043

Chesterfield Imaging Center
13636 Hull Street Rd
Midlothian, VA 23112-2108
(804)639-5489
FAX: (866)451-0096

Virginia Physicians - Westchester
15769 Wc Main St, Midlothian Family Practice
Midlothian, VA 23113-7327
(504)560-5859
FAX: (804)272-2909

Virginia Physicians For Women
13801 St Francis Blvd Ste 150
Midlothian, VA 23114-3206
(804)897-2100
FAX: (804)897-9074

Virginia Women's Center
13801 St Francis Blvd Ste 100
Midlothian, VA 23114-3206
(804)545-6858
FAX: (804)545-9548

New Canton

Central Virginia Community Health Ctr Mammography Dept.
25892 N James Madison Hwy
New Canton, VA 23123-2234
(434)581-3271
FAX: (434)581-1105

Newport News

Dorothy G. Hoefer Comprehensive Breast Center
11803 Jefferson Ave Ste 130
Newport News, VA 23606-4390
(757)594-1899
FAX: (757)594-1901

Mid-Atlantic Imaging Centers
808 Triton Ct, Ste 102
Newport News, VA 23606-4538
(757)223-5059
FAX: (757)223-5664

Riverside Diagnostic And Breast Imaging Center
895 City Center Blvd, Ste 104
Newport News, VA 23606-3080
(757)989-8830
FAX: (757)594-4072

The Breast Center Of Tpmg
860 Omni Blvd Ste 109
Newport News, VA 23606-4430
(757)873-0848
FAX: (757)223-7760

Norfolk

Bon Secours Depaul Women's Imaging A Dept Of Maryview Mc
100 Kingsley Ln, Ste 306
Norfolk, VA 23505-4613
(757)889-5200
FAX: (757)398-2288

Branch Health Clinic Naval Station Norfolk
1721 Taussig Blvd
Norfolk, VA 23511
(757)953-8773
FAX: (757)953-8295

Fort Norfolk Diagnostic Center
301 Riverview Ave, Ste 830 Ste 830B
Norfolk, VA 23510-1065
(757)252-9100
FAX: (757)252-9133

Mid-Atlantic Imaging Centers
844 Kempsville Rd Ste 210
Norfolk, VA 23502-3927
(757)461-6131
FAX: (757)461-3897

Sentara McLeskey Comprehensive Breast Center
6251 E Virginia Beach Blvd, Ste 105
Norfolk, VA 23502-2824
(757)264-0138
FAX: (757)962-7716

Sentara Norfolk General Hospital
600 Gresham Dr
Norfolk, VA 23507-1999
(757)388-5525
FAX: (757)388-2795

North Chesterfield

Women's Cancer And Wellness Institute
1401 Johnston Willis Dr Ste 1100
North Chesterfield, VA 23235-4730
(804)323-5040
FAX: (804)323-5070

Norton

Norton Community Hospital Mammography Department
100 15th St NW
Norton, VA 24273-1616
(276)439-1380
FAX: (276)439-1381

Onancock

Riverside Shore Memorial Hospital
20480 Market St
Onancock, VA 23417-4309
(757)302-2321
FAX: (757)789-0614

Orange

Orange Family Physicians
13198 James Madison Hwy
Orange, VA 22960-2851
(540)672-3010
FAX: (540)434-9700

Pearisburg

Carilion Giles Community Hospital
159 Hartley Way
Pearisburg, VA 24134-2471
(540)922-4182
FAX: (540)921-5230

Petersburg

Southside Regional Medical Center Women's Imaging Center
210 Medical Park Blvd, Ste 225
Petersburg, VA 23805-0003
(804)765-6035
FAX: (804)765-5525

Portsmouth

Naval Medical Center - Portsmouth
620 John Paul Jones Cir Bldg 2
Portsmouth, VA 23708-2197
(757)953-4900
FAX: (757)953-0505

Prince George

Virginia Physicians For Women
1775 Lake Harley Dr
Prince George, VA 23875-1259
(804)897-2100
FAX: (804)897-9074

Pulaski

Lewisgale Hospital Pulaski
2400 Lee Hwy N
Pulaski, VA 24301-2326
(540)994-8480
FAX: (540)994-8392

Reston

Kaiser Permanente Reston
1890 Metro Center Dr
Reston, VA 20190-5222
(877)390-0033
FAX: (301)548-5849

Women's Imaging Center Of Reston
1860 Town Center Dr Ste 400
Reston, VA 20190-5901
(703)689-9005
FAX: (703)639-9404

Richlands

Clinch Valley Medical Center
6801 Governor Gc Peery Hwy
Richlands, VA 24641-2194
(276)596-6601
FAX: (276)596-6602

Richmond

Advanced Diagnostic Breast Center At Henrico Doctors Sarah C
7607 Forest Ave, Ste 210
Richmond, VA 23229-4913
(804)200-7035
FAX: (804)289-5679

Bon Secours - Richmond Community Hospital
1500 N 28th St
Richmond, VA 23223-5396
(804)627-5660
FAX: (804)225-1758

Bon Secours Imaging Center Reynolds Crossing
6605 W Broad St, Ste. B Ground Fl.
Richmond, VA 23230-1714
(804)287-3500
FAX: (804)285-1405

Bon Secours St. Mary's Hospital Women's Imaging Center
5875 Bremo Rd Ste 105MOB
Richmond, VA 23226-1934
(804)287-7501
FAX: (804)287-7504

Chippenham Medical Center
7101 Jahnke Rd
Richmond, VA 23225-4044
(804)327-8706
FAX: (804)483-0551

Cjw Johnston-Willis Medical Center
1401 Johnston Willis Dr, Ste 1101
Richmond, VA 23235-4730
(804)327-8706
FAX: (804)483-6291

Independence Park Imaging Center
9930 Independence Park Dr Ste 100
Richmond, VA 23233-1475
(804)217-9729
FAX: (804)217-9531

Laburnum Diagnostic Imaging Center
4630 S Laburnum Ave, Ste C
Richmond, VA 23231-2441
(804)226-4637
FAX: (804)222-7551

Paredes Institute For Womens Imaging
2530 Gaskins Rd Ste C
Richmond, VA 23238-1483
(804)523-2303
FAX: (804)934-0342

Retreat Doctors' Hosp-A Campus Of Henrico Doctors' Hospital
2621 Grove Ave
Richmond, VA 23220-4308
(804)254-5444
FAX: (804)254-5293

St. Marys Short Pump Emergency Center
12320 W Broad St
Richmond, VA 23233-7603
(804)923-1415
FAX: (804)360-0871

Vcu Health At Nelson Clinic - Breast Imaging
401 N 11th St, Third Floor, Room 300
Richmond, VA 23219-1901
(804)237-6666
FAX: (804)237-6663

Vcu Health At Stony Point - Breast Imaging
9000 Stony Point Pkwy
Richmond, VA 23235-1900
(804)237-6666
FAX: (804)237-6663

Virginia Physicians For Women
10710 Midlothian Tpke Ste 200
Richmond, VA 23235-4759
(804)897-2100
FAX: (804)897-9074

Virginia Physicians For Women
1630 Wilkes Ridge Pkwy Ste 200
Richmond, VA 23233-7460
(804)897-2100
FAX: (804)897-9074

Virginia Women's Center
12129 Graham Meadows Dr
Richmond, VA 23233-6661
(804)545-6858
FAX: (804)559-2046

Virginia Womens Center
6600 W Broad St Ste 100
Richmond, VA 23230-1709
(804)545-6858
FAX: (804)545-9345

Roanoke

Carilion Breast Care Center
102 Highland Ave SE Ste 202
Roanoke, VA 24013-2254
(540)985-9885
FAX: (540)224-6946

Carilion Breast Care Center
1211 S Jefferson St
Roanoke, VA 24016-4705
(540)985-9885
FAX: (540)983-1254

Carilion North Roanoke, Screening Mammography
6415 Peters Creek Rd
Roanoke, VA 24019-4021
(540)265-5545
FAX: (540)366-6563

Lewis Gale Imaging At Brambleton
4330 Brambleton Ave
Roanoke, VA 24018-3405
(540)283-3700
FAX: (540)283-3701

Physicians To Women, Inc.
21 Highland Ave SE Ste 202
Roanoke, VA 24013-2201
(540)982-8881
FAX: (877)502-7991

Rocky Mount

Carilion Franklin Memorial Hospital
180 Floyd Ave
Rocky Mount, VA 24151-1318
(540)484-8594
FAX: (540)484-8549

Salem

Lewisgale Breast Center Salem
1900 Electric Rd
Salem, VA 24153-7494
(540)776-4983
FAX: (540)769-2471

South Boston

Sentara Halifax Regional Hospital
2204 Wilborn Ave
South Boston, VA 24592-1645
(434)517-8994
FAX: (434)517-3686

South Hill

Vcu Health Community Memorial Hospital
1755 N Mecklenburg Ave
South Hill, VA 23970-4080
(434)584-5219
FAX: (434)584-5215

Springfield

Ifrc, Llc Dba Fairfax Radiology Center Of Springfield
5510 Alma Ln Ste 100
Springfield, VA 22151-4028
(703)698-4488
FAX: (703)698-0864

Kaiser Permanente - Springfield
6501 Loisdale Ct
Springfield, VA 22150-1885
(703)359-7878
FAX: (301)548-5849

Stafford

Colonial Forge Medical Center
125 Hospital Center Blvd Ste 110
Stafford, VA 22554-6202
(877)390-0033
FAX: (301)548-5849

Imaging Center For Women At North Stafford
125 Woodstream Blvd, Ste 101
Stafford, VA 22556-4630
(540)741-9729
FAX: (540)657-9730

Staunton

Augusta Health Outpatient Center
851 Statler Blvd
Staunton, VA 24401-4894
(540)932-4053
FAX: (540)932-5378

Sterling

Ifrc, Llc D/B/A Fairfax Radiology Center At Sterling
4 Pidgeon Hill Dr
Sterling, VA 20165-6173
(703)450-5800
FAX: (703)450-0495

Washington Radiology Associates
21351 Ridgetop Cir, Ste 100
Sterling, VA 20166-6608
(571)434-0140
FAX: (571)434-0144

Stuarts Draft

Augusta Health Stuarts Draft Outpatient Center
2570 Stuarts Draft Hwy
Stuarts Draft, VA 24477-3237
(540)932-4053
FAX: (540)932-5387

Suffolk

Bayview Physicians Services,P.C.-Suffolk
2000 Meade Pkwy, Ste 160
Suffolk, VA 23434-4259
(757)934-9308
FAX: (757)539-7582

Bon Secours Millie Lancaster Womens Center
5838 Harbour View Blvd, Ste 210
Suffolk, VA 23435-3602
(757)541-1914
FAX: (757)673-5969

Mid-Atlantic Imaging Centers
2050 Hillpoint Blvd N
Suffolk, VA 23434-7181
(757)290-6190
FAX: (757)461-3897

Sentara Belleharbour
3920A Bridge Rd, Ste 300
Suffolk, VA 23435-1117
(757)983-0010
FAX: (757)983-0011

Sentara Louise Obici Memorial Hospital
2800 Godwin Blvd
Suffolk, VA 23434-8038
(757)934-4973
FAX: (757)934-4735

Tappahannock

Vcu Health Tappahannock Hospital
618 Hospital Rd
Tappahannock, VA 22560-5000
(804)443-6044
FAX: (804)443-6045

Tazewell

Carilion Tazewell Community Hospital
388 Ben Bolt Ave
Tazewell, VA 24651-5386
(276)988-8730
FAX: (276)988-8735

Troy

Fluvanna Correctional Center For Women
144 Prison Ln
Troy, VA 22974-3761
(434)422-3496
FAX: (434)984-7610

Vienna

Ifrc, Llc Dba Fairfax Radiology Center Of Vienna
115 Park St SE Ste 203
Vienna, VA 22180-4653
(703)698-4488
FAX: (703)242-4474

Virginia Beach

Aici-Mammo
800 Independence Blvd, Radiology Department
Virginia Beach, VA 23455-6011
(757)363-6383
FAX: (757)363-6474

Mid-Atlantic Imaging Centers
1181 First Colonial Rd Ste 101
Virginia Beach, VA 23454-2437
(757)228-1600
FAX: (757)228-1727

Mid-Atlantic Imaging Centers
3300 Princess Anne Rd Ste 743
Virginia Beach, VA 23456-2605
(757)301-2500
FAX: (757)301-2003

Sentara Princess Anne Comprehensive Breast Center
1950 Glenn Mitchell Dr Ste 206
Virginia Beach, VA 23456-0047
(757)507-0665
FAX: (757)507-0103

Sentara Princess Anne Mammography Center
1975 Glenn Mitchell Dr Ste 100
Virginia Beach, VA 23456-0167
(757)507-0663
FAX: (757)507-0103

Sentara Virginia Beach Comprehensive Breast Center
1080 First Colonial Rd Ste 100
Virginia Beach, VA 23454-2406
(757)388-2030
FAX: (757)395-6490

Tricare Prime Boone Clinic
1035 Nider Blvd Ste 100
Virginia Beach, VA 23459-8701
(866)645-4584
FAX: (757)953-8246

Tricare Prime Clinic Virginia Beach
2100 Lynnhaven Pkwy Ste 201
Virginia Beach, VA 23456-1492
(757)953-6676
FAX: (757)953-6657

Warrenton

Fauquier Hospital
500 Hospital Dr
Warrenton, VA 20186-3099
(540)316-5800
FAX: (540)316-4501

Williamsburg

Riverside Diagnostic Center - Williamsburg
120 Kings Way, Ste 1200
Williamsburg, VA 23185-2508
(757)989-8830
FAX: (757)345-2241

Sentara Williamsburg Women's Imaging Pavilion
400 Sentara Cir
Williamsburg, VA 23188-5716
(757)345-4024
FAX: (757)345-4001

Tpmg Breast Center Williamsburg
5424 Discovery Park Blvd, Ste 102
Williamsburg, VA 23188
(757)873-0848
FAX: (757)223-7760

Winchester

Progressive Radiology
1867 Amherst St, Ste 103
Winchester, VA 22601-2869
(540)931-0139
FAX: (540)931-0142

Winchester Medical Center - Diagnostic Center
300 Campus Blvd
Winchester, VA 22601-6903
(540)536-8988
FAX: (540)536-3196

Winchester Women's Specialists
1870 Amherst St Ste 2E
Winchester, VA 22601-2847
(540)667-4546
FAX: (540)667-6893

Woodbridge

Association Of Alexandria Radiologists Woodbridge Va
4001 Prince William Pkwy Ste 302
Woodbridge, VA 22192-7667
(703)824-3260
FAX: (703)357-9636

Kaiser Permanente - Woodbridge
14139 Potomac Mills Rd
Woodbridge, VA 22192-4644
(877)390-0033
FAX: (301)548-5849

Sentara Northern Virginia Medical Center
2300 Opitz Blvd
Woodbridge, VA 22191-3311
(703)523-1995
FAX: (703)583-4923

Woodstock

Shenandoah Memorial Hospital
759 S Main St
Woodstock, VA 22664-1154
(540)459-1207
FAX: (540)459-1205

Wytheville

Wythe County Community Hospital
600 W Ridge Rd
Wytheville, VA 24382-1099
(276)228-0233
FAX: (276)228-1720

Zion Crossroads

University Of Virginia Imaging, Llc
1015 Spring Creek Pkwy Ste 130
Zion Crossroads, VA 22942-7019
(434)243-0321
FAX: (434)243-0307

WASHINGTON

Aberdeen

Grays Harbor Imaging
1108 Basich Blvd
Aberdeen, WA 98520-1066
(360)533-0400
FAX: (360)533-5633

Anacortes

Island Hospital
1211 24th St, Radiology Department
Anacortes, WA 98221-2562
(360)299-1315
FAX: (360)299-1349

Arlington

Skagit Regonial Health / Cascade Valley Hospital
330 S Stillaguamish Ave
Arlington, WA 98223-1642
(360)435-2133
FAX: (360)435-0587

Auburn

Center For Diagnostic Imaging
1268 E Main St Ste 1
Auburn, WA 98002-5708
(253)735-1991
FAX: (253)735-8837

Franciscan Breast Imaging At Auburn
205 10th St NE, Ste 106
Auburn, WA 98002-4045
(253)944-4025
FAX: (253)351-5269

Bainbridge Island

Virginia Mason Bainbridge Island Medical Center
1344 Wintergreen Ln NE
Bainbridge Island, WA 98110-5147
(206)842-5632
FAX: (206)842-5992

Bellevue

Bellevue Medical Imaging
1400 116th Ave NE
Bellevue, WA 98004-3816
(425)454-1700
FAX: (425)454-0600

Center For Diagnostic Imaging
1810 116th Ave NE Ste 101
Bellevue, WA 98004-3058
(425)974-1045
FAX: (425)974-1033

Kaiser Permanente Bellevue Medical Center
11511 NE 10th St, Breast Imaging 4th Fl
Bellevue, WA 98004-8578
(425)502-3090
FAX: (425)502-3092

Overlake Breast Health Center
1135 116th Ave. NE St. 200
Bellevue, WA 98004
(425)688-5985
FAX: (425)467-3685

The Everett Clinic At Eastside Family Medicine
1200 112th Ave NE Ste C160
Bellevue, WA 98004-3742
(425)453-1039
FAX: (425)453-8955

University Of Washington /Eastside Specialty Center
3100 Northup Way
Bellevue, WA 98004-1467
(206)598-2388
FAX: (206)598-6758

Virginia Mason Bellevue Medical Center
11695 NE 4th St
Bellevue, WA 98004-5268
(425)637-1855
FAX: (425)344-7970

Bellingham

Mt. Baker Imaging - Women's Diagnostic Center
4029 Northwest Ave Ste 101
Bellingham, WA 98226-9078
(360)647-2422
FAX: (360)752-0979

Bonney Lake

Diagnostic Imaging Northwest Bonney Lake Imaging Ctr
21110 State Route 410 E Ste 110
Bonney Lake, WA 98391-8457
(253)841-4353
FAX: (253)862-1656

Franciscan Medical Pavilion Bonney Lake
9230 Sky Island Dr E
Bonney Lake, WA 98391-7385
(253)573-7320
FAX: (253)750-6065

Bothell

Pacmed Clinics Dba Pacific Medical Center - Canyon Park
1909 214th St SE Ste 300
Bothell, WA 98021-4418
(425)412-6322
FAX: (425)412-6334

Bremerton

Center For Diagnostic Imaging
2601 Cherry Ave, Ste 105
Bremerton, WA 98310-4214
(360)627-9024
FAX: (360)813-1375

Naval Hospital Bremerton
1 Boone Rd 55 Code
Bremerton, WA 98312-1898
(360)475-4220
FAX: (360)475-4197

Brewster

Okanogan Douglas District Hospital Dba Three Rivers Hospital
507 Hospital Way
Brewster, WA 98812-0019
(509)689-2517
FAX: (509)689-2876

Burien

Franciscan Breast Center-Burien
16045 1st Ave S
Burien, WA 98148-1401
(206)248-8900
FAX: (206)965-4289

Centralia

Providence Health & Services-Washington Dba Prov Imag Ctr
908 S Scheuber Rd
Centralia, WA 98531-9027
(360)330-8507
FAX: (360)330-8882

Chelan

Lake Chelan Community Hospital
503 E Highland Ave, Chelan Co. Public Hosp. Dist 2, PO Box
Chelan, WA 98816-8631
(509)682-3300
FAX: (509)682-3432

Chewelah

Providence Health & Services-Washington Dba Prov St Joseph
500 E Webster Ave
Chewelah, WA 99109-9523
(509)935-5250
FAX: (509)935-5295

Clarkston

Tri-State Memorial Hospital
1221 Highland Ave
Clarkston, WA 99403-2829
(509)751-4557
FAX: (509)254-0076

Clinton

Whidbey General Hospital - South
11245 State Route 525
Clinton, WA 98236-8638
(360)678-7607
FAX: (360)678-7670

Colfax

Whitman Hospital & Medical Clinics
1200 W Fairview St
Colfax, WA 99111-9579
(509)397-5713
FAX: (509)397-5780

Colville

Providence Health & Services Dba Prov Mount Carmel
982 E Columbia Ave
Colville, WA 99114-3316
(509)685-5280
FAX: (509)685-2087

Coupeville

Whidbey General Hospital
101 N Main St, Mammography Department
Coupeville, WA 98239-3413
(360)678-7607
FAX: (360)678-7652

Covington

Multicare Covington Medical Center
17700 SE 272nd St Ste 130, Ms: 177-11-Bhs
Covington, WA 98042-4951
(253)372-7240
FAX: (253)372-7246

Uw/Vmc The Breast Center At Covington Clinic North
16850 SE 272nd St Ste 250
Covington, WA 98042-4931
(425)656-5588
FAX: (425)656-5563

Davenport

Lincoln Hospital District 3
10 Nicholls St
Davenport, WA 99122-9729
(509)725-2975
FAX: (509)725-7107

Edmonds

Swedish Edmonds Breast Center
7320 216th St SW Ste 120
Edmonds, WA 98026-8006
(425)673-3930
FAX: (425)673-3948

The Everett Clinic Edmonds
21401 72nd Ave W
Edmonds, WA 98026-7702
(425)317-3400
FAX: (425)339-5403

Virginia Mason Edmonds Family Medicine
7315 212th St SW Ste 101
Edmonds, WA 98026-7610
(425)775-9474
FAX: (425)670-3554

Ellensburg

Kittitas Valley Healthcare
603 S Chestnut St
Ellensburg, WA 98926-3897
(509)962-7385
FAX: (509)925-8481

Elma

Summit Pacific Wellness Center
610 E Main St.
Elma, WA 98541
(360)346-2347
FAX: (360)346-2156

Enumclaw

St. Elizabeth Hospital
1455 Battersby Ave
Enumclaw, WA 98022-3634
(360)802-8577
FAX: (360)802-8589

Ephrata

Columbia Basin Hospital
200 Nat Washington Way
Ephrata, WA 98823-1997
(509)717-5216
FAX: (509)754-1367

Everett

Kaiser Permanente Everett Medical Center
2930 Maple St, Mammography Dept
Everett, WA 98201-3832
(425)261-1542
FAX: (425)261-1555

Providence Health & Services-Washington Dba Prmce-Brst Cr
900 Pacific Ave, Ste 120
Everett, WA 98201-4188
(425)258-7788
FAX: (425)258-7531

Providence Health & Services-Washington Dba Prmce-Millcrk
12800 Bothell Everett Hwy
Everett, WA 98208-6642
(425)258-7900
FAX: (425)258-7531

Swedish - Mill Creek Medical Imaging
13020 Meridian Ave S
Everett, WA 98208-6468
(425)357-3960
FAX: (425)357-3961

The Everett Clinic
3901 Hoyt Ave
Everett, WA 98201-4988
(425)317-3400
FAX: (425)339-5403

Federal Way

Center For Diagnostic Imaging
909 S 336th St Ste B101
Federal Way, WA 98003-7394
(253)839-8779
FAX: (253)874-0409

Franciscan Breast Center At St. Francis
34503 9th Ave S Ste 320
Federal Way, WA 98003-8726
(253)944-4143
FAX: (253)944-4074

Virginia Mason Federal Way Clinic
33501 1st Way S
Federal Way, WA 98003-6208
(253)874-1620
FAX: (253)874-1761

Forks

Forks Community Hospital
530 Bogachiel Way
Forks, WA 98331-9120
(360)374-6271
FAX: (360)374-6084

Friday Harbor

Peace Island Medical Center
1117 Spring St
Friday Harbor, WA 98250-9782
(360)738-6345
FAX: (360)856-7557

Gig Harbor

Multicare Breast Health Services-Gig Harbor
4545 Point Fosdick Dr MS 4545-1-Whw, Multicare Gig Harbor Med Park
Gig Harbor, WA 98335-1700
(253)792-6220
FAX: (253)530-8126

St Anthony Hospital Mammography
11511 Canterwood Blvd Ste 230
Gig Harbor, WA 98332-5819
(253)530-2655
FAX: (253)530-2659

Goldendale

Klickitat Valley Health
310 S Roosevelt St, Diagnostic Imaging
Goldendale, WA 98620-9201
(509)773-4022
FAX: (509)773-6497

Grand Coulee

Coulee Medical Center
411 Fortuyn Rd
Grand Coulee, WA 99133-8718
(509)633-6385
FAX: (509)633-0284

Ilwaco

Ocean Beach Hospital
174 1st Ave N
Ilwaco, WA 98624-9137
(360)642-6382
FAX: (360)998-3412

Issaquah

Overlake Breast Screening Center - Issaquah
1740 NW Maple St Ste 207
Issaquah, WA 98027-8127
(425)688-5985
FAX: (425)557-0148

Swedish/Issaquah Imaging
751 NE Blakely Dr
Issaquah, WA 98029-6201
(425)313-5400
FAX: (425)313-5401

Virginia Mason Issaquah Medical Center
100 NE Gilman Blvd
Issaquah, WA 98027-2925
(425)557-8013
FAX: (425)557-8051

Kenmore

Evergreen Breast Center-Kenmore
18151 68th Ave NE Ste 100
Kenmore, WA 98028-2835
(425)899-3800
FAX: (425)899-1846

Kennewick

Inland Imaging Tri Cities
7221 W Deschutes Ave Ste A
Kennewick, WA 99336-7807
(509)374-4030
FAX: (509)374-8690

Rcch Trios Health Llc, Dba Trios Health
3730 Plaza Way
Kennewick, WA 99338-2718
(509)221-5441
FAX: (509)221-6132

Kirkland

Evergreen Breast Center
12303 NE 130th Ln Ste 100
Kirkland, WA 98034-3058
(425)899-2831
FAX: (425)899-1846

Virginia Mason Kirkland
11800 NE 128th St Ste 300
Kirkland, WA 98034-7211
(425)814-5114
FAX: (425)814-5122

Lakewood

Tra Medical Imaging - Lakewood
5919 100th St SW, Lakewood Office
Lakewood, WA 98499-2731
(253)761-4200
FAX: (253)588-3870

Leavenworth

Cascade Medical
817 Commercial St
Leavenworth, WA 98826-1316
(509)548-2512
FAX: (509)548-3437

Longview

Kearney Breast Center Peacehealth St. John
1615 Delaware St
Longview, WA 98632-2367
(360)414-2701
FAX: (360)414-2705

Longview-Kelso Medical Office
1230 7th Ave
Longview, WA 98632-3198
(503)571-5645
FAX: (503)571-8469

Lynden

Mt. Baker Imaging- Lynden Mammography
1610 Grover St Bldg C Ste 4
Lynden, WA 98264-1539
(360)647-2422
FAX: (360)752-0979

Lynnwood

Virginia Mason Lynnwood
19116 33rd Ave W
Lynnwood, WA 98036-4706
(425)712-7900
FAX: (425)712-7905

Marysville

The Everett Clinic At Smokey Point
2901 174th St NE
Marysville, WA 98271-4743
(425)317-3400
FAX: (425)339-5403

Mill Creek

The Everett Clinic Mill Creek
15418 Main St Ste 200
Mill Creek, WA 98012-9030
(425)317-3400
FAX: (425)339-5403

Monroe

Evergreen Health Monroe Breast Program
14701 179th Ave SE
Monroe, WA 98272-1108
(360)863-4654
FAX: (360)863-4673

Providence Medical Group Monroe
19200 N Kelsey St
Monroe, WA 98272-1431
(425)258-7900
FAX: (425)258-7531

Morton

Lewis County Hospital District No. 1
521 Adams Ave
Morton, WA 98356-9323
(360)496-3520
FAX: (360)496-5054

Moses Lake

Confluence Health - Moses Lake
840 E Hill Ave
Moses Lake, WA 98837-2238
(509)764-6432
FAX: (509)764-6464

Samaritan Healthcare
801 E Wheeler Rd
Moses Lake, WA 98837-1899
(509)793-9651
FAX: (509)764-3232

Mount Vernon

Skagit Digital Imaging
1320 E Division St
Mount Vernon, WA 98274-4133
(360)428-7270
FAX: (360)424-3756

Newport

Newport Hospital And Health Services
714 W Pine St
Newport, WA 99156-9046
(509)447-9317
FAX: (509)447-7925

Oak Harbor

Whidbeyhealth Primary Care Oak Harbor
1300 NE Goldie St
Oak Harbor, WA 98277-4832
(360)678-7607
FAX: (360)678-7652

Olympia

Capital Mammography
3920 Capital Mall Dr SW Ste 401
Olympia, WA 98502-8700
(360)570-3025
FAX: (360)570-3007

Kaiser Permanente Olympia Medical Center
700 Lilly Rd NE
Olympia, WA 98506-5196
(360)923-7645
FAX: (360)923-7677

South Sound Radiologists, Inc., P.S.
3417 Ensign Rd NE
Olympia, WA 98506-5075
(360)252-9301
FAX: (360)486-6611

Tra Medical Imaging On Lilly
500 Lilly Rd NE Ste 160
Olympia, WA 98506-9107
(360)413-8383
FAX: (360)413-8775

Omak

Confluence Health-Omak Clinic
916 Koala Dr
Omak, WA 98841-9759
(509)826-1800
FAX: (509)826-7915

Mid Valley Hospital, Okanogan Co. Public Health
810 Jasmine St
Omak, WA 98841-9578
(509)826-1760
FAX: (509)826-7644

Othello

Othello Community Hospital
315 N 14th Ave
Othello, WA 99344-1297
(509)331-2682
FAX: (509)331-2619

Pasco

Lourdes Medical Center
PO Box 2568, 520 N Fourth Ave
Pasco, WA 99302-2568
(509)546-2225
FAX: (509)546-2223

Lourdes West Pasco Diagnostic Imaging
7425 Wrigley Dr Ste 102
Pasco, WA 99301-5292
(509)543-7583
FAX: (509)543-7326

Port Angeles

Olympic Medical Center
939 Caroline St
Port Angeles, WA 98362-3997
(360)565-9003
FAX: (360)565-9001

Olympic Medical Imaging Center
1102 E Front St
Port Angeles, WA 98362-4308
(360)417-7736
FAX: (360)565-9001

Port Orchard

Center For Diagnostic Imaging
463 Tremont St W, Ste 130
Port Orchard, WA 98366-3743
(360)876-3141
FAX: (360)876-3142

Harrison Imaging Centers - Port Orchard Mammography
450 S Kitsap Blvd Ste 110
Port Orchard, WA 98366-3709
(360)337-6500
FAX: (360)337-6504

Port Townsend

Jefferson Healthcare
834 Sheridan St
Port Townsend, WA 98368-2499
(360)379-9235
FAX: (360)379-2251

Poulsbo

Center For Diagnostic Imaging
20700 Bond Rd NE Bldg B
Poulsbo, WA 98370-9099
(360)598-3141
FAX: (360)598-3431

Harrison Imaging Centers - Poulsbo Mammography
22180 Olympic College Way NW Ste 101
Poulsbo, WA 98370-6664
(360)337-6500
FAX: (360)662-5501

Prosser

Prosser Memorial Health Prosser Public Hospital District
723 Memorial St
Prosser, WA 99350-1524
(509)786-6650
FAX: (509)788-6003

Pullman

Pullman Regional Hospital
835 SE Bishop Blvd
Pullman, WA 99163-5512
(509)336-7446
FAX: (509)336-7447

Puyallup

Center For Diagnostic Imaging
2930 S Meridian, Ste 160
Puyallup, WA 98373-1654
(253)286-2092
FAX: (253)848-2161

Diagnostic Imaging Northwest Sunrise Imaging Center
11212 Sunrise Blvd E Ste 200
Puyallup, WA 98374-8847
(253)841-4353
FAX: (253)445-0314

Diagnostic Imaging Nw - Puyallup Imaging Center
222 15th Ave SE
Puyallup, WA 98372-3754
(253)841-4353
FAX: (253)845-3680

Kaiser Permanente Puyallup Medical Center - Mobile
1007 39th Ave SE
Puyallup, WA 98374-2192
(206)561-6273
FAX: (360)923-7677

Redmond

Swedish - Redmond Medical Imaging
18100 NE Union Hill Rd
Redmond, WA 98052-3330
(425)498-2031
FAX: (425)498-2032

Renton

Uw/Vmc The Breast Center
4033 Talbot Rd S Ste 470
Renton, WA 98055-5700
(425)656-5588
FAX: (425)656-5563

Richland

Outpatient Imaging Center-Kadlec
945 Goethals Dr Ste 100
Richland, WA 99352-3552
(509)942-2655
FAX: (509)942-2203

Seattle

Diagnostic And Wellness Center For Women
1200 12th Ave S
Seattle, WA 98144-2712
(206)568-3833
FAX: (206)568-3837

Kaiser Permanente Central Hospital
201 16th Ave E, Mammography Department
Seattle, WA 98112-5226
(206)326-3600
FAX: (206)326-3651

Seattle Cancer Care Alliance Breast Imaging
825 Eastlake Ave E G3-303
Seattle, WA 98109-4405
(206)606-6733
FAX: (206)606-6719

Swedish Ballard Breast Center
5300 Tallman Ave NW
Seattle, WA 98107-3932
(307)760-0034
FAX: (206)781-6020

Swedish Breast Imaging Center
1101 Madison St Ste 310
Seattle, WA 98104-1320
(206)215-8100
FAX: (206)386-3777

Swedish Imaging Center For Comprehensive Care
515 Minor Ave Ste 110
Seattle, WA 98104-2145
(206)386-9699
FAX: (206)386-9529

Swedish Mobile Mammography Program - Mobile
1101 Madison St, Ste 350
Seattle, WA 98104-3599
(206)320-2500
FAX: (206)233-7377

The Polyclinic Madison Center
904 7th Ave
Seattle, WA 98104-1132
(206)860-5496
FAX: (206)860-4451

The Polyclinic Northgate
9709 3rd Ave NE
Seattle, WA 98115-2062
(206)860-5496
FAX: (206)720-8420

Univ. Of Wash. Medical Ctr. Roosevelt II Radiology
4245 Roosevelt Way NE, Xb-45
Seattle, WA 98105-6008
(206)606-7800
FAX: (206)606-6644

Uw Medical Center- Northwest Breast Imaging Clinic
1560 N 115th St Ste 104
Seattle, WA 98133-8414
(206)668-1749
FAX: (206)668-1790

Virginia Mason Medical Center
1100 9th Ave, Mailstop Xii-Mam
Seattle, WA 98101-2756
(206)625-7250
FAX: (206)223-6376

Virginia Mason University Village
2671 NE 46th St
Seattle, WA 98105-5041
(206)525-8000
FAX: (206)525-8070

Sedro Woolley

Breast Care Suite
2000 Hospital Dr
Sedro Woolley, WA 98284-4327
(360)856-7244
FAX: (360)856-7557

Sequim

Olympic Medical Imaging Sequim
840 N 5th Ave Ste 1100
Sequim, WA 98382-3045
(360)565-9003
FAX: (360)565-9001

Shelton

Mason General Hospital & Family Of Clinics
901 Mountain View Dr
Shelton, WA 98584-4401
(360)427-9590
FAX: (360)427-0103

Silverdale

Harrison Imaging Centers - Silverdale Mammography
1780 NW Myhre Rd Ste 1220
Silverdale, WA 98383-8676
(360)337-6500
FAX: (360)337-6553

Kaiser Permanente Silverdale Medical Center
10452 Silverdale Way NW
Silverdale, WA 98383-9411
(360)307-7349
FAX: (360)307-7449

South Bend

Willapa Harbor Hospital
800 Alder St
South Bend, WA 98586-4900
(360)875-4505
FAX: (360)875-5797

Spokane

Inland Imaging At Holy Family
5715 N Lidgerwood St
Spokane, WA 99208-1225
(509)455-4455
FAX: (509)363-7999

Inland Imaging At South Center
525 S Cowley St
Spokane, WA 99202-1389
(509)455-4455
FAX: (509)624-6900

Inland Imaging Valley Center
12420 E Mission Ave
Spokane, WA 99216-1051
(509)455-4455
FAX: (509)363-7297

Inland Imaging, Llc At Sacred Heart
105 W 8th Ave Ste 100C
Spokane, WA 99204-2302
(509)455-4455
FAX: (509)363-7869

Rockwood Clinic P.S.
400 E 5th Ave, Frnt
Spokane, WA 99202-1336
(509)838-2531
FAX: (509)342-3571

Spokane Valley

Inland Imaging At Providence Medical Park
16528 E Desmet Ct Ste A1300
Spokane Valley, WA 99216-3522
(509)455-4455
FAX: (509)363-7297

Multicare Rockwood Clinic Spokane Primary Care
1215 N McDonald Rd Ste 001
Spokane Valley, WA 99216-1557
(509)598-7935
FAX: (509)924-3572

Sunnyside

Astria Sunnyside Hospital
10th Ave & Tacoma Ave, Radiology Department
Sunnyside, WA 98944
(509)837-1760
FAX: (509)837-1593

Tacoma

Carol Milgard Breast Center
4525 S 19th St
Tacoma, WA 98405-1106
(253)759-2622
FAX: (253)759-0168

Kaiser Permanente Tacoma Medical Center
209 Martin Luther King Jr Way
Tacoma, WA 98405-4265
(253)596-3480
FAX: (253)596-3369

Madigan Army Medical Center
9040 Fitzsimmons Dr
Tacoma, WA 98431-1000
(253)968-3669
FAX: (253)968-2024

Tonasket

North Valley Hospital
203 S Western Ave
Tonasket, WA 98855-8803
(509)486-2151
FAX: (509)486-3102

Toppenish

Astria Toppenish Hospital
502 W 4th Ave
Toppenish, WA 98948-1616
(509)865-1650
FAX: (509)865-1667

Tukwila

Assured Imaging Womens Wellness Of Washington Llc - Mobile
565 Andover Park W, Ste 110
Tukwila, WA 98188-3357
(206)467-1949
FAX: (206)467-1912

Vancouver

Kaiser Cascade Park Medical Office
12607 SE Mill Plain Blvd
Vancouver, WA 98684-4098
(503)571-5645
FAX: (503)571-8469

Kaiser Permanente-Salmon Creek
14406 NE 20th Ave
Vancouver, WA 98686-1448
(503)571-5645
FAX: (503)571-8469

Legacy Salmon Creek Breast Center
2101 NE 139th St Ste 155
Vancouver, WA 98686-2309
(360)487-1800
FAX: (360)487-1494

Peacehealth Sw Medical Center - Kearney Breast Center
200 NE Mother Joseph Pl Ste 420
Vancouver, WA 98664-3203
(360)514-1234
FAX: (360)514-6140

The Vancouver Clinic
700 NE 87th Ave Ste 170
Vancouver, WA 98664-4896
(360)397-2539
FAX: (360)604-1694

The Vancouver Clinic - Columbia Tech Center
501 SE 172nd Ave
Vancouver, WA 98684-9542
(360)253-1236
FAX: (360)604-1694

The Vancouver Clinic - Salmon Creek
2525 NE 139th St
Vancouver, WA 98686-2719
(360)882-2778
FAX: (360)604-1694

Vancouver Radiologists
4816 NE Thurston Way Ste A
Vancouver, WA 98662-6661
(360)449-4958
FAX: (360)892-1533

Walla Walla

Providence St Mary Medical Center
401 W Poplar St, Diagnostic Imaging Department
Walla Walla, WA 99362-2862
(509)897-2572
FAX: (509)897-5163

Walla Walla Clinic
55 W Tietan St
Walla Walla, WA 99362-4498
(509)525-3720
FAX: (509)522-1571

Wenatchee

Confluence Health- Wenatchee Valley Hospital And Clinics
820 N Chelan Ave
Wenatchee, WA 98801-2028
(509)663-4868
FAX: (509)664-7176

White Salmon

Skyline Hospital
PO Box 99, 211 Skyline Dr
White Salmon, WA 98672-0099
(509)637-2957
FAX: (509)493-1251

Yakima

ohana Memorials Mammography Services
1515 W Yakima Ave
Yakima, WA 98902-2950
(509)574-3863
FAX: (509)249-5319

WEST VIRGINIA

Alderson

Fpc Alderson
Glen Ray Road Box A
Alderson, WV 24910
(304)445-3300
FAX: (304)445-3312

Beckley

Beckley Appalachian Regional Hospital
306 Stanaford Rd
Beckley, WV 25801-3186
(304)255-5679
FAX: (304)255-3545

Beckley Oncology Assoc.Inc., Dba Raleigh X-Ray Diagnostics
275 Dry Hill Rd
Beckley, WV 25801-2605
(304)253-6066
FAX: (304)253-6086

Professional Medical Ultrasonics
200 Carriage Dr
Beckley, WV 25801-2876
(304)252-0609
FAX: (304)252-0646

Raleigh General Hospital
1717 Harper Rd, Radiology Department
Beckley, WV 25801-3373
(304)254-3000
FAX: (304)461-3809

Berkeley Springs

War Memorial Hospital
1 Healthy Way
Berkeley Springs, WV 25411-7463
(304)258-6508
FAX: (304)258-7423

Bridgeport

United Hospital Center
327 Medical Park Dr
Bridgeport, WV 26330-9006
(681)624-2250
FAX: (681)342-1335

Buckhannon

St. Joseph's Hospital
1 Amalia Dr
Buckhannon, WV 26201-2200
(304)473-2053
FAX: (304)473-2052

Charleston

Advanced Women's Imaging By Saint Francis Hospital
400 Court St Ste 201A
Charleston, WV 25301-1653
(304)347-6166
FAX: (304)347-6167

Camc - The Breast Center
3415 Maccorkle Ave SE, Third Floor
Charleston, WV 25304-1334
(304)388-9677
FAX: (304)388-2723

David J Patton MD Inc
108 Washington St W, Ste 101
Charleston, WV 25302-2344
(304)345-4525
FAX: (304)345-4527

Imaging Center Charleston Area Medical Center
3416 Maccorkle Ave SE
Charleston, WV 25304-1335
(304)388-1659
FAX: (304)388-1663

Elkins

Davis Medical Center
PO Box 1484, Gorman And Reed St
Elkins, WV 26241-1484
(304)637-3185
FAX: (304)637-3344

Fairmont

Fairmont Clinic Gateway Uha
100 Stoney Hill Rd
Fairmont, WV 26554-1589
(304)293-1223
FAX: (304)293-6703

Mon Health Obstetrics And Gynecology Fairmont
1703 Locust Ave
Fairmont, WV 26554-1320
(304)366-6100
FAX: (304)366-2220

Franklin

Pendleton Community Care Inc
82 Pine St
Franklin, WV 26807
(304)358-2355
FAX: (304)358-3054

Gassaway

Wvu Medicine - Braxton County Memorial Hospital
100 Hoylman Dr, Radiology Department
Gassaway, WV 26624-9318
(304)364-1106
FAX: (304)364-1209

Glen Dale

Wvu Medicine Reynolds Memorial Hospital
800 Wheeling Ave
Glen Dale, WV 26038-1697
(304)843-3310
FAX: (304)843-3316

Grafton

Grafton City Hospital
1 Hospital Plz
Grafton, WV 26354-1283
(304)265-0400
FAX: (304)265-6437

Grantsville

Minnie Hamilton Health System
186 Hospital Dr
Grantsville, WV 26147-7100
(304)354-9244
FAX: (304)354-5958

Huntington

Breast Health Center At Cabell Huntington Hospital, Inc.
1415 Hal Greer Blvd
Huntington, WV 25701-4113
(304)526-2270
FAX: (304)526-2436

Edwards Comprehensive Cancer Center
1400 Hal Greer Blvd
Huntington, WV 25701-4114
(304)399-6556
FAX: (304)399-6554

St. Mary's Medical Center
2900 1st Ave
Huntington, WV 25702-1271
(304)526-8221
FAX: (304)399-7476

St. Mary's Medical Center Dba Himg
5170 US Route 60
Huntington, WV 25705-2004
(304)528-4690
FAX: (304)399-2385

Hurricane

Camc - Teays Valley Hospital
1400 Hospital Dr
Hurricane, WV 25526-9202
(304)757-1882
FAX: (304)757-1845

Keyser

Potomac Valley Hospital
100 Pin Oak Ln
Keyser, WV 26726-5908
(304)597-3692
FAX: (304)597-3549

Kingwood

Preston Memorial Hospital
150 Memorial Dr
Kingwood, WV 26537-1141
(304)329-4713
FAX: (304)329-2807

Madison

Boone Memorial Hospital Inc.
701 Madison Ave
Madison, WV 25130-1699
(304)369-8805
FAX: (304)307-2601

Martinsburg

Spring Mills Mammography
61 Campus Dr
Martinsburg, WV 25404-7542
(304)264-1297
FAX: (304)264-1003

Valley Health Spring Mills Imaging Center
120 Campus Dr, Ste 121
Martinsburg, WV 25404-7552
(540)536-8988
FAX: (681)247-1271

Womens Imaging Center Mob 3
880 N Tennessee Ave
Martinsburg, WV 25401-9401
(304)264-1297
FAX: (304)350-3284

Montgomery

Montgomery General Hospital
401 6th Ave
Montgomery, WV 25136-2199
(304)442-7417
FAX: (304)442-1347

Moorefield

Love Memorial Clinic
112 Kuykendall Ln
Moorefield, WV 26836-1167
(304)530-7755
FAX: (304)530-7756

Morgantown

Betty Puskar Breast Care Center
1 Medical Center Dr, Radiology Box 8062
Morgantown, WV 26506-1200
(304)293-1223
FAX: (304)293-6703

Monongalia General Hospital
1200 J D Anderson Dr
Morgantown, WV 26505-3486
(304)285-1642
FAX: (304)607-3672

West Virginia University Hospitals- Mobile
1 Medical Center Dr, Radiology Box 8062
Morgantown, WV 26506-1200
(304)293-1223
FAX: (304)293-6703

Wvu Cheat Lake Physicians
608 Cheat Rd
Morgantown, WV 26508-4210
(304)293-1223
FAX: (304)293-6703

Wvu Medicine University Town Center
6040 University Town Centre Dr
Morgantown, WV 26501-2421
(304)293-1223
FAX: (304)293-6703

New Martinsville

Wetzel County Hospital, Inc.
3 E Benjamin Dr
New Martinsville, WV 26155-2758
(304)455-8090
FAX: (304)455-8019

Oak Hill

Plateau Medical Center
430 Main St W
Oak Hill, WV 25901-3455
(304)469-8655
FAX: (304)929-2461

Oceana

Princeton Community Hospital - Medical Imaging Center
930 Cook Pkwy.
Oceana, WV 24870
(304)324-2740
FAX: (304)487-7849

Parkersburg

Wvu Medicine Camden Clark Medical Center
705 Garfield Ave, Medical Office Building B
Parkersburg, WV 26101-5444
(304)424-2778
FAX: (304)424-2722

Petersburg

Grant Memorial Hospital
Route 28 & Route 55, 117 Hospital Drive
Petersburg, WV 26847
(304)257-1026
FAX: (304)257-9783

Philippi

Broaddus Hospital
1 Healthcare Dr
Philippi, WV 26416-9405
(304)457-8162
FAX: (304)457-8589

Point Pleasant

Pleasant Valley Hospital
2520 Valley Dr, Radiology Dept
Point Pleasant, WV 25550-2092
(304)675-4340
FAX: (304)675-4341

Princeton

Women's Diagnostic Imaging
Parkview Center - Morrison Drive
Princeton, WV 24740
(304)324-2627
FAX: (304)487-7849

Rainelle

Rainelle Medical Center, Inc.
176 Medical Center Dr
Rainelle, WV 25962-1064
(304)438-6188
FAX: (304)438-4037

Ranson

Jefferson Medical Center Womens Imaging Ctr
207 S Preston St
Ranson, WV 25438-1628
(304)728-1648
FAX: (304)728-8809

Ripley

Jackson General Hospital
122 Pinnell St
Ripley, WV 25271-9101
(304)373-1525
FAX: (304)373-1543

Romney

Hampshire Memorial Hospital, Inc.
363 Sunrise Blvd
Romney, WV 26757-4607
(304)822-4929
FAX: (304)822-4956

Ronceverte

Greenbrier Physicians Inc.
1322 Maplewood Ave
Ronceverte, WV 24970-8016
(304)647-1102
FAX: (304)781-3485

Greenbrier Valley Medical Center
1320 Maplewood Ave
Ronceverte, WV 24970-8016
(304)647-6505
FAX: (304)739-3544

Scott Depot

Marshall Health - Teays Valley
300 Corporate Center Drive
Scott Depot, WV 25560
(304)691-1800
FAX: (304)691-5372

Sistersville

Marietta Memorial Hospital Of Tyler County, Inc.
314 S Wells St
Sistersville, WV 26175-1098
(304)447-2433
FAX: (304)652-9930

South Charleston

Charleston Area Medical Center
60 R H L Blvd
South Charleston, WV 25309-8278
(304)720-9729
FAX: (304)720-9730

Thomas Imaging Center
4800 Maccorkle Ave SW
South Charleston, WV 25309-1332
(304)766-3726
FAX: (304)766-3840

Spencer

Roane General Hospital
200 Hospital Dr, Radiology Department
Spencer, WV 25276-1050
(304)927-6231
FAX: (304)927-3721

Summersville

Summersville Regional Medical Center
400 Fairview Heights Rd
Summersville, WV 26651-9308
(304)872-8464
FAX: (304)872-6497

Weirton

Weirton Medical Center
651 Colliers Way, Ste 207
Weirton, WV 26062-5055
(304)797-6008
FAX: (304)797-6601

Welch

Welch Community Hospital
454 McDowell St
Welch, WV 24801-2097
(304)436-8610
FAX: (304)436-4749

Weston

Stonewall Jackson Memorial Hospital
230 Hospital Plz
Weston, WV 26452-8558
(304)269-8075
FAX: (304)269-8155

Wheeling

Wheeling Hospital
1 Medical Park
Wheeling, WV 26003-6300
(304)243-3032
FAX: (304)243-7170

White Sulphur Springs

The Greenbrier Clinic, Inc.
40823 Midland Trl E
White Sulphur Springs, WV 24986-5064
(304)536-4870
FAX: (304)536-8019

WISCONSIN

Altoona

Sacred Heart Hospital D/B/A Prevea Health-Mobile
3119 Woodman Dr
Altoona, WI 54720-2668
(715)717-5288
FAX: (715)717-5275

Amery

Amery Hospital And Clinic
265 Griffin St E
Amery, WI 54001-1439
(715)268-0476
FAX: (715)268-0481

Antigo

Aspirus Langlade Hospital
112 E 5th Ave
Antigo, WI 54409-2710
(715)623-9276
FAX: (715)623-9414

Appleton

Ascension St. Elizabeth Hospital
1506 S Oneida St
Appleton, WI 54915-1396
(920)831-1200
FAX: (920)831-1220

Encircle Health
2500 E Capitol Dr
Appleton, WI 54911-8735
(920)358-1554
FAX: (920)358-1556

Primary Care Associates Of Appleton, Ltd
3916 N Intertech Ct, Ste A
Appleton, WI 54913-6957
(920)996-1000
FAX: (920)996-1052

Thedacare Physicians Darboy
W5282 Amy Ave
Appleton, WI 54915-7233
(920)454-8609
FAX: (920)358-1985

Ashland

Chequamegon Clinic - A St. Luke's Clinic
2201 Lake Shore Dr E
Ashland, WI 54806-2331
(715)685-6600
FAX: (715)685-6677

Essentia Health Ashland Clinic
1615 Maple Ln Ste 1
Ashland, WI 54806-3630
(715)685-7500
FAX: (715)685-7077

Memorial Medical Center
1615 Maple Ln
Ashland, WI 54806-3689
(715)685-5415
FAX: (715)685-5423

Baldwin

Western Wisconsin Health
1100 Bergslien St
Baldwin, WI 54002-2600
(715)684-1380
FAX: (715)684-1369

Baraboo

Ssm Health St Clare Hospital
707 14th St
Baraboo, WI 53913-1597
(608)356-1477
FAX: (608)356-1341

Barron

Mayo Clinic Health System Northland
1222 E Woodland Ave
Barron, WI 54812-1765
(715)537-6747
FAX: (715)537-9949

Beaver Dam

Beaver Dam Community Hospitals, Inc.
707 S University Ave
Beaver Dam, WI 53916-3089
(920)887-4006
FAX: (920)887-4084

Beloit

Beloit Memorial Hospital
1969 W Hart Rd
Beloit, WI 53511-2230
(608)364-5266
FAX: (608)364-5312

Berlin

Thedacare Medical Center-Berlin, Inc.
225 Memorial Dr
Berlin, WI 54923-1243
(920)361-5304
FAX: (920)361-5486

Black River Falls

Krohn Clinic
610 W Adams St
Black River Falls, WI 54615-9110
(715)284-4311
FAX: (715)284-2568

Bloomer

Mayo Clinic Health System Chippewa Valley - Bloomer
1501 Thompson St
Bloomer, WI 54724-1257
(715)568-6126
FAX: (715)568-6829

Boscobel

Gundersen Boscobel Area Hospital And Clinics
205 Parker St
Boscobel, WI 53805-1642
(608)375-6321
FAX: (608)375-6319

Brookfield

Ascension Elmbrook Pavlic Ctr
19305 W North Ave
Brookfield, WI 53045-4132
(414)527-5000
FAX: (414)527-5005

Aurora Health Center - Brookfield
16985 W Bluemound Rd
Brookfield, WI 53005-5909
(262)236-8787
FAX: (262)236-8789

Froedtert Calhoun Health Center
1905 N Calhoun Rd
Brookfield, WI 53005-5036
(262)532-3083
FAX: (262)532-8697

Prohealth Waukesha Memorial Hospital-Brookfield
195 Discovery Dr
Brookfield, WI 53045-2862
(262)928-3000
FAX: (262)513-7111

Brown Deer

Ascension Se Wisconsin At Brown Deer
9252 N Green Bay Rd
Brown Deer, WI 53209-1104
(414)527-5000
FAX: (414)527-5005

Burlington

Aurora Health Center Southern Lakes
709 Spring Valley Rd
Burlington, WI 53105-7614
(262)767-6440
FAX: (262)971-9573

Chilton

Ascension Calumet Hospital
614 Memorial Dr
Chilton, WI 53014-1568
(920)849-7502
FAX: (920)849-7534

Chippewa Falls

Marshfield Clinic, Chippewa Falls Center
2655 County Highway I
Chippewa Falls, WI 54729-1423
(715)726-4140
FAX: (715)726-0620

Mayo Clinic Health System Chippewa Valley - Chippewa Falls
611 1st Ave
Chippewa Falls, WI 54729-1242
(715)720-4453
FAX: (715)720-4471

St. Joseph's Hospital Of The Hospital Sisters Of The Third
2661 County Highway I
Chippewa Falls, WI 54729-5407
(715)717-7280
FAX: (715)717-7669

Columbus

Prairie Ridge Health, Inc.
1515 Park Ave, Medical Imaging Dept.
Columbus, WI 53925-2402
(920)623-2200
FAX: (920)623-6440

Crandon

Forest County Potawatomi Health And Wellness Center
8201 Mish Ko Swen Dr
Crandon, WI 54520-8631
(715)478-4339
FAX: (715)478-4769

Cudahy

Aurora St. Luke's South Shore
5900 S Lake Dr, Radiology Dept
Cudahy, WI 53110-3171
(414)489-4579
FAX: (414)489-4169

Cumberland

Cumberland Memorial Hospital-Extended Care Unit, Inc.
1110 7th Ave
Cumberland, WI 54829-9138
(715)822-7392
FAX: (715)822-7391

Darlington

Memorial Hospital Of Lafayette County
800 Clay St
Darlington, WI 53530-1228
(608)776-5726
FAX: (608)776-5784

De Pere

Aurora Health Center - Depere
1881 Chicago St
De Pere, WI 54115-3770
(920)403-8167
FAX: (920)403-8203

St Vincent Hospital Dba Prevea Health - Depere Site
3860 Monroe Rd
De Pere, WI 54115-8399
(920)496-4700
FAX: (920)272-1527

Dodgeville

Upland Hills Health
800 Compassion Way
Dodgeville, WI 53533-1956
(608)930-7145
FAX: (608)930-7281

Durand

Adventhealth Durand
PO Box 224
Durand, WI 54736-0224
(715)672-3517
FAX: (715)672-3801

Eagle River

Ascension Eagle River Hospital
201 Hospital Rd
Eagle River, WI 54521-8835
(715)479-0262
FAX: (715)479-0364

Eau Claire

Marshfield Medical Center- Eau Claire
2116 Craig Rd
Eau Claire, WI 54701-6118
(715)858-4644
FAX: (715)858-4959

McHs-Northwest Wisconsin Region,Inc-Clairemont
733 W Clairemont Ave
Eau Claire, WI 54701-6101
(715)838-3926
FAX: (715)838-6207

McHs-Northwest Wisconsin Region.Inc- Hers Breast Center
1400 Bellinger St
Eau Claire, WI 54703-5222
(715)838-3926
FAX: (715)838-3456

Oakleaf Clinics, S.C.
3802 Oakwood Mall Dr
Eau Claire, WI 54701-3016
(715)839-8020
FAX: (715)839-7440

Sacred Heart Hospital Of The Hospital Sisters Of The Third O
900 W Clairemont Ave, Radiology Department
Eau Claire, WI 54701-6122
(715)717-4151
FAX: (715)717-3005

Edgerton

Edgerton Hospital And Health Services, Inc.
11101 N Sherman Rd
Edgerton, WI 53534-9002
(608)884-1380
FAX: (608)884-1612

Fitchburg

Group Health Cooperative
3051 Cahill Main
Fitchburg, WI 53711-7109
(608)661-7200
FAX: (608)661-7210

Fond Du Lac

Aurora Health Center - Fdl
210 Wisconsin American Dr
Fond Du Lac, WI 54937-2999
(920)907-7055
FAX: (920)907-7413

St. Agnes Hospital Breast Screening Center
430 E Division St
Fond Du Lac, WI 54935-4560
(920)926-5594
FAX: (920)926-8824

Fort Atkinson

Fort Health Care
611 Sherman Ave E
Fort Atkinson, WI 53538-1960
(920)568-5420
FAX: (920)568-6026

Franklin

Ascension Se Wisconsin-Franklin
10101 S 27th St
Franklin, WI 53132-7209
(414)325-3834
FAX: (414)325-3831

Aurora Health Center-Franklin W Oakwood Park Ct
4202 W Oakwood Park Ct Ste 330
Franklin, WI 53132-9565
(414)747-7474
FAX: (414)423-0615

Aurora Health Center-Franklin-Loomis Rd
9200 W Loomis Rd, Radiology Department
Franklin, WI 53132-8887
(414)747-7474
FAX: (414)427-3298

Friendship

Gundersen Moundview Hospital & Clinics
402 W Lake St, Radiology Department
Friendship, WI 53934-9699
(608)339-8373
FAX: (608)339-8329

Germantown

Aurora Health Care - Germantown
W180N11070 River Ln
Germantown, WI 53022-3109
(262)236-8787
FAX: (262)532-8405

Glendale

Columbia St. Mary's River Woods Outpatient Center
375 W River Woods Pkwy
Glendale, WI 53212-1080
(414)326-1670
FAX: (414)326-1571

Grafton

Aurora Health Center - Cedar Creek
215 Washington St
Grafton, WI 53024-1700
(262)387-8281
FAX: (262)387-8258

Aurora Medical Center - Grafton
975 Port Washington Rd, Women's Imaging Ctr
Grafton, WI 53024-9204
(262)329-4600
FAX: (262)329-4601

Grantsburg

Burnett Medical Center
257 W Saint George Ave
Grantsburg, WI 54840-7827
(715)463-7292
FAX: (715)463-7347

Green Bay

Aurora Bay Care Health Center
PO Box 8930, 2253 W Mason St
Green Bay, WI 54308-8930
(920)288-3300
FAX: (920)288-4577

Aurora Baycare Medical Center
2845 Greenbrier Rd
Green Bay, WI 54311-6519
(920)288-3300
FAX: (920)288-4577

Bellin Health Hospital Site
744 S Webster Ave
Green Bay, WI 54301-3581
(920)445-7272
FAX: (920)433-5811

St. Vincent Hosp Dba Prevea Hlth Allouez Site
1821 S Webster Ave
Green Bay, WI 54301-2253
(920)496-4789
FAX: (920)496-4732

St. Vincent Hospital Dba Prevea Health - St. Mary's
1860 Shawano Ave
Green Bay, WI 54303-2667
(920)496-4700
FAX: (920)431-1816

Greenfield

Center For Diagnostic Imaging - Greenfield Highlands
4455 S 108th St Ste 140
Greenfield, WI 53228-2504
(414)409-7593
FAX: (414)409-7594

Hartford

Aurora Advocate Hartford Clinic
1640 E Sumner St
Hartford, WI 53027-2684
(262)670-7734
FAX: (262)670-4451

Hayward

Hayward Area Memorial Hospital
11040 N State Road 77
Hayward, WI 54843-3606
(715)934-4237
FAX: (715)934-4279

Lac Courte Oreilles Health Center
13380 W Trepania Rd
Hayward, WI 54843-2186
(715)638-5166
FAX: (715)634-0484

Hillsboro

St. Joseph's Health Services, Inc.
PO Box 527, 400 Water Ave
Hillsboro, WI 54634-0527
(608)489-8230
FAX: (608)489-8191

Hudson

Hudson Hospital & Clinics
405 Stageline Rd
Hudson, WI 54016-1793
(715)531-6434
FAX: (715)531-6439

Janesville

Mercy Health
1000 Mineral Point Ave
Janesville, WI 53548-2982
(608)741-6999
FAX: (608)756-6688

Ssm Health Dean Medical Group - Janesville East Clinic
3200 E Racine St
Janesville, WI 53546-2343
(608)371-8850
FAX: (608)371-8915

Kaukauna

Aurora Baycare Health Center-Kaukauna
1500 Arbor Way
Kaukauna, WI 54130-7305
(920)288-3300
FAX: (920)288-4577

Kenosha

Kenosha Radiology Center
10117 74th St Ste 150
Kenosha, WI 53142-7533
(262)697-7770
FAX: (262)697-7771

La Crosse

Gundersen Health System - Lacrosse
1900 South Ave
La Crosse, WI 54601-5467
(608)775-5337
FAX: (608)775-6674

Mayo Clinic Health System - Franciscan Healthcare
700 West Ave S
La Crosse, WI 54601-4783
(608)392-9822
FAX: (608)392-9041

Lac Du Flambeau

Peter Christensen Health Center
129 Old Abe Rd
Lac Du Flambeau, WI 54538-9386
(715)588-3371
FAX: (715)588-2039

Ladysmith

Marshfield Medical Center - Ladysmith
900 College Ave W
Ladysmith, WI 54848-2116
(715)532-5561
FAX: (715)532-0270

Lake Geneva

Mercy Walworth Hospital And Medical Center
N2950 State Road 67
Lake Geneva, WI 53147-2655
(262)245-2240
FAX: (262)245-7710

Lancaster

Grant Regional Health Center
507 S Monroe St
Lancaster, WI 53813-2099
(608)723-3246
FAX: (608)723-3243

Madison

Associated Physicians, L.L.P.
4410 Regent St, Radiology Dept.
Madison, WI 53705-4994
(608)233-9746
FAX: (608)233-9993

Ssm Health Dean Medical Group - East Clinc
1821 S Stoughton Rd
Madison, WI 53716-2257
(608)250-1560
FAX: (608)260-6101

Ssm Health Dean Medical Group - Fish Clinic
1313 Fish Hatchery Rd, Department Of Mammography
Madison, WI 53715-1911
(608)250-1560
FAX: (608)283-7361

Ssm Health Dean Medical Group - West Clinic
752 N High Point Rd
Madison, WI 53717-2236
(608)250-1560
FAX: (608)824-4931

U.W. Health Medical Imaging
1 S Park St
Madison, WI 53715-1375
(608)287-2050
FAX: (608)287-2377

U.W. Health Union Corners
2402 Winnebago St
Madison, WI 53704-5341
(608)245-6122
FAX: (608)504-4404

University Of Wisconsin Hosp & Clinics - East Clinic
5249 E Terrace Dr, Mammography
Madison, WI 53718-8339
(608)265-1260
FAX: (608)265-1284

University Of Wisconsin Hosp. & Clinics - West Clinic
451 Junction Rd 9901
Madison, WI 53717-2656
(608)265-7539
FAX: (608)265-7538

University Of Wisconsin Hospital And Clinics
600 Highland Ave, Radiology/Mammography G3-140
Madison, WI 53792-3284
(608)266-6400
FAX: (608)262-7400

Uw Health Odana Atrium
5618 Odana Rd
Madison, WI 53719-1208
(608)287-2050
FAX: (608)287-2343

Wildwood Family Clinic
4901 Cottage Grove Rd
Madison, WI 53716-1392
(608)221-1501
FAX: (608)223-3540

Manitowoc

Holy Family Memorial, Inc.
2300 Western Ave, Women's Imaging Center
Manitowoc, WI 54220-3712
(920)320-3700
FAX: (920)320-3710

Marinette

Aurora Medical Center -Bay Area
3003 University Dr
Marinette, WI 54143-4110
(715)735-4200
FAX: (715)735-8029

Bellin Health Marinette
2820 Roosevelt Rd
Marinette, WI 54143-3834
(715)735-2226
FAX: (715)735-2227

Marshfield

Marshfield Clinic
1000 N Oak Ave
Marshfield, WI 54449-5702
(715)387-5261
FAX: (715)387-9282

Marshfield Medical Center
1000 N Oak Ave
Marshfield, WI 54449-5702
(715)387-5261
FAX: (715)387-9282

Mauston

Mile Bluff Medical Center
1050 Division St
Mauston, WI 53948-1931
(608)847-6161
FAX: (608)847-3841

Medford

Aspirus Medford Hospital
135 S Gibson St
Medford, WI 54451-1622
(715)748-8136
FAX: (715)748-8195

Menasha

Thedacare Physicians-Menasha
2005 Midway Rd, Family Medicine Midway
Menasha, WI 54952-7002
(920)380-4863
FAX: (920)380-4840

Menomonee Falls

Aurora Health Center - Menomonee Falls
N84W16889 Menomonee Ave
Menomonee Falls, WI 53051-2810
(262)236-8787
FAX: (262)250-1828

Center For Diagnostic Imaging
W129N7055 Northfield Dr, Ste 101
Menomonee Falls, WI 53051-0538
(262)251-5305
FAX: (262)251-5207

F&Mcw Community Memorial Hospital
W180N8085 Town Hall Rd
Menomonee Falls, WI 53051-3558
(262)257-5024
FAX: (262)257-1724

Froedtert And The Med. College Wi Community Physicians
W180N8000 Town Hall Rd
Menomonee Falls, WI 53051-4002
(262)532-3081
FAX: (262)532-8697

Menomonie

Mayo Clinic Health System Red Cedar
2321 Stout Rd
Menomonie, WI 54751-7003
(715)233-7228
FAX: (715)233-7795

Mequon

Aurora Health Center - East Mequon
12203 Corporate Pkwy
Mequon, WI 53092-3388
(262)236-8787
FAX: (262)387-8258

Columbia St. Mary's Hospital Ozaukee, Inc
13111 N Port Washington Rd
Mequon, WI 53097-2416
(262)243-7525
FAX: (262)243-7512

Mequon Health Center
11430 N Port Washington Rd
Mequon, WI 53092-3414
(262)836-8388
FAX: (262)836-5541

Merrill

Ascension Good Samaritan Hospital
601 S Center Ave
Merrill, WI 54452-3404
(715)539-2124
FAX: (715)539-2134

Milwaukee

Ascension Se Hospital-St. Joseph
5000 W Chambers St
Milwaukee, WI 53210-1650
(414)527-5000
FAX: (414)527-5005

Ascension-St Francis-Women's Imaging
3237 S 16th St Ste 300, St. Francis Outpatient Center
Milwaukee, WI 53215-4526
(414)527-5000
FAX: (414)527-5005

Aurora Health Center - 84south
PO Box 20858
Milwaukee, WI 53220-0858
(414)747-7474
FAX: (262)827-2280

Aurora Health Center - Good Hope
3003 W Good Hope Rd
Milwaukee, WI 53209-2042
(262)236-8787
FAX: (414)247-4890

Aurora Medical Group-Rivercenter
1575 N Rivercenter Dr
Milwaukee, WI 53212-3978
(414)747-7474
FAX: (414)274-4044

Aurora Sinai Medical Center Of Aurora Health Care Metro Inc.
945 N 12th St
Milwaukee, WI 53233-1305
(414)747-7474
FAX: (414)643-6555

Aurora St. Luke's Medical Center Breast Imaging Center
2900 W Oklahoma Ave
Milwaukee, WI 53215-4330
(414)649-6095
FAX: (414)649-5482

Froedtert Memorial Lutheran Hospital Inc.
9200 W Wisconsin Ave
Milwaukee, WI 53226-3596
(414)805-4950
FAX: (414)805-4955

Isaac Coggs Heritage Health Center
8200 W Silver Spring Dr
Milwaukee, WI 53218-2552
(414)267-2026
FAX: (414)267-3709

Mbccap-Southside Health Center
1639 S 23rd St
Milwaukee, WI 53204-2550
(414)286-6654
FAX: (414)286-6670

Mlk-Heritage Health Center
2555 N Dr Martin Luther King Jr Dr
Milwaukee, WI 53212-2709
(414)372-8080
FAX: (414)464-6245

Progressive Community Health Center
PO Box 80257
Milwaukee, WI 53208-8004
(414)935-8000
FAX: (414)344-3381

Van Dyke Haebler Center For Womens Imaging
2323 N Lake Dr
Milwaukee, WI 53211-4508
(414)326-1800
FAX: (414)326-1802

Wisconsin Health Fund
6200 W Bluemound Rd
Milwaukee, WI 53213-4145
(414)870-0360
FAX: (414)431-0139

Minocqua

Marshfield Medical Center - Minocqua
9576 State Highway 70
Minocqua, WI 54548-9067
(715)847-3507
FAX: (715)358-1128

Monona

Unitypoint Health - Meriter - Monona Clinic
6408 Copps Ave
Monona, WI 53716-3702
(608)417-3000
FAX: (608)417-3109

Uw Health Yahara
1050 E Broadway
Monona, WI 53716-4023
(608)222-8779
FAX: (608)222-8944

Monroe

Monroe Clinic
2005 5th St
Monroe, WI 53566-1546
(608)324-1183
FAX: (608)324-1208

Mt Pleasant

Premier Radiology Mt. Pleasant
10180 Washington Ave, Ste 101
Mt Pleasant, WI 53177-1604
(414)973-7830
FAX: (414)973-7831

Mukwonago

Prohealth Waukesha Mem. Hosp Dba D.N.Greenwald Ctr-Mukwonago
240 Maple Ave
Mukwonago, WI 53149-8475
(262)928-3000
FAX: (262)928-1804

Neenah

Aurora Medical Group, Inc. - Neenah
1136 Westowne Dr
Neenah, WI 54956-2175
(920)720-8200
FAX: (920)720-8017

Thedacare Physicians Neenah
333 N Green Bay Rd
Neenah, WI 54956-1954
(920)729-3363
FAX: (920)729-2112

Thedacare Regional Medical Center Neenah
130 2nd St
Neenah, WI 54956-2883
(920)729-3363
FAX: (920)729-2112

Neillsville

Marshfield Medical Center-Neillsville
N3708 River Ave
Neillsville, WI 54456-7218
(715)819-8330
FAX: (715)819-8482

New Berlin

Aurora Health Center-New Berlin- W National Ave
14555 W National Ave Ste 1
New Berlin, WI 53151-4494
(262)236-8787
FAX: (262)827-3186

Froedtert & Med College Community Physicians
4805 S Moorland Rd
New Berlin, WI 53151-7401
(414)777-1900
FAX: (262)798-7312

Prohealth Waukesha Memorial Hospital - New Berlin
13900 W National Ave Ste 200
New Berlin, WI 53151-9515
(262)928-3000
FAX: (262)696-0739

New London

Thedacare Medical Center - New London
1405 Mill St
New London, WI 54961-2155
(920)531-2054
FAX: (920)531-2418

New Richmond

Westfields Hospital
535 Hospital Rd
New Richmond, WI 54017-1449
(715)243-2735
FAX: (715)243-2732

Oak Creek

Drexel Town Square Health Center
7901 S 6th St
Oak Creek, WI 53154-2010
(262)532-3081
FAX: (262)532-9517

Oconomowoc

Prohealth Oconomowoc Memorial Hospital
791 Summit Ave
Oconomowoc, WI 53066-3896
(262)928-3000
FAX: (262)560-4528

Onalaska

Gundersen Health System - Onalaska
3111 Gundersen Dr
Onalaska, WI 54650-8447
(608)775-2886
FAX: (608)775-6674

Mayo Clinic Health System Onalaska Clinic
191 Theater Rd
Onalaska, WI 54650-8679
(608)392-5000
FAX: (608)791-7882

Oneida

Oneida Community Health Center
PO Box 365, 525 Airport Rd
Oneida, WI 54155-0365
(920)869-2711
FAX: (920)869-1699

Osceola

Osceola Medical Center
2600 65th Ave
Osceola, WI 54020-4370
(715)294-4756
FAX: (715)294-5697

Oshkosh

Aurora Medical Center
855 N Westhaven Dr
Oshkosh, WI 54904-7668
(920)456-7040
FAX: (920)303-5698

Mercy Oakwood Breast Center
2700 W 9th Ave, Ste 201
Oshkosh, WI 54904-7864
(920)236-1880
FAX: (920)236-1881

Thedacare Physicians Oshkosh
600 N Westhaven Dr
Oshkosh, WI 54904-6926
(920)237-5000
FAX: (920)237-5697

Osseo

Mayo Clinic Health System - Oakridge
13025 8th St
Osseo, WI 54758-7634
(715)597-8755
FAX: (507)422-1051

Park Falls

Marshfield Medical Center - Park Falls
98 Sherry Ave
Park Falls, WI 54552-1467
(715)762-7311
FAX: (715)762-7545

Platteville

Southwest Health
1400 Eastside Rd
Platteville, WI 53818-9800
(608)348-2331
FAX: (608)342-4791

Pleasant Prairie

Aurora Health Center Pleasant Prairie
12500 Aurora Dr
Pleasant Prairie, WI 53158-1227
(262)857-5037
FAX: (262)857-5031

Froedtert South,Inc - Pleasant Prairie Hospital
9555 76th St, Froedtert South,Inc - Pleasant Prairie H
Pleasant Prairie, WI 53158-1984
(262)656-2508
FAX: (262)577-8764

Plover

Ascension St. Michael's Hospital At Plover
2401 Plover Rd
Plover, WI 54467-3916
(715)295-3800
FAX: (715)295-3814

Plymouth

Aurora Sheboygan Clinic
2600 Kiley Way
Plymouth, WI 53073-5020
(920)451-5545
FAX: (920)449-7331

Portage

Divine Savior Healthcare
2817 New Pinery Rd, Ste 202
Portage, WI 53901-9296
(608)745-6275
FAX: (608)745-5097

Prairie Du Chien

Gundersen Health System - Prairie Du Chien
610 E Taylor St
Prairie Du Chien, WI 53821-2109
(608)326-6466
FAX: (608)326-6273

Pdc Memorial Hospital Assoc, Inc.,Dba Crossing Rivers Health
37868 US Highway 18
Prairie Du Chien, WI 53821-8416
(608)357-2000
FAX: (608)357-2280

Prairie Du Sac

Sauk Prairie Healthcare
260 26th St
Prairie Du Sac, WI 53578-1599
(608)643-7274
FAX: (608)643-7502

Racine

Ahc Racine Dept. Of Amc-Kenosha, Wi.
8400 Washington Ave
Racine, WI 53406-3735
(262)321-3025
FAX: (262)321-3031

Ascension All Saints Healthcare-Women's Imaging- Spring Stre
3821 Spring St
Racine, WI 53405-1667
(262)687-2600
FAX: (262)687-3926

Reedsburg

Reedsburg Area Medical Center
2000 N Dewey Ave
Reedsburg, WI 53959-1049
(608)768-6229
FAX: (608)524-7897

Rhinelander

Ascension St. Mary's Hospital
2251 N Shore Dr Ste 100
Rhinelander, WI 54501-6710
(715)361-2699
FAX: (715)361-2795

Rice Lake

Diagnostic Radiology Associates Of Wi
1024 N Main St
Rice Lake, WI 54868-1288
(715)234-7776
FAX: (715)234-9750

Marshfield Medical Center - Rice Lake
1700 W Stout St
Rice Lake, WI 54868-5000
(715)236-8484
FAX: (715)236-8194

Mayo Clinic Health System Northland
331 S Main St Ste H
Rice Lake, WI 54868-2253
(715)537-6747
FAX: (715)537-9949

Richland Center

The Richland Hospital, Inc.
333 E 2nd St
Richland Center, WI 53581-1914
(608)647-6321
FAX: (608)647-2990

Ripon

Ripon Community Hospital
845 Parkside St
Ripon, WI 54971-8505
(920)745-3036
FAX: (920)745-7916

River Falls

River Falls Area Hospital
1629 E Division St
River Falls, WI 54022-1571
(715)307-6400
FAX: (715)307-6245

Shawano

Thedacare Medical Center Shawano
100 County Road B
Shawano, WI 54166-7072
(715)526-7224
FAX: (715)851-7461

Sheboygan

Aurora Sheboygan Clinic
2414 Kohler Memorial Dr
Sheboygan, WI 53081-3170
(920)453-3885
FAX: (920)453-3972

Marsho Family Medical Group
1703 N Taylor Dr
Sheboygan, WI 53081-1933
(920)457-4438
FAX: (920)451-3269

St. Nicholas Hospital
3100 Superior Ave, Radiology Department
Sheboygan, WI 53081-1994
(920)459-5171
FAX: (920)459-5183

Shell Lake

Indianhead Med Center Inc -Shell Lake
113 4th Ave
Shell Lake, WI 54871-4457
(715)468-7833
FAX: (715)468-7303

Sparta

Gundersen Health System - Sparta
1111 W Wisconsin St
Sparta, WI 54656-2233
(608)269-6731
FAX: (608)269-1537

Mayo Clinic Health System Sparta Campus
310 W Main St
Sparta, WI 54656-2170
(608)366-5242
FAX: (608)791-7882

Spooner

Spooner Health System
1180 Chandler Dr
Spooner, WI 54801-2204
(715)939-1594
FAX: (715)939-1564

St Croix Falls

St. Croix Regional Medical Center
235 E State St
St Croix Falls, WI 54024-4117
(715)483-0270
FAX: (715)483-0274

St Francis

Aurora Health Center-St Francis-Layton Ave
2000 E Layton Ave Ste 130
St Francis, WI 53235-6067
(414)747-7474
FAX: (414)747-6676

Stanley

Ascension Our Lady Of Victory Hospital
1120 Pine St
Stanley, WI 54768-1297
(715)644-6112
FAX: (715)644-6150

Stevens Point

Ascension Medical Group Part Of St. Michael's Hospital
824 Illinois Ave
Stevens Point, WI 54481-3112
(715)342-6482
FAX: (715)346-0709

Ascension St. Michael's Hospital At Hoover
3500 Hoover Rd
Stevens Point, WI 54481-5600
(715)346-0222
FAX: (715)346-0280

Aspirus Stevens Point Clinic
5409 Vern Holmes Dr
Stevens Point, WI 54482-8853
(715)847-2947
FAX: (715)342-1188

Stoughton

Stoughton Hospital
900 Ridge St
Stoughton, WI 53589-1897
(608)873-2299
FAX: (608)873-2364

Sturgeon Bay

Aurora Health Care
1910 Alabama St
Sturgeon Bay, WI 54235-3532
(920)746-7200
FAX: (920)746-7299

Door County Memorial Hospital
323 S 18th Ave
Sturgeon Bay, WI 54235-1401
(920)746-3540
FAX: (920)746-3797

Summit

Aurora Medical Center Summit
36500 Aurora Dr
Summit, WI 53066-4899
(262)434-1400
FAX: (262)434-1450

Sun Prairie

Ssm Health Dean Medical Group - Sun Prairie Clinic
10 Tower Dr
Sun Prairie, WI 53590-1239
(608)825-3504
FAX: (608)825-3791

Superior

Essentia Health St. Mary's Hospital Superior
3500 Tower Ave
Superior, WI 54880-5395
(218)786-4427
FAX: (715)395-5324

Mariner Medical Clinic
109 N 28th St E
Superior, WI 54880-6598
(715)395-3902
FAX: (715)395-3962

Tomah

Gundersen Health System - Tomah
505 Gopher Dr
Tomah, WI 54660-4513
(608)372-4111
FAX: (608)372-4330

Mayo Clinic Health System - Tomah Clinic
325 Butts Ave
Tomah, WI 54660-1412
(608)372-5951
FAX: (608)791-7882

Tomahawk

Ascension Sacred Heart Hospital
401 W Mohawk Dr Ste 100
Tomahawk, WI 54487-2273
(715)453-7736
FAX: (715)453-7706

Two Rivers

Aurora Health Center Manitowoc County
5300 Memorial Dr
Two Rivers, WI 54241-3923
(920)793-6520
FAX: (920)793-6521

Viroqua

Vernon Memorial Hospital
507 S Main St
Viroqua, WI 54665-2096
(608)637-4350
FAX: (608)637-4283

Watertown

Watertown Regional Medical Center, Center For Women's Health
128 Hospital Dr
Watertown, WI 53098-3304
(920)262-4825
FAX: (920)206-3066

Waukesha

Aurora Health Center Waukesha
W231N1440 Corporate Ct
Waukesha, WI 53186-1503
(262)896-6078
FAX: (262)896-3925

Center For Diagnostic Imaging
2315 E Moreland Blvd Ste 1500
Waukesha, WI 53186-2939
(262)646-5199
FAX: (262)646-5788

Prohealth Medical Group Delafield Street
1111 Delafield St, Ste 112
Waukesha, WI 53188-3402
(262)696-5693
FAX: (262)696-0739

Prohealth Waukesha Memorial Hospital-Pewaukee
N16W24131 Riverwood Dr
Waukesha, WI 53188-1106
(262)928-3000
FAX: (262)696-0739

Waupaca

Thedacare Physicians Waupaca
710 Riverside Dr
Waupaca, WI 54981-1941
(715)256-2088
FAX: (715)258-1155

Waupun

Agnesian Healthcare-Waupun Memorial Hospital
620 W Brown St
Waupun, WI 53963-1799
(920)324-5581
FAX: (920)324-0172

Wausau

Ascension Medical Group-Westwood
1901 Westwood Center Blvd
Wausau, WI 54401-2892
(715)355-9539
FAX: (715)355-9512

Aspirus Wausau Hospital
333 Pine Ridge Blvd
Wausau, WI 54401-4187
(715)847-2586
FAX: (715)847-2151

Marshfield Clinic- Wausau Center
2727 Plaza Dr
Wausau, WI 54401-4192
(715)847-3507
FAX: (715)847-3513

Wautoma

Aurora Health Center Wautoma
900 E Division St
Wautoma, WI 54982-6944
(920)787-6900
FAX: (920)787-6903

Wauwatosa

Ascension- Wauwatosa
201 N Mayfair Rd
Wauwatosa, WI 53226-4216
(414)527-5000
FAX: (414)527-5005

Aurora Health Center - Mayfair North
3289 N Mayfair Rd
Wauwatosa, WI 53222-3203
(262)236-8787
FAX: (414)607-6336

West Allis

Aurora West Allis Medical Center
8901 W Lincoln Ave
West Allis, WI 53227-2477
(414)329-4332
FAX: (414)329-5652

Gateway Medical Clinic
801 S 70th St
West Allis, WI 53214-3147
(414)773-6680
FAX: (414)773-6695

West Bend

Aurora Health Care West Bend Valley Avenue
205 Valley Ave
West Bend, WI 53095-5312
(262)670-4040
FAX: (262)670-4451

Froedtert & The Medical College Of Wi Community Physicians
1700 W Paradise Dr
West Bend, WI 53095-9795
(262)532-3081
FAX: (262)532-9517

St. Josephs Community Hospital Of West Bend
3200 Pleasant Valley Rd
West Bend, WI 53095-9274
(414)805-4959
FAX: (414)805-4955

West Salem

Coulee Diagnostic Radiology
1580 Heritage Blvd
West Salem, WI 54669-9418
(608)518-3406
FAX: (608)518-3405

Weston

Aspirus Weston Clinic
4005 Community Center Dr
Weston, WI 54476-4139
(715)847-2914
FAX: (715)847-2640

Whitehall

Gundersen Tri-County Hospital And Clinics
18606 Ervin St
Whitehall, WI 54773-8613
(715)538-4355
FAX: (715)538-4340

Wild Rose

Thedacare Medical Center- Wild Rose
601 Grove Ave
Wild Rose, WI 54984-6903
(920)622-6005
FAX: (920)622-5499

Windsor

Uw Health Deforest - Windsor
4131 Meridian Dr
Windsor, WI 53598-9699
(608)287-2050
FAX: (608)846-7898

Wisconsin Rapids

Aspirus Doctors Clinic
2031 Peach St
Wisconsin Rapids, WI 54494-5181
(715)421-7432
FAX: (715)422-6663

Aspirus Riverview Hospital And Clinics
410 Dewey St
Wisconsin Rapids, WI 54494-4715
(715)421-7430
FAX: (715)421-7554

Woodruff

Howard Young Medical Center
240 Maple St
Woodruff, WI 54568-9190
(715)356-8020
FAX: (715)356-8254

WYOMING

Afton

Star Valley Health
PO Box 579, 901 Adams
Afton, WY 83110-0579
(307)885-5940
FAX: (307)885-3842

Basin

Three Rivers Health Dba
388 US Highway 20 S
Basin, WY 82410-8902
(307)568-3311
FAX: (307)568-2139

Buffalo

Johnson County Healthcare Center
497 W Lott St
Buffalo, WY 82834-1658
(307)684-6179
FAX: (307)684-0906

Casper

Outpatient Radiology Llc
419 S Washington St Ste 101
Casper, WY 82601-2951
(307)232-5012
FAX: (307)237-1074

Summit Medical Center
6350 E 2nd St
Casper, WY 82609-4264
(307)232-6590
FAX: (307)333-6083

Cheyenne

Cheyenne Rad Grp Dba Cheyenne Women's Imaging Pav
2003 Bluegrass Cir
Cheyenne, WY 82009-7329
(307)633-8992
FAX: (307)634-7760

Cheyenne Rad Grp Dba Cheyenne Women's Imaging Pavilion
5050 Powderhouse Rd
Cheyenne, WY 82009-4800
(307)433-8282
FAX: (307)433-8870

Cody

West Park Hospital
707 Sheridan Ave
Cody, WY 82414-3409
(307)578-2857
FAX: (307)578-2880

Douglas

Memorial Hospital Of Converse County
111 S 5th St
Douglas, WY 82633-2434
(307)358-1438
FAX: (307)358-1489

Evanston

Evanston Regional Hospital
190 Arrowhead Dr, Radiology Department
Evanston, WY 82930-9266
(307)783-8196
FAX: (307)783-8274

Gillette

Campbell County Memorial Hospital
501 S Burma Ave
Gillette, WY 82716-3426
(307)688-1600
FAX: (307)688-1640

Jackson

St. John's Medical Health
625 E Broadway Ave
Jackson, WY 83001-8642
(307)739-7531
FAX: (307)739-7674

Kemmerer

South Lincoln Medical Center
711 Onyx St
Kemmerer, WY 83101-3214
(307)800-8665
FAX: (307)877-2214

Lander

Sagewest Lander
1320 Bishop Randall Dr
Lander, WY 82520-3939
(307)335-6259
FAX: (307)335-6467

Laramie

Ivinson Memorial Hospital
255 N 30th St
Laramie, WY 82072-5195
(307)755-4640
FAX: (307)721-4713

Lovell

North Big Horn Hospital
1115 Lane 12, Radiology Department
Lovell, WY 82431-9537
(307)548-5245
FAX: (307)548-5248

Newcastle

Weston County Health Services
1124 Washington Blvd
Newcastle, WY 82701-2972
(307)746-3704
FAX: (307)746-3729

Powell

Powell Hospital District 1 Dba Powell Valley Healthcare
777 Avenue H
Powell, WY 82435-2260
(307)754-1220
FAX: (307)754-7727

Rawlins

Memorial Hospital Of Carbon County
2221 Elm St
Rawlins, WY 82301-5108
(307)324-8381
FAX: (307)324-8382

Riverton

Riverton Memorial Hospital, Llc, D/B/A
Sagewest Health Care.
2100 W Sunset Dr
Riverton, WY 82501-2274
(307)857-3462
FAX: (307)857-3478

Rock Springs

Aspen Mountain Medical Center
4401 College Dr
Rock Springs, WY 82901-3507
(307)352-8900
FAX: (307)352-8936

Memorial Hospital Of Sweetwater County
1200 College Dr
Rock Springs, WY 82901-5868
(307)352-8386
FAX: (307)352-8151

Rock Creek Medical Imaging
2620 Commercial Way Ste 10
Rock Springs, WY 82901-4705
(307)382-4282
FAX: (307)382-4291

Sheridan

Sheridan Memorial Hospital
1401 W 5th St
Sheridan, WY 82801-2799
(307)672-1046
FAX: (307)672-1149

Thermopolis

Hot Springs Health
150 E Arapahoe St
Thermopolis, WY 82443-2498
(307)864-5047
FAX: (307)864-5028

Torrington

Torrington Community Hospital
2000 Campbell Dr
Torrington, WY 82240-1597
(307)532-3184
FAX: (307)532-5584

Wheatland

Platte County Memorial Hospital
201 14th St
Wheatland, WY 82201-3201
(307)322-3636
FAX: (307)322-4826

Worland

Washakie Medical Center-Radiology
Department
400 S 15th St
Worland, WY 82401-3531
(307)347-5744
FAX: (307)347-6966

Apo

31 Medical Group Aviano Ab, Italy
Unit 6180, 31 Medical Group
Apo, AE 09604-6180
(390)434-3050
FAX: (390)434-0000

35th Medical Group Misawa Ab Japan
Unit 5024
Apo, AP 96319-5024
(813)117-7766
FAX: (811)767-0000

48th Medical Group 48 Msgs/Sgcr
Unit 5115, 48 Msgs/Sgcr
Apo, AE 09461-5115
(011)441-6385
FAX: (441)638-8000

Landstuhl Regional Medical Center
CMR 402, McEul-R
Apo, AE 09180
(011)496-3719
FAX: (496)371-8000

Fpo

U.S. Naval Hospital - Naples,Italy
PSC 808 Box 19
Fpo, AE 09618-0001
(011)390-8181
FAX: (390)818-0001

U.S. Naval Hospital - Sigonella [italy]
PSC 836 Box 2670
Fpo, AE 09636-9998
(390)955-6470
FAX: (390)955-0006

U.S. Naval Hospital - Yokosuka, Japan
PSC 475, Box 1 Usnh
Fpo, AP 96350-1200
(011)814-6816
FAX: (814)686-0016

U.S. Naval Hospital Rota, Spain
PSC 819, Box 18
Fpo, AE 09645-0001
(349)568-2343
FAX: (349)568-0002

US POSSESSIONS

Christiansted

Governor Juan F Luis Hospital & Medical
Center
4007 Estate Diamond Ruby
Christiansted, VI 00820-4435
(340)778-6311
FAX: (340)772-7375

Imaging Center, P.C.
4500 Sion Farm, Island Medical Center Ste 4B
Christiansted, VI 00820
(340)778-5305
FAX: (340)778-2778

Oka, Tamuning

Guam Memorial Hospital Authority
850 Governor Carlos G. Camacho Rd.
Oka, Tamuning, GU 96911
(671)647-2137
FAX: (671)647-2900

Pago Pago

Lbj Tropical Medical Center
PO Box Lbj, Mammography Department
Pago Pago, AS 96799-0010
(684)633-1222
FAX: (684)633-1869

Saipan

Commonwealth Healthcare Corporation
1 Lower Navy Hill
Saipan, MP 96950
(670)236-8325
FAX: (670)234-8930

St Thomas

Roy Lester Schneider Hospital
9048 Sugar Est
St Thomas, VI 00802-3634
(340)776-8311
FAX: (340)714-6336

St. Thomas Radiology Associates, Llc
9149 Estate Thomas, Ste 103
St Thomas, VI 00802-3132
(340)774-0265
FAX: (340)776-0228

Tamuning

Fhp Health Center
548 S Marine Corps Dr Main Bldg, Radiology
Department
Tamuning, GU 96913-3539
(671)646-5824
FAX: (671)647-3527

Guam Radiology Consultants
633 Gov Carlos G Camacho Rd Ste 210, Guam
Medical Plaza
Tamuning, GU 96913-3195
(671)649-1001
FAX: (671)647-4600

Guam Seventh Day Adventist Clinic
388 Ypao Rd
Tamuning, GU 96913-3701
(671)646-8881
FAX: (671)648-2554

Mdx Imaging Center
643 Chalan San Antonio, Ste 109
Tamuning, GU 96913-3644
(671)648-6390
FAX: (671)648-6398

U.S. Naval Hospital - Guam
50 Farenholt Ave
Tamuning, GU 96913-3106
(671)344-9706
FAX: (671)344-9702

Alphabetical Index

A Woman's View	Hickory	NC
A Womans Place Naples, Llc	Naples	FL
A. O. Fox Memorial Hospital	Oneonta	NY
Abbeville Area Medical Center	Abbeville	SC
Abbeville General Hospital	Abbeville	LA
Abbott Northwestern Hospital Piper Breast Center	Minneapolis	MN
Abercrombie Radiological Consultants	Knoxville	TN
Abington Health - Mary T Sachs Breast Imaging Ctr	Willow Grove	PA
Abington Health Center - Warminster Campus	Warminster	PA
Abington Health Center At Blue Bell	Blue Bell	PA
Abington Health Lansdale Hospital	Lansdale	PA
Abington Memorial Hospital	Abington	PA
Abraham Lincoln Memorial Hospital	Lincoln	IL
Abrom Kaplan Memorial Hospital	Kaplan	LA
Acadian Plaza Diagnostic Ctr - Memorial Hosp Gulfport	Gulfport	MS
Ackerman Cancer Center	Amelia Island	FL
Ackerman Cancer Center	Jacksonville	FL
Acp Northwest Imaging Center	Tucson	AZ
Ad Hospital East, Llc	Houston	TX
Ad Hospital East, Llc	Houston	TX
Adair County Health Center, Inc. Dba Physicians Clinic	Stilwell	OK
Adair County Memorial Hospital	Greenfield	IA
Adams County Regional Medical Center	Seaman	OH
Adams Memorial Hospital	Decatur	IN
Addison Gilbert Hospital	Gloucester	MA
Adena Fayette Medical Center	Washington Court House	OH
Adena Health Center	Chillicothe	OH
Adena Health Center - Waverly	Waverly	OH
Adena Health Center - Western Avenue	Chillicothe	OH
Adirondack Health At Saranac Lake	Saranac Lake	NY
Advance Cardiovascular Imaging Inc	Miami	FL
Advance Technological Radiology Pa	Lake Wales	FL
Advance Technological Radiology, P.A.	Davenport	FL
Advance Technological Radiology, P.A.	Winter Haven	FL
Advanced Diagnostic Breast Center At Henrico Doctors Sarah C	Richmond	VA
Advanced Diagnostic Radiology, Llc	Cumberland	MD
Advanced Imaging	Stevensville	MT
Advanced Imaging Center	Palmdale	CA
Advanced Imaging Center	Missoula	MT
Advanced Imaging Center	Missoula	MT
Advanced Imaging Center At Adventist Health Lodi Memorial	Lodi	CA
Advanced Imaging Center, Llc	Moline	IL
Advanced Imaging Concepts Pl	Brooksville	FL
Advanced Imaging Of Alabama	Anniston	AL
Advanced Imaging Of Gadsden	Gadsden	AL
Advanced Imaging Specialists	Dunmore	PA
Advanced Medical Imaging	Kokomo	IN
Advanced Medical Imaging	Bozeman	MT
Advanced Medical Imaging	Lincoln	NE
Advanced Medical Imaging	McAllen	TX
Advanced Medical Imaging Northpointe	Fresno	CA
Advanced Medical Img. Of Englewood Hosp & Med. Ctr	Emerson	NJ
Advanced Mri & Ct Institute	Vega Baja	PR
Advanced Radiology - Cross Roads	Ellicott City	MD
Advanced Radiology - Aiello	Glen Burnie	MD
Advanced Radiology - Annapolis	Annapolis	MD
Advanced Radiology - Arundel Mills	Hanover	MD
Advanced Radiology - Dundalk	Baltimore	MD
Advanced Radiology - Eldersburg	Eldersburg	MD
Advanced Radiology - Gbmc Pavilion	Towson	MD
Advanced Radiology - Glen Burnie	Glen Burnie	MD
Advanced Radiology - Harford	Bel Air	MD
Advanced Radiology - Lutherville	Lutherville	MD
Advanced Radiology - Medical Arts	Baltimore	MD
Advanced Radiology - Owings Mills	Owings Mills	MD
Advanced Radiology - Perry Hall	Baltimore	MD
Advanced Radiology - St. Joe's	Towson	MD
Advanced Radiology - Timonium	Timonium	MD
Advanced Radiology Consultants - Fairfield	Fairfield	CT
Advanced Radiology Consultants - Stamford	Stamford	CT
Advanced Radiology Consultants Stratford	Stratford	CT
Advanced Radiology Imaging Associates, Llc	Ft Myers	FL
Advanced Radiology Medical Group, Inc.	Rosemead	CA
Advanced Radiology- Maiden Choice	Baltimore	MD
Advanced Radiology- Pomona	Baltimore	MD
Advanced Radiology-Fisher	Westminster	MD
Advanced Radiology-Knoll Imaging	Columbia	MD
Advanced Radiology-Shipley's Choice	Millersville	MD
Advanced Radiology-Wilton	Wilton	CT
Advanced Shore Imaging Associates	Northfield	NJ
Advanced Southern Imaging Llc	Conyers	GA
Advanced Southern Imaging- Conyers	Conyers	GA
Advanced Women's Imaging By Saint Francis Hospital	Charleston	WV
Advanced Womens Imaging Center	Trumbull	CT
Advantage Radiology	Brooklyn	NY
Advent Health - Lenexa	Lenexa	KS
Advent Health Heart Of Florida	Davenport	FL
Advent Health North Pinellas	Tarpon Springs	FL
Advent Health Tampa- Kay Meyer Breast Care Center	Tampa	FL
Advent Health Waterman	Tavares	FL
Advent Health West Florida Imaging Inc.	Tampa	FL
Adventhealth Apopka	Apopka	FL
Adventhealth Breast Surgery At Davenport	Davenport	FL
Adventhealth Carrollwood	Tampa	FL
Adventhealth Central Texas	Killeen	TX
Adventhealth Durand	Durand	WI
Adventhealth Gordon	Calhoun	GA
Adventhealth Hendersonville	Hendersonville	NC
Adventhealth Imaging Altamonte Springs	Altamonte Springs	FL
Adventhealth Imaging Celebration	Celebration	FL
Adventhealth Imaging Center Apopka	Apopka	FL
Adventhealth Imaging Center Roeland Park	Roeland Park	KS
Adventhealth Imaging Center-Westchase	Tampa	FL
Adventhealth Imaging Deltona	Deltona	FL
Adventhealth Imaging East Orlando	Orlando	FL
Adventhealth Imaging Lake Mary	Lake Mary	FL
Adventhealth Imaging Lake Nona	Orlando	FL
Adventhealth Imaging Ormond Beach	Ormond Beach	FL
Adventhealth Imaging Oviedo	Oviedo	FL
Adventhealth Imaging Palm Coast	Palm Coast	FL
Adventhealth Imaging Partin Settlement	Kissimmee	FL
Adventhealth Imaging Princeton	Orlando	FL
Adventhealth Imaging Sebring	Sebring	FL
Adventhealth Imaging South Asheville	Arden	NC
Adventhealth Imaging Waterford Lakes	Orlando	FL
Adventhealth Imaging Winter Garden	Winter Garden	FL
Adventhealth Imaging Womens Center Deland	Deland	FL
Adventhealth Imaging-New Smyrna Health Park	New Smyrna Beach	FL
Adventhealth Kissimmee	Kissimmee	FL
Adventhealth Lake Wales	Lake Wales	FL
Adventhealth Manchester	Manchester	KY
Adventhealth Murray	Chatsworth	GA
Adventhealth New Smyrna Beach	New Smyrna Beach	FL
Adventhealth Palm Coast	Palm Coast	FL
Adventhealth Rollins Brook	Lampasas	TX
Adventhealth Sebring	Sebring	FL
Adventhealth Shawnee Mission	Shawnee Mission	KS
Adventhealth South Overland Park Women's Imaging	Overland Park	KS
Adventhealth Wauchula	Wauchula	FL
Adventhealth Women's Center Winter Park	Winter Park	FL
Adventhealth Zephyrhills	Zephyrhills	FL
Adventist Health Adventist Medical Center	Portland	OR
Adventist Health And Rideout Center For Women's Imaging	Yuba City	CA
Adventist Health Bakersfield	Bakersfield	CA
Adventist Health Bakersfield	Bakersfield	CA
Adventist Health Breast Care Center - Hanford	Hanford	CA
Adventist Health Castle	Kailua	HI
Adventist Health Clear Lake Hospital	Clearlake	CA
Adventist Health Delano	Delano	CA
Adventist Health Glendale	Glendale	CA
Adventist Health Medical Imaging Oakhurst	Oakhurst	CA
Adventist Health Physicians Network 821 S St. Helena Hwy 2	Saint Helena	CA
Adventist Health Reedley Dba Adventist Med Ctr Reedley	Reedley	CA
Adventist Health Simi Valley Nancy Reagan Breast Center	Simi Valley	CA
Adventist Health Sonora Health Pavilion	Sonora	CA
Adventist Health Tehachapi Valley	Tehachapi	CA
Adventist Health Tillamook	Tillamook	OR
Adventist Health Tulare	Tulare	CA

Name	City	State
Adventist Health Ukiah Valley	Ukiah	CA
Adventist Health Ukiah Valley	Ukiah	CA
Adventist Health-Bakersfield	Bakersfield	CA
Adventist Healthcare Fort Washington Medical Center	Fort Washington	MD
Adventist Medical Center-Selma	Selma	CA
Adventist Mendocino Coast Hospital	Fort Bragg	CA
Adventist Plainfield Imaging And Outpatient Center	Plainfield	IL
Advocate Aurora Health	Oak Lawn	IL
Advocate Christ Center For Breast Care	Oak Lawn	IL
Advocate Condell Medical Center	Gurnee	IL
Advocate Condell Medical Center	Libertyville	IL
Advocate Good Samaritan OP Ctr Downers Grove	Downers Grove	IL
Advocate Good Shepherd OP Ctr - Crystal Lake	Crystal Lake	IL
Advocate Good Shepherd OP Ctr-Lake Zurich	Lake Zurich	IL
Advocate Illinois Masonic Medical Center	Chicago	IL
Advocate Medical Group - Irving And Western	Chicago	IL
Advocate Medical Group - Sykes	Chicago	IL
Advocate Medical Group Orland Park	Orland Park	IL
Advocate Medical Group-Beverly	Chicago	IL
Advocate Medical Nesset Radiology	Park Ridge	IL
Advocate Outpatient Center	Des Plaines	IL
Advocate Outpatient Center Radiology	Huntley	IL
Advocate Sherman Hospital	Elgin	IL
Advocate Sherman Imaging Center - Randall	Elgin	IL
Advocate Sherman Outpatient Center - Algonquin	Algonquin	IL
Advocate Sherman Outpatient Center - South Elgin	South Elgin	IL
Advocate South Suburban Hospital	Hazel Crest	IL
Advocate Trinity Hospital	Chicago	IL
Ag Radiology Imaging Center, Llc	Katy	TX
Agnesian Healthcare-Waupun Memorial Hospital	Waupun	WI
Aguada Medical Radiology	Aguada	PR
Ahc Racine Dept. Of Amc-Kenosha, Wi.	Racine	WI
Ahn Hempfield Imaging	Greensburg	PA
Ahn Outpatient Center Waterworks	Pittsburgh	PA
Ahs Pryor Hospital,Llc Dba Hillcrest Hospital Pryor	Pryor	OK
Aici-Mammo	Virginia Beach	VA
Aid System Llc	Rio Piedras	PR
Aims Diagnostic Imaging Of South Jersey, Llc	Cape May Court House	NJ
Akmc Dba Allegheny Valley Hospital, Radiological Imaging	Natrona Heights	PA
Akron Gen. Reflections Breast Hlth Ctr - Akron	Akron	OH
Akumin	Ft Lauderdale	FL
Akumin	Jacksonville	FL
Akumin	Jacksonville	FL
Akumin	Jacksonville	FL
Akumin	Orange Park	FL
Akumin Langhorne	Langhorne	PA
Akumin Northeast	Philadelphia	PA
Akumin - Coral Springs Women's Center	Coral Springs	FL
Akumin Boot Ranch	Palm Harbor	FL
Akumin Downingtown	Downingtown	PA
Akumin Haverford	Havertown	PA
Akumin Hollywood	Hollywood	FL
Akumin Imaging Texas, Llc	El Paso	TX
Akumin Imaging Texas, Llc	El Paso	TX
Akumin Imaging Texas, Llc	El Paso	TX
Akumin Imaging Texas, Llc	El Paso	TX
Akumin Lake Worth	Lake Worth	FL
Akumin Largo	Largo	FL
Akumin Pines	Pembroke Pines	FL
Akumin Plantation	Plantation	FL
Akumin Riverview	Riverview	FL
Akumin Royal Palm	Coral Springs	FL
Akumin Sarasota	Sarasota	FL
Akumin Springfield	Springfield	PA
Akumin Tampa	Tampa	FL
Akumin Trinity	Trinity	FL
Akumin Wellington	Wellington	FL
Akumin Wesley Chapel	Wesley Chapel	FL
Akumin Zephyrhills	Zephyrhills	FL
Akumin, Pembroke Pines East	Pembroke Pines	FL
Akumin, Plantation East	Plantation	FL
Akumin- Boca Raton	Boca Raton	FL
Akumin- Deltona	Deltona	FL
Akumin- Mount Dora	Mount Dora	FL
Akumin- Palm Harbor	Palm Harbor	FL
Akumin- Port Charlotte	Port Charlotte	FL
Akumin- St Petersburg	St Petersburg	FL
Akumin-Clearwater	Clearwater	FL
Akumin-Fleming Island	Fleming Island	FL
Akumin-Kissimmee West	Kissimmee	FL
Akumin-Winter Haven	Winter Haven	FL
Alabama Medical Group, P.C.	Mobile	AL
Alameda Health System Dba Alameda Hospital	Alameda	CA
Alamogordo Imaging Center	Alamogordo	NM
Alaska Imaging	Wasilla	AK
Alaska Native Medical Center	Anchorage	AK
Alaska Regional Hospital	Anchorage	AK
Albany Medical Center South Clinical Campus	Albany	NY
Albert Einstein Med Ctr-Marion-Louise Saltzman Womens Ctr	Philadelphia	PA
Alexandria Cdi	Alexandria	MN
Alexandria Clinic A Service Of Alomere Health	Alexandria	MN
Alexandria Women's Center	Alexandria	LA
Alexian Bros. Immediate Care Center	Addison	IL
Alexian Brothers Medical Center - Women's Ctr	Elk Grove Village	IL
Alfa Diagnostic, Llc	Aventura	FL
Alice Gorman Imaging - Oneida Healthcare Center	Oneida	NY
Alice Hyde Medical Center	Malone	NY
Alice Peck Day Memorial Hospital	Lebanon	NH
Alinea Medical Imaging	Pomona	CA
Alinea Medical Imaging-Mobile	Pomona	CA
All Women Ob/Gyn	Louisville	KY
Alle-Kiski Medical Center, Dba Allegheny Valley Hospital	Natrona Heights	PA
Alleghany Memorial Hospital	Sparta	NC
Allegheny Clinic Radiology-Sewickley	Sewickley	PA
Allegheny General Breast Care Center	Pittsburgh	PA
Allegheny Imaging Of Robinson	Mc Kees Rocks	PA
Allen Memorial Hospital	Waterloo	IA
Allendale County Hospital	Fairfax	SC
Alliance Community Hospital	Alliance	OH
Alliance Health Durant	Durant	OK
Alliance Health Woodward	Woodward	OK
Alliance Healthcare System	Holly Springs	MS
Alliance Imaging	Saint Cloud	MN
Alliance Medical Group	San Pablo	CA
Alliancehealth Clinton	Clinton	OK
Alliancehealth Ponca City	Ponca City	OK
Allina Health - Apple Valley	Apple Valley	MN
Allina Health Bandana Square Clinic	Saint Paul	MN
Allina Health Coon Rapids Clinic	Coon Rapids	MN
Allina Health Elk River Clinic	Elk River	MN
Allina Health Forest Lake Clinic	Forest Lake	MN
Allina Health Richfield Clinic	Richfield	MN
Allina Health Woodbury Clinic	Woodbury	MN
Allina Medical Clinic - Northfield, Part Of Allina Health	Northfield	MN
Allium Diagnostic Imaging	Ridgewood	NY
Allwood Imaging Pa	Clifton	NJ
Alma C. Kinn Mammo Ctr Promedica Fostoria Community Hospital	Fostoria	OH
Alta Bates Summit Med. Ctr-Lafayette Womens Hlth	Lafayette	CA
Alta View Hospital	Sandy	UT
Alta Vista Regional Hospital	Las Vegas	NM
Alton Memorial Hospital	Alton	IL
Alton Multispecialists Physicians	Alton	IL
Altru Clinic - Crookston	Crookston	MN
Altru Clinic - Devils Lake	Devils Lake	ND
Altru Health System	Grand Forks	ND
Altus Women's Center Of Baytown, Lp	Baytown	TX
Amberwell Hiawatha	Hiawatha	KS
Amboy Medical Practice	Staten Island	NY
Ambulatory Diagnostic Center	Coral Gables	FL
Ambulatory Diagnostic Center	Miami	FL
Ambulatory Imaging Center-Johnston Medical Center	Smithfield	NC
American Fork Hospital	American Fork	UT
American Imaging Of Southwest Florida	Port Charlotte	FL
American Multispecialty Group Dba Esse Health Excel Imaging	Saint Louis	MO
American Radiology Services At Fleet Street	Baltimore	MD
American Radiology Services At Howard County	Columbia	MD
American Radiology Services At Waldorf	Waldorf	MD
Amery Hospital And Clinic	Amery	WI
Amesbury Health Center	Amesbury	MA
Amg Via Christi On Murdock	Wichita	KS
Amherst Community Health Ctr. Cooley Dickinson Hosp.	Amherst	MA
Amherst Medical Center-Valley Medical Group	Amherst	MA
Amherst Radiology/Breast Screening Center Of Western Ny	Buffalo	NY
Ami - Atlanticare Partners In Imaging	Hammonton	NJ
Ami-Atlanticare	Manahawkin	NJ
Amita Healing Arts Pavilion	New Lenox	IL
Amita Health - Westmont Imaging Center	Westmont	IL
Amita Health Adventist Medical Center, Glenoaks	Glendale Heights	IL
Amita Health Cancer Institute & Outpatient Center	Hinsdale	IL
Amita Health Holy Family Medical Center Des Plaines	Des Plaines	IL
Amita Health Medical Imaging Bourbonnais	Bourbonnais	IL
Amita Health Saints Mary And Elizabeth Medical Center	Chicago	IL
Amita Health St. Joseph Hospital Elgin	Elgin	IL

Alphabetical Index

Name	City	State
Amita Health Willowbrook Mammography Center	Willowbrook	IL
Amita Healthcare Woodridge Ambulatory Center	Woodridge	IL
Amita Plainfield Healing Arts Pavilion	Plainfield	IL
Amita St. Joseph Medical Center	Joliet	IL
Anchorage Native Primary Care Clinic	Anchorage	AK
Anchorage Neighborhood Health Center	Anchorage	AK
Andalusia Health	Andalusia	AL
Anderson County Hospital	Garnett	KS
Anderson Diagnostic Imaging, Inc.	Anderson	SC
Anderson Regional Breast Center	Meridian	MS
Andrew A. Roth, M.D., S.C.	Lombard	IL
Andrew Shimer, M.D., P.A.	McKinney	TX
Androscoggin Valley Hospital	Berlin	NH
Androscoggin Valley Medical Arts Ctr	Livermore Falls	ME
Angel Medical Center	Franklin	NC
Angel Williamson Imaging Center	Pensacola	FL
Anmed Health Women's & Children Hospital	Anderson	SC
Ann Baroco Center At Pace Of Optimal Imaging	Pace	FL
Ann L. Baroco Center At Optimal Imaging	Pensacola	FL
Anna Hospital Corp Dba Union County Hospital	Anna	IL
Anna Jaques Hospital	Newburyport	MA
Anna Jaques Hospital At Parkway Imaging	Haverhill	MA
Anne Arundel Diagnostic Imaging, Easton	Easton	MD
Anne Arundel Diagnostics	Odenton	MD
Anne Arundel Diagnostics Breast Center	Annapolis	MD
Anne Arundel Diagnostics, Imaging	Chester	MD
Anne Arundel Diagnostics, Inc.	Bowie	MD
Anne C. Pappas Center For Breast Imaging	Providence	RI
Annie Jeffrey Memorial County Health Center	Osceola	NE
Annie Penn Hospital	Reidsville	NC
Anniston Ob-Gyn Associates, P.A.	Anniston	AL
Antelope Memorial Hospital	Neligh	NE
Anthony Breast Center - St Joseph Hospital	Fort Wayne	IN
Antioch Health Center	Antioch	CA
Antioch Medical Imaging	Antioch	CA
Apollo Imaging Management Llc	Elmhurst	NY
Apollo Medical Diagnostic Services Pllc	Jamaica	NY
Appling Healthcare System	Baxley	GA
Appomattox Imaging Center	Colonial Heights	VA
Ara - St. David's Imaging, Lp	Georgetown	TX
Ara/St. David's Imaging, L.P.	Austin	TX
Ara/St. David's Imaging, L.P.	Austin	TX
Ara/St. David's Imaging, L.P.	Round Rock	TX
Arcadia Radiology Imaging	Arcadia	CA
Arcadia Radiology Women's Imaging	Arcadia	CA
Archbold Women's Center	Thomasville	GA
Arh Our Lady Of The Way	Martin	KY
Arizona Breastnet, L.L.C.	Scottsdale	AZ
Arizona Community Physicians- Eastside Imaging Center	Tucson	AZ
Arizona Diagnostic Radiology Group	Tempe	AZ
Arizona Diagnostic Radiology Group, Llc.	Apache Junction	AZ
Arizona Diagnostic Radiology Group, Llc.	Casa Grande	AZ
Arizona Diagnostic Radiology Group, Llc.	Gilbert	AZ
Arizona Diagnostic Radiology Group, Llc.	Maricopa	AZ
Arizona Diagnostic Radiology Group, Llc.	Phoenix	AZ
Arizona Diagnostic Radiology Group, Llc.	Phoenix	AZ
Arkansas Methodist Medical Center	Paragould	AR
Arkansas Valley Regional Medical Center	La Junta	CO
Arlene M. Weinshelbaum, M.D. P.A.	Gainesville	FL
Arlington Heights Health Center	Arlington Heights	IL
Armstrong County Memorial Hospital	Kittanning	PA
Armstrong Out Patient Imaging Center	Kittanning	PA
Arnot Health - Corning Medical Office Building	Corning	NY
Arnot Ogden Med. Ctr. - Horseheads Medical Office Bldg.	Horseheads	NY
Arnot Ogden Medical Center - Health Center For Women	Elmira	NY
Arraiza Radiology Psc Dba Arecibo Radiology	Arecibo	PR
Arrowhead McKee Family Health Center	San Bernardino	CA
Arrowhead Regional Medical Center	Colton	CA
Arroyo Vista Family Health Center	Los Angeles	CA
Ars An Affiliate Of Maryland Imaging Network	Prince Frederick	MD
Artesia General Hospital	Artesia	NM
Asante Ashland Community Hospital, Llc	Ashland	OR
Asante Imaging	Medford	OR
Asante Women's Imaging		
Asante Three Rivers Medical Ctr. Llc	Grants Pass	OR
Ascension - Macomb Breast Center	Warren	MI
Ascension All Saints Healthcare-Women's Imaging-Spring Stre	Racine	WI
Ascension Allegan Hospital	Allegan	MI
Ascension Borgess At Woodbridge Hills	Portage	MI
Ascension Borgess Hospital Breast Imaging Center	Kalamazoo	MI
Ascension Borgess Westside Radiology	Kalamazoo	MI
Ascension Borgess, Promed Physicians Three Rivers	Three Rivers	MI
Ascension Borgess-Lee Hospital	Dowagiac	MI
Ascension Calumet Hospital	Chilton	WI
Ascension Eagle River Hospital	Eagle River	WI
Ascension Elmbrook Pavlic Ctr	Brookfield	WI
Ascension Genesys Ambulatory Imaging	Burton	MI
Ascension Genesys Ambulatory Imaging	Clio	MI
Ascension Genesys Ambulatory Imaging	Grand Blanc	MI
Ascension Good Samaritan Hospital	Merrill	WI
Ascension Livingston Ambulatory Medical Center	Howell	MI
Ascension Medical Center Livonia	Livonia	MI
Ascension Medical Group Part Of St. Michael's Hospital	Stevens Point	WI
Ascension Medical Group St. Vincent - Brownsburg Imaging	Brownsburg	IN
Ascension Medical Group St. Vincent - Crawfordsville Imaging	Crawfordsville	IN
Ascension Medical Group St. Vincent - Plainfield Imaging	Plainfield	IN
Ascension Medical Group St. Vincent Frankfort	Frankfort	IN
Ascension Medical Group-Founders Circle	Wichita	KS
Ascension Medical Group-Westwood	Wausau	WI
Ascension Our Lady Of Victory Hospital	Stanley	WI
Ascension Providence	Waco	TX
Ascension Providence Farmington Hills	Farmington Hills	MI
Ascension Providence Hospital - Novi Campus	Novi	MI
Ascension Providence Hospital Imaging At S. Washington	Oxford	MI
Ascension Providence Hospital Southfield Campus	Southfield	MI
Ascension Providence Rochester Barclay Imaging Center	Rochester Hills	MI
Ascension Providence Rochester Center For Breast Health	Auburn Hills	MI
Ascension Providence Rochester Hospital	Rochester	MI
Ascension River District Hospital	East China	MI
Ascension Sacred Heart Emerald Coast	Santa Rosa Beach	FL
Ascension Sacred Heart Hospital	Tomahawk	WI
Ascension Se Hospital-St. Joseph	Milwaukee	WI
Ascension Se Wisconsin At Brown Deer	Brown Deer	WI
Ascension Se Wisconsin-Franklin	Franklin	WI
Ascension Seton	Austin	TX
Ascension Seton	Bastrop	TX
Ascension Seton	Kyle	TX
Ascension Seton	Luling	TX
Ascension Seton	Marble Falls	TX
Ascension Seton	Smithville	TX
Ascension St John Outpatient Radiology	Tulsa	OK
Ascension St John Sapulpa	Sapulpa	OK
Ascension St Vincent Carmel Breast Center	Carmel	IN
Ascension St Vincent Fishers Breast Center	Fishers	IN
Ascension St Vincent Indianapolis Breast Center And Mobile	Indianapolis	IN
Ascension St. Elizabeth Hospital	Appleton	WI
Ascension St. John Hospital Health Center At 12 Mile	St Clair Shores	MI
Ascension St. John Hospital Health Center At 23 Mile	Macomb Township	MI
Ascension St. John Hospital Health Center At Kercheval	Grosse Pointe	MI
Ascension St. John Hospital, Liggett Breast Center	Grosse Pointe Woods	MI
Ascension St. Joseph Hospital	Tawas City	MI
Ascension St. Mary's Hospital	Rhinelander	WI
Ascension St. Mary's Of Michigan Bay City	Bay City	MI

Name	City	State
Ascension St. Mary's Of Michigan Towne Centre	Saginaw	MI
Ascension St. Michael's Hospital At Hoover	Stevens Point	WI
Ascension St. Michael's Hospital At Plover	Plover	WI
Ascension St. Vincent Anderson Women's Center	Anderson	IN
Ascension St. Vincent Clay	Brazil	IN
Ascension St. Vincent Evansville Breast Center	Newburgh	IN
Ascension St. Vincent Jennings	North Vernon	IN
Ascension St. Vincent Mercy	Elwood	IN
Ascension St. Vincent Randolph	Winchester	IN
Ascension St. Vincent Salem	Salem	IN
Ascension St. Vincent Westside Crossing	Evansville	IN
Ascension St. Vincent Williamsport	Williamsport	IN
Ascension St. Vincent Women's Center Kokomo	Kokomo	IN
Ascension St. Vincent's Clay County	Middleburg	FL
Ascension St. Vincent's Mobile Mammography	Jacksonville	FL
Ascension St. Vincent's Riverside	Jacksonville	FL
Ascension St. Vincent's Southside	Jacksonville	FL
Ascension St.John Jane Phillips	Bartlesville	OK
Ascension St.John Jane Phillips Imaging Center	Bartlesville	OK
Ascension St.Vincent Dunn	Bedford	IN
Ascension St.Vincent Evansville Breast Center - Mobile	Newburgh	IN
Ascension Via Christi Hospital Pittsburg, Inc.	Pittsburg	KS
Ascension Via Christi Imaging L.L.C.	Wichita	KS
Ascension Via Christi Imaging Wichita, Llc	Wichita	KS
Ascension Via Christi St Joseph	Wichita	KS
Ascension- Wauwatosa	Wauwatosa	WI
Ascension-St Francis-Women's Imaging	Milwaukee	WI
Ascension-Standish Hospital	Standish	MI
Ascesnion Borgess-Pipp Hospital	Plainwell	MI
Ashe Memorial Hospital	Jefferson	NC
Asheville Women's Diagnostic Center	Asheville	NC
Ashford Presbyterian Community Hospital	San Juan	PR
Ashley County Medical Center	Crossett	AR
Ashley Medical Center	Ashley	ND
Ashley Regional Medical Center	Vernal	UT
Ashtabula County Medical Center	Ashtabula	OH
Aspen Mountain Medical Center	Rock Springs	WY
Aspen Valley Hospital	Aspen	CO
Aspirus Doctors Clinic	Wisconsin Rapids	WI
Aspirus Houghton Clinic	Houghton	MI
Aspirus Iron River Hospital And Clinics	Iron River	MI
Aspirus Ironwood Hospital	Ironwood	MI
Aspirus Keweenaw Hospital	Laurium	MI
Aspirus Langlade Hospital	Antigo	WI
Aspirus Medford Hospital	Medford	WI
Aspirus Ontonagon Hospital	Ontonagon	MI
Aspirus Riverview Hospital And Clinics	Wisconsin Rapids	WI
Aspirus Stevens Point Clinic	Stevens Point	WI
Aspirus Wausau Hospital	Wausau	WI
Aspirus Weston Clinic	Weston	WI
Associated Clinicians Of East Texas, Pllc Dba: Dcol	Longview	TX
Associated Physicians, L.L.P.	Madison	WI
Associates For Womens Medicine	North Syracuse	NY
Associates In Women's Health	Baton Rouge	LA
Associates In Women's Healthcare, Pa	Raleigh	NC
Association Of Alexandria Radiologists Alexandria Va	Alexandria	VA
Association Of Alexandria Radiologists Woodbridge Va	Woodbridge	VA
Assured Imaging Womens Wellness Of Washington Llc - Mobile	Tukwila	WA
Assured Imaging Women's Wellness Of Southern Arizona, Llc	Tucson	AZ
Assured Imaging Women's Wellness Of Southern Arizona, Llc	Clovis	NM
Assured Imaging Women's Wellness Of Southern Arizona, Llc	Las Cruces	NM
Assured Imaging Women's Wellness Of Southern Arizona, Llc	Los Lunas	NM
Assured Imaging Women's Wellness Of Southern Arizona- Mobile	Ft Worth	TX
Assured Imaging Women's Wellness Of Southern Az Llc-Mobile	Tucson	AZ
Assured Imaging Women's Wellness Of Southern Az, Llc	Scottsdale	AZ
Assured Imaging Womens Wellness Of California Inc - Mobile	Tucson	AZ
Astria Sunnyside Hospital	Sunnyside	WA
Astria Toppenish Hospital	Toppenish	WA
Atchison Hospital	Atchison	KS
Athens Hospital, Llc	Athens	TX
Athens Hospital, Llc	Gun Barrel City	TX
Athens Limestone Hospital	Athens	AL
Athens Ob-Gyn L.L.C.	Athens	GA
Athens-Limestone Hospital Limestone Medical Village	Athens	AL
Athol Memorial Hospital	Athol	MA
Atlanta Women's Healthcare Specialists	Atlanta	GA
Atlantic General Hospital	Berlin	MD
Atlantic General Women's Imaging	Ocean City	MD
Atlantic Imaging Services At Clark	Clark	NJ
Atlantic Medical Center	Barceloneta	PR
Atlantic Medical Imaging	Bridgeton	NJ
Atlantic Medical Imaging	Cape May Court House	NJ
Atlantic Medical Imaging	Egg Harbor Township	NJ
Atlantic Medical Imaging	Galloway	NJ
Atlantic Medical Imaging	Manasquan	NJ
Atlantic Medical Imaging	Old Bridge	NJ
Atlantic Medical Imaging	Toms River	NJ
Atlantic Medical Imaging	Vineland	NJ
Atlantic Medical Imaging Llc	Somers Point	NJ
Atlantic Medical Imaging Toms River Women's Center	Toms River	NJ
Atlantic Medical Imaging Women's Imaging Center	Brick	NJ
Atlanticare Regional Medical Center - City Division	Atlantic City	NJ
Atlanticare Regional Medical Center - Mainland Div	Pomona	NJ
Atmore Community Hospital	Atmore	AL
Atrium Diagnostic Imaging	Manalapan	NJ
Atrium Health - Cleveland Imaging	Shelby	NC
Atrium Health Anson	Wadesboro	NC
Atrium Health Lincoln	Lincolnton	NC
Atrium Health Lincoln Imaging Denver	Denver	NC
Atrium Health Stanly- The Breast Center	Albemarle	NC
Atrium Health-Cabarrus Breast Health Center	Concord	NC
Atrium Health-Cabarrus Outreach Health Services-Mobile	Concord	NC
Atrium Medical Center	Middletown	OH
Atrium Ob/Gyn Inc.	Canton	OH
Atriumhealth Kings Mtn, A Facility Of Atriumhealth Cleveland	Kings Mountain	NC
Atrius Health	Chelmsford	MA
Atrius Health	Somerville	MA
Atrius Health, Inc - Imaging Dept	Weymouth	MA
Au Health Imaging	Augusta	GA
Au Medical Center, Inc.	Augusta	GA
Auburn Community Hospital	Auburn	NY
Auburn Diagnostic Imaging	Auburn	AL
Audrain Community Hospital	Mexico	MO
Audubon County Memorial Hospital	Audubon	IA
Augusta Health	Fishersville	VA
Augusta Health Outpatient Center	Staunton	VA
Augusta Health Stuarts Draft Outpatient Center	Stuarts Draft	VA
Aultman Carrollton Facility	Carrollton	OH
Aultman Hospital	Canton	OH
Aultman Massillon Stark County Facility	Massillon	OH
Aultman North Stark County Facility	North Canton	OH
Aultman Orrville Hospital	Orrville	OH
Aurora Advocate Hartford Clinic	Hartford	WI
Aurora Bay Care Health Center	Green Bay	WI
Aurora Baycare Health Center-Kaukauna	Kaukauna	WI
Aurora Baycare Medical Center	Green Bay	WI
Aurora Health Care	Sturgeon Bay	WI
Aurora Health Care - Germantown	Germantown	WI
Aurora Health Care West Bend Valley Avenue	West Bend	WI
Aurora Health Center - 84south	Milwaukee	WI
Aurora Health Center - Brookfield	Brookfield	WI
Aurora Health Center - Cedar Creek	Grafton	WI
Aurora Health Center - Depere	De Pere	WI
Aurora Health Center - East Mequon	Mequon	WI
Aurora Health Center - Fdl	Fond Du Lac	WI
Aurora Health Center - Good Hope	Milwaukee	WI
Aurora Health Center - Mayfair North	Wauwatosa	WI
Aurora Health Center - Menomonee Falls	Menomonee Falls	WI
Aurora Health Center Manitowoc County	Two Rivers	WI
Aurora Health Center Pleasant Prairie	Pleasant Prairie	WI
Aurora Health Center Southern Lakes	Burlington	WI
Aurora Health Center Waukesha	Waukesha	WI
Aurora Health Center Wautoma	Wautoma	WI
Aurora Health Center-Franklin W Oakwood Park Ct	Franklin	WI
Aurora Health Center-Franklin-Loomis Rd	Franklin	WI

Name	City	State
Aurora Health Center-New Berlin- W National Ave	New Berlin	WI
Aurora Health Center-St Francis-Layton Ave	St Francis	WI
Aurora Medical Center	Oshkosh	WI
Aurora Medical Center - Grafton	Grafton	WI
Aurora Medical Center -Bay Area	Marinette	WI
Aurora Medical Center Summit	Summit	WI
Aurora Medical Group, Inc. - Neenah	Neenah	WI
Aurora Medical Group-Rivercenter	Milwaukee	WI
Aurora Sheboygan Clinic	Plymouth	WI
Aurora Sheboygan Clinic	Sheboygan	WI
Aurora Sinai Medical Center Of Aurora Health Care Metro Inc.	Milwaukee	WI
Aurora St. Luke's Medical Center Breast Imaging Center	Milwaukee	WI
Aurora St. Luke's South Shore	Cudahy	WI
Aurora West Allis Medical Center	West Allis	WI
Austin Area Breast Imaging Llc	Austin	TX
Austin Breast Imaging, Llc	Austin	TX
Austin Breast Imaging, Llc	Austin	TX
Austin Radiological Association	Austin	TX
Austin Radiological Association	Austin	TX
Austin Radiological Association	Austin	TX
Austin Radiological Association	Austin	TX
Austin Radiological Association	Austin	TX
Austin Radiological Association	Cedar Park	TX
Austin Radiological Association	Dripping Springs	TX
Austin Radiological Association	Kyle	TX
Austin Radiological Association	Manor	TX
Austin Radiological Association	San Marcos	TX
Austin Regional Clinic, Pa	Austin	TX
Austin Regional Clinic, Pa	Austin	TX
Aventura Breast Diagnostic Center	Aventura	FL
Avera Breast Center	Aberdeen	SD
Avera Breast Center	Sioux Falls	SD
Avera Breast Center - Mitchell	Mitchell	SD
Avera Breast Center - Mobile	Sioux Falls	SD
Avera Breast Center West	Sioux Falls	SD
Avera Creighton Hospital	Creighton	NE
Avera Dells Area Hospital	Dell Rapids	SD
Avera Granite Falls	Granite Falls	MN
Avera Gregory Hospital	Gregory	SD
Avera Holy Family	Estherville	IA
Avera Marshall Regional Medical Center	Marshall	MN
Avera Medical Group Brookings	Brookings	SD
Avera Medical Group McGreevy 69th And Western	Sioux Falls	SD
Avera Medical Group McGreevy 69th And Cliff	Sioux Falls	SD
Avera Medical Group McGreevy 7th Avenue	Sioux Falls	SD
Avera Medical Group Windom	Windom	MN
Avera Medical Group Worthington	Worthington	MN
Avera Merrill Pioneer Hospital	Rock Rapids	IA
Avera Sacred Heart Hospital	Yankton	SD
Avera St Anthony's Hospital	Oneill	NE
Avera St. Benedict	Parkston	SD
Avera St. Mary's Hospital	Pierre	SD
Avery Center Ob-Gyn	Westport	CT
Avestee Women's Imaging Center Of Alamo Heights	San Antonio	TX
Avestee Women's Imaging Center Of Boerne	Boerne	TX
Avestee Women's Imaging Center Of Westover Hills	San Antonio	TX
Avh Outpatient Care Center-New Kensington	New Kensington	PA
Avina Womens Care	Westerville	OH
Avina Womens Care- Dublin	Dublin	OH
Avita Bucyrus Hospital	Bucyrus	OH
Avita Ontario	Ontario	OH
Avon Comprehensive Breast Center Mgh	Boston	MA
Avon Foundation Breast Imaging Center	New York	NY
Avoyelles Hospital	Marksville	LA
B & G Diagnostic Services	Hialeah	FL
Baaxten, Llc	Brownsville	TX
Baaxten, Llc	Harlingen	TX
Backus Outpatient Care Center	Norwich	CT
Bacon County Hospital	Alma	GA
Bailey Medical Center	Owasso	OK
Ballad Health	Rogersville	TN
Ballad Health Coach - Mobile	Kingsport	TN
Ballad Health Dba Sycamore Shoals Hospital	Elizabethton	TN
Ballad Health Lonesome Pine Hospital	Big Stone Gap	VA
Ballinger Memorial Hospital District	Ballinger	TX
Banner Baywood Medical Center - Women's Services	Mesa	AZ
Banner Churchill Community Hospital	Fallon	NV
Banner Del E Webb Women's Diagnostic Services	Sun City West	AZ
Banner Fort Collins Medical Center	Fort Collins	CO
Banner Health Center-Maricopa	Maricopa	AZ
Banner Imaging Baywood Breast Center	Mesa	AZ
Banner Imaging Chandler	Chandler	AZ
Banner Imaging Dobson Breast Center	Mesa	AZ
Banner Imaging Gilbert	Gilbert	AZ
Banner Imaging Management Serviced Llc, Estrella Breast	Phoenix	AZ
Banner Imaging Management Services Llc, Camino Del Sol	Sun City West	AZ
Banner Imaging Management Services Llc, Arrowhead Commons	Glendale	AZ
Banner Imaging Management Services Llc, New River Trails	Glendale	AZ
Banner Imaging Management Services Llc, Paradise Valley	Phoenix	AZ
Banner Imaging Management Services Llc, Peoria	Peoria	AZ
Banner Imaging Management Services Llc, Sunwest Breast	Glendale	AZ
Banner Imaging Management Services Llc, Union Hills	Phoenix	AZ
Banner Imaging Services Colorado	Greeley	CO
Banner Imaging Services Colorado	Loveland	CO
Banner Imaging Tempe	Tempe	AZ
Banner Imaging, Casa Grande	Casa Grande	AZ
Banner Lassen Medical Center	Susanville	CA
Banner M.D. Anderson Cancer Center	Gilbert	AZ
Banner Payson Medical Center	Payson	AZ
Banner University Medicine - Advanced Breast Imaging	Tucson	AZ
Baptist Beaumont Hospital	Orange	TX
Baptist Breast Center	San Antonio	TX
Baptist Breast Center At Westover Hills	San Antonio	TX
Baptist Breast Center Downtown	San Antonio	TX
Baptist Breast Health Center	Montgomery	AL
Baptist Collierville	Collierville	TN
Baptist Crestwood	Crestwood	KY
Baptist Diagnostic Ctr At West Kendall Hosp	Miami	FL
Baptist Diagnostic Imaging At Clay	Fleming Island	FL
Baptist Health	Bardstown	KY
Baptist Health Breast Center	Little Rock	AR
Baptist Health Breast Center North Little Rock	North Little Rock	AR
Baptist Health Corbin	Corbin	KY
Baptist Health Diagnostic Imaging At Plantation	Plantation	FL
Baptist Health Diagnostics At Brandenburg	Brandenburg	KY
Baptist Health Eastpoint Diagnostic Center	Louisville	KY
Baptist Health Floyd	New Albany	IN
Baptist Health Hardin Diagnostic Main Campus	Elizabethtown	KY
Baptist Health Hardin Elizabethtown	Elizabethtown	KY
Baptist Health Imaging	Corydon	IN
Baptist Health Imaging Center - Saline County	Benton	AR
Baptist Health Lagrange	Lagrange	KY
Baptist Health Lexington Breast Imag. Services At Georgetown	Georgetown	KY
Baptist Health Lexington Breast Imaging Services	Lexington	KY
Baptist Health Lexington Breast Imaging Services Hamburg	Lexington	KY
Baptist Health Lexington Breast Imaging Services At Beaumont	Lexington	KY
Baptist Health Lexington Breast Imaging Services At Richmond	Richmond	KY
Baptist Health Louisville	Louisville	KY
Baptist Health Medical Center Hot Spring County	Malvern	AR
Baptist Health Medical Center-Arkadelphia	Arkadelphia	AR
Baptist Health Medical Center-Conway	Conway	AR
Baptist Health Medical Center-Stuttgart	Stuttgart	AR
Baptist Health Medical Group - Medeast	Louisville	KY
Baptist Health Medical Group Louisville Ob/Gyn	Louisville	KY
Baptist Health Medical Group/Partners In Womens Health	Louisville	KY
Baptist Health Middletown Diagnostic Imaging Center	Louisville	KY
Baptist Health Paducah - Baptist Imaging Ctr	Paducah	KY
Baptist Health Richmond	Richmond	KY
Baptist Health Services-Women's Imaging	Fort Smith	AR
Baptist Health Women's Care	Madisonville	KY
Baptist Healthcare Of Ok Dba Integris Bass Baptist Hlth Ctr	Enid	OK
Baptist Healthplace At Nocatee	Ponte Vedra Beach	FL
Baptist Hlth Lexington Breast Img Services Brannon Crossing	Nicholasville	KY
Baptist Hospital Women's Imaging	Pensacola	FL
Baptist Hospitals Of Southeast Texas	Beaumont	TX

Name	City	State
Baptist Hospitals Of Southeast Texas	Beaumont	TX
Baptist Imaging Hoover	Hoover	AL
Baptist M & S Imaging - Mission Trail	San Antonio	TX
Baptist M&S Imaging - Legacy Oaks	San Antonio	TX
Baptist M&S Imaging New Braunfels	New Braunfels	TX
Baptist M&S Imaging Schertz	Schertz	TX
Baptist Mammography Center In Macy's, The Falls	Miami	FL
Baptist Medical Center - Beaches	Jacksonville Beach	FL
Baptist Medical Center - Yazoo, Inc.	Yazoo City	MS
Baptist Medical Center Attala	Kosciusko	MS
Baptist Medical Center Heber Springs	Heber Springs	AR
Baptist Medical Center Nassau	Fernandina Beach	FL
Baptist Medical Center South	Jacksonville	FL
Baptist Medical Hub At Miami Beach	Miami Beach	FL
Baptist Medical Park Navarre-Diagnostic Center	Navarre	FL
Baptist Medical Plaza At Brickell	Miami	FL
Baptist Medical Plaza At Coral Gables	Coral Gables	FL
Baptist Medical Plaza At Coral Springs	Coral Springs	FL
Baptist Medical Plaza At Doral	Miami	FL
Baptist Medical Plaza At Palmetto Bay	Miami	FL
Baptist Medical Plaza At Pembroke Pines	Pembroke Pines	FL
Baptist Medical Plaza At Tamiami Trail	Miami	FL
Baptist Medical Plaza At Westchester	Miami	FL
Baptist Memorial Hospital - Booneville	Booneville	MS
Baptist Memorial Hospital - Carroll County	Huntingdon	TN
Baptist Memorial Hospital - Desoto Womens Center	Southaven	MS
Baptist Memorial Hospital - North Mississippi	Oxford	MS
Baptist Memorial Hospital - Tipton	Covington	TN
Baptist Memorial Hospital - Union City	Union City	TN
Baptist Memorial Hospital - Union County	New Albany	MS
Baptist Memorial Hospital Carroll County, OP Diagnostic Cent	Mc Kenzie	TN
Baptist Memorial Hospital Crittenden	West Memphis	AR
Baptist Memorial Hospital For Women - Mobile	Memphis	TN
Baptist Memorial Hospital-Golden Triangle	Columbus	MS
Baptist Memorial Leake	Carthage	MS
Baptist North Medical Campus	Jacksonville	FL
Baptist Outpatient Center	Miami	FL
Baptist Outpatient Services, Inc. Med. Plaza At Miami Lakes	Miami Lakes	FL
Baptist Womens Health Center	Memphis	TN
Baraga County Memorial Hospital	Lanse	MI
Barbara Brodsky Comprehensive Breast Ctr At Bryn Mawr Hosp.	Bryn Mawr	PA
Barbara Edelstein, MD Women's Radiology, Pc	New York	NY
Barbara Kort Women's Imaging Ctr. At Ucla Santa Monica	Santa Monica	CA
Barbara L. Moersch, M.D. - Obgyn	Anniston	AL
Barbourville Arh	Barbourville	KY
Barnabas Health Ambulatory Care Center	Livingston	NJ
Barnes - Jewish Hospital	Saint Louis	MO
Barnes Jewish Hospital, Center For Advanced Medicine-South	Saint Louis	MO
Barnes-Jewish Hospital At Highlands Plaza 3	Saint Louis	MO
Barnes-Jewish St. Peter's Hospital	St Peters	MO
Barnes-Jewish West County Hospital	Saint Louis	MO
Barnesville Hospital	Barnesville	OH
Barranquitas Ultrasound And Mammography Center	Barranquitas	PR
Barrett Hospital & Healthcare	Dillon	MT
Barrington Radiologic Services	Indianapolis	IN
Barstow Community Hospital	Barstow	CA
Bartlett Regional Hospital	Juneau	AK
Barton Memorial Hospital	South Lake Tahoe	CA
Basha Diagnostics, P.C.	Dearborn	MI
Basha Diagnostics, P.C.	Royal Oak	MI
Basha Diagnostics, P.C.	Sterling Heights	MI
Bass Imaging	Walnut Creek	CA
Bassett Army Community Hospital	Ft Wainwright	AK
Bassett Healthcare Network	Cooperstown	NY
Bassett Healthcare Network - Herkimer	Herkimer	NY
Bassett Healthcare Network Little Falls Hospital	Little Falls	NY
Bassett Hospital Of Schoharie County	Cobleskill	NY
Bates County Memorial Hospital	Butler	MO
Bath Community Hospital	Hot Springs	VA
Baton Rouge General Ascension	Prairieville	LA
Baton Rouge General Imaging Center	Baton Rouge	LA
Baton Rouge General Medical Center - Bluebonnet	Baton Rouge	LA
Baton Rouge General Medical Center Mid - City	Baton Rouge	LA
Baxter Regional Medical Center	Mountain Home	AR
Bay Area Healthcare Group, Ltd.	Corpus Christi	TX
Bay Area Hospital	Coos Bay	OR
Bay Area Hospital Women's Imaging Ctr	Coos Bay	OR
Bay Park Community Hospital	Oregon	OH
Bay Radiology Llc	Severna Park	MD
Bay Radiology Women's Imaging Center, Llc	Panama City	FL
Bay Ridge Medical Imaging At Dyker Heights	Brooklyn	NY
Bay Ridge Medical Imaging, Pc	Brooklyn	NY
Bay Ridge Medical Imaging, P.C.	Brooklyn	NY
Bay Valley Medical Group, Inc.	Hayward	CA
Bayamon Medical Center	Bayamon	PR
Bayamon Radiology Llc/ Dba Santa Juanita Radiology	Bayamon	PR
Baycare OP Imaging - Van Dyke	Lutz	FL
Baycare Outpatient Imaging	Largo	FL
Baycare Outpatient Imaging - Big Bend	Riverview	FL
Baycare Outpatient Imaging Bloomingdale	Valrico	FL
Baycare Outpatient Imaging Carillon	St Petersburg	FL
Baycare Outpatient Imaging South Tampa	Tampa	FL
Baycare Outpatient Imaging St. Anthony's	St Petersburg	FL
Baycare Outpatient Imaging Trinity	Trinity	FL
Baycare Outpatient Imaging-Countryside	Safety Harbor	FL
Baycare Outpatient Imaging-Hampton Lakes	Tampa	FL
Bayfront Health Brooksville	Brooksville	FL
Bayfront Health Port Charlotte	Port Charlotte	FL
Bayfront Health Seven Rivers	Crystal River	FL
Bayfront Health Spring Hill	Spring Hill	FL
Bayhealth Hospital - Sussex Campus	Milford	DE
Bayhealth Medical Center, Kent General Hospital	Dover	DE
Bayhealth Outpatient Center - Sussex	Milford	DE
Baylor Medical Center At Irving	Irving	TX
Baylor Medical Center At Irving	Irving	TX
Baylor Medical Center At Waxahachie	Waxahachie	TX
Baylor Medical Centers At Garland And McKinney	McKinney	TX
Baylor Regional Medical Center At Grapevine	Grapevine	TX
Baylor Regional Medical Center At Plano	Plano	TX
Baylor Regional Medical Center At Plano	Richardson	TX
Baylor Scott & White Medical Center - College Station	College Station	TX
Baylor Scott & White Medical Center - Taylor	Taylor	TX
Baylor Scott & White Medical Centers-Capitol Area	Pflugerville	TX
Baylor St. Luke's Medical Center	Houston	TX
Baylor University Medical Center	Dallas	TX
Baylor University Medical Center	Dallas	TX
Bayne-Jones Army Community Hospital	Fort Polk	LA
Bayonne Medical Center	Bayonne	NJ
Bayshore Medical Center Women's Center	Holmdel	NJ
Baystate Breast & Wellness Center	Springfield	MA
Baystate Franklin Medical Center	Greenfield	MA
Baystate Mary Lane Outpatient Center	Ware	MA
Baystate Radiology & Imaging	Longmeadow	MA
Baystate Radiology & Imaging	South Hadley	MA
Baystate Radiology And Imaging - Northampton	Northampton	MA
Baystate Radiology And Imaging, Inc.	Enfield	CT
Bayview Physicians Services,P.C.-Suffolk	Suffolk	VA
Bayview Radiology	Tampa	FL
Bbh -Walker Breast Center	Jasper	AL
Bchc Family Medicine Oelwein	Oelwein	IA
Bear Lake Memorial Hospital	Montpelier	ID
Bear Valley Community Hospital	Big Bear Lake	CA
Bearden Josey Center For Breast Health	Spartanburg	SC
Bearden Josey Center For Breast Health - North Grove	Spartanburg	SC

Alphabetical Index

Alphabetical Index

Alphabetical Index

Name	City	State
Elizabeth Pusey Md, Inc Dba Women's Medical Imaging	Newport Beach	CA
Elizabeth Wende Breast Care	Geneseo	NY
Elizabeth Wende Breast Care	Webster	NY
Elizabeth Wende Breast Care Llc	Rochester	NY
Elizabeth Wende Breast Care Llc	Victor	NY
Elizabeth Wende Breast Care, L.L.C.	Batavia	NY
Elizabeth Wende Breast Care, L.L.C.	Carthage	NY
Elizabeth Wende Breast Care, Lcc	Rochester	NY
Elkhart General Hospital	Elkhart	IN
Elkview General Hospital	Hobart	OK
Ellenville Regional Hospital	Ellenville	NY
Elliot Breast Imaging Center At River's Edge	Manchester	NH
Elliot Imaging Center At Londonderry	Londonderry	NH
Elliott Breast Clinic	Baton Rouge	LA
Ellis Fischel Cancer Center	Columbia	MO
Ellis Medicine Bellevue Women's Center	Niskayuna	NY
Ellis Medicine McClellan Street Health Center	Schenectady	NY
Ellsworth Municipal Hospital Dba Hansen Family Hospital	Iowa Falls	IA
Elmendorf Air Force Base, 673d Medical Group	Jber	AK
Elmhurst Hospital Center	Elmhurst	NY
Elmhurst Memorial Addison Center For Health	Addison	IL
Elmhurst Memorial Center For Health	Elmhurst	IL
Elmhurst Memorial Lombard Health Care	Lombard	IL
Elmore Community Hospital	Wetumpka	AL
Ely Bloomenson Community Hospital	Ely	MN
Emanate Health -Foothill Presbyterian Hospital	Glendora	CA
Emanate Health Inter-Community Hospital	Covina	CA
Emanate Health Medical Group	Glendora	CA
Emanuel Medical Center	Swainsboro	GA
Emanuel Outpatient Diagnostic Center	Portland	OR
Emerald Coast Obgyn Of The Panhandle	Panama City	FL
Emerson Hospital Health Center-Westford	Westford	MA
Emery Medical Solutions, Inc.	Apopka	FL
Emory Clark-Holder Clinic	Lagrange	GA
Emory Decatur Hospital	Decatur	GA
Emory Hillandale Hospital	Lithonia	GA
Emory Johns Creek Hospital	Johns Creek	GA
Emory University Hospital - Midtown	Atlanta	GA
Emory University Hospital Breast Imaging Center	Atlanta	GA
Emusc, Llc	Glendale	NY
Encircle Health	Appleton	WI
Encompass Medical Group - Hickman Mills	Grandview	MO
Encompass Medical Group - Premier Imaging	Kansas City	MO
Encompass Medical Group - Premier Imaging - Independence	Independence	MO
Encompass Medical Group - Premier Imaging Lenexa	Lenexa	KS
Encompass Medical Group Lee's Summit Clinic	Lees Summit	MO
Encompass Medical Group-Premier Imaging Englewood	Gladstone	MO
Endless Mountains Health System	Montrose	PA
Englewood Hospital Imaging At Fair Lawn	Fair Lawn	NJ
Envision Diagnostic Center Pllc	Novi	MI
Envision Imaging At Pennsylvania	Fort Worth	TX
Envision Imaging At Southlake	Southlake	TX
Envision Imaging Of Dallas	Dallas	TX
Envision Imaging Of Frisco	Frisco	TX
Envision Imaging Of North Arlington	Arlington	TX
Envision Imaging Of South Arlington	Arlington	TX
Ephraim McDowell Diagnostic Center	Danville	KY
Ephraim McDowell James B. Haggin Hospital	Harrodsburg	KY
Ephrata Community Hospital	Ephrata	PA
Epic Imaging P.C.	Clackamas	OR
Epic Imaging, P.C.	Beaverton	OR
Epic Imaging, P.C.	Portland	OR
Epic Imaging, P.C. Bethany	Beaverton	OR
Epic Primary Care	Southfield	MI
Erlanger Bledsoe Hospital	Pikeville	TN
Erlanger East Breast Center	Chattanooga	TN
Erlanger Imaging Mammography Center	Chattanooga	TN
Erlanger Murphy Medical Center	Murphy	NC
Erlanger North Breast Center	Chattanooga	TN
Escorial Mri & Ct Imaging Center	Carolina	PR
Espanola Hospital - Radiology Department	Espanola	NM
Essentia Health	Fargo	ND
Essentia Health	Wahpeton	ND
Essentia Health Ashland Clinic	Ashland	WI
Essentia Health Duluth Clinic	Duluth	MN
Essentia Health Hermantown Breast Ctr	Hermantown	MN
Essentia Health Hibbing Clinic	Hibbing	MN
Essentia Health Holy Trinity Hospital	Graceville	MN
Essentia Health International Falls Clinic	International Falls	MN
Essentia Health Sandstone	Sandstone	MN
Essentia Health St Joseph's Baxter Clinic	Baxter	MN
Essentia Health St. Joseph's Medical Center	Brainerd	MN
Essentia Health St. Mary's Detroit Lakes	Detroit Lakes	MN
Essentia Health St. Mary's Hospital Superior	Superior	WI
Essentia Health Virginia, Llc	Virginia	MN
Essentia Health West Duluth Clinic	Duluth	MN
Essentia Health-Deer River	Deer River	MN
Essentia Health-Grand Rapids Clinic	Grand Rapids	MN
Essentia Health-Moose Lake	Moose Lake	MN
Estes Park Health	Estes Park	CO
Evans Memorial Hospital	Claxton	GA
Evans U.S. Army Community Hospital	Fort Carson	CO
Evanston Regional Hospital	Evanston	WY
Evergreen Breast Center	Kirkland	WA
Evergreen Breast Center-Kenmore	Kenmore	WA
Evergreen Health Monroe Breast Program	Monroe	WA
Evergreen Medical Center	Evergreen	AL
Excel Imaging Center	Garden Grove	CA
Excel Medical Imaging	New Port Richey	FL
Excela Health Frick Hospital	Mount Pleasant	PA
Excela Health Westmoreland Hospital	Greensburg	PA
Excela Square At Latrobe	Latrobe	PA
Excela Square At Norwin	North Huntingdon	PA
Excelsior Integrated Medical Group, Pllc	Brooklyn	NY
Excelsior Springs Hospital	Excelsior Springs	MO
Executive Health Exams	New York	NY
Executive Imaging, Llc	Marion	OH
Executive Medical Services/Greenwich, Pc	New York	NY
Exeter Hospital	Exeter	NH
Exeter Hospital	Plaistow	NH
Express Medical Imaging	Palatka	FL
F&Mcw Community Memorial Hospital	Menomonee Falls	WI
Facey Medical Foundation Mission Hills	Mission Hills	CA
Facey Medical Foundation-Valencia Specialty	Valencia	CA
Facey Medical Foundation: Northridge-Corbin	Northridge	CA
Facey Medical Group Canyon Country	Santa Clarita	CA
Fair Lawn Imaging	Fair Lawn	NJ
Fair Oaks Imaging Center	Fairfax	VA
Fairbanks Memorial Hospital	Fairbanks	AK
Fairchild Medical Center	Yreka	CA
Fairfax Health Center	Fairfax	VA
Fairfield Hospital District	Fairfield	TX
Fairfield Medical Center - River Valley	Lancaster	OH
Fairfield Memorial Hospital	Fairfield	IL
Fairmont Clinic Gateway Uha	Fairmont	WV
Fairview Breast Health Center	Cleveland	OH
Fairview Center For Women-Edina	Edina	MN
Fairview Clinics-Bloomington Oxboro	Bloomington	MN
Fairview Clinics-Eagan	Eagan	MN
Fairview Fridley Clinic	Fridley	MN
Fairview Fridley Clinic - Mobile	Brooklyn Park	MN
Fairview Hospital	Great Barrington	MA
Fairview Hospital Westlake Ptc-Women's Radiology Services	Westlake	OH
Fairview Oxboro Clinic - Mobile	Apple Valley	MN
Faith Regional Health Services	Norfolk	NE
Faith Regional Health Services South	Norfolk	NE
Fajardo Imaging Inc.	Fajardo	PR
Fallon Medical Complex	Baker	MT
Falmouth Hospital - Seifer Imaging Center	Falmouth	MA
Family Health Center Of Worcester, Inc.	Worcester	MA
Family Medcenters Diagnostics	Derby	KS
Family Medical Center Of Hastings	Hastings	NE
Family Medicine Of White Hall	White Hall	AR
Fannin County Hospital Authority Dba Tmc Bonham Hopsital	Bonham	TX
Fannin Regional Hospital	Blue Ridge	GA
Farmbrook Radiology	Southfield	MI
Farmington Health Center	Farmington	UT
Fauquier Hospital	Warrenton	VA
Fawcett Memorial Hospital	Port Charlotte	FL
Fayette County Hospital	Vandalia	IL
Fayette Medical Center	Fayette	AL
Federal Bureau Of Prisons Fci Dublin-Hsa	Dublin	CA
Federal Medical Center Carswell	Fort Worth	TX
Fenway Health	Boston	MA

Name	City	State
Fern Feldman Anolick Center For Breast Health	Kingston	NY
Ferrell Hospital	Eldorado	IL
Fhn Memorial Hospital	Freeport	IL
Fhp Health Center	Tamuning	GU
Field Health System	Centreville	MS
Fillmore Community Hospital	Fillmore	UT
Fillmore County Hospital	Geneva	NE
Finger Lakes Breast Care	Clifton Springs	NY
Finley Hospital	Dubuque	IA
Firelands Regional Medical Center The Center For Breast Care	Sandusky	OH
First Care Medical Services Dba Essentia Health-Fosston	Fosston	MN
First Health Montgomery Memorial Hospital	Troy	NC
First Health Richmond Memorial Hospital	Rockingham	NC
First Medical Care	Decatur	GA
Firsthealth Imaging Lee	Sanford	NC
Firsthealth Moore Regional Hospital-Hoke Campus	Raeford	NC
Firsthealth Of The Carolinas - Moore Regional Hospital	Pinehurst	NC
Fisher-Titus Medical Center	Norwalk	OH
Fishermen's Community Hospital	Marathon	FL
Fitzgibbon Hospital	Marshall	MO
Fiu Herbert Wertheim College Of Medicine	Miami	FL
56th Medical Group/Sgss, Luke Afb	Luke Afb	AZ
Flaget Memorial Hospital	Bardstown	KY
Flagler Health Plus Imaging	Ponte Vedra	FL
Flagler Health Plus Imaging	Saint Augustine	FL
Flagler Health Plus Imaging	St Augustine	FL
Fleming County Hospital	Flemingsburg	KY
Florida Diagnostic Imaging	Palm Bay	FL
Florida Hospital Wesley Chapel	Wesley Chapel	FL
Florida Medical Center A Campus Of North Shore	Ft Lauderdale	FL
Florida Medical Clinic	Wesley Chapel	FL
Florida Medical Clinic	Zephyrhills	FL
Flower Mound Hospital Partners, Llc	Flower Mound	TX
Flowers Hospital Breast Health Center	Dothan	AL
Floyd County Medical Center	Charles City	IA
Floyd Valley Healthcare	Lemars	IA
Flushing Hospital Medical Center	Flushing	NY
Flushing Pet/Ct & Biopsy Services, Pc	Flushing	NY
Fluvanna Correctional Center For Women	Troy	VA
Foley Hospital Corp Dba South Baldwin Regional Med Ctr Gs	Gulf Shores	AL
Fontaine Medical Center	Harwich	MA
Forbes Hospital	Monroeville	PA
Forest City Diagnostic Imaging, Llc	Rockford	IL
Forest County Potawatomi Health And Wellness Center	Crandon	WI
Forest Hills Hospital - Long Island Jewish	Forest Hills	NY
Forest Park Imaging, Llc	Mason City	IA
Forks Community Hospital	Forks	WA
Forrest City Medical Center	Forrest City	AR
Forsyth Imaging Center	Forsyth	IL
Fort Bend Imaging, Inc.	Sugar Land	TX
Fort Collins Mammography Center	Fort Collins	CO
Fort Duncan Medical Center, Inc	Eagle Pass	TX
Fort Hamilton Hospital	Hamilton	OH
Fort Health Care	Fort Atkinson	WI
Fort Jesse Imaging Center	Normal	IL
Fort Logan Hospital	Stanford	KY
Fort Loudoun Medical Center	Lenoir City	TN
Fort Madison Community Hospital	Fort Madison	IA
Fort Norfolk Diagnostic Center	Norfolk	VA
Fort Sanders Obstetrical & Gynecological Group Pc	Knoxville	TN
Fort Walton Beach Medical Center	Fort Walton Beach	FL
Fortunato Breast Health Ctr Mather Hospital Northwell Health	Port Jefferson	NY
Foundcare, Inc	West Palm Beach	FL
48th Medical Group 48 Msgs/Sgcr	Apo	AE
Fox Chase Cancer Center	Philadelphia	PA
Foxcare Center Medical Imaging	Oneonta	NY
Fpc Alderson	Alderson	WV
Frances Mahon Deaconess Hospital	Glasgow	MT
Franciscan Alliance Inc Dba Franciscan Health Crown Point	Crown Point	IN
Franciscan Beacon Hospital	Laporte	IN
Franciscan Breast Center At St. Francis	Federal Way	WA
Franciscan Breast Center-Burien	Burien	WA
Franciscan Breast Imaging At Auburn	Auburn	WA
Franciscan Health - Dyer	Dyer	IN
Franciscan Health Crawfordsville	Crawfordsville	IN
Franciscan Health Indianapolis	Indianapolis	IN
Franciscan Health Lafayette Breast Center	Lafayette	IN
Franciscan Health Lafayette Screening Breast Center	Lafayette	IN
Franciscan Health Mc Breast Center	Michigan City	IN
Franciscan Health Mooresville	Mooresville	IN
Franciscan Health Munster	Munster	IN
Franciscan Health Olympia Fields	Olympia Fields	IL
Franciscan Health Rensselaer	Rensselaer	IN
Franciscan Medical Pavilion Bonney Lake	Bonney Lake	WA
Franciscan Plainfield Health Center	Plainfield	IN
Franciscan Stones Crossing	Greenwood	IN
Frank Aguirre, MD	Newark	NJ
Frank J. Voralik, M.D.	Honolulu	HI
Frankfort Regional Medical Center	Frankfort	KY
Franklin County Medical Center	Preston	ID
Franklin Foundation Hospital	Franklin	LA
Franklin General Hospital	Hampton	IA
Franklin Hospital	Benton	IL
Franklin Medical Center	Winnsboro	LA
Franklin Memorial Hospital	Farmington	ME
Franklin Primary Health Center, Inc.-Mobile	Mobile	AL
Frederick Health Imaging	Frederick	MD
Frederick Health Imaging	Frederick	MD
Fredonia Regional Hospital	Fredonia	KS
Freeman Health System, Freeman Women's Pavilion	Joplin	MO
Freeman Regional Health Services	Freeman	SD
Freeman Women's Pavilion - Neosho	Neosho	MO
Fresno Diagnostic Center	Fresno	CA
Frio Regional Hospital	Pearsall	TX
Froedtert Calhoun Health Center	Brookfield	WI
Froedtert & Med College Community Physicians	New Berlin	WI
Froedtert & The Medical College Of Wi Community Physicians	West Bend	WI
Froedtert And The Med. College Wi Community Physicians	Menomonee Falls	WI
Froedtert Memorial Lutheran Hospital Inc.	Milwaukee	WI
Froedtert South,Inc - Pleasant Prairie Hospital	Pleasant Prairie	WI
Frontera, Colon & Suarez - Radiologos	Mayaguez	PR
Frontera, Colon, And Suarez Radiologos	Mayaguez	PR
Fryecare Mammography	Hickory	NC
Fsah - Chesterton Health And Er Center	Chesterton	IN
Ft Belvoir Community Hospital	Fort Belvoir	VA
Ft Sanders West Diag Ctr Div Of Ft Sanders Regional Med Ctr	Knoxville	TN
Ft. Belknap Center Ihs	Harlem	MT
Fulton County Health Center	Wauseon	OH
Fulton County Medical Center	McConnellsburg	PA
Fulton Medical Imaging An Affilate Of Oswego Health	Fulton	NY
Funnell & Strebel Inc.	Oklahoma City	OK
Future Diagnostics Group	Joliet	IL
G & G Medical Center.	Miami	FL
Gadsden Regional Medical Center	Gadsden	AL
Gainesville Community Hospital, Inc.	Gainesville	TX
Galeria Radiologica Digital Llc	Bayamon	PR
Galesburg Cottage Hospital	Galesburg	IL
Galion Hospital	Galion	OH
Gallup Indian Medical Center	Gallup	NM
Garden Spot Imaging	New Holland	PA
Garfield Memorial Hosp Mobile Mammo Unit Mobile	Panguitch	UT
Garnet Health Medical Center - Catskills Grover Hermann Div	Callicoon	NY
Garnet Health Medical Center Ray W. Moody,MD Breast Center	Middletown	NY
Garnet Health Medical Center-Catskills Women's Imaging	Harris	NY
Gateway Imaging Of Waterloo	Waterloo	IL
Gateway Medical Clinic	West Allis	WI
Gateway Radiology Consultants P.A.	Pinellas Park	FL
Gateway Radiology Consultants, Pa	St Petersburg	FL
Gateway Regional Medical Center	Granite City	IL
Geary Community Hospital	Junction City	KS
Geisinger Bloomsburg Hospital	Bloomsburg	PA
Geisinger Clinic Lewistown	Lewistown	PA
Geisinger Gray's Woods Clinic	Port Matilda	PA
Geisinger Jersey Shore Hospital	Jersey Shore	PA
Geisinger Lycoming Clinic	Montoursville	PA
Geisinger Medical Center	Danville	PA
Geisinger Medical Group - Philipsburg	Philipsburg	PA
Geisinger Medical Group Mt. Pocono	Mount Pocono	PA
Geisinger Medical Group Tunkhannock	Tunkhannock	PA
Geisinger Mobile Mammography-Mobile	Pottsville	PA
Geisinger Mount Pleasant	Scranton	PA
Geisinger Shamokin Area Community Hospital	Coal Township	PA
Geisinger St. Luke's	Orwigsburg	PA
Geisinger-Lewistown Hospital	Lewistown	PA

Alphabetical Index

Name	City	State
Geisinger-Lewistown Hospital Outpatient Center - Jvm	Mifflintown	PA
Geisinger-Viewmont Imaging	Scranton	PA
General Leonard Wood Army Community Hospital	Fort Leonard Wood	MO
Genesis - Kenneth H. McKay, M.D. Center For Breast Health	Davenport	IA
Genesis Health System Dba Genesis Medical Ctr Silvis Campus	Silvis	IL
Genesis Healthcare System	Zanesville	OH
Genesis Imaging Center 53rd St	Davenport	IA
Genesis Imaging Center Bettendorf	Bettendorf	IA
Genesis Imaging Center, Moline	Moline	IL
Genesis Medical Center - Aledo	Aledo	IL
Genesis Medical Center - Dewitt Campus	Dewitt	IA
Genesis Ob/Gyn La Cholla	Tucson	AZ
Genesis Ob/Gyn Wyatt	Tucson	AZ
Genesiscare USA Landmark, Llc	Muskogee	OK
Genesiscare USA Landmark, Llc	Mesquite	TX
Genesiscare USA Landmark, Llc	Plano	TX
Geneva General Hospital Women's Health Services	Geneva	NY
Gentle Touch Breast Diagnostics, Inc	Coral Springs	FL
George C. Grape Community Hospital	Hamburg	IA
George L. Mee Memorial Hospital	King City	CA
George Regional Hospital	Lucedale	MS
George Washington Hospital	Washington	DC
George Washington Imaging Center At 19th Street	Washington	DC
Georgetown Community Hospital	Georgetown	KY
Georgetown Memorial Hospital	Georgetown	SC
Gessler Clinic, P. A.	Winter Haven	FL
Gibson Area Hospital & Health Services	Gibson City	IL
Gibson General Hospital, Inc.	Princeton	IN
Gifford Medical Center	Randolph	VT
Gila Regional Medical Center	Silver City	NM
Girard Medical Center	Girard	KS
Girltalk & Gynecology	Morehead City	NC
Glacial Ridge Health System	Glenwood	MN
Glencoe Regional Health Services	Glencoe	MN
Glendive Medical Center	Glendive	MT
Glens Falls Hospital - Breast Center At Baybrook	Queensbury	NY
Glens Falls Hospital Breast Center	Glens Falls	NY
Glenwood Regional Medical Center A Steward Family Hospital	West Monroe	LA
Global Imaging Llp	Sugar Land	TX
Gmg Health Systems Ltd.	San Antonio	TX
Gmg Health Systems, Ltd.	San Antonio	TX
Golden Valley Medical Warsaw	Warsaw	MO
Golden Valley Memorial Healthcare - Osceola	Osceola	MO
Golden Valley Memorial Hospital	Clinton	MO
Goleta Valley Cottage Hospital	Santa Barbara	CA
Gonzales Healthcare Systems	Gonzales	TX
Good Samaritan Breast Care Center	Los Gatos	CA
Good Samaritan Breast Care Center	Vincennes	IN
Good Samaritan Hospital	Greensboro	GA
Good Samaritan Hospital	Suffern	NY
Good Samaritan Hospital	Cincinnati	OH
Good Samaritan Hospital Women's Imaging Center	West Islip	NY
Good Samaritan Hospital-Advocate	Downers Grove	IL
Good Samaritan Medical Center	West Palm Beach	FL
Good Samaritan Medical Center - Womens Imaging	North Easton	MA
Good Samaritan Medical Center Outpatient Imaging Lake Worth	Lake Worth	FL
Good Samaritan Outpatient Center	Cincinnati	OH
Good Samaritan Western Ridge	Cincinnati	OH
Good Shepherd Healthcare Llc	Riverside	CA
Good Shepherd Hospital Breast Care Center	Barrington	IL
Good Shepherd Medical Center	Hermiston	OR
Goodland Regional Medical Center	Goodland	KS
Goppert Center For Breast Care	Overland Park	KS
Gordon Memorial Health Services	Gordon	NE
Goshen Health The Retreat Women's Health Center	Goshen	IN
Gotham Health Vanderbilt	Staten Island	NY
Gothenburg Health	Gothenburg	NE
Gottlieb Community Health Services Corporation D/B/A Macneal	Berwyn	IL
Gottlieb Memorial Hospital	Melrose Park	IL
Gouverneur Healthcare Services	New York	NY
Gouverneur Hospital	Gouverneur	NY
Governor Juan F Luis Hospital & Medical Center	Christiansted	VI
Gpch Llc	Borger	TX
Gptlhb-Oyate Health Center	Rapid City	SD
Grady Comprehensive Care Center At Camp Creek	Atlanta	GA
Grady General Hospital	Cairo	GA
Grady Health System Breast Imaging	Atlanta	GA
Grady Memorial Hospital Womens Imaging Center	Chickasha	OK
Grafton City Hospital	Grafton	WV
Graham Hospital	Canton	IL
Graham Hospital District	Graham	TX
Grand Avenue Imaging	Los Angeles	CA
Grand Island Regional Medical Center	Grand Island	NE
Grand Itasca Clinic And Hospital	Grand Rapids	MN
Grand Junction Diagnostics	Grand Junction	CO
Grand River Hospital District	Rifle	CO
Grand River Medical Group	Dubuque	IA
Grand View Hospital OP Ctr At Quakertown	Quakertown	PA
Grand View Hospital Outpatient Center At Lansdale	Lansdale	PA
Grand View Hospital Outpatient Center At Sellersville	Sellersville	PA
Grand View Hospitals Harleysville Outpatient Center	Harleysville	PA
Grand View Outpatient Center At Chalfont	Chalfont	PA
Grande Ronde Hospital	La Grande	OR
Grande Ronde Hospital Regional Medical Plaza	La Grande	OR
Grandview Hospital And Medical Center	Dayton	OH
Grandview Imaging Trussville	Birmingham	AL
Granger Family Medicine	Granger	IN
Grant Memorial Hospital	Petersburg	WV
Grant Regional Health Center	Lancaster	WI
Granville Medical Center	Oxford	NC
Graves Gilbert Clinic	Bowling Green	KY
Graves Gilbert Clinic Family Care Center	Bowling Green	KY
Graybill Medical Group Inc	Fallbrook	CA
Graybill Medical Group, Inc.	Escondido	CA
Grays Harbor Imaging	Aberdeen	WA
Great Falls Clinic Hospital	Great Falls	MT
Great Lakes Medical Imaging	Orchard Park	NY
Great Lakes Medical Imaging Llc	Williamsville	NY
Great Plains Health Imaging Center	North Platte	NE
Great Plains Regional Medical Center	Elk City	OK
Great River Medical Center	Blytheville	AR
Greater Maryland Health System, Inc.	Lanham	MD
Greater Regional Medical Center	Creston	IA
Green Clinic Breast Center	Ruston	LA
Green Hospital Of Scripps Clinic	La Jolla	CA
Green Valley Ob/Gyn	Greensboro	NC
Greenbrier Physicians Inc.	Ronceverte	WV
Greenbrier Valley Medical Center	Ronceverte	WV
Greene Co. Health Care - Snow Hill Medical Center	Snow Hill	NC
Greene County General Hospital	Linton	IN
Greene County Medical Center	Jefferson	IA
Greene Medical Imaging	Catskill	NY
Greene Memorial Hospital, Inc.	Xenia	OH
Greeneville Community Hospital-East Campus	Greeneville	TN
Greensboro Ob/Gyn Associates	Greensboro	NC
Greenview Regional Hospital	Bowling Green	KY
Greenwich Hospital Breast Center	Greenwich	CT
Greenwich Hospital Diagnostic Center	Stamford	CT
Greenwich Regional Medical Center	Greenwich	NY
Greenwood Leflore Hospital	Greenwood	MS
Gresham Imaging Center	Gresham	OR
Griffin Obgyn Clinic	Griffin	GA
Grinnell Regional Medical Center	Grinnell	IA
Grosse Pointe Physicians X-Ray Center, P.C.	Grosse Pointe Woods	MI
Grossman Imaging Center	Oxnard	CA
Grossman Imaging Center	Ventura	CA
Grossmont Imaging Llc	La Mesa	CA
Group Health Cooperative	Fitchburg	WI
Grove City Medical Center	Grove City	PA
Grove Hill Memorial Hospital	Grove Hill	AL
Grundy County Memorial Hospital	Grundy Center	IA
Guadalupe Regional Medical Center	Seguin	TX
Guam Memorial Hospital Authority	Oka, Tamuning	GU
Guam Radiology Consultants	Tamuning	GU
Guam Seventh Day Adventist Clinic	Tamuning	GU
Guaynabo Medical Mall	Guaynabo	PR
Guild Imaging Center Of Norwood Hospital	Norwood	MA
Guilford Radiology	Guilford	CT
Gulf Coast Cancer & Diagnostic Center @ South East, Inc.	Houston	TX
Gulf Coast Obstetrics And Gynecology Of Sarasota	Sarasota	FL
Gundersen Boscobel Area Hospital And Clinics	Boscobel	WI
Gundersen Health System - Decorah	Decorah	IA

Name	City	State
Gundersen Health System - Lacrosse	La Crosse	WI
Gundersen Health System - Onalaska	Onalaska	WI
Gundersen Health System - Prairie Du Chien	Prairie Du Chien	WI
Gundersen Health System - Sparta	Sparta	WI
Gundersen Health System - Tomah	Tomah	WI
Gundersen Moundview Hospital & Clinics	Friendship	WI
Gundersen Palmer Lutheran Hospital And Clinics	West Union	IA
Gundersen St Elizabeth's Hospital And Clinics	Wabasha	MN
Gundersen Tri-County Hospital And Clinics	Whitehall	WI
Gundersen Winona Campus	Winona	MN
Gunnison Valley Hospital	Gunnison	CO
Gunnison Valley Hospital	Gunnison	UT
Guthrie Corning Hospital Breast Care Center	Corning	NY
Guthrie Cortland Medical Center	Cortland	NY
Guthrie County Hospital	Guthrie Center	IA
Guthrie Medical Group Big Flats	Horseheads	NY
Guthrie Medical Group Ithaca	Ithaca	NY
Guthrie Medical Group Owego	Owego	NY
Guthrie Medical Group Southport	Elmira	NY
Guthrie Medical Group Wellsboro	Wellsboro	PA
Guthrie Robert Packer Hospital	Sayre	PA
Guttenberg Municipal Hospital	Guttenberg	IA
Gwinette's Progressive Healthcare For Women	Lawrenceville	GA
Gwinnett Clinic Ltd	Lawrenceville	GA
Gynecology & Laparoscopic Surgeons, Pc	Raleigh	NC
H. B. Magruder Memorial Hospital	Port Clinton	OH
H. Claude Hudson Comprehensive Health Center	Los Angeles	CA
Habersham County Medical Center	Demorest	GA
Hackensack Meridian Health Palisades Medical Center	North Bergen	NJ
Hackensack Meridian Health Pascack Valley Medical Center	Westwood	NJ
Hackensack Meridian Mountainside Medical Center	Montclair	NJ
Hackettstown Medical Center	Hackettstown	NJ
Hallmark Health Medical Center Reading	Reading	MA
Halo Medical Group Dba Halo Breast Care Center	Chico	CA
Hamilton County Hospital Dba Van Diest Family Health Clinic	Webster City	IA
Hamilton County Hospital District	Hamilton	TX
Hamilton Memorial Hospital	McLeansboro	IL
Hammond Henry Hospital	Geneseo	IL
Hampshire Memorial Hospital, Inc.	Romney	WV
Hampton Regional Medical Center	Varnville	SC
Hancock County Memorial Hospital	Britt	IA
Hannibal Clinic Operations	Hannibal	MO
Hannibal Regional Hospital	Hannibal	MO
Hanover Imaging Center	Mechanicsville	VA
Harbin Clinic Cartersville Imaging Center	Cartersville	GA
Harbor Beach Community Hospital	Harbor Beach	MI
Harbor Ucla Medical Center	Torrance	CA
Harbor-Ucla Diagnostic Imaging	Torrance	CA
Hardin County General Hospital	Rosiclare	IL
Hardin Medical Center	Savannah	TN
Hardin Memorial Hospital	Kenton	OH
Hardtner Medical Center	Olla	LA
Harford Healthcare Health Center At Winsted	Winsted	CT
Harlan Appalachian Regional Hospital	Harlan	KY
Harlan County Health System	Alma	NE
Harlan Medical Clinic	Harlan	KY
Harlem Hospital Center	New York	NY
Harlingen Medical Center L.P.	Harlingen	TX
Harnett Health Breast Care Ctr	Dunn	NC
Harney District Hospital	Burns	OR
Harrington Healthcare At Charlton	Charlton	MA
Harrington Healthcare At Webster	Webster	MA
Harrington Memorial Hospital	Southbridge	MA
Harris County Hospital District	Houston	TX
Harris County Hospital District	Houston	TX
Harris County Hospital District	Houston	TX
Harris County Hospital District	Houston	TX
Harris County Hospital District	Houston	TX
Harris County Hospital District	Houston	TX
Harris County Hospital District	Houston	TX
Harris County Hospital District	Pasadena	TX
Harris Medical Park	Sylva	NC
Harrisburg Medical Center, Inc.	Harrisburg	IL
Harrison Community Hospital	Cadiz	OH
Harrison County Community Hospital	Bethany	MO
Harrison County Hospital	Corydon	IN
Harrison Imaging Centers - Port Orchard Mammography	Port Orchard	WA
Harrison Imaging Centers - Poulsbo Mammography	Poulsbo	WA
Harrison Imaging Centers - Silverdale Mammography	Silverdale	WA
Harrison Memorial Hospital	Cynthiana	KY
Harrisonburg Obgyn	Harrisonburg	VA
Hartford Hospital	Hartford	CT
Hartsdale Imaging	Hartsdale	NY
Harvard Vanguard Medical Assoc - Kenmore Practice	Boston	MA
Hastings Medical Imaging	Hastings	NE
Hato Rey X-Ray & Imaging Center	San Juan	PR
Hato Tejas X Rays	Bayamon	PR
Havasu Regional Medical Center	Lake Havasu City	AZ
Hawaii Diagnostic Radiology Services, Llc	Waipahu	HI
Hawaii Radiologic Associates, Ltd.	Kailua Kona	HI
Hawarden Regional Healthcare	Hawarden	IA
Hawthorne Obgyn Associates	Winston Salem	NC
Hays Medical Center Inc.	Hays	KS
Hayward Area Memorial Hospital	Hayward	WI
Hazard Arh Imaging Ctr. Llc - Med. Mall Imaging Ctr	Hazard	KY
Hazel Hawkins Memorial Hospital	Hollister	CA
Hca Health Srv Of Tn Inc Dba Tristar Centennial Med Ctr	Nashville	TN
Hca John Randolph Medical Center	Hopewell	VA
Hcmc Whittier Clinic	Minneapolis	MN
Healdsburg Hospital OP Services	Healdsburg	CA
Health Alliance - Clinton Hospital, Clinton Campus	Clinton	MA
Health Alliance-Clinton Hospital, Burbank Campus	Fitchburg	MA
Health Alliance-Clinton Hospital, Leominster Campus	Leominster	MA
Health And Wellness Pavilion	Wexford	PA
Health Center At Bath Breast Health Services	Bath	PA
Health Central Hospital	Ocoee	FL
Health Diagnostics Of California, A Professional Corporation	Daly City	CA
Health Diagnostics Of California, A Professional Corporation	San Bernardino	CA
Health Diagnostics Of California, A Professional Corporation	San Francisco	CA
Health Diagnostics Of California, A Professional Corporation	San Francisco	CA
Health Diagnostics Of California, Pc - Laguna Hills	Laguna Hills	CA
Health First Breast Center	Melbourne	FL
Health First Diagnostic Center Merritt Island	Merritt Island	FL
Health First Diagnostic Ctr - Viera Medical Plaza	Melbourne	FL
Health First Palm Bay Hospital	Palm Bay	FL
Health Image Diagnostics/Senos Puerto Rico	San Juan	PR
Health Images At South Potomac	Aurora	CO
Health Images Breast Center At Diamond Hill	Denver	CO
Health Partners - Arden Hills	Arden Hills	MN
Health Partners - Woodbury Clinic	Woodbury	MN
Health Partners Bloomington Clinic	Bloomington	MN
Health Pointe	Grand Haven	MI
Health Village Imaging	Jackson	NJ
Health Village Imaging	Manahawkin	NJ
Healthcare Imaging Center At Day Street	Riverside	CA
Healthcare Imaging Of Kendall	Miami	FL
Healtheast Rice Street Clinic	Saint Paul	MN
Healthpartners - St. Paul Clinic	Saint Paul	MN
Healthpartners Brooklyn Center Clinic	Brooklyn Center	MN
Healthpartners Como Clinic	Saint Paul	MN
Healthpartners Coon Rapids Clinic	Coon Rapids	MN
Healthpartners Health Center For Women	Saint Paul	MN
Healthpartners Maplewood Clinic	Maplewood	MN
Healthpartners Mobile	Arden Hills	MN
Healthpartners Riverway Anoka Clinic	Anoka	MN
Healthpartners White Bear Clinic	White Bear Lake	MN
Healthstar Physicians, P.C.	Morristown	TN
Healthtexas Provider Network	Dallas	TX
Healthway Park	New Palestine	IN
Heart Institute Of Brownsville, Llp	Brownsville	TX
Heart Of America Medical Center	Rugby	ND
Heart Of Texas Healthcare System	Brady	TX

Alphabetical Index

Name	City	State
Heart Of The Rockies Regional Medical Center	Salida	CO
Heartland Imaging	Louisville	KY
Heartland Regional Medical Center	Marion	IL
Heber Valley Hospital	Heber	UT
Hedrick Medical Center	Chillicothe	MO
Hegg Health Center	Rock Valley	IA
Helen Keller Hospital	Sheffield	AL
Helen Newberry Joy Hospital	Newberry	MI
Helena Imaging Center	Helena	MT
Helena Regional Medical Center	Helena	AR
Hemet Valley Imaging Medical Group, Inc.	Hemet	CA
Henderson And Walton Women's Center	Birmingham	AL
Henderson And Walton Women's Center Cullman	Cullman	AL
Henderson Co Community Hosp Lexington Tennessee	Lexington	TN
Henderson Health Care Services Inc.	Henderson	NE
Henderson Hospital,Llc	Henderson	TX
Hendrick Medical Center	Abilene	TX
Hendrick Medical Center	Abilene	TX
Hendrick Medical Center Brownwood	Brownwood	TX
Hendricks Community Hospital	Hendricks	MN
Hendricks Regional Health	Danville	IN
Hendricks Regional Health Brownsburg Hospital	Brownsburg	IN
Hendricks Regional Health-Plainfield	Plainfield	IN
Hendry Regional Convenient Care Center	Labelle	FL
Hendry Regional Medical Center	Clewiston	FL
Hennepin County Medical Center	Minneapolis	MN
Hennepin Healthcare Brooklyn Park	Brooklyn Park	MN
Hennepin Healthcare Richfield	Richfield	MN
Henrietta Medical Campus	Henrietta	NY
Henry County Diagnostic Center	Paris	TN
Henry County Health Center Inc	Mount Pleasant	IA
Henry County Hospital	New Castle	IN
Henry County Hospital, Inc.	Napoleon	OH
Henry Ford Allegiance Diagnostic Center- Professional Bldg	Jackson	MI
Henry Ford Allegiance Health	Jackson	MI
Henry Ford Allegiance Mobile Health-Mobile	Jackson	MI
Henry Ford Allegiance Women's Health Center	Jackson	MI
Henry Ford Cancer Center	Detroit	MI
Henry Ford Health Center Brownstown	Brownstown	MI
Henry Ford Hospital	Detroit	MI
Henry Ford Hospital -		
Hacomb Chesterfield Hlth Ctr	Chesterfield Township	MI
Henry Ford Macomb - Washington Township	Washington Twp	MI
Henry Ford Macomb Health Center Fraser	Clinton Township	MI
Henry Ford Macomb Hospital	Clinton Township	MI
Henry Ford Medical Center - Livonia	Livonia	MI
Henry Ford Medical Center Bloomfield Township	Bloomfield Hills	MI
Henry Ford Medical Center Cottage	Grosse Pointe Farms	MI
Henry Ford Medical Center-Detroit Northwest	Detroit	MI
Henry Ford Medical Center-Fairlane	Dearborn	MI
Henry Ford Medical Center-Lakeside	Sterling Heights	MI
Henry Ford Medical Center-Sterling Heights	Sterling Heights	MI
Henry Ford Medical Center-Taylor	Taylor	MI
Henry Ford Mobile Mammography	Clinton Township	MI
Henry Ford West Bloomfield Hospital	West Bloomfield	MI
Herington Municipal Hospital	Herington	KS
Heritage Medical Associates	Brentwood	TN
Heritage Medical Associates	Hermitage	TN
Heritage Medical Associates	Nashville	TN
Heritage Valley Diagnostic Center - Chippewa	Beaver Falls	PA
Heritage Valley Diagnostic Center Robinson	Pittsburgh	PA
Heritage Valley Edgeworth	Sewickley	PA
Heritage Valley Ellwood City	Ellwood City	PA
Heritage Valley Health System - East Liverpool	Calcutta	OH
Heritage Valley Health System Women's Health Center	Aliquippa	PA
Heritage Valley Kennedy	McKees Rocks	PA
Hermann Area District Hospital	Hermann	MO
Hermel Breast Health Center Emerson Hospital	Concord	MA
Heywood Hospital	Gardner	MA
Hh / Killeen Health System, Llc	Harker Heights	TX
Hi-Desert Medical Center	Joshua Tree	CA
Hialeah Hospital	Hialeah	FL
Hibbing Family Medical Clinic	Hibbing	MN
Higgins General Hospital	Bremen	GA
High Desert Imaging	Elko	NV
High Desert Regional Health Center	Lancaster	CA
High Point Regional Health Dba High Point Regional Hospital	High Point	NC
High Resolution	Albuquerque	NM
High Resolution Rust	Rio Rancho	NM
High Resolution Santa Fe	Santa Fe	NM
High Tech Medical Park	Palos Heights	IL
High Tech Medical Park	Tinley Park	IL
Highland Breast Imaging	Penfield	NY
Highland Breast Imaging	Rochester	NY
Highland Breast Imaging At Anthony Jordan Health Center	Rochester	NY
Highland Community Hospital	Picayune	MS
Highland District Hospital	Hillsboro	OH
Highland Hospital	Oakland	CA
Highland Hospital Highland Breast Imaging	Rochester	NY
Highlands - Cashiers Hospital	Highlands	NC
Highlands Breast And Imaging Center	Sebring	FL
Highlands Hospital	Connellsville	PA
Highlands Regional Medical Center	Sebring	FL
Hill Country Memorial Hospital	Fredericksburg	TX
Hill Imaging Center, Inc.	Glendora	CA
Hillcrest Baptist Medical Center	Waco	TX
Hillcrest Hospital	Mayfield Heights	OH
Hillcrest Hospital / Claremore	Claremore	OK
Hillcrest Hospital Cushing	Cushing	OK
Hillcrest Hospital Henryetta	Henryetta	OK
Hillcrest Hospital South	Tulsa	OK
Hillcrest Radiology	Mayfield Heights	OH
Hillcrest South Diagnostic Center	Tulsa	OK
Hills & Dales General Hospital	Cass City	MI
Hillsboro Area Hospital	Hillsboro	IL
Hillsborough Radiology Centers, Llc	Hillsborough	NJ
Hillsdale Hospital	Hillsdale	MI
Hillside Medical Center	Hanover	PA
Hilton Head Hospital	Hilton Head Island	SC
Hima-San Pablo Humacao	Humacao	PR
Hirsch And Ratakonda, M.D. P.A.	Morristown	NJ
Hirsch, Ratakonda, M.D. P.A.	Morristown	NJ
Hmfp Radiology	Brookline	MA
Hmh Hospitals Corporation	Hackensack	NJ
Hmh Hospitals Corporation	Maywood	NJ
Hoag Breast Care And Imaging Center	Newport Beach	CA
Hoag Clinic	Laguna Hills	CA
Hoag Clinic- San Clemente	San Clemente	CA
Hoag Clinic-Irvine	Irvine	CA
Hoag Health Center Irvine - Sand Canyon	Irvine	CA
Hoag Health Center-Foothill Ranch	Foothill Ranch	CA
Hoag Imaging Center - Costa Mesa	Costa Mesa	CA
Hoag Imaging Center Aliso Viejo	Aliso Viejo	CA
Hoag Imaging Center Huntington Beach	Huntington Beach	CA
Hoag Imaging Center Irvine	Irvine	CA
Hoboken University Medical Center	Hoboken	NJ
Hocking Valley Community Hospital	Logan	OH
Hoke Imaging, Llc	Raeford	NC
Holland Hospital Breast Health Services	Holland	MI
Holland Hospital Breast Health Services-Hmic	Holland	MI
Holland Hospital Breast Health Services-Zeeland	Zeeland	MI
Hollings Cancer Center Breast Imaging Program	Charleston	SC
Hollywood Diagnostics Center	Hollywood	FL
Holmdel Imaging Llc	Holmdel	NJ
Holmes County Hospital And Clinics	Lexington	MS
Holton Community Hospital	Holton	KS
Holy Cross Hospital	Nogales	AZ
Holy Cross Hospital	Chicago	IL
Holy Cross Hospital Of Silver Spring, Inc	Silver Spring	MD
Holy Cross Medical Center	Taos	NM
Holy Family Hospital	Methuen	MA
Holy Family Memorial, Inc.	Manitowoc	WI
Holy Name Medical Center	Teaneck	NJ
Holy Redeemer Healthcare	Philadelphia	PA
Holy Redeemer Healthcare At 821	Huntingdon Valley	PA
Holy Redeemer Healthcare At Bensalem	Bensalem	PA
Holy Redeemer Healthcare At Feasterville	Feasterville	PA
Holy Redeemer Women's Healthcare At Southampton	Southampton	PA
Holy Rosary Healthcare	Miles City	MT
Holyoke Medical Center Women's Center	Holyoke	MA
Holzer	Athens	OH
Holzer	Gallipolis	OH

Name	City	State
Holzer	Jackson	OH
Holzer	Pomeroy	OH
Homestead Diagnostic Center	Homestead	FL
Homestead Hospital	Homestead	FL
Honorhealth Breast Health And Research Center - Jcl	Phoenix	AZ
Honorhealth Breast Health And Research Center- Dv	Phoenix	AZ
Honorhealth Breast Health And Research Center- Sonoran	Phoenix	AZ
Hoopeston Community Memorial Hospital	Hoopeston	IL
Hopedale Medical Complex	Hopedale	IL
Horizon Medical Center Dba Natchez Imaging Center	Dickson	TN
Horn Memorial Hospital	Ida Grove	IA
Hospital Auxilio Mutuo	Hato Rey	PR
Hospital Bella Vista Mamografia	Mayaguez	PR
Hospital Buen Samaritano	Aguadilla	PR
Hospital Centro Comprensivo De Cancer Upr	San Juan	PR
Hospital De La Concepcion	San German	PR
Hospital Del Maestro	Hato Rey	PR
Hospital District 6 Of Harper County Kansas	Anthony	KS
Hospital Episcopal San Lucas Ponce	Ponce	PR
Hospital For Special Surgery, Llc Dba Onecore-Cdi Location	Oklahoma City	OK
Hospital Hima San Pablo Caguas	Caguas	PR
Hospital Hima San Pablo Fajardo	Fajardo	PR
Hospital Menonita Caguas	Caguas	PR
Hospital Menonita Guayama	Guayama	PR
Hospital Metropolitano	San Juan	PR
Hospital Metropolitano - South West Health Corp.	San German	PR
Hospital Metropolitano Cabo Rojo	Cabo Rojo	PR
Hospital Metropolitano Dr. Susoni Inc.	Arecibo	PR
Hospital Metropolitano Dr.Pila	Ponce	PR
Hospital Of Central Connecticut	New Britain	CT
Hospital Of Central Connecticut Breast Imaging	Southington	CT
Hospital Of University Of Pennsylvania-Perelman Ctr	Philadelphia	PA
Hospital Pavia Arecibo	Arecibo	PR
Hospital Pavia Hato Rey	Hato Rey	PR
Hospital Pavia Yauco	Yauco	PR
Hospital Perea-Clinica De La Mujer	Mayaguez	PR
Hospital Ryder Memorial	Humacao	PR
Hospital San Carlos Borromeo	Moca	PR
Hospital San Cristobal	Coto Laurel	PR
Hospital San Francisco, Centro De Imagenes	San Juan	PR
Hot Springs Health	Thermopolis	WY
Houlton Regional Hospital	Houlton	ME
Houston Health Pavilion Diagnostic Center	Warner Robins	GA
Houston Medical Imaging	Houston	TX
Houston Medical Imaging, Llc.	Houston	TX
Houston Methodist Clear Lake Hospital	Houston	TX
Houston Methodist Hospital	Houston	TX
Houston Methodist Hospital	Houston	TX
Houston Methodist Sugar Land Hospital	Sugar Land	TX
Houston Methodist The Woodlands Hospital	The Woodlands	TX
Houston Methodist West Hospital	Houston	TX
Houston Methodist Willowbrook Hospital	Houston	TX
Howard County Medical Center	St Paul	NE
Howard Memorial Hospital	Nashville	AR
Howard University Faculty Practice Plan	Washington	DC
Howard University Hospital	Washington	DC
Howard Young Medical Center	Woodruff	WI
Hpm Foundation Inc Centro De Imagenes	Santurce	PR
Hshs Good Shepherd Hospital	Shelbyville	IL
Hshs Holy Family Hospital, Inc.	Greenville	IL
Hshs Imaging Center, Belleville	Belleville	IL
Hshs St. Anthony's Diagnostic Center- Mattoon	Mattoon	IL
Hshs St.Anthony's Womens Wellness Center	Effingham	IL
Huber Health Center	Huber Heights	OH
Hubert H. Humphrey Comprehensive Health Center	Los Angeles	CA
Hudson Headwaters Health Network	Warrensburg	NY
Hudson Hospital & Clinics	Hudson	WI
Hudson Regional Hospital	Secaucus	NJ
Hudson River Radiology Center	Jersey City	NJ
Hudson River Radiology Center	Union City	NJ
Hudson River Radiology Center	Wayne	NJ
Hudson Valley Imaging	Monroe	NY
Hudson Valley Imaging	New Windsor	NY
Hudson Valley Radiology Associates Of Westchester	Tuckahoe	NY
Huggins Hospital	Wolfeboro	NH
Hugh Chatham Memorial Hospital	Elkin	NC
Humacao X-Ray Imaging Center	Humacao	PR
Humboldt County Memorial Hospital	Humboldt	IA
Humboldt General Hospital	Winnemucca	NV
Humboldt Park Health	Chicago	IL
Hunt Memorial Hospital District	Greenville	TX
Hunterdon Advanced Imaging At Bridgewater	Bridgewater	NJ
Hunterdon Radiological Associates Pa	Annandale	NJ
Hunterdon Womens Imaging Center	Flemington	NJ
Huntington Beach Diagnostic Imaging And Breast Center	Huntington Beach	CA
Huntington Hill Imaging	Pasadena	CA
Huntington-Hill Breast Center	Arcadia	CA
Huntsman Comprehensive Breast Care Center	Salt Lake City	UT
Huntsville Community Hospital,Dba Huntsville Memorial Hosp.	Huntsville	TX
Huntsville Hospital Breast Center	Huntsville	AL
Huron Memorial Hospital Dba McLaren Thumb Region	Bad Axe	MI
Huron Regional Medical Center	Huron	SD
Huron Valley - Sinai Hospital	Commerce	MI
Hutchinson Clinic, P.A.	Hutchinson	KS
Hutchinson Health	Hutchinson	MN
Hvra Of Yonkers	Yonkers	NY
Hyatt Imaging Center	Tipp City	OH
Iberia Medical Center	New Iberia	LA
Idaca Llc	Doral	FL
Idaca, Llc	Hialeah	FL
Idaho Medical Imaging Portneuf Medical Center	Pocatello	ID
Ide Imaging Partners Inc Dba Borg & Ide Imaging Pc	Brockport	NY
Ide Imaging Partners Inc Dba Borg & Ide Imaging Pc	Rochester	NY
Ide Imaging Partners Inc Dba Borg & Ide Imaging Pc	Rochester	NY
Ide Imaging Partners Inc Dba Borg And Ide Imaging	Rochester	NY
Ide Imaging Partners, Inc., Dba/Borg & Ide Imaging, Pc	Rochester	NY
Ifrc, Llc D/B/A Fairfax Radiology Center At Sterling	Sterling	VA
Ifrc, Llc Dba Fairfax Radiology Breast Center Of Loudoun	Lansdowne	VA
Ifrc, Llc Dba Fairfax Radiology Breast Center Of Reston/Hern	Herndon	VA
Ifrc, Llc Dba Fairfax Radiology Center At Heritage	Clinton	MD
Ifrc, Llc Dba Fairfax Radiology Center At Patuxent	Prince Frederick	MD
Ifrc, Llc Dba Fairfax Radiology Center Of Fairfax City	Fairfax	VA
Ifrc, Llc Dba Fairfax Radiology Center Of Springfield	Springfield	VA
Ifrc, Llc Dba Fairfax Radiology Center Of Vienna	Vienna	VA
Ifrc,Llc Dba Fairfax Radiology Breast Center Of Fairfax	Fairfax	VA
Ifrc,Llc Dba Fairfax Radiology Center At Pembrooke	Waldorf	MD
Ifrc,Llc Dba Fairfax Radiology Center Of Ballston	Arlington	VA
Ifrc,Llc Dba Fairfax Radiology Center Of Centreville	Centreville	VA
Ifwh Austin Breast Imaging, Llc	San Antonio	TX
Image Care Morristown	Morristown	NJ
Image Care Of West Orange Llc	West Orange	NJ
Imagecare Balltown	Schenectady	NY
Imagecare Center At Millburn	Millburn	NJ
Imagecare Clifton Park	Clifton Park	NY
Imagecare Guilderland	Schenectady	NY
Imagecare Latham	Latham	NY
Imagecare Saratoga	Saratoga Springs	NY
Imagenes Radiology And Breast Diagnostic Center	Caguas	PR
Images - Trinity Health System	Steubenville	OH
Imaging Associates	Anchorage	AK
Imaging Associates	Palmer	AK
Imaging Associates Of Hazleton Pc	Hazleton	PA
Imaging Associates Of Nw Ar At Fountain Plaza	Bentonville	AR
Imaging Center At Baxter Village	Fort Mill	SC
Imaging Center Braselton	Braselton	GA
Imaging Center Charleston Area Medical Center	Charleston	WV
Imaging Center Dawsonville	Dawsonville	GA
Imaging Center For Women At North Stafford	Stafford	VA
Imaging Center Of Baxter Regional Medical Center-Mobile	Mountain Home	R
Imaging Center Of Columbus	Columbus	MS
Imaging Center Of Idaho	Caldwell	ID
Imaging Center Of Plymouth	Plymouth	MN
Imaging Center Placentia Linda Hospital	Placentia	CA
Imaging Center, P.C.	Christiansted	VI
Imaging For Women At Sumner Station A Dept Of Srmc	Gallatin	TN
Imaging For Women, Llc	Kansas City	MO
Imaging Healthcare Specialists - Alvarado	San Diego	CA
Imaging Healthcare Specialists - Encinitas	Encinitas	CA
Imaging Healthcare Specialists - Golden Triangle	La Jolla	CA
Imaging Healthcare Specialists - National City	National City	CA
Imaging Healthcare Specialists - South Bay	Chula Vista	CA

Alphabetical Index

Alphabetical Index

Alphabetical Index

Alphabetical Index

Name	City	State
Newyork-Presbyterian/Hudson Valley Hospital	Cortlandt Manor	NY
Newyork-Presbyterian/Lower Manhattan Hospital	New York	NY
Newyork-Presbyterian/Queens	Flushing	NY
Nhci Of Hillsboro Inc., Dba Hill Regional Hospital	Hillsboro	TX
Nicholas H. Noyes Memorial Hospital	Dansville	NY
Njin Of Clifton	Clifton	NJ
Njin Of Cranford	Cranford	NJ
Njin Of Edison	Edison	NJ
Njin Of Hackensack	Hackensack	NJ
Njin Of Haddon Heights	Haddon Heights	NJ
Njin Of Randolph	Randolph	NJ
Njin Of Rutherford	Rutherford	NJ
Njin Of Toms River West & Women's Imaging	Toms River	NJ
Njin Of Union City	Union City	NJ
Njin Of Union Women's Imaging	Union	NJ
Njin Of Washington Township	Turnersville	NJ
Njin Of Woodbridge	Avenel	NJ
Nk - Kfh - San Rafael	San Rafael	CA
Nk Kfh Richmond	Richmond	CA
Nk Kfh South Sacramento	Sacramento	CA
Nk Kfh Vacaville Mob B	Vacaville	CA
Nk The Permanente Medical Group San Francisco	San Francisco	CA
Nk Tpmg San Rafael Park Medical Center	San Rafael	CA
Nk Tpmg Campbell Mob	Campbell	CA
Nk Tpmg Clovis	Clovis	CA
Nk Tpmg Dublin	Dublin	CA
Nk Tpmg Elk Grove	Elk Grove	CA
Nk Tpmg Elk Grove - Promenade	Elk Grove	CA
Nk Tpmg Martinez	Martinez	CA
Nk Tpmg Milpitas Mob	Milpitas	CA
Nk Tpmg Mountain View Mob	Mountain View	CA
Nk Tpmg Napa Mob2	Napa	CA
Nk Tpmg Novato	Novato	CA
Nk Tpmg Petaluma	Petaluma	CA
Nk Tpmg Pinole	Pinole	CA
Nk Tpmg Redwood City Marshall Mob	Redwood City	CA
Nk Tpmg Rohnert Park	Rohnert Park	CA
Nk Tpmg Sacramento Point West	Sacramento	CA
Nk Tpmg San Francisco Mission Bay	San Francisco	CA
Nk Tpmg San Jose - Skyport	San Jose	CA
Nk Tpmg San Mateo Mob	San Mateo	CA
Nk Tpmg Santa Clara M.O.B.	Santa Clara	CA
Nk Tpmg Santa Rosa Mob5	Santa Rosa	CA
Nk Tpmg Santa Rosa Mob6	Santa Rosa	CA
Nk Tpmg Scotts Valley	Scotts Valley	CA
Nk Tpmg Selma	Selma	CA
Nk Tpmg Union City Mob B	Union City	CA
Nk Tpmg Watsonville	Watsonville	CA
Nk-Kfh Fremont	Fremont	CA
Nktpmg San Rafael	San Rafael	CA
Nm Cdh Diagnostic Imaging - Glen Ellyn	Glen Ellyn	IL
Nm Cdh Diagnostic Imaging- Naperville	Naperville	IL
Nm Cdh Diagnostic Imaging-Bloomingdale	Bloomingdale	IL
Nm Central Dupage Hospital	Winfield	IL
Nmmc Pontotoc	Pontotoc	MS
Nmmc-West Point	West Point	MS
Noble Mammography Unit	Canton	NY
Nolan County Hospital District	Sweetwater	TX
Noms Fremont Imaging	Fremont	OH
Noms Imaging Sandusky	Sandusky	OH
Noms Premium Imaging	Elyria	OH
Nor-Lea General Hospital	Lovington	NM
Norcal Healthconnect Dba Petaluma Valley Hospital	Petaluma	CA
Norcal Imaging - Concord	Concord	CA
Norcal Imaging - Walnut Creek	Walnut Creek	CA
Norcal Imaging Fremont	Fremont	CA
Norcal Imaging Oakland	Oakland	CA
Norcal Imaging Pleasanton	Pleasanton	CA
Norcal Imaging Sanleandro	San Leandro	CA
Norman Regional Breast Care Center	Norman	OK
Norman Regional Hlth Sys. Dba Norman Regional Moore	Moore	OK
North Arkansas Regional Medical Center	Harrison	AR
North Atlanta Women's Specialists- Johns Creek	Johns Creek	GA
North Atlanta Women's Specialists-East Cobb	Marietta	GA
North Baldwin Infirmary	Bay Minette	AL
North Bay Diagnostics	Biloxi	MS
North Big Horn Hospital	Lovell	WY
North Brevard County Hospital District Dba Parrish Medical C	Cocoa	FL
North Brevard County Hospital District Dba Parrish Medical C	Titusville	FL
North Caddo Medical Center	Vivian	LA
North Canyon Medical Center	Gooding	ID
North Carolina Correctional Institute For Women Hcf	Raleigh	NC
North Central Bronx Hospital	Bronx	NY
North Central Imaging Llc	Enfield	CT
North Country Hospital	Newport	VT
North Country Imaging Ctr. Adirondack Radiology Assoc, P.C.	Glens Falls	NY
North East Alabama Regional Medical Center	Anniston	AL
North East Medical Services	San Francisco	CA
North East Medical Services	San Francisco	CA
North East Medical Services	San Jose	CA
North Florida Ob-Gyn	Orange Park	FL
North Florida Obgyn, Llc	Jacksonville	FL
North Florida Regional Medical Center	Gainesville	FL
North Florida Regional Medical Center Starke Campus	Starke	FL
North Hawaii Community Hospital, Inc.	Kamuela	HI
North Jefferson Imaging	Gardendale	AL
North Kansas City Hospital	North Kansas City	MO
North Kansas City Hospital Dba Medical Imaging	Kansas City	MO
North Lancaster Medical Office	Salem	OR
North Memorial Health Breast Center	Robbinsdale	MN
North Memorial Health Clinic - Minnetonka Medical Center	Minnetonka	MN
North Memorial Health Clinic Fridley	Fridley	MN
North Mississippi Medical Center - Eupora	Eupora	MS
North Mississippi Medical Gilmore-Amory	Amory	MS
North Ms Medical Center Breast Care Center	Tupelo	MS
North Ms Medical Center Breast Care Suite	Tupelo	MS
North Oaks Medical Center, Llc	Hammond	LA
North Okaloosa Medical Center	Crestview	FL
North Ottawa Community Health Systems	Grand Haven	MI
North Shore Health	Grand Marais	MN
North Shore Medical Center	Miami	FL
North Shore Physicians Group Imaging Services	Rowley	MA
North Star Fm, Lp	Flower Mound	TX
North Star Mri Of Frisco, Lp	Frisco	TX
North Star Mri, Lp	Allen	TX
North Suburban Medical Center	Thornton	CO
North Texas Imaging/Hampton Center Ii, Ltd.	Dallas	TX
North Valley Breast Clinic	Redding	CA
North Valley Hospital	Whitefish	MT
North Valley Hospital	Tonasket	WA
Northcrest Medical Center	Springfield	TN
Northeast Alabama Regional Medical Center-Tyler Center	Anniston	AL
Northeast Diagnostic Imaging	Columbia	SC
Northeast Georgia Diagnostic Associates And Clinic, Llc	Gainesville	GA
Northeast Georgia Medical Center Barrow	Winder	GA
Northeast Health Imaging Center Albany Memorial Hosp	Rensselaer	NY
Northeast Montana Health Services, Inc.	Wolf Point	MT
Northeast Radiology	Danbury	CT
Northeast Radiology	Brewster	NY
Northeast Radiology	Mount Kisco	NY
Northeast Regional Medical Center	Kirksville	MO
Northeastern Health Systems	Tahlequah	OK
Northeastern Nevada Regional Hospital	Elko	NV
Northeastern Tribal Health System	Miami	OK
Northeastern Vermont Regional Hospital	St Johnsbury	VT
Northern Arizona Radiology, P.C.	Flagstaff	AZ
Northern Berkshire Health Center Of Berkshire Medical Center	North Adams	MA
Northern California Women's Imaging Center	Palo Alto	CA
Northern Cochise Community Hospital	Willcox	AZ
Northern Dutchess Hospital	Rhinebeck	NY
Northern Inyo Hospital Healthcare District	Bishop	CA
Northern Light Charles A. Dean Hospital	Greenville	ME
Northern Light Mayo Hospital Imaging Center For Women	Dover Foxcroft	ME
Northern Light Mercy Hospital Mammography Center	Portland	ME
Northern Maine Medical Center	Fort Kent	ME
Northern Michigan Medical Management	Rogers City	MI
Northern Montana Hospital	Havre	MT
Northern Navajo Medical Center	Shiprock	NM
Northern Nevada Med. Ctr - Diagnostic Breast Care Ctr	Sparks	NV
Northern Radiology Imaging	Watertown	NY
Northern Regional Hospital	Mount Airy	NC
Northern Westchester Hospital	Mount Kisco	NY
Northern Westchester Hospital At Yorktown Imaging	Yorktown Heights	NY
Northfield Hospital	Northfield	MN
Northgate Medical Imaging Llc Dba Priority Radiology	New Albany	IN
Northland Radiology, Inc.	Southfield	MI
Northpoint Health & Wellness Center	Minneapolis	MN
Northpointe Health And Wellness Campus	Roscoe	IL
Northport Medical Center - Dch	Northport	AL
Northridge Diagnostic Med Group	Reseda	CA
Northshore - Gurnee - Rollins Rd	Gurnee	IL
Northshore At 680	Chicago	IL
Northshore At Northbrook Court	Northbrook	IL
Northshore Evanston Hospital	Evanston	IL

Name	City	State
Paredes Institute For Women's Imaging	Glen Allen	VA
Paredes Institute For Womens Imaging	Richmond	VA
Paris Community Hospital	Paris	IL
Paris Regional Medical Center	Paris	TX
Park Avenue Diagnostic Center	Memphis	TN
Park Avenue Imaging	Orange Park	FL
Park City Hospital	Park City	UT
Park Nicollet Bloomington	Bloomington	MN
Park Nicollet Clinic Burnsville	Burnsville	MN
Park Nicollet Clinic Chanhassen	Chanhassen	MN
Park Nicollet Clinic Jane Brattain Breast Center	St Louis Park	MN
Park Nicollet Clinic Maple Grove	Maple Grove	MN
Park Nicollet Hvc Women's Center	St Louis Park	MN
Park Nicollet Mobile Mammography	St Louis Park	MN
Park Nicollet Wayzata	Wayzata	MN
Park Plaza Radiology	Flint	MI
Park West Imaging	Pueblo	CO
Parkland Health Center - Bjc	Farmington	MO
Parkland Moody Center For Breast Health	Dallas	TX
Parkridge East Hospital	East Ridge	TN
Parkridge Medical Center, Inc. Dba Parkridge Medical Center	Chattanooga	TN
Parkridge West Hospital	Jasper	TN
Parkview Cancer Institute	Fort Wayne	IN
Parkview Dekalb Hospital	Auburn	IN
Parkview Huntington Hospital	Huntington	IN
Parkview Lagrange Hospital	Lagrange	IN
Parkview Medical Center	Pueblo	CO
Parkview Noble Hospital	Kendallville	IN
Parkview Outpatient Radiology	Riverside	CA
Parkview Phys Group Ohio McHa	Bryan	OH
Parkview Wabash Hospital	Wabash	IN
Parkview Warsaw Medical Complex	Warsaw	IN
Parkview Whitley Hospital Breast Diagnostic Center	Columbia City	IN
Parkway Imaging Center	Greenfield	IN
Parkway Medical Center - Women's Diagnostic Center	Myrtle Beach	SC
Parkwest Comprehensive Breast Center	Knoxville	TN
Parrish Medical Group	Titusville	FL
Partners Imaging Center Of Bradenton	Bradenton	FL
Partners Imaging Center Of Sarasota	Sarasota	FL
Partners In Womens Healthcare Pc	Lemoyne	PA
Pasco Imaging And Open Mri	Hudson	FL
Passavant Memorial Area Hospital	Jacksonville	IL
Paul B. Hall Regional Medical Center	Paintsville	KY
Paulding County Hospital	Paulding	OH
Pavilion Imaging St Marys Hospital	Grand Junction	CO
Pawnee County Memorial Hospital	Pawnee City	NE
Pawnee Indian Health Center	Pawnee	OK
Pawnee Valley Community Hospital	Larned	KS
Pdc Memorial Hospital Assoc, Inc.,Dba Crossing Rivers Health	Prairie Du Chien	WI
Peace Harbor Medical Center	Florence	OR
Peace Island Medical Center	Friday Harbor	WA
Peacehealth Cottage Grove Community Medical Center	Cottage Grove	OR
Peacehealth Ketchikan Medical Center	Ketchikan	AK
Peacehealth Sw Medical Center - Kearney Breast Center	Vancouver	WA
Peachtree City Obstetrics And Gynecology, Pc	Peachtree City	GA
Peachtree Women's Clinic	Atlanta	GA
Peachtree Women's Clinic	Cumming	GA
Pearland Mri & Imaging Center	Pearland	TX
Pearlie Harris Center For Breast Health	Greenville	SC
Peeples Cancer Institute	Dalton	GA
Pella Regional Health Center	Pella	IA
Pella Regional Health Center - Ottumwa	Ottumwa	IA
Pembroke Pink Imaging	Pembroke Pines	FL
Pender Community Hospital	Pender	NE
Pender Health And Diagnostics	Rocky Point	NC
Pendleton Community Care Inc	Franklin	WV
Peninsula Breast Center Of Tidalhealth Peninsula Regional	Salisbury	MD
Peninsula Diagnostic Imaging, Inc.	San Mateo	CA
Peninsula Imaging, L.L.C	Salisbury	MD
Penn Highlands Brookville	Brookville	PA
Penn Highlands Elk	St Marys	PA
Penn Highlands Huntingdon	Huntingdon	PA
Penn Med. Princeton Med.Ctr. Breast Health Center	East Windsor	NJ
Penn Medicine At Radnor	Radnor	PA
Penn Medicine At Valley Forge	Berwyn	PA
Penn Medicine Cherry Hill	Cherry Hill	NJ
Penn Medicine Lancaster General Health Parkesburg	Parkesburg	PA
Penn Medicine Princeton Medical Center	Plainsboro	NJ
Penn Medicine Southern Chester County	West Grove	PA
Penn Medicine Woodbury	Woodbury Heights	NJ
Penn State Health Camp Hill Outpatient Center	Camp Hill	PA
Penn State Health Carlisle Outpatient Center	Carlisle	PA
Penn State Health Century Drive Outpatient Center	Mechanicsburg	PA
Penn State Health Dillsburg Outpatient Center	Dillsburg	PA
Penn State Health Duncannon Outpatient Center	Duncannon	PA
Penn State Health Medical Group - Lime Spring	Lancaster	PA
Penn State Health Medical Group Union Deposit Diagnostic Ce	Harrisburg	PA
Penn State Health Progress Outpatient Center	Harrisburg	PA
Penn State Health Silver Creek Outpatient Center	Mechanicsburg	PA
Penn State Health Trindle Road Outpatient Center	Mechanicsburg	PA
Penn State Medical Group Camp Hill	Camp Hill	PA
Penn State Milton S Hershey Medical Center	Hershey	PA
Pennsburg Outpatient Center Of Grand View Hospital	Pennsburg	PA
Pennsville Radiology	Pennsville	NJ
Pennsylvania Hospital Center For Breast Imaging	Philadelphia	PA
Penobscot Valley Hospital	Lincoln	ME
Penrad Imaging	Colorado Springs	CO
Penrad Imaging At Broadmoor	Colorado Springs	CO
Penrad Imaging At Sisters Grove Pavilion	Colorado Springs	CO
Penrad Imaging At Tri-Lakes Pavilion	Monument	CO
People's Health Centers, Inc.	Saint Louis	MO
Pepino Health Group Inc.	San Sebastian	PR
Pequot Health Center	Groton	CT
Perham Health	Perham	MN
Perkins County Health Services	Grant	NE
Permian Regional Medical Center	Andrews	TX
Perry County Memorial Hospital	Tell City	IN
Perry County Memorial Hospital	Perryville	MO
Perry Hospital	Perry	GA
Perry Memorial Hospital	Princeton	IL
Pershing Memorial Hospital	Brookfield	MO
Person Memorial Hospital	Roxboro	NC
Perth Amboy Diagnostic Imaging	Perth Amboy	NJ
Perth Broadalbin Primary Care	Perth	NY
Pet-Ct & Mri Of Miami Llc	Miami	FL
Peter Christensen Health Center	Lac Du Flambeau	WI
Petersburg Medical Center	Petersburg	AK
Peterson Afb 21 Mdg Mdss/Sgsar	Peterson Afb	CO
Phc-Cleveland Dba Bolivar Medical Center	Cleveland	MS
Phelps Health	Rolla	MO
Phelps Health	Waynesville	MO
Phelps Hospital At Dobbs Ferry	Dobbs Ferry	NY
Phelps Hospital Croton On Hudson	Croton On Hudson	NY
Phelps Memorial Breast Center	Sleepy Hollow	NY
Phelps Memorial Health Center	Holdrege	NE
Phila. Dept. Of Health District 2	Philadelphia	PA
Philadelphia Department Of Public Health, Health Center 10	Philadelphia	PA
Philadelphia Department Of Public Health, Health Center 4	Philadelphia	PA
Philadelphia Department Of Public Health, Health Center 5	Philadelphia	PA
Phillips County Hospital	Phillipsburg	KS
Phoebe Sumter Medical Center	Americus	GA
Phoenix Indian Medical Center	Phoenix	AZ
Phoenixville Hospital	Phoenixville	PA
Phoenixville Hospital Outpatient Center At Limerick	Limerick	PA
Physicians East P.A. Greenville Women's Clinic	Greenville	NC
Physicians East - Greenville Obstetrics And Gynecology	Greenville	NC
Physicians East Diagnostic Center	Greenville	NC
Physicians East Farmville	Farmville	NC
Physicians East Pa Kinston	Kinston	NC
Physicians For Women Of Greensboro	Greensboro	NC
Physicians For Women's Health Dba Central Ct Ob/Gyn	Southington	CT
Physicians For Women's Health, Llc	Worcester	MA
Physicians Imaging-Lake City, Llc	Lake City	FL
Physicians Regional Healthcare System	Naples	FL
Physicians Regional Medical Center Collier Blvd.	Naples	FL
Physicians To Women Pa	Port St Lucie	FL
Physicians To Women Pa	Stuart	FL
Physicians To Women, Inc.	Roanoke	VA
Pickens County Primary Care, Pc	Reform	AL

Name	City	State
Piedmont Athens Regional Medical Center Inc.	Athens	GA
Piedmont Comprehensive Women's Center	High Point	NC
Piedmont Fayette Women's Imaging	Fayetteville	GA
Piedmont Healthcare Imaging Center	Statesville	NC
Piedmont Healthcare Mooresville Mammography	Mooresville	NC
Piedmont Henry Breast Health Center	Stockbridge	GA
Piedmont Henry Hospital	Stockbridge	GA
Piedmont Imaging	Winston Salem	NC
Piedmont Imaging At Kennesaw	Kennesaw	GA
Piedmont Imaging Brookhaven	Atlanta	GA
Piedmont Mountainside Hospital	Jasper	GA
Piedmont Mountainside Hospital OP Diagnostic Center	East Ellijay	GA
Piedmont Mountainside Hospital Outpt Imaging Ctr Canton	Canton	GA
Piedmont Newnan Faye Hendrix-Ware Breast Health Center	Newnan	GA
Piedmont Newton Hospital	Covington	GA
Piedmont Oconee Health Campus	Watkinsville	GA
Piedmont Outpatient Center	Newnan	GA
Piedmont Rockdale Hospital	Conyers	GA
Piedmont Royston Health Campus	Royston	GA
Piedmont Walton Hospital	Monroe	GA
Piedmont West Mammography Center	Atlanta	GA
Pih Health Breast Center Whittier	Whittier	CA
Pih Health Hospital-Downey	Downey	CA
Pih Health Mammography Hacienda Heights	Hacienda Heights	CA
Pike County Medical Center	Hawley	PA
Pike County Memorial Hospital	Louisiana	MO
Pikeville Medical Ctr Diagnostic Ctr	Pikeville	KY
Pinckneyville Community Hospital	Pinckneyville	IL
Pine Ridge Reservation Comprehensive Health Care Ctr	Pine Ridge	SD
Pinehurst Radiology Associates	Pinehurst	NC
Pinehurst Surgical Clinic	Pinehurst	NC
Pineville Community Health Center	Pineville	KY
Pineywoods Healthcare System, Lp	Lufkin	TX
Pink Breast Center	Flemington	NJ
Pink Breast Center	Paterson	NJ
Pink Monarch Breast Center	Columbus	GA
Pink Monarch Breast Center North	Columbus	GA
Pink Ribbon Mammography Woman's Clinic	Jackson	TN
Pinnacle Diagnostic Radiology At Bay Parkway	Brooklyn	NY
Pinnacle Hospital	Crown Point	IN
Pinnacle Imaging Center	Miami	FL
Pinnacle Medical Group	Rialto	CA
Pioneer Medical Group - Artesia Facility	Bellflower	CA
Pioneers Memorial Healthcare District	Brawley	CA
Pipeline East Dallas, Llc	Dallas	TX
Piper Breast Center - Mercy Hospital	Coon Rapids	MN
Piper Breast Center Westhealth	Plymouth	MN
Piper Breast Center-United	Saint Paul	MN
Pipestone County Medical Center	Pipestone	MN
Pittsburg Health Center	Pittsburg	CA
Placer Center For Health	Rocklin	CA
Plainfield Backus Emergency Care Center	Plainfield	CT
Plains Regional Medical Center - Clovis	Clovis	NM
Plains Regional Mob	Clovis	NM
Plainview Radiology, Llc	Plainview	TX
Plant City Imaging	Plant City	FL
Plateau Medical Center	Oak Hill	WV
Platte County Memorial Hospital	Wheatland	WY
Platte Health Center Avera	Platte	SD
Platte Valley Medical Center	Brighton	CO
Pleasant Valley Hospital	Point Pleasant	WV
Pleasanton Diagnostic Imaging	Pleasanton	CA
Plg Breast Imaging Services,Psc	Guaynabo	PR
Plumas District Hospital	Quincy	CA
Pmc Hospital, Llc	Pasadena	TX
Pocahontas Community Hospital	Pocahontas	IA
Pocahontas Medical Clinic	Pocahontas	AR
Poinciana Medical Center	Kissimmee	FL
Pointe Coupee General Hospital	New Roads	LA
Policlinica Bella Vista	Mayaguez	PR
Polk Medical Center	Cedartown	GA
Pom Mri & Imaging Center Of Cooper City	Cooper City	FL
Pom Mri & Imaging Center Of Plantation	Plantation	FL
Pom Mri & Radiology Center Of Fort Lauderdale	Fort Lauderdale	FL
Pomerene Hospital	Millersburg	OH
Pomona Valley Imaging Center At Chino Hills	Chino Hills	CA
Pomona Valley Imaging Center At Laverne	La Verne	CA
Pomona Valley Imaging Ctr Claremont	Claremont	CA
Port Orange Imaging Center	Port Orange	FL
Port Royal Medical Center	Port Royal	SC
Porter Breast Care	Denver	CO
Portneuf Medical Center	Pocatello	ID
Portsmouth Imaging Center	Portsmouth	RI
Potomac Valley Hospital	Keyser	WV
Pottstown Hospital	Pottstown	PA
Poudre Valley Hospital - Breast Diagnostic Center	Fort Collins	CO
Poudrevalley Medical Group Llc Dba Colo Health Medical Group	Longmont	CO
Powell Hospital District 1 Dba Powell Valley Healthcare	Powell	WY
Prairie Parkway Imaging	Cedar Falls	IA
Prairie Ridge Health, Inc.	Columbus	WI
Pratt Regional Medical Center	Pratt	KS
Prattville Imaging Center	Prattville	AL
Preble County Medical Center	Eaton	OH
Precise Radiological Associates, Inc.	Yuba City	CA
Precision Health Center	Miami	FL
Precision Imaging Centers	Fleming Island	FL
Precision Imaging Centers	Fleming Island	FL
Precision Imaging Centers - St. Augustine	St Augustine	FL
Precision Imaging Centers-Beach	Jacksonville	FL
Premier Diagnostic Imaging, L.L.C.	Cookeville	TN
Premier Imaging	High Point	NC
Premier Medical Associates	Monroeville	PA
Premier Medical Group, P.C.	Clarksville	TN
Premier Obgyn Of Minnesota Pa	Minnetonka	MN
Premier Physicians Center	Westlake	OH
Premier Radiology Antioch	Antioch	TN
Premier Radiology Belle Meade	Nashville	TN
Premier Radiology Bellevue	Nashville	TN
Premier Radiology Brentwood	Brentwood	TN
Premier Radiology Briarville	Madison	TN
Premier Radiology Cool Springs	Franklin	TN
Premier Radiology Gallatin	Gallatin	TN
Premier Radiology Hendersonville	Hendersonville	TN
Premier Radiology Hermitage	Hermitage	TN
Premier Radiology Lenox Village	Nashville	TN
Premier Radiology Mt Juliet	Mt Juliet	TN
Premier Radiology Mt. Pleasant	Mt Pleasant	WI
Premier Radiology Nashville	Nashville	TN
Premier Radiology New Salem	Murfreesboro	TN
Premier Radiology Smyrna	Smyrna	TN
Premier Womens Care	Cape Coral	FL
Premier Womens Care	Fort Myers	FL
Premium Heath Group Clinic	Carolina	PR
Prescott Medical Imaging	Prescott	AZ
Presence Healing Arts Pavilion Romeoville	Romeoville	IL
Presence Mercy Medical Center	Aurora	IL
Presence St. Mary's Hospital	Kankakee	IL
Presentation Medical Center	Rolla	ND
Preston Memorial Hospital	Kingwood	WV
Prevost Memorial Hospital	Donaldsonville	LA
Prhc - Ennis, Lp Dba Ennis Regional Medical Ctr	Ennis	TX
Price, Hoffman, Stone And Associates, M.D.'s, P.A.	St Petersburg	FL
Primacare Diagnostic Center	Fall River	MA
Primary Care Associates Of Appleton, Ltd	Appleton	WI
Primary Care Centers Of Eastern Kentucky	Hazard	KY
Primary Care Physicians Of Joliet Sc	Joliet	IL
Prime Care Medical Center	Selmer	TN
Prime Health Care Services-Lower Bucks Hospital	Bristol	PA
Prime Healthcare Services - Mesquite, Llc	Mesquite	TX
Prime Healthcare Services - Pampa, Llc	Pampa	TX
Prime Healthcare Services - Roxborough Memorial Hospital	Philadelphia	PA
Prime Healthcare Services - St. Mary's Passaic, Llc	Passaic	NJ
Prime Healthcare Services Garden City Llc	Garden City	MI
Prime Healthcare Services-Landmark,Llc	Woonsocket	RI
Prime Healthcare Women's Center At Spivey Station	Jonesboro	GA
Prime Imaging And Vein Center	Chattanooga	TN
Prime Imaging Battlefield	Ringgold	GA
Prime Imaging Chattanooga Outpatient Ctr.	Chattanooga	TN
Prime Imaging Hixson	Hixson	TN
Prime Medical Imaging	Mokena	IL
Primehealtcare Services- St Francis, Llc Dba St. Francis Med	Lynwood	CA
Princeton Baptist Medical Center	Birmingham	AL
Princeton Community Hospital - Medical Imaging Center Oceana		WV
Princeton Radiology	Freehold	NJ
Princeton Radiology	Mercerville	NJ
Princeton Radiology Associates	Englishtown	NJ
Princeton Radiology Associates, P.A.	Monroe	NJ
Princeton Radiology Associates, P.A.	Princeton	NJ
Prisma Health - Oconee Memorial Hospital	Seneca	SC
Prisma Health Baptist Easley Hospital	Easley	SC
Prisma Health Baptist Parkridge	Columbia	SC

Alphabetical Index

Name	City	State
Prisma Health Breast Center	Columbia	SC
Prisma Health Breast Center	Sumter	SC
Prisma Health Greer Memorial Hospital	Greer	SC
Prisma Health Hillcrest Hospital	Simpsonville	SC
Prisma Health Laurens County Hospital	Clinton	SC
Prisma Health North Greenville Hospital	Travelers Rest	SC
Prisma Health Outpatient Radiology	Greenville	SC
Prisma Health Patewood Medical Campus	Greenville	SC
Prisma Health Richland Breast Center	Columbia	SC
Pro Healthcare Associates, Llp	Huntington	NY
Pro-Life Imaging Llc	Long Beach	CA
Professional Imaging Centers	Kissimmee	FL
Professional Imaging Centers	Orlando	FL
Professional Imaging Of Lvmc	Lompoc	CA
Professional Medical Ultrasonics	Beckley	WV
Professional Radiology, Pllc	El Paso	TX
Professionals For Women's Health	Columbus	OH
Progress West Hospital	Ofallon	MO
Progressive Community Health Center	Milwaukee	WI
Progressive Radiology	Winchester	VA
Prohealth Medical Group Delafield Street	Waukesha	WI
Prohealth Oconomowoc Memorial Hospital	Oconomowoc	WI
Prohealth Radiology Behtpage	Bethpage	NY
Prohealth Radiology Of Plainview	Plainview	NY
Prohealth Radiology Rockville Centre	Rockville Centre	NY
Prohealth Waukesha Mem. Hosp Dba D.N.Greenwald Ctr-Mukwonago	Mukwonago	WI
Prohealth Waukesha Memorial Hospital - New Berlin	New Berlin	WI
Prohealth Waukesha Memorial Hospital-Brookfield	Brookfield	WI
Prohealth Waukesha Memorial Hospital-Pewaukee	Waukesha	WI
Prohealth Women's Imaging & Bone Densitometry	Lake Success	NY
Project Health Inc Dba Langley Health Services Ocala	Ocala	FL
Project Health, Inc.	Sumterville	FL
Project Renewal Scan Van - Mobile	New York	NY
Promedica Bixby Hospital	Adrian	MI
Promedica Breast Care	Toledo	OH
Promedica Defiance Regional Hospital	Defiance	OH
Promedica Flower Hospital A Division Of Promedica Toledo Hos	Sylvania	OH
Promedica Hickman Hosp - Women's Health Center	Adrian	MI
Promedica Monroe Regional Hospital Womens Health Center	Monroe	MI
Promedica Perrysburg	Perrysburg	OH
Proscan Imaging	Naples	FL
Proscan Pink Ribbon Center Tri-County	Cincinnati	OH
Proscan Women's Imaging	Cincinnati	OH
Prospect Chartercare,Sjhsri,Llc Dba Our Lady Of Fatima Hosp	North Providence	RI
Prospect Ct Medical Foundation	Waterbury	CT
Prospect Diagnostic Imaging	Prospect	CT
Prospect Manchester Memorial Hospital	Manchester	CT
Prospect Rockville General Hospital	Rockville	CT
Prospect Rockville Hosp Inc D/B/A Womens Center For Wellness	South Windsor	CT
Prosser Memorial Health Prosser Public Hospital District	Prosser	WA
Providence Canby Health Center	Canby	OR
Providence Cedars-Sinai Tarzana Outpatient Women's Center	Tarzana	CA
Providence Health	Columbia	SC
Providence Health & Services Dba Prov Mount Carmel	Colville	WA
Providence Health & Services-Washington Dba Prmce-Brst Cr	Everett	WA
Providence Health & Services-Washington Dba Prmce-Millcrk	Everett	WA
Providence Health & Services-Washington Dba Prov Imag Ctr	Centralia	WA
Providence Health & Services-Washington Dba Prov Ki Med Ctr	Kodiak	AK
Providence Health & Services-Washington Dba Prov St Joseph	Chewelah	WA
Providence Holy Cross Health Ctr - Porter Ranch	Porter Ranch	CA
Providence Hood River Memorial Hospital	Hood River	OR
Providence Hospital	Washington	DC
Providence Imaging Center	Anchorage	AK
Providence Imaging Center, Inc.	Hendersonville	NC
Providence Imaging Center, Inc.-South Asheville	Asheville	NC
Providence Imaging Center-Mars Hill	Mars Hill	NC
Providence Little Co. Of Mary Women's Imaging Center	Torrance	CA
Providence Little Company Of Mary San Pedro	San Pedro	CA
Providence Medical Center	Kansas City	KS
Providence Medical Center	Wayne	NE
Providence Medical Foundation	Diamond Bar	CA
Providence Medical Foundation C/O St Joseph Heritage Medical	Orange	CA
Providence Medical Group Monroe	Monroe	WA
Providence Medical Imaging Center	Kansas City	KS
Providence Milwaukie Hospital	Milwaukie	OR
Providence Mission Hospital-Laguna Beach	Laguna Beach	CA
Providence Mission Imaging Center	Mission Viejo	CA
Providence Newberg Medical Center	Newberg	OR
Providence Saint John's Health Center	Santa Monica	CA
Providence Saint Joseph Breast Health Center	Burbank	CA
Providence Seaside Hospital	Seaside	OR
Providence Southeast Diagnostic Imaging	Portland	OR
Providence St Mary Medical Center	Walla Walla	WA
Providence St. Joseph Medical Center	Polson	MT
Providence St.Vincent Medical Center	Portland	OR
Providence Willamette Falls Medical Center	Oregon City	OR
Provident Hospital Of Cook County	Chicago	IL
Prowers Medical Center	Lamar	CO
Pueblo Medical Imaging	Henderson	NV
Pueblo Medical Imaging	Las Vegas	NV
Pueblo Medical Imaging	Las Vegas	NV
Pueblo Medical Imaging	Las Vegas	NV
Puerto Rico Imaging Center	Bayamon	PR
Pulaski Memorial Hospital	Winamac	IN
Pullman Regional Hospital	Pullman	WA
Punxsutawney Area Hospital	Punxsutawney	PA
Putnam County Hospital	Greencastle	IN
Putnam County Memorial Hospital	Unionville	MO
Putnam Diagnostic Imaging Center	Palatka	FL
Putnam General Hospital	Eatonton	GA
Putnam Hospital Center	Carmel	NY
Putnam Radiology Group	Palatka	FL
Pwh, Llc D/B/A Women's Health Breast Imaging Of Waterbury	Waterbury	CT
Qualcare Medical Group	Pembroke Pines	FL
Queen Of The Valley Medical Center	Napa	CA
Queens Hospital Center	Jamaica	NY
Queens Physicians Office Bldg., III	Honolulu	HI
Quentin N. Burdick Mem. Hlth Care Fac. - Phs Indian Hospital	Belcourt	ND
Quincy Medical Group	Pittsfield	IL
Quincy Medical Group	Quincy	IL
Radiation Oncology Of The South Plains Pa	Lubbock	TX
Radiation Oncology Of The South Plains, Pa	Live Oak	TX
Radilogia Del Turabo, C.S.P. D/B/A Quadrangle Imaging Center	Caguas	PR
Radioimagenes Diagnosticas	Moca	PR
Radiologic Associates Of Northern New Jersey, P.A. Vernon	Vernon	NJ
Radiology & Imaging Of South Texas	Corpus Christi	TX
Radiology & Imaging Of South Texas	Corpus Christi	TX
Radiology Affiliates Imaging/Capital Health Imaging, Llc	Hamilton Township	NJ
Radiology Affiliates Lawrenceville	Lawrenceville	NJ
Radiology And Imaging Specialists	Lakeland	FL
Radiology And Mri Of Bethlehem	Bethlehem	PA
Radiology Associates P.A.-Searcy	Searcy	AR
Radiology Associates Imaging Deltona	Deltona	FL
Radiology Associates Llp	Corpus Christi	TX
Radiology Associates Llp	Portland	TX
Radiology Associates Of Brooklyn	Brooklyn	NY
Radiology Associates Of Brooklyn Llp	Brooklyn	NY
Radiology Associates Of Brooklyn, Llp	Brooklyn	NY
Radiology Associates Of Hackettstown Llc	Hackettstown	NJ
Radiology Associates Of Hartford P.C	Bloomfield	CT
Radiology Associates Of Hartford P.C.	Enfield	CT
Radiology Associates Of Hartford P.C.	Glastonbury	CT
Radiology Associates Of Hartford, P. C. - Avon, Ct	Avon	CT
Radiology Associates Of Ridgewood, P.A.	Waldwick	NJ
Radiology Associates Of Venice & Englewood	Englewood	FL
Radiology Associates Of Venice & Englewood	Sarasota	FL

Name	City	State
Radiology Associates Of Venice & Englewood	Venice	FL
Radiology Associates, L.L.P.	Alice	TX
Radiology Associates, L.L.P.	Corpus Christi	TX
Radiology Associates, Llp	Corpus Christi	TX
Radiology Clinics Of Laredo	Laredo	TX
Radiology Consultants	Hollywood	FL
Radiology Consultants Of Iowa, Plc	Cedar Rapids	IA
Radiology Diagnostic Center	Templeton	CA
Radiology Group, P.C.	Branford	CT
Radiology Group, P.C.	Hamden	CT
Radiology Imaging Associates	Fort Pierce	FL
Radiology Imaging Associates	Port Saint Lucie	FL
Radiology Imaging Associates	Stuart	FL
Radiology Imaging Specialists Llc	Ocala	FL
Radiology Ltd La Cholla Center For Diagnostic Imaging	Tucson	AZ
Radiology Ltd Midvale Imaging Center	Tucson	AZ
Radiology Ltd Wilmot Ctr For Women's Imaging	Tucson	AZ
Radiology Ltd. Green Valley Casa Verde	Green Valley	AZ
Radiology Ltd. Green Valley Continental	Green Valley	AZ
Radiology Ltd. St. Mary's Medical Plaza	Tucson	AZ
Radiology Ltd., Rancho Vistoso Diagnostic Imaging	Oro Valley	AZ
Radiology Ltd., Rincon Imaging Center	Tucson	AZ
Radiology Medical Group Of Santa Cruz County, Inc.	Santa Cruz	CA
Radiology Muskegon, P.C. Breast Imaging Center	Muskegon	MI
Radiology Regional Center	Bonita Springs	FL
Radiology Regional Center	Cape Coral	FL
Radiology Regional Center	Cape Coral	FL
Radiology Regional Center	Cape Coral	FL
Radiology Regional Center	Estero	FL
Radiology Regional Center	Fort Myers	FL
Radiology Regional Center	Fort Myers	FL
Radiology Regional Center	Lehigh Acres	FL
Radiology Regional Center	Lehigh Acres	FL
Radiology Regional Center	Naples	FL
Radiology Regional Center	Naples	FL
Radiology Regional Center	Port Charlotte	FL
Radiology Regional Center - Mobile Unit	Fort Myers	FL
Rainelle Medical Center, Inc.	Rainelle	WV
Rainy Lake Medical Center	International Falls	MN
Raleigh General Hospital	Beckley	WV
Raleigh Radiology Clayton	Clayton	NC
Raleigh Radiology Fuquay Varina	Fuquay Varina	NC
Raleigh Radiology Knightdale	Knightdale	NC
Raleigh Radiology Oberlin	Raleigh	NC
Raleigh Radiology Wake Forest	Wake Forest	NC
Raleigh Radiology- Cary	Cary	NC
Raleigh Radiology-Blue Ridge	Raleigh	NC
Ralph Lauren Center For Cancer Care And Prevention	New York	NY
Ramapo Diagnostics Imaging	Suffern	NY
Rancho San Antonio Medical Center	Rancho Cucamonga	CA
Rancho Springs Medical Center	Murrieta	CA
Randolph Air Force Base 359th Med Group	Randolph Afb	TX
Randolph Hospital	Asheboro	NC
Range Regional Health Services Mesaba Clinic Hibbing	Hibbing	MN
Rangely District Hospital	Rangely	CO
Ransom Memorial Hospital	Ottawa	KS
Rapid City Medical Center, Llp	Rapid City	SD
Rapides Breast Imaging Center	Alexandria	LA
Rapides Regional Medical Center	Alexandria	LA
Raritan Bay Medical Center Old Bridge Division	Old Bridge	NJ
Raritan Bay Medical Center Pad	Perth Amboy	NJ
Raulerson Hospital	Okeechobee	FL
Ravenswood Family Health Center	East Palo Alto	CA
Ray County Memorial Hospital	Richmond	MO
Rayos X Centro 4	Trujillo Alto	PR
Rcch Trios Health Llc, Dba Trios Health	Kennewick	WA
Reading Hospital At Spring Ridge, Breast Health Center	Wyomissing	PA
Reading Hospital Imaging Center At Exeter	Reading	PA
Reagan Medical Center, L.L.C., Dba/Georgia Diagnostic Center Lawrenceville		GA
Red Bank Radiologists, P.A.	Little Silver	NJ
Red Bay Hospital	Red Bay	AL
Red Bud Regional Hospital	Red Bud	IL
Red Lake Indian Hospital	Redlake	MN
Red Rock Radiology A Department Of Mountainview Hosp.	Las Vegas	NV
Redington-Fairview General Hospital	Skowhegan	ME
Redlandsfamily practice medical group, Inc.	San Bernardino	CA
Redmond Regional Medical Center	Rome	GA
Redstone Mammography Center	Park City	UT
Redwood Health Center	Salt Lake City	UT
Redwood Memorial Hospital	Fortuna	CA
Reedsburg Area Medical Center	Reedsburg	WI
Reeves County Hospital District	Pecos	TX
Regenstein Breast Imaging Center	Chicago	IL
Regina Hospital, Part Of Allina Health	Hastings	MN
Regional Breast Care Center	Bangor	ME
Regional Family Medicine, Pa	Mountain Home	AR
Regional Health Medical Clinic-Dpt Reg Health Spearfish Hosp	Spearfish	SD
Regional Health Services Of Howard County	Cresco	IA
Regional Management Service Organization,Llc	Staten Island	NY
Regional Management Service Organization,Llc	Staten Island	NY
Regional Medical Center	Manchester	IA
Regional Medical Center Mediplex - Oxford	Oxford	AL
Regional Medical Center Of Central Alabama	Greenville	AL
Regional Medical Imaging	Davison	MI
Regional Medical Imaging	Fenton	MI
Regional Medical Imaging	Flint	MI
Regional Medical Imaging	Flint	MI
Regional Medical Imaging	Grand Blanc	MI
Regional Medical Imaging	Lapeer	MI
Regional Medical Imaging	Royal Oak	MI
Regional Medical Imaging Pc	Southgate	MI
Regional Medical Imaging, Pc	Novi	MI
Regional One Health	Memphis	TN
Regional One Health East	Memphis	TN
Regional West Medical Center	Scottsbluff	NE
Regional Women's Health Group, Llc - Bridgewater	Bridgewater	NJ
Regional Women's Health Group, Llc - East Brunswick	East Brunswick	NJ
Regional Women's Health Group, Llc - Haverford	Haverford	PA
Regional Women's Health Group, Llc - Limerick	Limerick	PA
Regional Women's Health Group, Llc - West Orange	West Orange	NJ
Regional Women's Health Group,Llc-Paoli	Paoli	PA
Regional Womens Health Group Llc - Langhorne	Langhorne	PA
Regions Breast Health Center	Saint Paul	MN
Rehoboth McKinley Christian Hospital	Gallup	NM
Reid Health Mammography	Richmond	IN
Reid Health-Connersville	Connersville	IN
Reliant Medical Group	Leominster	MA
Reliant Medical Group	Southborough	MA
Reliant Medical Group	Worcester	MA
Renaissance Health Care Network	New York	NY
Renaissance Austin Breast Imaging, Llc	Austin	TX
Renaissance Imaging Ctr At Antelope Valley Hospital [avoic]	Lancaster	CA
Renaissance Imaging Medical Associates, Inc.	Los Angeles	CA
Renaissance Imaging Medical Associates, Inc.	Northridge	CA
Renaissance Imaging Medical Associates, Inc.	Westlake Village	CA
Reno Diagnostic Center	Reno	NV
Reno Diagnostic Centers	Reno	NV
Renown Breast Health Center	Reno	NV
Renown Health X-Ray And Imaging Services At South McCarran	Reno	NV
Renown Imaging And X-Ray At Vista	Sparks	NV
Republic County Hospital	Belleville	KS
Research Medical Center	Kansas City	MO
Research Medical Center Brookside Campus	Kansas City	MO
Resolute Health Hospital	New Braunfels	TX
Resurrection Medical Center Women's Imaging Center	Chicago	IL
Retreat Doctors' Hosp-A Campus Of Henrico Doctors' Hospital	Richmond	VA
Revere Health Imaging St. George	St George	UT
Revere Health Imaging, American Fork	American Fork	UT
Revere Health Imaging, Provo	Provo	UT
Revere Health Imaging, Salem	Salem	UT
Rexville Radiology	Bayamon	PR
Reynolds Army Health Clinic	Fort Sill	OK
Rgh Mobile Mammography Center	Rochester	NY
Rghs Imaging At Alexander Park	Rochester	NY
Rghs Imaging At Cross Keys	Fairport	NY
Rghs Imaging At Mob	Rochester	NY
Rhea Medical Center	Dayton	TN
Rhode Island Medical Imaging	Cranston	RI
Rhode Island Medical Imaging	East Providence	RI
Rhode Island Medical Imaging	Johnston	RI
Rhode Island Medical Imaging	Lincoln	RI

Name	City	State
Rhode Island Medical Imaging	North Providence	RI
Rhode Island Medical Imaging	Warwick	RI
Rhode Island Medical Imaging, Inc	Providence	RI
Rhode Island Medical Imaging, Inc.	East Greenwich	RI
Rhode Island Medical Imaging, Inc.	Pawtucket	RI
Rhode Island Medical Imaging, Inc.	Riverside	RI
Rhs-Clyburn Center For Primary Care	Aiken	SC
Ricardo T. Baldonado, M.D., North Jersey Imaging Center	West New York	NJ
Riceland Diagnostic Health	Port Arthur	TX
Richardson Medical Center	Rayville	LA
Richland Memorial Hospital, Inc.	Olney	IL
Richland Parish Hospital	Delhi	LA
Richmond Hill Radiology	Richmond Hill	NY
Richmond Hill Radiology Pc	Flushing	NY
Ridgecrest Regional Hospital Womens Imaging	Ridgecrest	CA
Ridgeview Le Sueur Medical Center	Le Sueur	MN
Ridgeview Medical Center	Waconia	MN
Ridgeview Sibley Medical Center	Arlington	MN
Riedman Health Center Imaging	Rochester	NY
Ringgold County Hospital	Mount Ayr	IA
Rio Pecos Medical Associates, Ltd.	Roswell	NM
Ripon Community Hospital	Ripon	WI
Ris & Lrh Pablo Campus	Lakeland	FL
River City Imaging Centers, Llc	New Braunfels	TX
River Falls Area Hospital	River Falls	WI
River Forest Breast Care Center	River Forest	IL
River Hospital Inc	Alexandria Bay	NY
River Radiology	Kingston	NY
River's Edge Hospital And Clinic	St Peter	MN
Rivero Diagnostic Center, Inc	Hialeah	FL
Riverpark Imaging Center	Vidalia	LA
Riverside Community Hospital Breast Imaging Center	Riverside	CA
Riverside Diagnostic And Breast Imaging Center	Newport News	VA
Riverside Diagnostic Center - Williamsburg	Williamsburg	VA
Riverside Diagnostic Center Hampton	Hampton	VA
Riverside Healthcare	Kankakee	IL
Riverside Medical Center	Franklinton	LA
Riverside Medical Center Bourbonnais Plaza	Bourbonnais	IL
Riverside Medical Center West Campus	Coal City	IL
Riverside Medical Clinic	Riverside	CA
Riverside Medical Clinic	Riverside	CA
Riverside Medical Clinic	Riverside	CA
Riverside Shore Memorial Hospital	Onancock	VA
Riverside University Health System - Medical Center	Moreno Valley	CA
Riverside Walter Reed Hospital	Gloucester	VA
Riverton Hospital	Riverton	UT
Riverton Memorial Hospital, Llc, D/B/A Sagewest Health Care.	Riverton	WY
Riverview Health	Crookston	MN
Riverview Health Westfield Hospital	Westfield	IN
Riverview Medical Center	Red Bank	NJ
Riverview Regional Medical Center	Carthage	TN
Riverview Women's Center	Noblesville	IN
Riverway Clinics Elk River	Elk River	MN
Riverwood Clinic McGregor	McGregor	MN
Riverwood Garrison Clinic	Garrison	MN
Riverwood Healthcare Center	Aitkin	MN
Riverwoods Advanced Diagnostic Imaging Center	Provo	UT
Rj Imaging	Panorama City	CA
Rm Imaging, Inc.	Boca Raton	FL
Roane General Hospital	Spencer	WV
Roane Medical Center	Harriman	TN
Robert And Audrey Luckow Pavillion	Paramus	NJ
Robert L. Bard, M.D., P.C.	New York	NY
Robert Packer Hospital Towanda Campus	Towanda	PA
Robert Stoico Fed Ctr For Breast Care St Anne's Hosp	Fall River	MA
Robert Wood Johnson University Hospital At Hamilton	Hamilton	NJ
Robert Wood Johnson University Hospital Rahway	Rahway	NJ
Robinwood Diagnostic Imaging Services Llc	Hagerstown	MD
Rochelle Community Hospital	Rochelle	IL
Rock County Hospital	Bassett	NE
Rock Creek Medical Imaging	Rock Springs	WY
Rockcastle Regional Hospital	Mount Vernon	KY
Rockland Diagnostic Imaging	West Nyack	NY
Rockledge Mri & Pet Center	Rockledge	FL
Rockwall Regional Hospital Llc	Rockwall	TX
Rockwood Clinic P.S.	Spokane	WA
Rocky Mount Family Medical Center	Rocky Mount	NC
Roger Williams Medical Center	Providence	RI
Rolling Oaks Imaging Center	Thousand Oaks	CA
Rolling Oaks Radiology - Camarillo	Camarillo	CA
Rolling Oaks Radiology Oxnard	Oxnard	CA
Rolling Oaks Radiology Ventura	Ventura	CA
Rolling Oaks Radiology-St. John's	Oxnard	CA
Rome Memorial Hospital	Rome	NY
Rooks County Health Center	Plainville	KS
Roosevelt General Hospital	Portales	NM
Roper Hospital	Charleston	SC
Roper Hospital Diagnostics & Er-Berkeley	Moncks Corner	SC
Roper St. Francis Hospital - Berkeley	Summerville	SC
Rosebud Ihs Hospital	Rosebud	SD
Roseland Community Hospital	Chicago	IL
Rosenbaum, Rosenfeld, M.D.'s	New York	NY
Roswell Imaging Center - Wellstar North Fulton Hospital	Roswell	GA
Roswell Park Cancer Institute Mammography Center	Buffalo	NY
Roswell Park Comprehensive Cancer Center, Park Club Lane	Williamsville	NY
Roy Lester Schneider Hospital	St Thomas	VI
Rrh Baycreek Imaging Center	Webster	NY
Rs Nuclear Medicine Pc	Brooklyn	NY
Ruby E Bergman Women's Diagnostic Center	Turlock	CA
Ruhs Medical Surgical Center	Moreno Valley	CA
Rumford Hospital	Rumford	ME
Rush Breast Imaging - Oak Brook	Oak Brook	IL
Rush Breast Imaging-South Loop	Chicago	IL
Rush Copley Health Center Diagnostic Imaging	Yorkville	IL
Rush Copley Medical Center Dba Midwest Ctr For Advanced Img.	Naperville	IL
Rush Imaging Center	Meridian	MS
Rush Memorial Hospital	Rushville	IN
Rush Oak Park Hospital	Oak Park	IL
Russell County Hospital	Russell Springs	KY
Russell Medical Women's Center	Alexander City	AL
Russell Regional Hospital	Russell	KS
Russellville Hospital	Russellville	AL
Rutland Regional Medical Center	Rutland	VT
Rye Radiology Associates, Llp	Rye Brook	NY
S Kfh Mission Viejo	Mission Viejo	CA
S Kfh - Bonita	Bonita	CA
S Kfh - Carlsbad	Carlsbad	CA
S Kfh - San Marcos	San Marcos	CA
S Kfh Clairemont Mesa	San Diego	CA
S Kfh Discovery	Bakersfield	CA
S Kfh Garden Grove	Garden Grove	CA
S Kfh Hesperia	Hesperia	CA
S Kfh Lancaster	Lancaster	CA
S Kfh Ming	Bakersfield	CA
S Kfh North Hollywood Medical Offices	N Hollywood	CA
S Kfh Palmdale	Palmdale	CA
S Kfh Santa Clarita	Santa Clarita	CA
S Kfh Stockdale	Bakersfield	CA
S Kfh West Covina Kaiser Permanente-West Covina	West Covina	CA
S Khf Euclid Medical Offices	Anaheim	CA
S Khf Santa Ana Harbor Macarthur Facility	Santa Ana	CA
Sabal Park Clinic	Tampa	FL
Sabetha Community Hospital	Sabetha	KS
Sacred Heart Hospital D/B/A Prevea Health- Mobile	Altoona	WI
Sacred Heart Hospital Of The Hospital Sisters Of The Third O	Eau Claire	WI
Sacred Heart Hospital On The Gulf	Port St Joe	FL
Safeway Foundation Breast Ctr, Providence Portland Med. Ctr	Portland	OR
Sage Women's Imaging And Specialty Ultrasound	Klamath Falls	OR
Sagewest Lander	Lander	WY
Sagoff Breast Imaging And Diagnostic Centre	Boston	MA
Saint Alphonsus Med Ctr Ontario	Ontario	OR
Saint Alphonsus Nampa Breast Care Center	Nampa	ID
Saint Alphonsus R.M.C. Breast Care Center	Boise	ID
Saint Alphonsus Rmc Mobile Health Screening Unit - Mobile	Boise	ID
Saint Clare's Hospital/Dover General	Dover	NJ
Saint Clare's Imaging Center At Parsippany Commons	Parsippany	NJ
Saint Francis Breast Health Services	Tulsa	OK
Saint Francis Broken Arrow Imaging Center	Broken Arrow	OK
Saint Francis Glenpool	Glenpool	OK
Saint Francis Hospital - Bartlett	Bartlett	TN
Saint Francis Hospital Muskogee Breast Care Center	Muskogee	OK
Saint Francis Hospital Vinita	Vinita	OK
Saint Francis Medical Center - Womancare	Cape Girardeau	MO
Saint Francis Medical Partners Kneibert Clinic	Poplar Bluff	MO
Saint Francis Outpatient Center - Pb	Poplar Bluff	MO
Saint Joseph - London	London	KY
Saint Joseph Breast Care At Saint Joseph East	Lexington	KY

Name	City	State
Saint Joseph Hospital Amita Health - Chicago	Chicago	IL
Saint Joseph Hospital Breast Care Center	Denver	CO
Saint Joseph Hospital Mobile Mammo Unit-Mobile	Denver	CO
Saint Joseph Jessamine	Nicholasville	KY
Saint Joseph Mercy Breast Imaging	Brighton	MI
Saint Joseph Mercy Breast Imaging	Howell	MI
Saint Joseph Mercy Breast Imaging	Ypsilanti	MI
Saint Joseph Mercy Chelsea, Inc	Chelsea	MI
Saint Joseph Mount Sterling	Mt Sterling	KY
Saint Joseph Regional Medical Center	Plymouth	IN
Saint Joseph Regional Medical Ctr-South Bend Campus, Inc	Mishawaka	IN
Saint Joseph's Imaging At Riverdale	Bronx	NY
Saint Luke's East Hospital	Lees Summit	MO
Saint Lukes Hospital Dba Wright Memorial Hospital	Trenton	MO
Saint Lukes's Mammography-Blue Springs	Blue Springs	MO
Saint Mary's Hospital	Waterbury	CT
Saint Mary's Medical Group Inc	Reno	NV
Saint Mary's Medical Group, Inc.	Reno	NV
Saint Mary's Outpatient Imaging Center	Reno	NV
Saint Mary's Southwest	Byron Center	MI
Saint Paul Place Specialists	Lutherville	MD
Saint Thomas Dekalb Hospital	Smithville	TN
Saint Thomas Highlands Hospital	Sparta	TN
Saint Thomas River Park Hospital	McMinnville	TN
Saint Thomas Stones River Hospital	Woodbury	TN
Saint Vincent East Side Imaging Center	Erie	PA
Saint Vincent Imaging Center	Erie	PA
Saint Vincent Women's Wellness Center	Worcester	MA
Sakakawea Medical Center	Hazen	ND
Salem Clinic, P.C.	Salem	OR
Salem Community Hospital-Firestone Town Center Mammography	Columbiana	OH
Salem Hospital Outpatient Services - Lynn	Lynn	MA
Salem Hospital Women's Imaging	Salem	OR
Salem Memorial District Hospital	Salem	MO
Salem Radiology A Department Of Parkland Medical Center	Salem	NH
Salem Radiology Consultants, P.C.	Salem	OR
Salem Regional Medical Center	Salem	OH
Salem Township Hospital	Salem	IL
Salina Regional Breast Diagnostic Center	Salina	KS
Salina Regional Health Center Dba Comcare	Salina	KS
Saline Memorial Hospital	Benton	AR
Salt Lake Regional Medical Center Breast Care Center	Salt Lake City	UT
Salud Integral De La Montana Corozal Pr	Corozal	PR
Salud Integral En La Montana, Comerio	Comerio	PR
Salud Y Vida	El Paso	TX
Sam & Jennie Bennett Breast Care Center	Lewiston	ME
Samaritan Corvallis Mammography	Corvallis	OR
Samaritan Healthcare	Moses Lake	WA
Samaritan Lebanon Community Hospital	Lebanon	OR
Samaritan North Lincoln Hospital	Lincoln City	OR
Samaritan Pacific Communities Hospital	Newport	OR
Samaritan Regional Health System	Ashland	OH
Samaritan Valley Imaging Services	Albany	OR
Samaritan Womens Health Service	Ashland	OH
Samc - Belvidere	Belvidere	IL
Samg/Stateline Clinic	Roscoe	IL
Sampson Regional Outpatient Diagnostic Center	Clinton	NC
Samuel Simmonds Memorial Hospital	Barrow	AK
Samuel U. Rodgers Community Health Center	Kansas City	MO
San Antonio Regional Women's Breast & Imaging Center Upland		CA
San Bernardino Advanced Imaging - Highland	San Bernardino	CA
San Carlos Apache Healthcare Corporation	Peridot	AZ
San Diego Imaging	Escondido	CA
San Diego Imaging	Oceanside	CA
San Diego Imaging, Chula Vista, Llc	Chula Vista	CA
San Dimas Community Hospital	San Dimas	CA
San Dimas Medical Group	Bakersfield	CA
San Francisco Imaging	Rio Piedras	PR
San German X-Ray And Body Imaging Center	San German	PR
San Gorgonio Memorial Hospital	Banning	CA
San Jacinto Imaging	San Jacinto	CA
San Jacinto Methodist Dba Houston Methodist Baytown Hosp	Baytown	TX
San Joaquin General Hospital	French Camp	CA
San Juan Regional Medical Center	Farmington	NM
San Juan Regional Medical Ctr Outpatient Diagnostic Ctr	Farmington	NM
San Leandro Hospital	San Leandro	CA
San Luis Valley Regional Medical Center	Alamosa	CO
San Manuel Indian Health	Grand Terrace	CA
San Mateo Medical Center	San Mateo	CA
San Ramon Regional Medical Center	San Ramon	CA
Sana Healthcare Carrollton, Llc	Carrollton	TX
Sand Lake Imaging	Lady Lake	FL
Sand Lake Imaging	Orlando	FL
Sand Lake Imaging- Maitland	Maitland	FL
Sanders Clinic For Women, P.A.	Tupelo	MS
Sandra Oneal Institute	Plano	TX
Sanford Canby Medical Center	Canby	MN
Sanford Chamberlain	Chamberlain	SD
Sanford Clinic - Bemidji	Bemidji	MN
Sanford Clinic Aberdeen	Aberdeen	SD
Sanford Clinic Detroit Lakes	Detroit Lakes	MN
Sanford Clinic Moorhead	Moorhead	MN
Sanford Clinic Southpointe	Fargo	ND
Sanford Clinic Watertown Breast Health Institute	Watertown	SD
Sanford Health Broadway Clinic	Alexandria	MN
Sanford Health East Grand Forks	East Grand Forks	MN
Sanford Health Jamestown Clinic	Jamestown	ND
Sanford Health Walker	Walker	MN
Sanford Health West Dickinson Clinic	Dickinson	ND
Sanford Hospital Webster	Webster	SD
Sanford Luverne Medical Center	Luverne	MN
Sanford Medical Center Fargo	Fargo	ND
Sanford Sheldon Medical Center	Sheldon	IA
Sanford Southpointe-Mobile	Fargo	ND
Sanford Thief River Falls Medical Center	Thief River Falls	MN
Sanford Vermillion Hospital	Vermillion	SD
Sanford Worthington Medical Center	Worthington	MN
Sanitas	Doral	FL
Sanitas Lauderdale Lakes	Lauderdale Lakes	FL
Sanitas Medical Center Of Tennessee - Murfreesboro	Murfreesboro	TN
Sanitas Miami Lakes	Miami	FL
Sanitas Plantation	Plantation	FL
Sanofi Us Breast Care Center	Somerville	NJ
Sanpete Valley Hospital	Mt Pleasant	UT
Sansum Clinic	Santa Barbara	CA
Santa Barbara Cottage Hospital	Santa Barbara	CA
Santa Clara Valley Medical Center	San Jose	CA
Santa Clara Valley Medical Center - Tully	San Jose	CA
Santa Clarita Imaging	Valencia	CA
Santa Cruz Valley Regional Hospital	Green Valley	AZ
Santa Fe Imaging, L.L.C.	Santa Fe	NM
Santa Paula Hospital	Santa Paula	CA
Santa Rosa Medical Center Medical Office Building	Milton	FL
Santa Rosa Memorial Hospital Outpatient Imaging	Santa Rosa	CA
Santa Ynez Valley Cottage Hospital	Solvang	CA
Santiam Hospital	Stayton	OR
Sarah Bush Lincoln Health Center	Mattoon	IL
Sarasota Memorial Health Care Center & Er At North Port	North Port	FL
Sarasota Memorial Ambulatory Ctr At University Pkwy Sarasota		FL
Sarasota Memorial Health Care Center At Blackburn Point	Osprey	FL
Sarasota Memorial Health Care Center At Clark Road	Sarasota	FL
Sarasota Memorial Hlth Care Ctr At Heritage Harbour	Bradenton	FL
Sarasota Memorial Urgent Care Center At Venice	Venice	FL
Saratoga Imaging Center	Saratoga Springs	NY
Sauk Prairie Healthcare	Prairie Du Sac	WI
Sault Ste Marie Tribe Of Chippewa Indians Health Center	Sault Sainte Marie	MI
Saunders Medical Center	Wahoo	NE
Savannah Health Services, Llc D/B/A Memorial Health Umc	Savannah	GA
Savoy Medical Center	Mamou	LA
Sbh Dba Absmc Carol Ann Read Breast Health Center	Oakland	CA
Sbh Dba Absmc Imaging & Mammography-5730 Telegraph	Oakland	CA
Sc Obgyn Associates	West Columbia	SC
Schaffer, Schonholz And Drossman, Llp	New York	NY
Schererville Imaging Center	Schererville	IN
Scheurer Hospital	Pigeon	MI
Schneck Medical Center	Seymour	IN

Schofield Barracks Health Clinic Schofield Barracks HI
Schoolcraft Memorial Hospital Manistique MI
Schuyler Hospital Montour Falls NY
Schuylkill Open Mri, Inc Dba Allentown Diagnostic Imaging Allentown PA
Scl Health Good Samaritan Medical Center Lafayette CO
Scl Health Montana St Vincent Breast Center Billings MT
Scotland County Hospital Memphis MO
Scotland Memorial Hospital Imaging Center Laurinburg NC
Scott & White Clinic Dba Baylor Scott & White -The Brenham Brenham TX
Scott & White Hospital - Round Rock Cedar Park TX
Scott & White Hospital - Marble Falls Marble Falls TX
Scott & White Hospital - Round Rock Georgetown TX
Scott & White Hospital - Round Rock Lakeway TX
Scott & White Hospital- Round Rock Round Rock TX
Scott & White Mem Hosp Dba Baylor S&W Clinic - Killeen Killeen TX
Scott & White Memorial Hosp Dba Baylor S&W Med Ctr - Temple Temple TX
Scott & White Memorial Hospital Dba Baylor S&W Clinic-Waco Waco TX
Scott County Hospital Scott City KS
Scott Memorial Health Scottsburg IN
Scottsville Medical Center Scottsville KY
Scripps Clinic Carmel Valley Gooding Imaging Center San Diego CA
Scripps Clinic Mission Valley San Diego CA
Scripps Clinic Rancho Bernardo San Diego CA
Scripps Clinic Rancho San Diego La Mesa CA
Scripps Coastal Medical Center Vista CA
Scripps Encinitas Imaging Center Encinitas CA
Scripps Medical Center Jefferson Oceanside CA
Scripps Mercy Imaging Center Chula Vista CA
Scripps Mercy O'Toole Breast Care Center San Diego CA
Scripps Polster Breast Care Center La Jolla CA
Scurry County Hospital District Snyder TX
Searhc Elmc, Juneau Juneau AK
Searhc Mt. Edgecumb Hospital Sitka AK
Searhc Wrangell Medical Center Wrangell AK
Searhc, Alicia Roberts Medical Center Klawock AK
Seattle Cancer Care Alliance Breast Imaging Seattle WA
Sebastian River Medical Center Sebastian FL
Segundo Ruiz Belvis Diagnostic Treatment Ctr Nychhc Bronx NY
Sekine, Rasner, And Brock Md, Pa - Ob/Gyn Jacksonville FL
Select Diagnostic Imaging Brooklyn NY
Selma A. Carlson Diagnostic Center San Luis Obispo CA
Seminole Hospital District Of Gaines County Seminole TX
Senior Health Radiology Manchester NH
Senos Puerto Rico Hato Rey PR
Sentara Albemarle Medical Center Elizabeth City NC
Sentara Belleharbour Suffolk VA
Sentara Careplex Hospital Hampton VA
Sentara Gloucester Imaging Ctr Gloucester VA
Sentara Greenbrier Healthplex At Advanced Imaging Ctr Chesapeake VA
Sentara Halifax Regional Hospital South Boston VA
Sentara Lake Ridge Advanced Imaging Center Lake Ridge VA
Sentara Lorton Station Women's Imaging Center Lorton VA
Sentara Louise Obici Memorial Hospital Suffolk VA
Sentara Martha Jefferson Comprehensive Breast Center Charlottesville VA
Sentara Martha Jefferson Occ At Proffit Road Charlottesville VA
Sentara McLeskey Comprehensive Breast Center Norfolk VA
Sentara Norfolk General Hospital Norfolk VA
Sentara Northern Virginia Medical Center Woodbridge VA
Sentara Princess Anne Comprehensive Breast Center Virginia Beach VA
Sentara Princess Anne Mammography Center Virginia Beach VA
Sentara Rmh Funkhouser Women's Center Harrisonburg VA
Sentara Spring Creek Family Medicine Gordonsville VA
Sentara St. Luke's Carrollton VA
Sentara Ultrasound Associates Womens Imaging Center Alexandria VA
Sentara Virginia Beach Comprehensive Breast Center Virginia Beach VA
Sentara Williamsburg Women's Imaging Pavilion Williamsburg VA
Sequoia Mri - California Medical Imaging Inc Porterville CA
Sequoia Whipple Radiology Redwood City CA
Sequoyah County-City Of Sallisaw Hospital Authority Sallisaw OK
Serene Diagnostic Imaging Corp Tavares FL
Serra Community Medical Clinic, Inc. Sun Valley CA
Servicios Preventivos Del Caribe - Mobile San Sebastian PR
Servicios Radiologicos Asociados San Juan PR
Servicios Radiologicos Asociados Imaging Center Carolina PR
Seton Breast Health Center Dba Ahmc Healthcare Inc. Daly City CA
Seton Family Of Doctors Kyle TX
Seton Family Of Doctors Temple TX
Seton Imaging Amherst NY
Seton Imaging Center Baltimore MD
Seton Imaging Route 40 Catonsville MD
Sevier Valley Medical Center Richfield UT
Sghs, Inc. Dba Southeast Georgia Health System - Brunswick Brunswick GA
Sghs, Inc. Dba Southeast Georgia Health System - Brunswick Brunswick GA
Sghs, Inc. Dba Southeast Georgia Health System - Brunswick Brunswick GA
Sghs, Inc.Dba Southeast Georgia Health System-Camden Saint Marys GA
Sgmc Berrien Campus Nashville GA
Sgmf Stockton Medical Plaza Imaging Center Stockton CA
Sgmf Turlock Medical Clinic Turlock CA
Shands Jacksonville Advanced Breast Ctr At Emerson Jacksonville FL
Shands Jacksonville Womens Center Jacksonville FL
Shane M. Sopp Md, Pc Syracuse NY
Shannon Medical Center San Angelo TX
Shannon Medical Center South San Angelo TX
Share Medical Center Alva OK
Sharon Hospital Sharon CT
Sharon Regional Health System-Diagnostic & Imaging Center Hermitage PA
Sharp Coronado Hospital Coronado CA
Sharp Memorial Outpatient Pavilion Imaging San Diego CA
Sharp Rees - Stealy Otay Ranch Chula Vista CA
Sharp Rees - Stealy/ Sorrento Mesa San Diego CA
Sharp Rees Stealy - Downtown San Diego CA
Sharp Rees Stealy Rancho Bernardo San Diego CA
Sharp Rees-Stealy Breast Imaging Center San Diego CA
Sharp Rees-Stealy Medical Centers-Santee Santee CA
Shaw Center For Women's Health, Pa Thomasville GA
Sheila R.Veloz Breast Imaging Ctr- H. M. Newhall Mem. Hosp. Valencia CA
Shelby Baptist Medical Center Alabaster AL
Shelby Medical Associates, P.A. Shelby NC
Shelby Ob/Gyn Pc Alabaster AL
Shenandoah Medical Center Shenandoah IA
Shenandoah Memorial Hospital Woodstock VA
Shenandoah Womens Healthcare Harrisonburg VA
Sheridan Community Hospital Sheridan MI
Sheridan Memorial Hospital Plentywood MT
Sheridan Memorial Hospital Sheridan WY
Sherman Grayson Hospital, Llc Sherman TX
Shields Imaging With Central Maine Health Llc Topsham ME
Shimberg Breast Center At St. Joseph's Hospital-South Riverview FL
Shin Imaging Center Buena Park CA
Shin Imaging Llc Fullerton CA
Shin Mri Llc Los Angeles CA
Shoals Hospital Muscle Shoals AL
Shore Imaging Pc Lakewood NJ
Shore Medical Center Somers Point NJ
Shore Medical Pavillion Ste 130 Imaging Queenstown MD
Shoshone Medical Center Kellogg ID
Sid Peterson Memorial Hospital Kerrville TX
Sidney Health Center Sidney MT
Sidney Regional Medical Center Sidney NE
Sierra Nevada Women's Imaging Center Grass Valley CA
Sierra View Medical Center Womens Imaging Dept Porterville CA
Sierra Vista Hospital Truth Or Consequences NM
Signature Healthcare Brockton Hospital 110 Liberty Street Brockton MA
Signature Healthcare - Brockton Hospital Brockton MA
Silicon Valley Medical Development San Jose CA
Siloam Springs Regional Hospital Siloam Springs AR
Silver Creek Radiology San Jose CA
Silver Cross Center For Women's Health New Lenox IL
Simedhealth Llc Gainesville FL
Simon-Williamson Clinic, P.C. Birmingham AL

Alphabetical Index

Alphabetical Index

Alphabetical Index

Name	City	State
St. Vincent Hospital At Auburn Grove Medical	Auburn	MA
St. Vincent Hospital Dba Prevea Health - St. Mary's	Green Bay	WI
St. Vincent's Blount	Oneonta	AL
St. Vincent's Chilton	Clanton	AL
St. Vincent's Hospital Comprehensive Breast Center	Birmingham	AL
St. Vincent's Medical Center	Bridgeport	CT
St. Vincent's One Nineteen Health & Wellness	Birmingham	AL
St. Vincent's St. Clair	Pell City	AL
St. Vincent's Trussville	Trussville	AL
St.Mary Corwin Medical Center Breast Center Of Excellence	Pueblo	CO
St.Thomas Midtown Hospital Center For Breast Health	Nashville	TN
Stamford Health Breast Imaging Center - Darien	Darien	CT
Stamford Health Breast Imaging Center - Tully	Stamford	CT
Stamford Health Breast Imaging Center - Wilton	Wilton	CT
Stamford Health Breast Imaging Center- Greenwich	Greenwich	CT
Stanford Cancer Center, South Bay	San Jose	CA
Stanford Health Care	Palo Alto	CA
Stanford Health Care	Palo Alto	CA
Stanford Health Care Emeryville	Emeryville	CA
Stanford Health Care Hoover	Palo Alto	CA
Stanford Health Care-Valleycare Breast Imaging Center	Pleasanton	CA
Stanislaus Surgical Hospital Precision Imaging	Modesto	CA
Star Valley Health	Afton	WY
Stark Womens Center	Canton	OH
Starling Diagnositcs	Bronx	NY
Starling Radiology	New Britain	CT
Starr County Hospital District	Rio Grande City	TX
Starr Regional Breast Center	Athens	TN
State Of Franklin Healthcare Assocs Comprehensive Breast Ctr	Johnson City	TN
Statesboro Imaging Center	Statesboro	GA
Steele Memorial Medical Center	Salmon	ID
Steeplechase Diagnostic Center, Inc.	Houston	TX
Stefanie Spielman Comprehensive Breast Center	Columbus	OH
Steinberg Diagnostic Medical Imaging	Henderson	NV
Steinberg Diagnostic Medical Imaging	Henderson	NV
Steinberg Diagnostic Medical Imaging	Las Vegas	NV
Steinberg Diagnostic Medical Imaging	Las Vegas	NV
Steinberg Diagnostic Medical Imaging	Las Vegas	NV
Steinberg Diagnostic Medical Imaging	Las Vegas	NV
Steinberg Diagnostic Medical Imaging	N Las Vegas	NV
Steinberg Diagnostic Medical Imaging Centers	Henderson	NV
Steinberg Diagnostic Medical Imaging Centers	Las Vegas	NV
Stellis Health, P.A.	Buffalo	MN
Stellis Health, Pa	Monticello	MN
Stephanie Tubbs Jones Community Health Ctr	East Cleveland	OH
Stephens County Hospital	Toccoa	GA
Stephens Memorial Hospital District	Breckenridge	TX
Stephenville Medical & Surgical Clinic, Pa	Stephenville	TX
Sterling Regional Medcenter	Sterling	CO
Stevens Community Medical Center	Morris	MN
Steward Carney Hospital	Dorchester	MA
Steward Imaging Center	Austintown	OH
Steward Medical Group Inc.	N Dartmouth	MA
Steward Melbourne Hospital, Inc.	Melbourne	FL
Steward Norwood Hospital, Inc.	Norwood	MA
Steward Rockledge Hospital, Inc	Rockledge	FL
Steward St Elizabeth Med Ctr	Boston	MA
Steward Texas Hospital Holdings, Llc	Big Spring	TX
Steward Trumbull Memorial Hospital, Inc.	Warren	OH
Stewardtrumbull Memorial Hospital, Inc. Center For Radiology	Cortland	OH
Stewart Memorial Community Hospital	Lake City	IA
Sths Er At Mission	Mission	TX
Sths Er At Weslaco	Weslaco	TX
Stillwater Billings Clinic	Columbus	MT
Stillwater Medical - Perry	Perry	OK
Stockdale Radiology	Bakersfield	CA
Stockton Diagnostic Imaging	Stockton	CA
Stone County Medical Center	Mountain View	AR
Stonebridge Diagnostic Center	New Freedom	PA
Stones Crossing Health Pavilion	Greenwood	IN
Stonesprings Hospital Center	Dulles	VA
Stonewall Jackson Memorial Hospital	Weston	WV
Stony Brook Eastern Long Island Hospital	Greenport	NY
Stony Brook Medicine Advanced Imaging	Stony Brook	NY
Stony Brook Medicine Advanced Imaging At Commack	Commack	NY
Stony Brook Medicine Advanced Imaging At Riverhead	Riverhead	NY
Stony Brook Medicine-Stony Brook University Hospital	Stony Brook	NY
Stormont Vail Women's Center	Topeka	KS
Stoughton Hospital	Stoughton	WI
Straub Clinic & Hospital	Kaneohe	HI
Straub Clinic & Hospital - Mililani Clinic	Mililani	HI
Straub Medical Center	Honolulu	HI
Straub Medical Center - Hawaii Kai Clinic	Honolulu	HI
Strong Memorial Hospital U Of R Medical Center	Rochester	NY
Sturdy Memorial Hospital	Attleboro	MA
Sturgis Hospital	Sturgis	MI
Suburban Community Hospital	Norristown	PA
Suffolk Breast Imaging, P.C.	Lake Grove	NY
Sugar House Health Center	Salt Lake City	UT
Sugar Mill Diagnostic Imaging	Homosassa	FL
Sullivan County Community Hospital	Sullivan	IN
Summa Health Center At Cuyahoga Falls	Cuyahoga Falls	OH
Summa Health Center At Green	Uniontown	OH
Summa Health Center At Lake Medina	Medina	OH
Summa Health Center At White Pond	Akron	OH
Summa Health Hudson Medical Center	Hudson	OH
Summa Health Stow Kent Medical Center	Stow	OH
Summa Health System - Summa Barberton Hospital	Barberton	OH
Summa Health System Breast And Imaging Center	Akron	OH
Summa Health Tallmadge Medical Center	Tallmadge	OH
Summa Health Wadsworth-Rittman Medical Center	Wadsworth	OH
Summerlin Hospital Medical Center	Las Vegas	NV
Summersville Regional Medical Center	Summersville	WV
Summerville Breast Center	Summerville	SC
Summit Diagnostic Imaging Center - Cedar Bluff	Knoxville	TN
Summit Diagnostic Imaging Center - Ft. City	Knoxville	TN
Summit Diagnostic Imaging Center - Wellington	Knoxville	TN
Summit Healthcare Reg Med Ctr Snowflake Outpatient Ctr	Snowflake	AZ
Summit Healthcare Regional Medical Center	Show Low	AZ
Summit Healthplex	Niagara Falls	NY
Summit Imaging	Brooksville	FL
Summit Imaging At Lebanon	Lebanon	TN
Summit Imaging Center In Mt. Juliet	Mt Juliet	TN
Summit Medical Center	Casper	WY
Summit Medical Group	Florham Park	NJ
Summit Medical Group	Livingston	NJ
Summit Medical Group	New Providence	NJ
Summit Medical Group	West Orange	NJ
Summit Medical Group	Westfield	NJ
Summit Medical Group Oregon/Bend Memorial Clinic	Bend	OR
Summit Medical Group Pa	Florham Park	NJ
Summit Medical Group, P.A.	Berkeley Hts	NJ
Summit Pacific Wellness Center	Elma	WA
Sun City Hospital Inc, Dba South Bay Hospital	Sun City Center	FL
Sun Imaging,Inc.	Los Angeles	CA
Sun Radiology	Glendale	AZ
Sun View Imaging Llc	Las Cruces	NM
Sunflower Diagnostic Center	Ruleville	MS
Sunrise Hospital And Medical Center	Las Vegas	NV
Sunset Radiology, Inc.	Miami	FL
Suny/Downstate Medical Center University Hospital	Brooklyn	NY
Surgical Care Of The Virginias, Llc	Bluefield	VA
Surgical Oncology Of North Georgia Dba Advanced Breast Care	Marietta	GA
Susan B. Allen Memorial Hospital	El Dorado	KS
Susan Cheek Needler Breast Center	Clearwater	FL
Susan Shepard McGillicuddy Breast Center At St. Anthony's	St Petersburg	FL
Susquehanna Health Imaging At Mansfield	Mansfield	PA
Susquehanna Valley Diagnostic Imaging Inc.	Bloomsburg	PA
Susquehanna Valley Imaging- A Service Of Geisinger Med Ctr	Lewisburg	PA
Sutter Amador Hospital	Jackson	CA
Sutter Bay Hospitals Dba Cpmc - Phoc	San Francisco	CA
Sutter Bay Hospitals Dba Novato Community Hospital	Novato	CA
Sutter Bay Medical Foundation	Santa Rosa	CA
Sutter Coast Hospital	Crescent City	CA
Sutter Delta Medical Center	Antioch	CA
Sutter East Bay Medical Foundation	Castro Valley	CA
Sutter Gould Medical Foundation	Modesto	CA
Sutter Imaging At Brookings Harbor	Brookings	OR
Sutter Lakeside Hospital	Lakeport	CA

Alphabetical Index

Alphabetical Index

Name	City	State
Welch Rd. Imaging	Menlo Park	CA
Welia Health	Mora	MN
Welia Health	Pine City	MN
Wellmont Bristol Regional Medical Center Leonard Breast Cent	Bristol	TN
Wellspan Adams Health Center	Gettysburg	PA
Wellspan Good Samaritan Hospital	Lebanon	PA
Wellspan Good Samaritan Hospital Ambulatory Services Center	Palmyra	PA
Wellspan Greencastle Health Center	Greencastle	PA
Wellspan Gsh Outpatient Radiology Center	Lebanon	PA
Wellspan Hayshire Health Center	York	PA
Wellspan Health & Surgery Center	Hanover	PA
Wellspan Rhonda Brake Shreiner Women's Center	Chambersburg	PA
Wellspan Shippensburg Health	Shippensburg	PA
Wellspan Washington Street Health Center	Gettysburg	PA
Wellspan Waynesboro Hospital	Waynesboro	PA
Wellspring Breast Care Center Uuh At Community General	Syracuse	NY
Wellstar -Vinings Health Park-Imaging	Smyrna	GA
Wellstar Acworth Health Park Mammography - Kennestone	Acworth	GA
Wellstar Atlanta Medical Center	Atlanta	GA
Wellstar Atlanta Medical Center South, Breast Center	East Point	GA
Wellstar Cherokee Health Park	Holly Springs	GA
Wellstar Cobb Hospital Mammography	Austell	GA
Wellstar Douglas Hospital	Douglasville	GA
Wellstar East Cobb Health Park Mammography	Marietta	GA
Wellstar Kennestone At Towne Lake Medical Imaging	Woodstock	GA
Wellstar Kennestone OP Womens Imaging Ctr	Marietta	GA
Wellstar Mammography At The Breast Center	Marietta	GA
Wellstar North Fulton Avalon Health Park Imaging Center	Alpharetta	GA
Wellstar Outpatient Imaging And Specialty Care At Campcreek	Atlanta	GA
Wellstar Paulding Imaging Center	Hiram	GA
Wellstar Primary Care Imaging Services	Atlanta	GA
Wellstar Spalding Regional Medical Center	Griffin	GA
Wellstar West Georgia Medical Center Women's Health Center	Lagrange	GA
Wellstar Windy Hill Hospital	Marietta	GA
Wendover Ob/Gyn And Infertility, Inc	Greensboro	NC
Wentworth-Douglass Hospital Breast Health Center	Portsmouth	NH
Weslaco Advanced Medical Imaging, Llc	Edinburg	TX
Wesley Medical Center	Wichita	KS
West Ann Arbor Health Center	Ann Arbor	MI
West Augusta Ob/Gyn	Augusta	GA
West Boca Diagnostic Imaging Center	Boca Raton	FL
West Calcasieu Cameron Hospital	Sulphur	LA
West Carroll Memorial Hospital	Oak Grove	LA
West Chester Hospital	West Chester	OH
West County Health Center	San Pablo	CA
West Feliciana Parish Hospital	Saint Francisville	LA
West Florida Hospital	Pensacola	FL
West Hernando Diagnostic Center	Spring Hill	FL
West Hernando Womens Imaging Center	Spring Hill	FL
West Hills Hospital & Medical Center/Women's Diagn. Ctr.	West Hills	CA
West Hills Open Mri And Imaging Center	Coraopolis	PA
West Holt Memorial Hospital	Atkinson	NE
West Kendall Obgyn	Miami	FL
West Open Mri & Radiology Services	Mayaguez	PR
West Park Hospital	Cody	WY
West Penn Hospital	Pittsburgh	PA
West River Regional Medical Center	Hettinger	ND
West Stanly Imaging	Locust	NC
West Tennessee Healthcare Bolivar Hospital	Bolivar	TN
West Tennessee Healthcare Dyersburg Hospital	Dyersburg	TN
West Tennessee Healthcare North Hospital	Jackson	TN
West Tennessee Imaging Center	Jackson	TN
West Valley Hospital	Dallas	OR
West Valley Medical Center	Caldwell	ID
West Virginia University Hospitals- Mobile	Morgantown	WV
West Wichita Family Physicians, P.A.	Wichita	KS
Westcare Medical Park Of Franklin	Franklin	NC
Westchester Advanced Imaging Center Med Group	Los Angeles	CA
Westchester General Hospital, Inc.	Miami	FL
Westchester Medical Center Advance Imaging	Hawthorne	NY
Westerly Hospital	Westerly	RI
Westerly Hospital - Wood River Health Services, Inc.	Hope Valley	RI
Western Arizona Regional Medical Center - Imaging Ctr.	Bullhead City	AZ
Western Connecticut Imaging	Ridgefield	CT
Western Ct Breast Imaging Center	Danbury	CT
Western Kentucky Diagnostic Img - Dept Of The Med Ctr	Bowling Green	KY
Western Missouri Medical Center	Warrensburg	MO
Western New York Breast Health - Mobile Mammography	Buffalo	NY
Western New York Mri	Buffalo	NY
Western New York Mri	Buffalo	NY
Western Plains Medical Complex	Dodge City	KS
Western Regional Medical Center Inc	Goodyear	AZ
Western Wisconsin Health	Baldwin	WI
Westerville Medical Campus	Westerville	OH
Westfield Memorial Hospital	Westfield	NY
Westfields Hospital	New Richmond	WI
Westmed Medical Group	Greenwich	CT
Westmed Medical Group	New Rochelle	NY
Westmed Medical Group	Purchase	NY
Westmed Medical Group	White Plains	NY
Westmed Medical Group	Yonkers	NY
Westmed Medical Group	Yonkers	NY
Weston County Health Services	Newcastle	WY
Westside Regional Medical Center	Plantation	FL
Westwood Womens Health	Waterbury	CT
Wetzel County Hospital, Inc.	New Martinsville	WV
Wewoka Indian Health Clinic	Wewoka	OK
Wheeling Hospital	Wheeling	WV
Whidbey General Hospital	Coupeville	WA
Whidbey General Hospital - South	Clinton	WA
Whidbeyhealth Primary Care Oak Harbor	Oak Harbor	WA
White Earth Phs Ihs	Ogema	MN
White Plains Hospital Center	White Plains	NY
White Plains Hospital Imaging At Armonk	Armonk	NY
White Plains Hospital Imaging At New Rochelle	New Rochelle	NY
White Plains Hospital Women's Imaging Ctr. At Rye Brook	Rye Brook	NY
White River Medical Center	Batesville	AR
White River Medical Center-North Complex Imaging Center	Cherokee Village	AR
White-Wilson Medical Center	Fort Walton Beach	FL
Whitesburg Arh	Whitesburg	KY
Whitman Hospital & Medical Clinics	Colfax	WA
Whs Greene	Waynesburg	PA
Wichita Ob/Gyn Associates	Wichita	KS
Wickenburg Community Hospital	Wickenburg	AZ
Wiinhealth Women's Imaging And Interventions	Sunrise	FL
Wilbarger County Hospital District	Vernon	TX
Wilcox Medical Center	Lihue	HI
Wildwood Family Clinic	Madison	WI
Wilford Hall Ambulatory Surgical Center	Jbsa Lackland	TX
Wilkes - Barre Hospital Co	Mountain Top	PA
Wilkes - Barre Hospital, Co Llc	Edwardsville	PA
Wilkes-Barre Hospital Co, Llc	Pittston	PA
Wilkins Mob At Grant Medical Center	Columbus	OH
Willamette Valley Mammography	Eugene	OR
Willamette Valley Medical Center	McMinnville	OR
Willapa Harbor Hospital	South Bend	WA
William Beaumont Army Medical Center	El Paso	TX
William Beaumont Hospital	Troy	MI
William Beaumont Hospital Rochester Hills	Rochester Hills	MI
William Bee Ririe Hospital	Ely	NV
William Newton Hospital	Winfield	KS
William W. Backus Hospital	Norwich	CT
Williamsburg Regional Hospital	Kingstree	SC
Williamson Imaging Llc Dba Cool Springs Imaging	Franklin	TN
Williamson Medical Ctr OP Imaging	Franklin	TN
Willis-Knighton Breast Center South	Shreveport	LA
Willis-Knighton Medical Center	Shreveport	LA
Williston Radiology Consultants Dba Fairlight Medical Center	Williston	ND
Willits Hospital, Inc., Dba Adventist Health Howard Memorial	Willits	CA
Wilma P. Mankiller Health Center	Stilwell	OK
Wilmington Health	Wilmington	NC
Wilmington Health , Leland Location	Leland	NC
Wilmington Health, Mayfaire	Wilmington	NC
Wilson Health	Sidney	OH

Name	City	State
Wilson Medical Center	Neodesha	KS
Wilson Medical Ctr OP Imaging	Wilson	NC
Wilton Medical Arts	Saratoga Springs	NY
Winchester Hospital Breast Care Center	Woburn	MA
Winchester Hospital Family Medical Center	Wilmington	MA
Winchester Medical Center - Diagnostic Center	Winchester	VA
Winchester Women's Specialists	Winchester	VA
Windham Community Memorial Hospital	Willimantic	CT
Windham Hospital Center For Women's Health At Mansfield	Mansfield	CT
Windom Area Hospital	Windom	MN
Windsong Radiology Group At Amherst	West Amherst	NY
Windsong Radiology Group At Hamburg	Hamburg	NY
Windsong Radiology Group At Lancaster	Depew	NY
Windsong Radiology Group At Williamsville	Williamsville	NY
Windsong Radiology Group, Pc-Mobile	Williamsville	NY
Windsor Diagnostic Center	Red Lion	PA
Windsor Imaging	Fort Pierce	FL
Windsor Radiology, Llc	East Windsor	NJ
Winn Army Community Hospital	Fort Stewart	GA
Winner Regional Health Care Center	Winner	SD
Winneshiek Medical Center	Decorah	IA
Winnie Community Hospital, Llp	Beaumont	TX
Winona Health Services	Winona	MN
Winston Medical Center	Louisville	MS
Winter Haven Women's Hospital	Winter Haven	FL
Wiregrass Medical Center	Geneva	AL
Wisconsin Health Fund	Milwaukee	WI
Wish Fresno Breast Center	Fresno	CA
Witham Health Services At Anson	Zionsville	IN
Witham Memorial Hospital Women's Center	Lebanon	IN
Wjmc Imaging At Ridgelake	Metairie	LA
Wk Breast Health Center	Shreveport	LA
Wk Palmetto Breast Clinic	Benton	LA
Wny Mri - Wny Womens Imaging	Williamsville	NY
Wnymri At Premier	Williamsville	NY
Woman's Breast Center - Advanced Imaging	Baton Rouge	LA
Woman's Care Ob/Gyn	Saratoga Springs	NY
Woman's Center Of Strhs-Winchester	Winchester	TN
Woman's Clinic Pllc	Houston	TX
Woman's Hospital Breast Center	Baton Rouge	LA
Woman's Hospital On-Site Mammography - Mobile	Baton Rouge	LA
Women & Infants Hospital	Providence	RI
Women & Infants Hospital - Eg East Greenwich Ri	East Greenwich	RI
Women & Infants Hospital - Providence Ri	Providence	RI
Women First Digital Breast Imaging	Stillwater	OK
Women First Of Louisville	Louisville	KY
Women Partners Austin Breast Imaging, Llc	Austin	TX
Women's And Children's Clinic	Springfield	IL
Women's Breast Health & Imaging Center	Aiken	SC
Women's Cancer And Wellness Institute	North Chesterfield	VA
Women's Care Center Of Memphis	Memphis	TN
Women's Care Florida - Lakeland Ob/Gyn	Lakeland	FL
Women's Care Florida Center For Breast Health	St Petersburg	FL
Women's Care Florida Contemporary Women's Care	Largo	FL
Women's Care Florida Division 1100 Partners In Ob/Gyn	Tampa	FL
Women's Care Florida Ob &Gyn Specialists	Winter Park	FL
Women's Care Florida Winter Park Ob-Gyn	Winter Park	FL
Women's Care Florida-Div 4400 Ob/Gyn Assoc., Riverview	Riverview	FL
Women's Care Imaging	Eugene	OR
Women's Care Of Lake Cumberland	Somerset	KY
Women's Care Phys Of Louisville A Part Of Norton Womens Care	Louisville	KY
Women's Care Specialists, P.C.	Birmingham	AL
Women's Care, Inc.	Mansfield	OH
Women's Center At Colorado Springs Imaging	Colorado Springs	CO
Women's Center For Radiology	Orlando	FL
Women's Center For Radiology	Orlando	FL
Women's Choice Mammography	Trumbull	CT
Women's Clinic Of Lincoln, P.C.	Lincoln	NE
Women's Diag Ctr-Community Hosp Of San Bernardino	San Bernardino	CA
Women's Diagnostic Center	Sparta	NJ
Women's Diagnostic Center Of St. Mary	Hobart	IN
Women's Diagnostic Center - Baptist Health Lagrange	Louisville	KY
Women's Diagnostic Center - Doctors Hospital Augusta	Augusta	GA
Women's Diagnostic Center - Piedmont Medical Center	Rock Hill	SC
Women's Diagnostic Center At Indian Path Hospital	Kingsport	TN
Women's Diagnostic Center Of Doylestown Hospital	Doylestown	PA
Women's Diagnostic Center Of St. Mary's	Valparaiso	IN
Women's Diagnostic Center Of Unitypoint Health-Pekin	Pekin	IL
Women's Diagnostic Center, Inc.	Birmingham	AL
Women's Diagnostic Imaging	Princeton	WV
Women's Diagnostic Imaging Medical Center Inc	Pasadena	CA
Women's Excellence	Lake Orion	MI
Women's Health & Imaging	Niceville	FL
Women's Health & Imaging Center	Johnson City	TN
Women's Health Advantage	Fort Wayne	IN
Women's Health Advantage	Ft Wayne	IN
Women's Health Associates	Aiken	SC
Women's Health Associates, Pllc	Flowood	MS
Women's Health Breast Imaging Center	Lynchburg	VA
Women's Health Center At Mt. Carmel Medical Center	Grove City	OH
Women's Health Center At Sebasticook Valley Health	Pittsfield	ME
Women's Health Center Mobile Services Unit - Mobile	Columbus	OH
Women's Health Center Mount Carmel Hilliard	Hilliard	OH
Women's Health Center New Albany	New Albany	OH
Women's Health Center Vestal	Vestal	NY
Women's Health Connecticut Obstetrics And Gynecology	Bridgeport	CT
Women's Health Medical & Arts Center	Beverly	MA
Women's Health Of Augusta, P.C.	Augusta	GA
Women's Health Services Of Bradenton Dba In A Woman's Image	Bradenton	FL
Women's Health Services, Chattanooga, P.C.	Chattanooga	TN
Women's Health Specialists	Jensen Beach	FL
Women's Health Specialists	Port Saint Lucie	FL
Women's Health Specialists	Park Ridge	IL
Women's Health Specialists Pllc	Germantown	TN
Women's Healthcare Associates	Athens	GA
Women's Healthcare Associates, Llc	Oregon City	OR
Women's Healthcare Center	Meridian	MS
Women's Healthcare Imaging Corp	Union	NJ
Women's Hlth Alliance Mammography & Specialty Svcs	Raleigh	NC
Women's Imaging & Breast Care Ctr	Marrero	LA
Women's Imaging & Mammography Center At Logan Hospital	Logan	UT
Women's Imaging At Apple Hill	York	PA
Women's Imaging Center	Los Angeles	CA
Women's Imaging Center	Orange	CA
Women's Imaging Center	Key West	FL
Women's Imaging Center	Lakeland	FL
Women's Imaging Center	Moscow	ID
Women's Imaging Center	Chelmsford	MA
Women's Imaging Center	Butler	PA
Women's Imaging Center - Hawaii Radiologic Associates, Ltd.	Hilo	HI
Women's Imaging Center - Munson Medical Center	Traverse City	MI
Women's Imaging Center - Penn Medicine University City	Philadelphia	PA
Women's Imaging Center / Dra Of Southbury	Southbury	CT
Women's Imaging Center At Bayhealth, Kent Campus	Dover	DE
Women's Imaging Center Longmont United Hospital Centura	Longmont	CO
Women's Imaging Center Of Reston	Reston	VA
Women's Imaging Center Tripler Army Medical Center	Tripler Amc	HI
Women's Imaging Ctr Chapin Lexington Med Ctr Chapin	Chapin	SC
Women's Imaging Ctr-Mobile Lexington Med. Ctr. - Mobile	West Columbia	SC
Women's Imaging Of South Jersey	Voorhees	NJ
Women's Imaging Specialists - Athens, Llc.	Watkinsville	GA
Women's Imaging Specialists - Cumming, Llc	Cumming	GA
Women's Imaging Specialists - Dublin, Llc	Dublin	GA
Women's Imaging Specialists - Eagles Landing, Llc.	Stockbridge	GA
Women's Imaging Specialists - Fairhope, Llc	Fairhope	AL
Women's Imaging Specialists - Foley, Llc	Foley	AL
Women's Imaging Specialists - Gwinnett, Llc	Lawrenceville	GA
Women's Imaging Specialists - Johns Creek, Llc	Suwanee	GA
Women's Imaging Specialists - Monroe, Llc	Monroe	GA
Women's Imaging Specialists - Warner Robins, Llc	Warner Robins	GA
Women's Imaging Specialists-Lawrenceville, Llc	Lawrenceville	GA

Women's Imaging- St Mary's Regional Medical Center Enid OK
Women's Imaging/Gulf Breeze Hospital Gulf Breeze FL
Women's Life Imaging Center Somersworth NH
Women's Mobile Medical Services, Llc-Mobile Geneva FL
Women's Pavilion Of South Mississippi Hattiesburg MS
Women's Services At Baptist Medical Park Pensacola FL
Women's Wellness Center Pa Fayetteville NC
Womencare Of Baldwin Park Orlando FL
Womens Care At Image Care Llc Columbia SC
Womens Care Florida Brandon FL
Womens Care Florida - Palm Beach Obgyn Lake Worth FL
Womens Care Ob/Gyn Glens Falls NY
Womens Diag Imaging Ctr At Salem Medical Center Salem NJ
Womens Diagnostic Center Marshall MI
Womens Diagnostic Imaging Ridgewood NJ
Womens Health And Menopause Center West Bloomfield MI
Womens Health Associates Pllc Boise ID
Womens Health Center Jersey City NJ
Womens Health Connecticut-Avon Avon CT
Womens Health Connecticut-Glastonbury Glastonbury CT
Womens Health Connecticut-West Hartford West Hartford CT
Womens Health Resource At Bristol Hospital Bristol CT
Womens Health Services Yuma AZ
Womens Healthcare Associates Pllc Amarillo TX
Womens Huron Valley Correctional Facility Ypsilanti MI
Womens Imaging And Intervention Llc Lake Oswego OR
Womens Imaging Center Mob 3 Martinsburg WV
Womens Imaging Ctr Amita Health Adventist Medical Center Bol Bolingbrook IL
Womens Imaging Pavilion At Ocean Medical Center Brick NJ
Womens Specialists Of Plano Pllc Plano TX
Womens's Diagnostic Svcs At Banner Lakes Imaging Ctr Sun City AZ
Wood County Hospital, Inc. Bowling Green OH
Woodburn Clinic Woodburn OR
Woodhull Medical & Mental Health Center Brooklyn NY
Woodland Clinic, A Service Of Dignity Health Medical Fdn Woodland CA
Woodlands Medical Specialists Pensacola FL
Woodlawn Hospital Rochester IN
Woodrow Wilson Keeble Memorial Health Care Center Sisseton SD
Wooster Community Hospital Women's Speciality Center Wooster OH
Wray Community District Hospital Wray CO
Wruble N D, M.D. Astoria NY
Wth Volunteer Hospital Martin TN
Wvu Cheat Lake Physicians Morgantown WV
Wvu Medicine - Braxton County Memorial Hospital Gassaway WV
Wvu Medicine Camden Clark Medical Center Parkersburg WV
Wvu Medicine Reynolds Memorial Hospital Glen Dale WV
Wvu Medicine Uniontown Hospital Uniontown PA
Wvu Medicine Uniontown Hospital Outpatient Diagnostic Center Uniontown PA
Wvu Medicine University Town Center Morgantown WV
Wyandot Memorial Hospital Upper Sandusky OH
Wyckoff Heights Medical Center Brooklyn NY
Wyckoff Heights Medical Center, Women's Health Center. Brooklyn NY
Wyoming County Community Hospital Warsaw NY
Wythe County Community Hospital Wytheville VA
X-Ray Associates Of Farmington Farmington NM
X-Ray Associates, Inc D/B/A Xra Medical Imaging Cranston RI
X-Ray Associates, Inc. D/B/A Xra Medical Imaging Smithfield RI
X-Ray Associates, Inc., D/B/A Xra Medical Imaging Johnston RI
X-Ray Associates, Inc., D/B/A Xra Medical Imaging Wakefield RI
Xray Associates At Santa Fe Santa Fe NM
Xxi Century Radiology And Imaging Brooklyn NY
Xxi Century Radiology And Imaging P.C. Brooklyn NY
Yale New Haven Hospital - Shoreline Medical Center Guilford CT
Yale New Haven Hospital Dept Of Diagnostic Imaging New Haven CT
Yale New Haven Radiology At Long Wharf New Haven CT
Yale-New Haven Hospital - Mobile New Haven CT
Yalobusha General Hospital Water Valley MS
Yankton Medical Clinic Yankton SD
Yavapai Regional Medical Center Breast Care Center Prescott Valley AZ
Yoakum Community Hospital Yoakum TX
York General Healthcare Services York NE
York Hospital York ME
York Hospital In Wells Wells ME
Yukon-Kuskokwim Delta Regional Hospital Bethel AK
Yuma District Hospital Yuma CO
Yuma Regional Foothills Imaging Center Yuma AZ
Yuma Regional Outpatient Diagnostic Imaging Ctr. Yuma AZ
Zuckerberg San Francisco General Hospital San Francisco CA
Zuni Comprehensive Community Health Center Zuni NM
Zwanger - Pesiri Radiology Stony Brook NY
Zwanger - Pesiri Radiology Group Plainview NY
Zwanger Pesiri Radiology Bayside NY
Zwanger Pesiri Radiology Bronx NY
Zwanger Pesiri Radiology Brooklyn NY
Zwanger Pesiri Radiology Coram NY
Zwanger Pesiri Radiology East Patchogue NY
Zwanger Pesiri Radiology Freeport NY
Zwanger Pesiri Radiology Great Neck NY
Zwanger Pesiri Radiology Huntington Station NY
Zwanger Pesiri Radiology Laurelton NY
Zwanger Pesiri Radiology Lawrence NY
Zwanger Pesiri Radiology Lynbrook NY
Zwanger Pesiri Radiology Massapequa NY
Zwanger Pesiri Radiology Port Jefferson Station NY
Zwanger Pesiri Radiology Sayville NY
Zwanger Pesiri Radiology Group Merrick NY
Zwanger-Pesiri Radiology Bay Shore NY
Zwanger-Pesiri Radiology Commack NY
Zwanger-Pesiri Radiology Elmont NY
Zwanger-Pesiri Radiology Hicksville NY
Zwanger-Pesiri Radiology Levittown NY
Zwanger-Pesiri Radiology Medford NY
Zwanger-Pesiri Radiology Shirley NY
Zwanger-Pesiri Radiology Smithtown NY
Zwanger-Pesiri Radiology Group West Islip NY
Zwanger-Pesiri Radiology Group, Llp Lindenhurst NY

readers service order card

detach, fill out and mail

MAMMOGRAPHY CENTERS DIRECTORY

Please send _____ copy (ies) of the MAMMOGRAPHY CENTERS DIRECTORY at $99.00 each.
Shipping and Handling $11.00.

❑ Check enclosed – Amount $ ______________ Date ________________________

Name ____ Title ________________________

Institution/Company ____ Dept. ______________________

Address ____

City/State/Zip ____ Phone ____________________

Email ____

Make check payable to: UNICOL, Inc.
Mail to: P.O. Box 260550, Pembroke Pines, FL 33026-7550
Call: (954) 430-7271 • Fax (954) 430-7227 • Web: www.Unicol-Publishing.com

readers service order card

detach, fill out and mail

MAMMOGRAPHY CENTERS DIRECTORY

Please send _____ copy (ies) of the MAMMOGRAPHY CENTERS DIRECTORY at $99.00 each.
Shipping and Handling $11.00.

❑ Check enclosed – Amount $ ______________ Date ________________________

Name ____ Title ________________________

Institution/Company ____ Dept. ______________________

Address ____

City/State/Zip ____ Phone ____________________

Email ____

Make check payable to: UNICOL, Inc.
Mail to: P.O. Box 260550, Pembroke Pines, FL 330260-7550
Call: (954) 430-7271 • Fax (954) 430-7227 • Web: www.Unicol-Publishing.com

readers service order card

detach, fill out and mail

MAMMOGRAPHY CENTERS DIRECTORY

Please send _____ copy (ies) of the MAMMOGRAPHY CENTERS DIRECTORY at $99.00 each.
Shipping and Handling $11.00.

❑ Check enclosed – Amount $ ______________ Date ________________________

Name ____ Title ________________________

Institution/Company ____ Dept. ______________________

Address ____

City/State/Zip ____ Phone ____________________

Email ____

Make check payable to: UNICOL, Inc.
Mail to: P.O. Box 260550, Pembroke Pines, FL 33026-7550
Call: (954) 430-7271 • Fax (954) 430-7227 • Web: www.Unicol-Publishing.com

CPSIA information can be obtained
at www.ICGtesting.com
Printed in the USA
BVHW010847201021
619084BV00012B/64

9 781880 973820